# Metabolic Syndrome: A Comprehensive Update with New Insights

Edited by

## Hafize Uzun

&

## Seyma Dumur

*Department of Medical Biochemistry*
*Istanbul Atlas University*
*Faculty of Medicine*
*Istanbul*
*Turkey*

**Metabolic Syndrome: A Comprehensive Update with New Insights**

Editors: Hafize Uzun & Seyma Dumur

ISBN (Online): 978-981-5322-13-2

ISBN (Print): 978-981-5322-14-9

ISBN (Paperback): 978-981-5322-15-6

First published in 2025.

need for a court order if at any point you breach any terms of this License Agreement. In no event will any delay or failure by Bentham Science Publishers in enforcing your compliance with this License Agreement constitute a waiver of any of its rights.

3. You acknowledge that you have read this License Agreement, and agree to be bound by its terms and conditions. To the extent that any other terms and conditions presented on any website of Bentham Science Publishers conflict with, or are inconsistent with, the terms and conditions set out in this License Agreement, you acknowledge that the terms and conditions set out in this License Agreement shall prevail.

**Bentham Science Publishers Pte. Ltd.**
80 Robinson Road #02-00
Singapore 068898
Singapore
Email: subscriptions@benthamscience.net

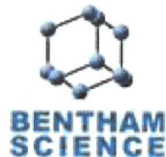

**BENTHAM SCIENCE**

# CONTENTS

# FOREWORD

Metabolic syndrome is an intricate condition characterized by a set of risk factors, including hyperglycemia, insulin resistance, hypertension, and obesity, which significantly elevate the risk of cardiovascular disease, stroke, and type 2 diabetes. Its growing prevalence worldwide poses a significant challenge to public health, necessitating a thorough understanding and innovative strategies for management. This book offers an in-depth exploration of metabolic syndrome, shielding a range of issues from functional changes and novel diagnostic methods to the interplay between metabolic syndrome and other health conditions like cancer, gastrointestinal disorders, and COVID-19. This complete text, featuring chapters on cutting-edge research and practical diagnosing and management strategies, is a valuable resource for healthcare professionals, researchers, and policymakers dedicated to addressing the multifaceted challenges of this syndrome.

**Era Gorica**
Department of Cardiology
Center for Translational and Experimental Cardiology (CTEC)
University Hospital Zürich, Wagistrasse 12, 8952 Schlieren
Switzerland

# PREFACE

Nowadays, metabolic syndrome (MetS) is a major health problem worldwide. MetS is characterized by high blood pressure, obesity, insulin resistance, and diabetes mellitus. Of these factors, insulin resistance is the main cause of MetS. It is very important for patients with MetS to change their lifestyle. Exercise, changes in dietary habits, and weight loss are necessary in the treatment of patients with MetS. As discussed in the light of current information about MetS in Chapter 13, exercise plays a very crucial role in controlling insulin activity, reducing the risk of cardiovascular disease, and maintaining weight control and Chapter 11 (Neutrogenomic strategies in metabolic syndrome) provides an update on our current understanding of the impact of neutrogenomic strategies on MetS. In the last few decades, many studies on the genetic and epigenetic screening of MetS in various populations have been published in the literature. The role of genetic and epigenetic mechanisms is discussed in Chapter 9.

Another important aspect is that MetS has been associated with psychiatric disorders. In those diagnosed with major depressive disorder and bipolar disorder in adulthood, the disruption of biological rhythms (sleep, social activities, and eating habits) has been associated with key components of MetS. MetS and its components have also been linked to a higher risk of suicide. It is clear that the relationship between behavior and MetS is bidirectional and that each component can influence the other. Awareness of factors related to MetS can help identify high-risk individuals and implement disease prevention and control strategies as well as lifestyle modifications. It is discussed in Chapter 10 (The Interplay between Metabolic Syndrome and Behavior) that lifestyle modification can help improve MetS status and behavior.

If patients with MetS fail to be treated with lifestyle changes, they should use certain medications. First, insulin resistance needs to be treated. Metformin, thiazolidinediones or glitazones should be used to treat insulin resistance and diabetes mellitus. Secondly, dyslipidemia and obesity need to be treated with statins and fibrates. Treatment of components of the MetS, such as cardiovascular disease, hypertension, and polycystic ovary syndrome, is often associated with the treatment of insulin resistance, obesity, and dyslipidemia. The MetS should be treated early because delayed treatment is ineffective and very expensive. In MetS and related diseases, rationalized and evidence-based pharmacotherapeutic strategies are cornerstones in reducing polypharmacy. The pharmacology network approach and advanced bioinformatics tools related to epigenetics, genomics, transcriptomics, proteomics, and metabolomics are recognized as useful bench-top tools for the search for molecular preventive and therapeutic multiple targets. Molecular multi-target therapy is recognized as a new pharmacological strategy underpinning personalized and precision medicine. This in turn will reduce socioeconomic burdens and improve health-related quality of life. In this context, Chapter 12 discusses perspectives on personalized medicine using a pharmacology network approach.

MetS is a cluster leading to increased cardiovascular morbidity and mortality as well as increased predisposition to other non-communicable diseases such as certain cancers. Although individual components of MetS have been linked to cancer, studies demonstrating a direct link between MetS and cancer are limited. Understanding this link will shed light on the process of oncogenesis in patients with MetS. Chapter 15 addresses the need to summarize the associated factors and mechanisms linking these two pathologies and to identify potential targets for treatment in patients with cancer and MetS. Furthermore, Chapter 15 focuses on the biological and physiological changes and specific factors associated with this process, including the insulin-like growth factor (IGF-1) pathway, estrogen signaling, visceral adiposity, hyperinsulinemia, hyperglycemia, aromatase activity, adipokinase production, angiogenesis, oxidative stress, DNA damage and pro-inflammatory cytokines, and their clinical implications in cancer therapy. A better understanding of this link will provide greater insight into the management of cancer patients by preventing MetS and related changes.

We would like to sincerely thank our team of authors from different countries who contributed excellent chapters that made the compilation of this book possible.

**Hafize Uzun**

&

**Seyma Dumur**
Department of Medical Biochemistry
Istanbul Atlas University
Faculty of Medicine
Istanbul
Turkey

# List of Contributors

**Abdulhalim Senyigit**    Department of Internal Medicine, Faculty of Medicine, Istanbul Atlas University, Istanbul, Turkey

**Ahmed Saber Shams**    Human Anatomy and Embryology Department, Faculty of Medicine, Suez Canal University, Ismailia, Egypt

**Asli Kutlu**    Department of Molecular Biology and Genetics, Faculty of Engineering and Natural Sciences, Istinye University, Istanbul, Turkiye

**Asmaa Seddek**    Department of Medical Physiology, Faculty of Medicine, Suez Canal University, Ismailia, Egypt

**Berrin Papila**    Istanbul University-Cerrahpasa, Cerrahpasa Medical Faculty, Istanbul, Turkey

**Dahlia Badran**    Medical Biochemistry & Molecular Biology department, Medicine faculty, Suez Canal University, Egypt
Medical Biochemistry & Molecular Biology department, Medicine faculty, Badr University in Cairo, Egypt

**Dina A Ali**    Clinical pharmacology Department, Faculty of Medicine, Suez Canal University, Ismailia, 41522, Egypt

**Demet Aygun**    Department of Neurology, Medicine Faculty, Istanbul Atlas University, Istanbul, Turkey

**Derya Aydın Sivri**    Department of Obstetrics and Gynecology, Faculty of Medicine, Istanbul Atlas University, İstanbul, Turkey

**Esra Bihter Gürler**    Department of Physiology, Faculty of Dentistry, İstanbul Galata University, İstanbul, Turkey

**Eman Mamdouh Kolieb**    Physiology Department, Faculty of Medicine, Suez Canal University, Ismailia, 41522, Egypt

**Esma Altinoglu**    Department of Internal Medicine, School of Medicine, Bahcesehir University, Istanbul, Turkey

**Fatma S. Samman**    Department of Clinical Pharmacology, Faculty of Medicine, Suez Canal University, 41522 Ismailia, Egypt

**Fatma Köksal Çakırlar**    stanbul University-Cerrahpasa, Cerrahpasa medicine Faculty, Istanbul, Turkey

**Hülya Çevik ARAS**    Department of Oral Medicine and Pathology, University of Gothenburg, Göteborg, Sweden

**Hurriyet Cetinok**    Faculty of Medicine, Istanbul Atlas University, Istanbul, Turkey

**Halit Eren Taşkın**    Department of General Surgery, Istanbul University-Cerrahpasa Cerrahpasa Medical Faculty, 34098, Istanbul, Fatih, Turkey

**Hafize Uzun**    Department of Medical Biochemistry, Faculty of Medicine, Istanbul Atlas University, Istanbul, Turkey

**Iskender Ekinci**    Department of Internal Medicine, Faculty of Medicine, Bezmialem Vakıf University, Istanbul, Turkey

**Marwa Mohamed Hosny**    Medical Biochemistry and Molecular Biology Department, Faculty of Medicine, Suez Canal University, Ismailia, Egypt
Oncology Diagnostic Unit, Faculty of Medicine, Suez Canal University, Ismailia, Egypt

**Marwa Mohamed Hosny**
Medical Biochemistry and Molecular Biology Department, Faculty of Medicine, Suez Canal University, Ismailia, Egypt
Oncology Diagnostic Unit, Faculty of Medicine, Suez Canal University, Ismailia, Egypt

**Mohamed Salah Rashwan**
Department of Otolaryngology, Faculty of Medicine, Suez Canal University, Ismailia, Egypt
Department of Otolaryngology, Queen's Hospital, Barking, Havering and Redbridge University Hospitals NHS Trust, Romford, UK

**Nagihan Bostanci**
Department of Dental Medicine, Karolinska Institutet, Stockholm, Sweden

**Nora Hosny**
Medical Biochemistry and Molecular Biology Department, Faculty of Medicine, Suez Canal University, Ismailia, Egypt

**Noura Ramadan Abdelhamid**
Department of Histology and Cell Biology, Faculty of Medicine, Suez Canal University, Ismailia, 41522, Egypt

**Naile Misirlioglu**
Department of Biochemistry, Gaziosmanpaşa Training and Research Hospital, University of Health Sciences, Istanbul, Turkey

**Neval Elgörmüş**
Department of Microbiology, Faculty of Medicine, Istanbul Atlas University, Istanbul, Turkey

**Omer Okuyan**
Istanbul Atlas University, Istanbul, Turkey

**Pelin Uysal**
Department of Pulmonary Medicine, Faculty of Medicine, Istanbul Atlas University, Istanbul, Turkey

**Ravindri Jayasinghe**
Department of Surgery, Faculty of Medicine, University of Colombo, Colombo, Sri Lanka

**Sinem Firtina**
Department of Medical Genetics, Cerrahpasa Faculty of Medicine, Istanbul University-Cerrahpasa, Istanbul, Turkiye

**Shimaa Mohammad Yousof**
Department of Medical Physiology, Faculty of Medicine in Rabigh, King Abdulaziz University, Rabigh, Saudi Arabia

**Samah M. Elaidy**
Department of Clinical Pharmacology, Faculty of Medicine, Suez Canal University, 41522 Ismailia, Egypt

**Samar Imbaby**
Department of Clinical Pharmacology, Faculty of Medicine, Suez Canal University, 41522 Ismailia, Egypt

**Seyma Dumur**
Department of Medical Biochemistry, Faculty of Medicine, Istanbul Atlas University, Istanbul, Turkey

**Sanjeewa Seneviratne**
Department of Surgery, Faculty of Medicine, University of Colombo, Colombo, Sri Lanka

**Umesh Jayarajah**
Department of Surgery, Faculty of Medicine, University of Colombo, Colombo, Sri Lanka

# CHAPTER 1

# General Aspects of Metabolic Syndrome: An Update on Diagnostic Criteria, Pathophysiology, and Management

## Abdulhalim Senyigit[1,*]

[1] *Department of Internal Medicine, Faculty of Medicine, Istanbul Atlas University, Istanbul, Turkey*

**Abstract:** Metabolic syndrome (MetS) is generally defined as a cluster/complex of factors that are risk factors for cardiovascular disease (CVD) and type 2 diabetes (T2DM), including hyperglycemia, insulin resistance, hypertension, hypertriglyceridemia, decreased HDL-cholesterol concentration and central obesity. MetS is a health problem whose prevalence is increasing worldwide and negatively affects people's lives. Although MetS is essentially insulin resistance (IR), is not considered a disease, it consists of a combination of many risk factors that force the body metabolism to work abnormally. In addition to factors such as sedentary lifestyle and nutrition, hereditary factors are also important in the formation of MetS. The main components of MetS can be listed as hyperglycemia, hypertension, obesity and dyslipidemia. MetS has different definitions for different organizations. The basic components of these definitions are waist circumference, IR, high blood pressure and dyslipidemia (high triglyceride, low HDL cholesterol). The most recently agreed upon diagnostic criteria for MetS are increased waist circumference (society and country specific), high triglycerides, low HDL cholesterol, high blood pressure and high fasting blood glucose. For diagnosis, the presence of at least 3 of these parameters is required. When countries are examined in terms of the prevalence of MetS, different results are obtained from each country. The most important factor affecting the incidence of MetS in a country is the percentage of obesity and abdominal obesity in that country. Although obesity and physical activity factors have an impact on the incidence of MetS, it is an undeniable fact that genetic factors also have a significant impact. Lifestyle changes are at the core of MetS treatment. People with this syndrome need to change their diet, increase their physical activity and lose weight. Determining MetS risk levels and predisposing risk factors, determining whether they meet diagnostic criteria, and raising awareness through education and consultancy activities will be effective in combating the prevalence of MetS and cardiovascular risk factors.

**Keywords:** Diagnostic criteria, Metabolic syndrome, Management, Pathophysiology.

---

<sup>*</sup> **Corresponding author Abdulhalim Senyigit:** Department of Internal Medicine, Faculty of Medicine, Istanbul Atlas University, Istanbul, Turkey; E-mail: abdulhalim.senyigit@atlas.edu.tr

# INTRODUCTION

Metabolic syndrome (MetS) is generally defined as a cluster/complex of factors, such as hyperglycaemia, insulin resistance (IR), hypertension (HT), hypertriglyceridemia, decreased HDL-cholesterol concentration and central obesity, which are risk factors for cardiovascular disease (CVD) and type 2 diabetes (T2DM) [1]. The association of MetS risk factors with T2DM and CVD began to be discussed in the 1970s and was first defined by Reaven in 1988 as a syndrome of metabolic abnormalities and named Syndrome X [2]. For the first time in 1988, Reaven defined "Syndrome X" as this complex disease in which various metabolic abnormalities (HT, hyperglycaemia, and hyperuricemia) coexist [1, 2]. MetS is also described by different terms such as IR syndrome, polymetabolic syndrome, deadly quartet, and civilisation syndrome [3]. MetS has also been given various names such as metabolic cardiovascular syndrome, dysmetabolic syndrome, plurimetabolic syndrome, and cardiometabolic risk syndrome. MetS is a major cause of morbidity, affecting an increasing number of people worldwide [4 - 6]. It is estimated that 3.2 million people die each year worldwide due to diabetes-related complications, and in countries with a high incidence of diabetes, such as the Pacific and the Middle East, diabetes accounts for a quarter of all causes of death in adults aged 35-64 years. CVD and its complications, a major component of the MetS, are also on the rise and have a major impact on global health systems. The estimated incidence of diabetes is projected to double by 2025 and cardiovascular diseases are expected to increase in parallel [7].

The National Cholesterol Education Program Adult Treatment Panel Working Group (NCEP-ATP III) introduced a new definition in 2001 and added abdominal obesity and waist circumference to the definition [8]. Today, the definition of MetS is widely used by various authorities such as the World Health Organization (WHO), American Heart Association (AHA), International Diabetes Federation (IDF), National Heart, Lung and Blood Institute (NHLBI), NCEP-ATP III).

## Prevalence of Metabolic Syndrome

The prevalence of MS is steadily increasing worldwide and has recently been identified as one of the major global public health problems. Although the prevalence of MetS varies according to different geographical and ethnic characteristics of societies (lifestyle), definitions used, population age and gender characteristics, it is considered a pandemic in the adult population in many countries. When countries are analysed in terms of the prevalence of MetS, different results are obtained from each country. The most important factor affecting the prevalence of MetS in a country is the percentage of obesity and abdominal obesity in that country. Although obesity and physical activity have an effect on the incidence of MetS, it is an undeniable fact that genetic factors also have an important effect. Prevalence is reported to increase with body mass index (BMI) and age. According to the National Health and Nutrition Examination Survey (NHANES), the prevalence of MetS was 34-35% in the period 1999-2012, and this rate was found to be 50% over the age of 60 years [9]. About a quarter of adults in the US, India and Europe have MetS [10]. It has been reported that the risk of death is 2 times higher and the risk of major cardiovascular events is 3-5 times higher in individuals with MetS. It is also reported that the risk of developing T2DM is 2-5 times higher in these individuals and that more than 80% of the world's 230 million people with T2DM are at risk of CVD-related death [8 - 10]. There is also an increased risk of other preventable chronic diseases such as cancer, neurodegenerative diseases, non-alcoholic fatty liver disease, circulatory disorders, dyslipidemia, and infertility [9].

The prevalence of MetS increases with age and is difficult to prevent as the ageing population expands [11]. Studies indicate that by 2050, approximately 83.7 million people in the US will be over 65 years of age, double the 2012 population of 43.1 million [12]. Although there is no consensus on age and gender studies in MetS, in 2023 Rus *et al.* [13] reported that both genders displayed a higher risk of developing MetS related to age. The most affected age groups were aged between 60-69 years old and the 70-79-year-old group, categories where women had a higher risk of developing the disease. For the rest of the age categories, the incidence and prevalence continued to be higher among men [13].

The MetS global prevalence varied from 12.5% to 31.4% depending on the diagnostic criteria in the meta-analysis prevalence of MetS. Despite the publication of numerous primary studies on MetS in various populations across the globe, little effort has been dedicated to summarizing data on the epidemiology of MetS at the global level. In this study, we aimed to determine the prevalence rates of MetS and its individual components according to different diagnostic criteria and cutoffs and to compare these rates across geographic regions and socioeconomic levels [14].

**Significance of Metabolic Syndrome**

MS is an important public health problem seen in the adult population worldwide [15]. It is a risk factor for cardiovascular diseases and T2DM. MetS is associated with CVDs and increases the risk of cardiovascular morbidity 3-fold, mortality 2-fold, and type 2 diabetes 5-fold [16]. The onset of MetS in children is a result of the increase in the prevalence of obesity and is defined as a comorbid condition [17, 18]. It has been reported that obesity and overweight in young people play an important role in MetS. MetS seen in children increases the risk of early death due to coronary heart disease in adults. It has been reported that atherosclerosis seen at an early age is associated with MetS and obesity seen in childhood [19]. With the spread of obesity, it is predicted that 10% of school children are obese and 60% of obese children older than 10 years will become obese adults [20].

The high correlation between obesity and T2DM has changed the approach to childhood obesity. Insulin resistance has been detected in some obese children and adolescents. Some of these children will develop MetS and T2DM, while others will not. However, it is reported that 60% of obese children and adolescents have at least one cardiovascular risk factor [21].

There is no consensus between the WHO and the National Cholesterol Education Program regarding the diagnosis of MetS in children. Accurate diagnosis in children is important for reducing or preventing the high morbidity related to chronic diseases seen in young adults [21].

**Pathogenesis of Metabolic Syndrome**

The pathophysiology of MetS involves many complex mechanisms that have not yet been fully clarified. No single genetic, infectious, or environmental factor has yet been identified to explain the etiopathogenesis of all components of the MetS. However, the etiology of MetS can be divided into three categories: Obesity/adipose tissue disorders, insulin resistance, and independent factors (such as molecules of vascular, hepatic, and immunologic origin). Although MetS is thought to develop as a result of a complex relationship between many environmental and genetic factors, the latest data suggest that obesity and insulin resistance are at the center of the development of the syndrome and play a key role in the development of chronic inflammatory and prothrombotic processes that accompany the syndrome.

Since insulin resistance is thought to be the main culprit in the development of the syndrome, subsequent studies have focused on revealing the common relationship between insulin resistance, obesity, and CVD development. As a result of these studies, it has been agreed that insulin resistance is insufficient as the only etiopathogenetic factor to explain the clustering of CVD risk factors in an individual - in this sense, the development of MetS - but it is the main underlying mechanism [1, 22 - 24].

**Diagnostic Criteria of Metabolic Syndrome**

Since 1998, many definitions have been made for MetS by many expert groups, and organizations, including WHO, have tried to improve these definitions [25,

26]. The definitions made by WHO in 1999, the European Group for the Study of Insulin Resistance (EGIR) in 1999, the American Association of Clinical Endocrinology (AACE) in 2003, NCEP-ATP III in 2001-2005, and IDF in 2005 are guiding in diagnosis and treatment. The most widely accepted definitions are those made by WHO, EGIR, and NCEP-ATP III [8].

According to the 2022 definition of MetS, considering the progress in understanding individual components of MetS and the most current guidance on the management of each individual condition, the authors propose that the definition of MetS encompasses the presence of obesity and two of the three following criteria: high blood pressure, impaired glucose metabolism, elevated non-high-density lipoprotein (non-HDL) cholesterol level (atherogenic dyslipidemia) [27]. The comparison of MetS diagnostic criteria between organizations is presented in Table **1**.

**Table 1. Diagnostic criteria of metabolic syndrome elucidated by different organizations [33].**

| | *Criteria* | | | | | | |
|---|---|---|---|---|---|---|---|
| **Organizations** | **Central Obesity** | **FBS** | **↑ TG** | **↓ HDL** | **↑ BP** | **Other** | **Diagnosed as MetS, If** |
| WHO (1998) [28] | Waist/hip ratio *Male* >0.90 cm *Female* >0.85 or BMI > 30 kg/m$^2$ | ≥110 mg/dL or IR or T2DM or Rx | ≥150 mg/dL | *Male* <40 mg/dL *Female* <50 mg/dL | *Diastolic ≥ 140 and Systolic ≥ 90 mmHg* | Microalbuminuria | Absolutely required IR plus ≥ 2 criteria |
| EGIR (1999) [30] | (WC *Male* ≥94 cm *Female* ≥80 cm | ≥108.11 mg/dL | ≥150 mg/dL | <39 mg/dL | Diastolic ≥ 140 and/or Systolic ≥ 90 mmHg or Rx | - | Absolutely required IR plus ≥ 2 criteria |
| IDF (2005) [29] | WC defined in terms of ethnicity specific values | ≥100 mg/dL or Rx | ≥150 mg/dL or Rx | Male: <40 mg/dL Female: <50 mg/dL | Diastolic ≥ 130 and/or systolic ≥ 85 mmHg or Rx | - | Absolutely required central obesity plus ≥ 2 criteria |
| AHA/NHLBI (2005) [31] | WC Male: ≥102 cm Female: ≥88 cm | ≥100 mg/dL or Rx | ≥150 mg/dL or Rx | Male: <40 mg/dL Female: <50 mg/dL | Diastolic ≥ 130 and/or systolic ≥ 85 mmHg or Rx | - | ≥3 criteria |

*(Table 1) cont.....*

| | | | | Criteria | | | |
|---|---|---|---|---|---|---|---|
| Organizations | Central Obesity | FBS | ↑ TG | ↓ HDL | ↑ BP | Other | Diagnosed as MetS, If |
| AHA/NHLBI and IDF:2009 [32] | WC defined in terms of population- and country-based specific definition | ≥100 mg/dL or Rx | ≥150 mg/dL or Rx | Male: <40 mg/dL Female: <50 mg/dL | Diastolic ≥ 130 and/or systolic ≥ 85 mmHg or Rx | - | ≥3 criteria |

**FBS,** Fasting blood sugar; **WHO,** World health organization; **Rx,** on medication; **EGIR,** Europe Group for the Study of IR; **IDF,** International Diabetes Federation; **IR,** insulin resistance; **WC,** waist circumference; **AHA** American Heart Association; NHLBI, National Heart, Lung, and Blood Institute.

## According to the WHO's 1998 Diagnostic Criteria for Metabolic Syndrome [28]

√ Having at least one of the diagnoses of insulin resistance, impaired glucose tolerance, and obvious diabetes mellitus.

√ High blood pressure (blood pressure above 140/90 mmHg or taking antihypertensive medication).

√ Abdominal obesity (Body Mass Index (BMI) over 30 kg/m$^2$ or waist/hip ratio greater than 0.90 cm in men and greater than 0.85 cm in women).

√ Dyslipidemia (Triglyceride (TG) level above 150 mg/dL or High-Density Lipoprotein (HDL) level less than 40 mg/dL in men and less than 50 mg/dL in women).

√ Microalbuminuria (urinary albumin excretion more than 20 µg/min or albumin/creatinine ratio more than 30 mg/g) in combination with at least two of the findings.

## According to the Diagnostic Criteria of NCEP-ATP III [8]

NCEP-ATP III is one of the most widely used definitions of MetS criteria in the world.

√ Abdominal obesity (waist circumference: >102 cm in men, >88 cm in women).

√ Hypertriglyceridemia (≥150 mg/dL).

√ Low HDL cholesterol (<40 mg/dL in men, <50 mg/dL in women).

√ Hypertension (blood pressure ≥ 130/85 mmHg).

√ Presence of at least three of the findings of hyperglycemia (fasting blood glucose > 100 mg/dL) makes the diagnosis of MetS.

### According to the IDF's 2005 Diagnostic Criteria for MetS [29]

√ Abdominal obesity (waist circumference of 94 cm and above in European men and 80 cm and above in women).

√ TG level≥150 mg/dL.

√ HDL level <40 mg/dL in men and <50 mg/dL in women.

√ Blood pressure≥130/85 mmHg.

√ A fasting blood glucose level of ≥100 mg/dL indicates the diagnosis of MetS.

Any patient diagnosed with MetS should at least be seen as a high cardiovascular-risk patient. A comprehensive assessment of the main and additional conditions of the MetS is advised, as well as implementing lifestyle modifications alongside appropriate medical treatment. Early intervention can prevent the development or slow the progression of individual components of the MetS [27].

### Risk Factors of Metabolic Syndrome

Although there is no consensus on the definition and diagnostic criteria of the syndrome, MetS is characterized by the coexistence of risk factors such as abdominal obesity, atherogenic dyslipidemia, high blood pressure, insulin resistance and high glucose levels [34] (Fig. **1**). Among these criteria, obesity is among the controllable risk factors as it is generally associated with excess calorie intake and insufficient physical activity [35].

There is currently significant research focusing on understanding the key pathways that control metabolism, which would be likely targets of risk factors (*e.g*, exposure to xenobiotics, genetics) and lifestyle factors (*e.g*, microbiome, nutrition, and exercise) that contribute to MetS [36]. In addition to genetic predisposition, environmental factors such as obesity, fat metabolism, high calorie intake, diet rich in cholesterol and atherogenic foods and low physical activity, aging and hormonal imbalances are separate risk factors affecting the development and progression of the syndrome. MetS is an important risk factor for CVD and T2DM and hepatosteatosis, steatohepatitis, and cirrhosis may develop in the same time period in patients with MetS. The frequency of MetS and its complications increases in proportion to the increase in the frequency of obesity in children and adolescents [24]. Cardiovascular risk factors associated with insulin resistance have been summarized in Table **2** [36].

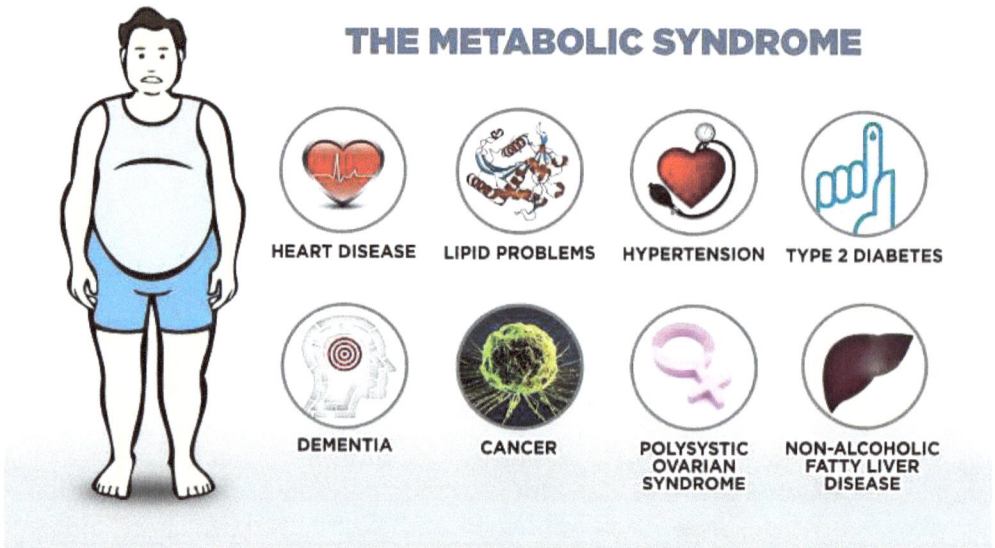

**THE METABOLIC SYNDROME**

HEART DISEASE    LIPID PROBLEMS    HYPERTENSION    TYPE 2 DIABETES

DEMENTIA    CANCER    POLYSYSTIC OVARIAN SYNDROME    NON-ALCOHOLIC FATTY LIVER DISEASE

**Fig. (1).** Risk factors of metabolic syndrome.

**Table 2. Cardiovascular risk factors associated with insulin resistance.**

| | |
|---|---|
| • High Blood Pressure. | • High fibrinogen level. |
| • Hyperinsulinemia. | • High PAI-1 level. |
| • Low HDL-C. | • Elevated CRP and other markers of inflammation. |
| • High triglyceride level. | • Increased blood viscosity. |
| • Small, dense LDL particles. | • Microalbuminuria. |
| • High Apo B. | • Hyperglycemia. |
| • Endothelial dysfunction. | |
| • Low Apo A-1 levels. | |

**Apo,** apolipoprotein; **PAI-1,** plasminogen activator inhibitor-1; **CRP,** C-reactive protein.

Instead of listing the causes of MetS one by one, it is more accurate to define all problems that increase the risk of heart attack as part of MetS.

## COMPONENTS OF METABOLIC SYNDROME

The main components of MetS are obesity, insulin resistance, T2DM, hypertension, dyslipidemia, and and prothrombotic state.

## Metabolic Syndrome and Obesity

Abdominal obesity is the most frequently occurring component of the MetS. The most important triggering factor in the development of insulin resistance is also abdominal obesity. Although obesity is caused by the intake of more food than the metabolism needs, it is estimated that obese people consume more energy than they need in addition to their sedentary life [27, 37].

The most important factor in the development of insulin resistance is abdominal obesity, which may not be present in every case of MetS [38] (Fig. **2**). Adipose tissue plays an active role in inflammation through hormones such as resistin, leptin, adiponectin and cytokines such as TNF-α, IL-6, IL-1 [39, 40]. Waist circumference measurement, which is an indicator of visceral adiposity, is used in the evaluation of MetS, and it is recommended to measure at the midpoint of the distance between the arcus costarium and spina iliaca anterior superior of the pelvis. for this measurement. The cut-off values for waist circumference defined by the WHO for the white race in overweight and obese people are 94 cm in overweight and 102 cm in obesity in men; 80 cm in overweight and 88 cm in obesity in women [38].

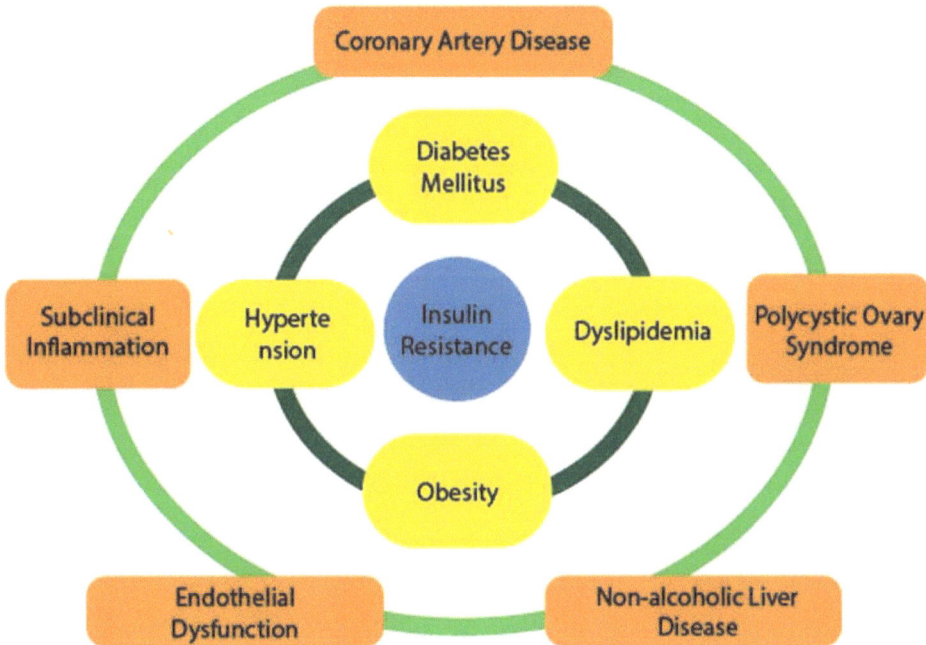

**Fig. (2).** Components of metabolic syndrome.

Free fatty acids (FFAs) formed by lipolysis from adipose tissues in the body increase according to the size of adipocytes. In visceral adipose tissue composed of large adipocytes, cytokine production increases with the intensity of lipolysis, while insulin sensitivity decreases. As a result, the excess in visceral adipose tissue leads to an increase in FFAs and thus insulin resistance [41]. Establishing the link between insulin resistance and obesity was made possible by the determination of the endocrine organ function of adipose tissues, where energy is stored, by adding peptide complement effector and cytokine secretion to the circulatory system [42]. It has been suggested that chronic inflammation is effective in the progression of insulin resistance. In studies, acute phase reactants and proinflammatory cytokines have been linked to MetS variables [43 - 45]. The inflammatory resilience phenotype of the overfed healthy males moved toward that of males diagnosed with MetS [44].

The IDF has accepted the inclusion of central obesity in the diagnostic criteria (it has been reported that it is unnecessary to measure insulin resistance because central obesity is strongly associated with insulin resistance) and the presence of at least two of the following: high triglycerides, low HDL, high blood pressure and high fasting glucose as the definition of MetS [46, 47]. While criteria for both ATP III and IDF consider central obesity (defined by waist circumference, with ethnicity- and gender-specific cut-off values), the IDF uses central obesity as a prerequisite for diagnosis, while the ATP III considers central obesity as one component out of several that could be present [48].

Studies have shown that individuals with predominant upper body obesity are more prone to MetS and that excess visceral adiposity is strongly associated with MetS [49, 50]. Obesity is known to promote the recruitment of excess fat to various organs or tissues, especially muscle and liver [51, 52]. Recent studies reveal that adipose tissue contributes adipokines that may influence metabolic risk factors [52 - 54]. These include adiponectin, interleukin-6, tumor necrosis factor alpha (TNF-α) resistin, leptin, angiotensinogen, and plasminogen activator inhibitor-1 [52, 55].

Normally, as fat cells expand, more leptin is released into the brain to signal the end of eating behavior. However, obese individuals can develop leptin resistance, similar to insulin resistance. In these individuals, even high leptin levels are not enough to induce satiety [56, 57]. Weight loss in patients with MetS can lead to improvements in multiple traits simultaneously, so a certain degree of adiposity seems to be necessary to reveal the abnormal pathophysiology. However, there are also patients who are obese but do not show any of the other components of the MetS, so both metabolic susceptibility to insulin resistance and obesity are necessary for the MetS phenotype to be observed [58, 59].

Ectopic adiposity resulting in adipocyte hypertrophy or adipose tissue enlargement and visceral obesity is the most important constituent of MetS. Ectopic adiposity is the accumulation of fat in visceral organs such as the omentum, liver, and muscle, in addition to subcutaneous adipose tissue. Today, visceral obesity, in other words, excessive fat in the intra-abdominal region, is known to increase the prevalence of MetS. It has been reported that there is a positive correlation between waist/hip ratio, which is used as a marker of visceral obesity, and plasma fasting glucose level and systolic-diastolic blood pressure, and that these factors are among the important risk factors for the development of CVD [60, 61]. This explains why obesity is a poorly identifiable CVD risk factor compared to others such as hypertension, smoking, and cholesterol (increased low-density lipoprotein (LDL)/decreased HDL). Although the accumulation of excess visceral fat is associated with various atherogenic and diabetogenic abnormalities, an important question is whether visceral fat is a causal factor or simply a marker of a dysmetabolic profile. Although obesity is not a major risk factor for insulin resistance, T2DM, and CVD, not all obese patients are insulin resistant or at high risk of diabetes and CVD [62].

## Metabolic Syndrome and Insulin Resistance

Individuals with MetS have a biological response to endogenous and exogenous insulin, and many factors such as genetic predisposition, nutritional disorders starting in the womb, malnutrition, malnutrition, concomitant obesity, inactivity, sedentary life, decreased body repair capacity with aging can lead to the development of insulin resistance. Although insulin resistance is accompanied by hyperglycemia, it is not always present [63].

Insulin resistance defined as an inadequate response to the required amount of insulin in the circulatory system, is a pathophysiology for the body and can be seen in obese, non-diabetic individuals and individuals with T2DM [64].

One of the hypotheses accepted to explain the pathophysiology of MetS is insulin resistance. MetS is, therefore, also known as insulin resistance syndrome. Insulin resistance is defined as a defect in the action of insulin, which is required to maintain euglycemia leading to hyperinsulinemia. Considering the main tissues targeted by insulin, it appears that insulin resistance in skeletal muscle leads to a reduction in glycogen synthesis and glucose transport, while insulin resistance in the liver leads to a reduction in the efficiency of insulin signaling. The exact mechanisms have not been fully confirmed and research in this area is ongoing [65, 66]. Hyperinsulinemia occurs to counteract this resistance and maintain euglycemia. While insulin resistance is usually associated with hyperinsulinemia, hyperglycemia may not always accompany insulin resistance. Hyperglycemia occurs in advanced stages of insulin resistance [67 - 69]. Abdominal obesity (visceral adiposity) is thought to be the main cause of insulin resistance. On the other hand, the increase in circulating FFA is thought to play an important role in the pathogenesis of MetS. With abdominal obesity, insulin-stimulated glucose uptake by cells is reduced, the non-esterified fatty acid is abnormally released from adipose tissue, muscle cells, and liver adiposity are formed, and these effects facilitate the development of insulin resistance and dyslipidemia [70, 71]. The increase in circulating FFAs has multiple effects on metabolism; FFAs reduce glucose uptake into muscles. They promote gluconeogenesis and lipogenesis in the liver. Acute skeletal muscle exposure to high FFA levels induces insulin resistance by inhibiting insulin-induced glucose uptake. Chronic exposure of the pancreas to high FFAs impairs pancreatic beta cell function. FFAs are also lipotoxic to pancreatic beta cells and cause impaired insulin secretion. As a result, insulin secretion is reduced [72, 73].

## Metabolic Syndrome and Prediabetes

Although the definitions of prediabetes, MetS and insulin resistance syndrome are closely related, they are recognized as separate entities that overlap each other. Different criteria for MetS developed by different groups are still widely used. Among these, the NCEP-ATP III criteria is one of the most widely used [74, 75].

The different definitions, interpretations and diagnostic criteria provided by each organization not only confuse clinicians but are also not similar in terms of determining cardiovascular risk. For example, in a survival analysis, it was found that NCEP diagnostic criteria were more in line with the risk of CVD than IDF diagnostic criteria [76]. In another study, it was shown that IDF diagnostic criteria were more sensitive than ATP III, WHO diagnostic criteria, impaired glucose tolerance, and impaired fasting glucose in predicting future diabetes development, but the false positive rate increased similarly with increasing sensitivity [77]. The fact that metformin treatment of patients with MetS in the diabetes prevention program has been shown to have little effect on the improvement of MetS compared to lifestyle changes is another indirect evidence that prediabetes and MetS are different entities. In conclusion, insulin resistance is a starting point for the presence of both prediabetes and MetS, approximately 75% of prediabetics may be associated with MetS, both insulin resistance, prediabetes and MetS are individually associated with increased cardiovascular risk, and prediabetes determines the future development of diabetes [77]. Accordingly, prediabetes and MetS are intertwined but separate concepts.

Beyond the fact that prediabetes is a condition that must be diagnosed correctly and closely monitored and treated in terms of both its conversion to diabetes and the many health problems it may cause, it is possible to prevent prediabetes by taking precautions to be taken by addressing risky individuals individually in order to prevent the aforementioned health problems from occurring, and today, it has been adopted by guidelines that prevention of prediabetes is the most accurate approach to reduce future health risks and expenditures [78].

## Metabolic Syndrome and Diabetes Mellitus

T2DM is becoming one of the most common chronic diseases after cancer and cardiovascular diseases. In recent years, the prevalence of this disease has been increasing significantly worldwide and is becoming one of the major societal social problems in the 21st century [79]. Although not all patients with T2DM have insulin resistance, the presence of overt DM or impaired glucose tolerance fulfills the first step of the diagnostic criteria for MetS and insulin resistance is not required. Insulin resistance increases the risk of atherosclerosis and cardiovascular disease independent of other risk factors [80]. In addition to fasting glucose levels, high postprandial glucose levels are risk factors for insulin resistance, prediabetes and overt diabetes, and this risk is present from the preclinical period [81 - 83].

DM is a metabolic disease characterized by hyperglycemia due to impaired insulin secretion/effectiveness. Long-term damage, dysfunction and failure of end organs such as kidneys, heart, and eyes may occur as a result of chronic hyperglycemia. Symptoms such as polyuria, polydipsia, polyphagia, nocturia, weight loss, numbness in hands and feet, burning, itching, and dry skin may be observed. Complications such as hyperglycemic hyperosmolar state or ketoacidosis may occur. Fasting plasma glucose, glycosylated hemoglobin A1c (HbA1c), or an oral glucose tolerance test (OGTT) may be used in the diagnosis [84].

## Metabolic Syndrome and Hypertension

Hypertension is common in individuals with T2DM, as it is often a component of the MetS. Other components of the MetS, such as central obesity and dyslipidemia (especially an atherogenic lipid profile) and associated oxidative stress, low-grade chronic inflammation, endothelial dysfunction, insulin resistance and hyperinsulinemia, are the most important underlying causes of hypertension in T2DM. Hypertension is one of the most influential components of MetS and is the sole risk factor for CVD. The strongest hypothesis about the causes of HT in MetS is the hyperinsulinemia-induced increase in sodium reabsorption. Although HT individuals do not have obesity, IR has been found to be present [85, 86]. Although insulin resistance is frequently found in the background of HT, insulin resistance is not only involved here but also in other vascular diseases. There may be an increase in sympathetic system activation and renal sodium retention through mediators such as nitric oxide (NO) [85]. There is a connection between hypertension, insulin resistance, hyperglycemia, and hyperinsulinemia [87].

High blood pressure is often associated with other CVD risk factors, including dyslipidemia and insulin resistance. Insulin resistance is one of the underlying causes of hypertension in individuals. The relationship between insulin resistance and hypertension is well known [88, 89]. Various mechanisms have been proposed to establish the relationship between hypertension and insulin resistance [88, 90]. For example, insulin is a vasodilator that has secondary effects in increasing sodium reabsorption by the kidney and can lead to hypertension. Insulin has a vasodilator effect, but in the case of insulin resistance, its vasodilator effect is reduced, while its effect on sodium reabsorption remains unchanged. Hyperinsulinemia activates the renin-angiotensin system (RAS) by increasing the expression of angiotensinogen, angiotensin II (AT-II), and angiotensin I (AT-I) receptors, which contribute to the development of vasoconstriction and hypertension [88, 91].

**Metabolic Syndrome and Dyslipidemia (Hyperlipidemia)**

Dyslipidemia is defined as raised triglycerides and decreased high-density lipoprotein (HDL) cholesterol levels. Dyslipidemia in MetS is characterized by high triglyceride values and is a common component in various diagnostic criteria made by international organizations [92, 93]. In addition, low levels of HDL cholesterol are another criterion associated with MetS. Low-Density Lipoprotein (LDL) levels, which have a potential atherogenic effect, are usually elevated. Similar to LDL cholesterol, Apolipoprotein B also has an atherogenic effect and increases the risk of cardiovascular disease. Apolipoprotein B measurement and monitoring are not yet widely used [94].

Muscle, fat, and other tissues may become less sensitive to insulin as we age, resulting in dysglycemia and dyslipidemia [95]. As a result of defects in lipoproteins, the amount of free fatty acids in circulation increases. Insulin resistance is caused by abdominal obesity and this increase in free fatty acids increases triglyceride synthesis in the liver. This dyslipidemia picture that emerges in MetS leads to cardiovascular disease predisposition and endothelial damage [96].

Dyslipidemia, which is the leading cause of young death in many countries, increases the likelihood of atherosclerotic CVDs [97, 98]. Among the factors that increase the likelihood of atherosclerotic CVD, dyslipidemia is the most likely to be prevented. In addition to directly affecting the pathogenesis of atherosclerosis, it is highly prevalent and asymptomatic in humans. In studies conducted on individuals living in North America and Europe, it has been reported that one in two adults has dyslipidemia [99, 100]. The rapid increase in T2DM and obesity today causes dyslipidemia to be seen frequently [101].

The claim that it is caused by lifestyle is not true for dyslipidemia. This is because the symptoms of familial hypercholesterolemia, which is an autosomal dominantly inherited single-gene disease and is very common worldwide, are associated with high cholesterol levels and early atherosclerotic CVDs, which do not occur due to lifestyle. Heterozygous familial hypercholesterolemia rates have been shown to range from 1/100 to 1/500 [102, 103].

There are many polygenic familial dyslipidemias with high lipid levels and the incidence in humans is 5-7%. Some of the polygenic familial dyslipidemias that are not related to lifestyle, such as familial hypercholesterolemia, are associated with TG alone, while others are associated with LDL and TG. Dyslipidemia is mostly investigated in association with the possibility of atherosclerotic CVD, and the increased risk of pancreatitis in case of excessive increase in TG levels should also be taken into consideration [104].

In many studies, it has been reported that the use of statins, a group of lipid-lowering drugs for primary and secondary prevention, reduces mortality from atherosclerotic CVDs [105, 106]. Research has shown that the magnitude of cardiovascular benefit is proportional to the reduction in LDL levels [107]. Based on this, several agents have been developed that provide strong reductions in LDL levels, and good results have been obtained [108].

## Metabolic Syndrome and Endothelial Dysfunction

Risk factors for oxidative stress such as hypertension, diabetes, smoking, and dyslipidemia cause vascular inflammation and endothelial dysfunction. In addition, a decrease in the level of vasodilator nitric oxide (NO) affects the increase in oxidative stress, leading to pathobiological consequences that open the door to vascular complexities [109 - 111].

With hyperinsulinemia and insulin resistance, endothelial function deteriorates and vascular damage progresses. One of the harms of insulin resistance is the inhibition of NO-induced vasodilation. In the presence of diabetes and MetS, NO levels decrease in the presence of excess synthesis of superoxide-like reactive oxygen radicals (ROS). Insulin resistance and the level of endothelial dysfunction are proportional to each other [112].

With the increase in insulin ratio in hyperinsulinemia, the nuclear effect caused by oxidative stress activates kappa B (NF-κB), leaving soluble vascular cell adhesion molecule-1 (sVCAM-1) and soluble intercellular adhesion molecule-1 (sICAM-1) in excess, which is recognized as the inflammatory phase of atherosclerosis. In addition, the regional concentration of C-reactive protein (CRP) leads to the production of interleukin-like pro-inflammatory cytokines [109]. In this way, hyperinsulinemia puts direct pressure on vascular smooth muscle and endothelial cells and supports the formation of atherosclerosis [113].

**Vascular Inflammation and Prothrombotic Status in Metabolic Syndrome**

In addition to inflammatory cytokines, many substances are produced from adipose tissue. Interleukin-6 (IL-6), which is the most potent cytokine involved in inflammatory activities, is one of the most important stimulators in CRP synthesis. Tumor necrosis alpha (TNF-α) can also be demonstrated from adipose tissue. TNF-α, which inhibits lipogenesis, prevents obesity formation by increasing apoptotic adipocyte formation and lipolysis. The best measures of the procoagulant or prothrombic pattern in these patients are the increase in plasminogen and plasminogen activator inhibitor-1 (PAI-1). As a result, it prepares the ground for the increase in atherogenesis and the formation of a thrombus that enables acute coronary progression [114, 115].

The variety of released adipokines includes hormones (*e.g.* leptin, adiponectin), peptides (*e.g.* angiotensinogen, apelin, resistin, and PAI-1, and inflammatory cytokines (IL-6, TNF-α, visfatin, omentin, and chemerin), all of which play a major role in the pathophysiology of insulin resistance and MetS [1, 115].

**Metabolic Syndrome and Non-alcoholic Fatty Liver Disease**

Non-alcoholic fatty liver disease (NAFLD) is a group of diseases characterized by marked macrovesicular steatosis in the liver without alcohol intake. Recent studies have shown that the relationship between NAFLD and MetS is reciprocal and bidirectional. For example, in the early 2000s, it became clear that surrogate indices of liver dysfunction predict T2DM and MetS [116, 117]. Taking these epidemiologic data further, it has been possible to conduct theoretical and meta-analytic studies showing that NAFLD is in fact a potential precursor of T2DM and MetS and that the fibrosis stage is a strong predictor of such a risk [118 - 120].

Metabolic dysfunction-associated steatotic liver disease (MASLD) is the latest term for steatotic liver disease associated with MetS. In July 2023, with the consensus of the International Liver Societies, terminology, and diagnostic criteria were revised under the main heading of 'steatotic liver disease (SLD)', and the name NAFLD was changed to 'metabolic associated steatotic liver disease (MASLD)' because the terms 'non-alcoholic' and 'fatty' did not fully reflect the pathophysiology [121].

MASLD is closely linked to MetS, as both conditions involve disturbances in metabolic processes that can lead to liver complications. Individuals with MetS often have a higher risk of developing MASLD. The accumulation of fat in the liver (steatosis) is a common feature of both conditions. In MetS, insulin resistance and dyslipidemia contribute to the accumulation of fat in the liver, leading to MASLD. The presence of MetS, T2DM, hypertension, dyslipidemia/hyperlipidemia, and hyperuricemia increases the risk of developing more severe forms of liver disease, such as MAFLD and metabolic dysfunction-associated steatohepatitis (MASH, former name NASH) [122 - 125].

The presence of NASH increases the risk of T2DM 2-5 times and the risk of cardiovascular disease 2-3 times [123, 125]. Insulin resistance is the most important responsible mechanism in comorbidities and NAFLD. In the association of NASH and T2DM, the risk of developing cirrhosis and HCC increases 2-4-fold [123 - 125]. The risk of death due to chronic liver disease is approximately 3 times higher in T2DM patients compared to non-diabetic patients [126]. Therefore, guidelines recommend that patients with obesity, insulin resistance, and/or MetS should be screened for NAFLD, and patients with prediabetes or T2DM should be evaluated for NAFLD every 6-12 months [127].

## TREATMENT

The primary treatment in MetS, which is a disease picture that emerges under the influence of genetic and environmental factors, should be a positive and permanent lifestyle modification. The general approach in treatment is to first establish lifestyle changes in the patient [128]. Lifestyle and dietary changes are encouraged to treat all of the components of MetS. Lifestyle and dietary changes are encouraged to treat all of the components of MetS. Since the majority of individuals with MetS are overweight, it is important to focus on dietary therapies that help individuals lose weight [129]. Weight loss provides many benefits. It is reported that a small decrease in body weight (5-10%) is sufficient to raise HDL-C and lower TG levels [130]. In addition, ideal weight loss has been shown to regulate blood pressure and reduce parameters associated with fasting blood glucose and insulin resistance [131]. Since the majority of individuals with MetS are overweight, it is important to focus on dietary therapies that help individuals lose weight [129]. Weight loss provides many benefits. It is reported that a small decrease in body weight (5-10%) is sufficient to raise HDL-C and lower TG levels [130]. In addition, ideal weight loss has been shown to regulate blood pressure and reduce parameters associated with fasting blood glucose and insulin resistance [131]. Baxheinrich *et al.* [132] suggested dietary food patterns with a low energy density and high intakes of monounsaturated fatty acid (MUFA) and α-linolenic acid may be a practical approach for long-term dietary treatment in patients with the MetS, leading to weight reduction and an improvement in the overall cardiovascular risk profile.

Lately, a consistent number of studies have been focusing on how to tailor medical nutrition therapy for individual patients within MetS populations. Indeed, personalized or tailored medical nutrition therapy (MNT) has gained increasing attention in the management of MetS. MetS is a complex condition with diverse underlying factors, including obesity, insulin resistance, dyslipidemia, and hypertension. Given this complexity and the variability among individuals, there's growing recognition that a one-size-fits-all approach to nutrition therapy may not be optimal for managing MetS effectively [133]. Nutrition practice based on scientific evidence is needed to promote an individual's global health.

## CONCLUSION

MetS is a major public health problem. The main component of MetS is insulin resistance. The cardiovascular risk associated with MetS is very high. The prevalence of MetS is increasing worldwide every year and is one of the most important causes of morbidity and mortality. Genetic variations and environmental factors contribute to the development of MetS by affecting abdominal adiposity, innate immunity, glucose, lipid and lipoprotein metabolism, and vascular function. The medical treatment of MetS and the resulting complications have become a major economic burden worldwide. It is therefore important to identify safe, effective, and feasible ways to prevent and reduce MetS. Although considerable progress has been made in understanding the etiology and mechanisms of MetS, more research is needed. The management of MetS involves lifestyle changes. Weight loss, proper nutrition, and adequate physical activity are the fundamental elements of treatment. Patients with MetS benefit greatly from lifestyle modifications. The goal of MetS treatment is to reduce the future risk of developing T2DM and cardiovascular disease. As seen in studies, the MetS brought about by changing eating habits and physical inactivity brought about by today's modern life is closely related to hormonal balance. In recent years, many diets with reported efficacy against T2DM, hypertension, dyslipidemia, and cardiovascular diseases can be applied in MetS in accordance with the findings.

## REFERENCES

[1]    Fahed G, Aoun L, Bou Zerdan M, *et al.* Metabolic Syndrome: Updates on Pathophysiology and Management in 2021. Int J Mol Sci 2022; 23(2): 786.

[http://dx.doi.org/10.3390/ijms23020786] [PMID: 35054972]

[2]     Parikh R, Mohan V. Changing definitions of metabolic syndrome. Indian J Endocrinol Metab 2012; 16(1): 7-12.
[http://dx.doi.org/10.4103/2230-8210.91175] [PMID: 22276247]

[3]     Micucci C, Valli D, Matacchione G, Catalano A. Current perspectives between metabolic syndrome and cancer. Oncotarget 2016; 7(25): 38959-72.
[http://dx.doi.org/10.18632/oncotarget.8341] [PMID: 27029038]

[4]     Hirode G, Wong RJ. Trends in the prevalence of metabolic syndrome in the United States, 2011-2016. JAMA 2020; 323(24): 2526-8.
[http://dx.doi.org/10.1001/jama.2020.4501] [PMID: 32573660]

[5]     McCracken E, Monaghan M, Sreenivasan S. Pathophysiology of the metabolic syndrome. Clin Dermatol 2018; 36(1): 14-20.
[http://dx.doi.org/10.1016/j.clindermatol.2017.09.004] [PMID: 29241747]

[6]     Sherling DH, Perumareddi P, Hennekens CH. Metabolic Syndrome. J Cardiovasc Pharmacol Ther 2017; 22(4): 365-7.
[http://dx.doi.org/10.1177/1074248416686187] [PMID: 28587579]

[7]     Alberti KGMM, Zimmet P, Shaw J. The metabolic syndrome-a new worldwide definition. Lancet 2005; 366(9491): 1059-62.
[http://dx.doi.org/10.1016/S0140-6736(05)67402-8] [PMID: 16182882]

[8]     Expert Panel on Detection, Evaluation, and Treatment of High Blood Cholesterol in Adults. Executive Summary of the Third Report of the National Cholesterol Education Program (NCEP) Expert Panel on Detection, Evaluation, and Treatment of High Blood Cholesterol in Adults (Adult Treatment Panel III). JAMA J Am Med Assoc [Internet]. 2001 [a.yer 13 Aralık 2022]; 285(19): 2486-97.
access address: http://jama.ama-assn.org/cgi/doi/10.1001/jama.285.19.2486

[9]     Castro-Barquero S, Ruiz-León AM, Sierra-Pérez M, Estruch R, Casas R. Dietary Strategies for Metabolic Syndrome: A Comprehensive Review. Nutrients 2020; 12(10): 2983.
[http://dx.doi.org/10.3390/nu12102983] [PMID: 33003472]

[10]    Mozumdar A, Liguori G. Persistent increase of prevalence of metabolic syndrome among U.S. adults: NHANES III to NHANES 1999-2006. Diabetes Care 2011; 34(1): 216-9.
[http://dx.doi.org/10.2337/dc10-0879] [PMID: 20889854]

[11]    Aguilar M, Bhuket T, Torres S, Liu B, Wong RJ. Prevalence of the metabolic syndrome in the United States, 2003-2012. JAMA 2015; 313(19): 1973-4.
[http://dx.doi.org/10.1001/jama.2015.4260] [PMID: 25988468]

[12]    Ortman JM, Velkoff VA, Hogan H. An Aging Nation: The Older Population in the United States, Current Population Reports. Washington, DC: U.S. Census Bureau 2014; pp. 25-1140.

[13]    Rus M, Crisan S, Andronie-Cioara FL, *et al.* Prevalence and Risk Factors of Metabolic Syndrome: A Prospective Study on Cardiovascular Health. Medicina (Kaunas) 2023; 59(10): 1711.
[http://dx.doi.org/10.3390/medicina59101711] [PMID: 37893429]

[14]    Noubiap JJ, Nansseu JR, Lontchi-Yimagou E, *et al.* Geographic distribution of metabolic syndrome and its components in the general adult population: A meta-analysis of global data from 28 million individuals. Diabetes Res Clin Pract 2022; 188: 109924.
[http://dx.doi.org/10.1016/j.diabres.2022.109924] [PMID: 35584716]

[15]    Ekelund U, Anderssen S, Andersen LB, *et al.* Prevalence and correlates of the metabolic syndrome in a population-based sample of European youth. Am J Clin Nutr 2009; 89(1): 90-6.
[http://dx.doi.org/10.3945/ajcn.2008.26649] [PMID: 19056570]

[16]    Misra A, Khurana L. The metabolic syndrome in South Asians: epidemiology, determinants, and prevention. Metab Syndr Relat Disord 2009; 7(6): 497-514.
[http://dx.doi.org/10.1089/met.2009.0024] [PMID: 19900153]

[17]   Bener A, Zirie M, Musallam M, Khader YS, Al-Hamaq AOAA. Prevalence of metabolic syndrome according to Adult Treatment Panel III and International Diabetes Federation criteria: a population-based study. Metab Syndr Relat Disord 2009; 7(3): 221-30.
[http://dx.doi.org/10.1089/met.2008.0077] [PMID: 19320557]

[18]   Grundy SM, Cleeman JI, Daniels SR, *et al.* Diagnosis and Management of the Metabolic Syndrome. Circulation 2005; 112(17): 2735-52.
[http://dx.doi.org/10.1161/CIRCULATIONAHA.105.169404] [PMID: 16157765]

[19]   Bokor S, Frelut ML, Vania A, *et al.* Prevalence of metabolic syndrome in European obese children. Int J Pediatr Obes 2008; 3(s2) (Suppl. 2): 3-8.
[http://dx.doi.org/10.1080/17477160802404509] [PMID: 18850405]

[20]   Iqbal Hydrie MZ, Shera AS, Fawwad A, Basit A, Hussain A. Prevalence of metabolic syndrome in urban Pakistan (Karachi): comparison of newly proposed International Diabetes Federation and modified Adult Treatment Panel III criteria. Metab Syndr Relat Disord 2009; 7(2): 119-24.
[http://dx.doi.org/10.1089/met.2008.0055] [PMID: 18928398]

[21]   Cizmecioğlu FM, Hatun S, Kalaça S. Metabolic syndrome in obese Turkish children and adolescents: comparison of two diagnostic models. Turk J Pediatr 2008; 50(4): 359-65.
[PMID: 19014050]

[22]   Lindsay RS, Howard BV. Cardiovascular risk associated with the metabolic syndrome. Curr Diab Rep 2004; 4(1): 63-8.
[http://dx.doi.org/10.1007/s11892-004-0013-9] [PMID: 14764282]

[23]   Moore KJ, Shah R. Introduction to the Obesity, Metabolic Syndrome, and CVD Compendium. Circ Res 2020; 126(11): 1475-6.
[http://dx.doi.org/10.1161/CIRCRESAHA.120.317240] [PMID: 32437304]

[24]   Mohamed SM, Shalaby MA, El-Shiekh RA, El-Banna HA, Emam SR, Bakr AF. Metabolic syndrome: risk factors, diagnosis, pathogenesis, and management with natural approaches. Food Chem Adv 2023; 3: 100335.
[http://dx.doi.org/10.1016/j.focha.2023.100335]

[25]   Grundy SM, Brewer HB Jr, Cleeman JI, Smith SC Jr, Lenfant C. Definition of metabolic syndrome: Report of the National Heart, Lung, and Blood Institute/American Heart Association conference on scientific issues related to definition. Circulation 2004; 109(3): 433-8.
[http://dx.doi.org/10.1161/01.CIR.0000111245.75752.C6] [PMID: 14744958]

[26]   Kassi E, Pervanidou P, Kaltsas G, Chrousos G. Metabolic syndrome: definitions and controversies. BMC Med 2011; 9(1): 48.
[http://dx.doi.org/10.1186/1741-7015-9-48] [PMID: 21542944]

[27]   Dobrowolski P, Prejbisz A, Kuryłowicz A, *et al.* Metabolic syndrome – a new definition and management guidelines A joint position paper by the Polish Society of Hypertension, Polish Society for the Treatment of Obesity, Polish Lipid Association, Polish Association for Study of Liver, Polish Society of Family Medicine, Polish Society of Lifestyle Medicine, Division of Prevention and Epidemiology Polish Cardiac Society, "Club 30" Polish Cardiac Society, and Division of Metabolic and Bariatric Surgery Society of Polish Surgeons. Arch Med Sci 2022; 18(5): 1133-56.
[http://dx.doi.org/10.5114/aoms/152921] [PMID: 36160355]

[28]   Alberti KGMM, Zimmet PZ. Definition, diagnosis and classification of diabetes mellitus and its complications. Part 1: diagnosis and classification of diabetes mellitus. Provisional report of a WHO Consultation. Diabet Med 1998; 15(7): 539-53.
[http://dx.doi.org/10.1002/(SICI)1096-9136(199807)15:7<539::AID-DIA668>3.0.CO;2-S]   [PMID: 9686693]

[29]   Zimmet P, Magliano D, Matsuzawa Y, Alberti G, Shaw J. The metabolic syndrome: a global public health problem and a new definition. J Atheroscler Thromb 2005; 12(6): 295-300.
[http://dx.doi.org/10.5551/jat.12.295] [PMID: 16394610]

[30]   Balkau B, Charles MA. Comment on the provisional report from the WHO consultation. Diabet Med 1999; 16(5): 442-3.
[http://dx.doi.org/10.1046/j.1464-5491.1999.00059.x] [PMID: 10342346]

[31]   Yamagishi K, Iso H. The criteria for metabolic syndrome and the national health screening and education system in Japan. Epidemiol Health 2017; 39: e2017003.
[http://dx.doi.org/10.4178/epih.e2017003] [PMID: 28092931]

[32]   Desroches S, Lamarche B. The evolving definitions and increasing prevalence of the metabolic syndrome. Appl Physiol Nutr Metab 2007; 32(1): 23-32.
[http://dx.doi.org/10.1139/h06-095] [PMID: 17332782]

[33]   Jha BK, Sherpa ML, Imran M, *et al.* Progress in Understanding Metabolic Syndrome and Knowledge of Its Complex Pathophysiology. Diabetology (Basel) 2023; 4(2): 134-59.
[http://dx.doi.org/10.3390/diabetology4020015]

[34]   Bovolini A, Garcia J, Andrade MA, Duarte JA. Metabolic syndrome pathophysiology and predisposing factors. Int J Sports Med 2021; 42(3): 199-214.
[http://dx.doi.org/10.1055/a-1263-0898] [PMID: 33075830]

[35]   Neeland IJ, Poirier P, Després JP. Cardiovascular and Metabolic Heterogeneity of Obesity. Circulation 2018; 137(13): 1391-406.
[http://dx.doi.org/10.1161/CIRCULATIONAHA.117.029617] [PMID: 29581366]

[36]   Mendrick DL, Diehl AM, Topor LS, *et al.* Metabolic Syndrome and Associated Diseases: From the Bench to the Clinic. Toxicol Sci 2018; 162(1): 36-42.
[http://dx.doi.org/10.1093/toxsci/kfx233] [PMID: 29106690]

[37]   Schoeller DA. Insights into energy balance from doubly labeled water. Int J Obes [Internet]. 2008 [a.yer 26 Aralık 2022];32(7):72-5. access address: http://www.nature.com/articles/ijo2008241
[http://dx.doi.org/10.1038/ijo.2008.241]

[38]   Obesity: preventing and managing the global epidemic. Report of a WHO consultation. World Health Organ Tech Rep Ser 2000; 894: i-xii, 1-253.
[PMID: 11234459]

[39]   Maury E, Brichard SM. Adipokine dysregulation, adipose tissue inflammation and metabolic syndrome. Mol Cell Endocrinol 2010; 314(1): 1-16.
[http://dx.doi.org/10.1016/j.mce.2009.07.031] [PMID: 19682539]

[40]   Andrade-Oliveira V, Câmara NOS, Moraes-Vieira PM. Adipokines as drug targets in diabetes and underlying disturbances. J Diabetes Res 2015; 2015: 1-11.
[http://dx.doi.org/10.1155/2015/681612] [PMID: 25918733]

[41]   Sears B, Perry M. The role of fatty acids in insulin resistance. Lipids Health Dis 2015; 14(1): 121.
[http://dx.doi.org/10.1186/s12944-015-0123-1] [PMID: 26415887]

[42]   Zatterale F, Longo M, Naderi J, *et al.* Chronic Adipose Tissue Inflammation Linking Obesity to Insulin Resistance and Type 2 Diabetes. Front Physiol 2020; 10: 1607.
[http://dx.doi.org/10.3389/fphys.2019.01607] [PMID: 32063863]

[43]   Olszanecka-Glinianowicz M, Kocełak P, Janowska J, Skorupa A, Nylec M, Zahorska-Markiewicz B. Plasma visfatin and tumor necrosis factor-alpha (TNF-α) levels in metabolic syndrome. Kardiol Pol 2011; 69(8): 802-7.
[PMID: 21850623]

[44]   Kardinaal AFM, Erk MJ, Dutman AE, *et al.* Quantifying phenotypic flexibility as the response to a high-fat challenge test in different states of metabolic health. FASEB J 2015; 29(11): 4600-13.
[http://dx.doi.org/10.1096/fj.14-269852] [PMID: 26198450]

[45]   van Dijk SJ, Mensink M, Esser D, Feskens EJM, Müller M, Afman LA. Responses to high-fat challenges varying in fat type in subjects with different metabolic risk phenotypes: a randomized trial.

PLoS One 2012; 7(7): e41388.
[http://dx.doi.org/10.1371/journal.pone.0041388] [PMID: 22844471]

[46]   Alberti KGMM, Zimmet P, Shaw J. Metabolic syndrome-a new world-wide definition. A Consensus Statement from the International Diabetes Federation. Diabet Med 2006; 23(5): 469-80.
[http://dx.doi.org/10.1111/j.1464-5491.2006.01858.x] [PMID: 16681555]

[47]   Alberti KGMM, Eckel RH, Grundy SM, *et al.* Harmonizing the Metabolic Syndrome. Circulation 2009; 120(16): 1640-5.
[http://dx.doi.org/10.1161/CIRCULATIONAHA.109.192644] [PMID: 19805654]

[48]   Zhu L, Spence C, Yang WJ, Ma GX. The IDF Definition Is Better Suited for Screening Metabolic Syndrome and Estimating Risks of Diabetes in Asian American Adults: Evidence from NHANES 2011–2016. J Clin Med 2020; 9(12): 3871.
[http://dx.doi.org/10.3390/jcm9123871] [PMID: 33260754]

[49]   Després JP. Is visceral obesity the cause of the metabolic syndrome? Ann Med 2006; 38(1): 52-63.
[http://dx.doi.org/10.1080/07853890500383895] [PMID: 16448989]

[50]   Tchernof A, Després JP. Pathophysiology of human visceral obesity: an update. Physiol Rev 2013; 93(1): 359-404.
[http://dx.doi.org/10.1152/physrev.00033.2011] [PMID: 23303913]

[51]   Shulman GI. Ectopic fat in insulin resistance, dyslipidemia, and cardiometabolic disease. N Engl J Med 2014; 371(12): 1131-41.
[http://dx.doi.org/10.1056/NEJMra1011035] [PMID: 25229917]

[52]   Grundy SM. Metabolic syndrome update. Trends Cardiovasc Med 2016; 26(4): 364-73.
[http://dx.doi.org/10.1016/j.tcm.2015.10.004] [PMID: 26654259]

[53]   Lehr S, Hartwig S, Lamers D, *et al.* Identification and validation of novel adipokines released from primary human adipocytes. Mol Cell Proteomics 2012; 11(1): M111.010504.
[http://dx.doi.org/10.1074/mcp.M111.010504]

[54]   Lehr S, Hartwig S, Sell H. Adipokines: A treasure trove for the discovery of biomarkers for metabolic disorders. Proteomics Clin Appl 2012; 6(1-2): 91-101.
[http://dx.doi.org/10.1002/prca.201100052] [PMID: 22213627]

[55]   Berg AH, Scherer PE. Adipose tissue, inflammation, and cardiovascular disease. Circ Res 2005; 96(9): 939-49.
[http://dx.doi.org/10.1161/01.RES.0000163635.62927.34] [PMID: 15890981]

[56]   Xu H, Li X, Adams H, Kubena K, Guo S. Etiology of Metabolic Syndrome and Dietary Intervention. Int J Mol Sci 2018; 20(1): 128.
[http://dx.doi.org/10.3390/ijms20010128] [PMID: 30602666]

[57]   Green M, Arora K, Prakash S. Microbial Medicine: Prebiotic and Probiotic Functional Foods to Target Obesity and Metabolic Syndrome. Int J Mol Sci 2020; 21(8): 2890.
[http://dx.doi.org/10.3390/ijms21082890] [PMID: 32326175]

[58]   Huang PL. A comprehensive definition for metabolic syndrome. Dis Model Mech 2009; 2(5-6): 231-7.
[http://dx.doi.org/10.1242/dmm.001180] [PMID: 19407331]

[59]   Pavone P, Polizzi A, Marino SD, *et al.* West syndrome: a comprehensive review. Neurol Sci 2020; 41(12): 3547-62.
[http://dx.doi.org/10.1007/s10072-020-04600-5] [PMID: 32827285]

[60]   Urbina EM, Gidding SS, Bao W, Elkasabany A, Berenson GS. Association of fasting blood sugar level, insulin level, and obesity with left ventricular mass in healthy children and adolescents: The Bogalusa Heart Study. Am Heart J 1999; 138(1): 122-7.
[http://dx.doi.org/10.1016/S0002-8703(99)70256-5] [PMID: 10385774]

[61]   Kim SH, Kang HW, Jeong JB, *et al.* Association of obesity, visceral adiposity, and sarcopenia with an

increased risk of metabolic syndrome: A retrospective study. PLoS One 2021; 16(8): e0256083.
[http://dx.doi.org/10.1371/journal.pone.0256083] [PMID: 34403431]

[62]    Després JP, Lemieux I. Abdominal obesity and metabolic syndrome. Nature 2006; 444(7121): 881-7.
[http://dx.doi.org/10.1038/nature05488] [PMID: 17167477]

[63]    Wang Y, Lam KSL, Kraegen EW, *et al.* Lipocalin-2 is an inflammatory marker closely associated with obesity, insulin resistance, and hyperglycemia in humans. Clin Chem 2007; 53(1): 34-41.
[http://dx.doi.org/10.1373/clinchem.2006.075614] [PMID: 17040956]

[64]    Savas HB, Gultekin F, Ciris IM. Positive effects of meal frequency and calorie restriction on antioxidant systems in rats. North Clin Istanb 2017; 4(2): 109-16.
[http://dx.doi.org/10.14744/nci.2017.21548] [PMID: 28971167]

[65]    Eckel RH, Grundy SM, Zimmet PZ. The metabolic syndrome. Lancet 2005; 365(9468): 1415-28.
[http://dx.doi.org/10.1016/S0140-6736(05)66378-7] [PMID: 15836891]

[66]    Liu Z, Zhang L, Qian C, *et al.* Recurrent hypoglycemia increases hepatic gluconeogenesis without affecting glycogen metabolism or systemic lipolysis in rat. Metabolism 2022; 136: 155310.
[http://dx.doi.org/10.1016/j.metabol.2022.155310] [PMID: 36063868]

[67]    Pyörälä M, Miettinen H, Halonen P, Laakso M, Pyörälä K. Insulin resistance syndrome predicts the risk of coronary heart disease and stroke in healthy middle-aged men: the 22-year follow-up results of the Helsinki Policemen Study. Arterioscler Thromb Vasc Biol 2000; 20(2): 538-44.
[http://dx.doi.org/10.1161/01.ATV.20.2.538] [PMID: 10669654]

[68]    Mirrakhimov E, Bektasheva E, Isakova J, *et al.* Association of leptin receptor gene Gln223Arg polymorphism with insulin resistance and hyperglycemia in patients with metabolic syndrome. Arch Med Sci 2023; 20(1): 54-60.
[http://dx.doi.org/10.5114/aoms/170121] [PMID: 38414477]

[69]    McCracken E, Monaghan M, Sreenivasan S. Pathophysiology of the metabolic syndrome. Clin Dermatol 2018; 36(1): 14-20.
[http://dx.doi.org/10.1016/j.clindermatol.2017.09.004] [PMID: 29241747]

[70]    Huang PL. A comprehensive definition for metabolic syndrome. Dis Model Mech 2009; 2(5-6): 231-7.
[http://dx.doi.org/10.1242/dmm.001180] [PMID: 19407331]

[71]    Luna-Luna M, Medina-Urrutia A, Vargas-Alarcón G, Coss-Rovirosa F, Vargas-Barrón J, Pérez-Méndez Ó. Adipose Tissue in Metabolic Syndrome: Onset and Progression of Atherosclerosis. Arch Med Res 2015; 46(5): 392-407.
[http://dx.doi.org/10.1016/j.arcmed.2015.05.007] [PMID: 26009250]

[72]    Boden G, Lebed B, Schatz M, Homko C, Lemieux S. Effects of acute changes of plasma free fatty acids on intramyocellular fat content and insulin resistance in healthy subjects. Diabetes 2001; 50(7): 1612-7.
[http://dx.doi.org/10.2337/diabetes.50.7.1612] [PMID: 11423483]

[73]    Ježek P, Jabůrek M, Holendová B, Plecitá-Hlavatá L. Fatty Acid-Stimulated Insulin Secretion *vs.* Lipotoxicity. Molecules 2018; 23(6): 1483.
[http://dx.doi.org/10.3390/molecules23061483] [PMID: 29921789]

[74]    Johnson RJ, Perez-Pozo SE, Sautin YY, *et al.* Hypothesis: could excessive fructose intake and uric acid cause type 2 diabetes? Endocr Rev 2009; 30(1): 96-116.
[http://dx.doi.org/10.1210/er.2008-0033] [PMID: 19151107]

[75]    Punthakee Z, Goldenberg R, Katz P. Definition, Classification and Diagnosis of Diabetes, Prediabetes and Metabolic Syndrome. Can J Diabetes 2018; 42 (Suppl. 1): S10-5.
[http://dx.doi.org/10.1016/j.jcjd.2017.10.003] [PMID: 29650080]

[76]    Lamond N, Tiggemann M, Dawson D. Factors predicting sleep disruption in Type II diabetes. Sleep 2000; 23(3): 1-2.
[http://dx.doi.org/10.1093/sleep/23.3.1i] [PMID: 10811386]

[77]   Tong PC, Kong AP, So WY, *et al.* The usefulness of the International Diabetes Federation and the National Cholesterol Education Program's Adult Treatment Panel III definitions of the metabolic syndrome in predicting coronary heart disease in subjects with type 2 diabetes. Diabetes Care 2007; 30(5): 1206-11.
[http://dx.doi.org/10.2337/dc06-1484] [PMID: 17259472]

[78]   5. Prevention or Delay of Type 2 Diabetes: *Standards of Medical Care in Diabetes-2018.* Diabetes Care 2018; 41 (Suppl. 1): S51-4.
[http://dx.doi.org/10.2337/dc18-S005] [PMID: 29222376]

[79]   He J, Zhang F, Han Y. Effect of probiotics on lipid profiles and blood pressure in patients with type 2 diabetes. Medicine (Baltimore) 2017; 96(51): e9166.
[http://dx.doi.org/10.1097/MD.0000000000009166] [PMID: 29390450]

[80]   Silveira Rossi JL, Barbalho SM, Reverete de Araujo R, Bechara MD, Sloan KP, Sloan LA. Metabolic syndrome and cardiovascular diseases: Going beyond traditional risk factors. Diabetes Metab Res Rev 2022; 38(3): e3502.
[http://dx.doi.org/10.1002/dmrr.3502] [PMID: 34614543]

[81]   Bhat SL, Abbasi FA, Blasey C, Reaven GM, Kim SH. Beyond fasting plasma glucose: The association between coronary heart disease risk and postprandial glucose, postprandial insulin and insulin resistance in healthy, nondiabetic adults. Metabolism 2013; 62(9): 1223-6.
[http://dx.doi.org/10.1016/j.metabol.2013.04.012] [PMID: 23809477]

[82]   Lorenzo C, Wagenknecht LE, D'Agostino RB Jr, Rewers MJ, Karter AJ, Haffner SM. Insulin resistance, β-cell dysfunction, and conversion to type 2 diabetes in a multiethnic population: the Insulin Resistance Atherosclerosis Study. Diabetes Care 2010; 33(1): 67-72.
[http://dx.doi.org/10.2337/dc09-1115] [PMID: 19808919]

[83]   Tura A, Göbl C, Moro E, Pacini G. Insulin resistance and beta-cell dysfunction in people with prediabetes according to criteria based on glycemia and glycosylated hemoglobin. Endocr J 2017; 64(1): 117-22.
[http://dx.doi.org/10.1507/endocrj.EJ16-0298] [PMID: 27628439]

[84]   American Diabetes Association. Glycemic Targets: Standards of Medical Care in Diabetes 2020. Diabetes Care [Internet]. 2020 [a.yer 23 Ocak 2023];43(Supplement_1):66-76. access address: https://diabetesjournals.org/care/article/43/Supplement_1/S66/30598/6- Glycemic-Targets-Standar-s-of-Medical-Care-in.

[85]   Reaven GM. Insulin resistance/compensatory hyperinsulinemia, essential hypertension, and cardiovascular disease. J Clin Endocrinol Metab 2003; 88(6): 2399-403.
[http://dx.doi.org/10.1210/jc.2003-030087] [PMID: 12788834]

[86]   Vijan S, Hayward RA. Treatment of hypertension in type 2 diabetes mellitus: blood pressure goals, choice of agents, and setting priorities in diabetes care. Ann Intern Med 2003; 138(7): 593-602.
[http://dx.doi.org/10.7326/0003-4819-138-7-200304010-00018] [PMID: 12667032]

[87]   Stanciu S, Rusu E, Miricescu D, *et al.* Links between Metabolic Syndrome and Hypertension: The Relationship with the Current Antidiabetic Drugs. Metabolites 2023; 13(1): 87.
[http://dx.doi.org/10.3390/metabo13010087] [PMID: 36677012]

[88]   Muniyappa R, Sowers JR. Role of insulin resistance in endothelial dysfunction. Rev Endocr Metab Disord 2013; 14(1): 5-12.
[http://dx.doi.org/10.1007/s11154-012-9229-1] [PMID: 23306778]

[89]   Castro L, Brant L, Diniz MF, *et al.* Association of hypertension and insulin resistance in individuals free of diabetes in the ELSA-Brasil cohort. Sci Rep 2023; 13(1): 9456.
[http://dx.doi.org/10.1038/s41598-023-35298-y] [PMID: 37301876]

[90]   De Boer MP, Meijer R, Wijnstok NJ, *et al.* Microvascular dysfunction: a potential mechanism in the pathogenesis of obesity-associated insulin resistance and hypertension. Microcirculation 2012; 19(1):

5-18.
[http://dx.doi.org/10.1111/j.1549-8719.2011.00130.x] [PMID: 21883642]

[91]    Anderson EA, Mark AL. The vasodilator action of insulin. Implications for the insulin hypothesis of hypertension. Hypertension 1993; 21(2): 136-41.
[http://dx.doi.org/10.1161/01.HYP.21.2.136] [PMID: 8428776]

[92]    Führer D, Reincke M. Fettstoffwechselstörungen und metabolisches Syndrom. Inn Med (Heidelb) 2023; 64(7): 609-10.
[http://dx.doi.org/10.1007/s00108-023-01545-7] [PMID: 37341737]

[93]    Ballard-Hernandez J, Sall J. Dyslipidemia Update. Nurs Clin North Am 2023; 58(3): 295-308.
[http://dx.doi.org/10.1016/j.cnur.2023.05.002] [PMID: 37536782]

[94]    Aquilante CL, Pharm D, Vande Griend JP, Pharm D, Cardiology AQ, Parra D, *et al.* Metabolic syndrome. 6th ed., Pharmacotherapy Self-Assessment Program 2019.

[95]    Cerezo C, Segura J, Praga M, Ruilope LM. Guidelines updates in the treatment of obesity or metabolic syndrome and hypertension. Curr Hypertens Rep 2013; 15(3): 196-203.
[http://dx.doi.org/10.1007/s11906-013-0337-4] [PMID: 23519746]

[96]    Therond P. Catabolism of lipoproteins and metabolic syndrome. Curr Opin Clin Nutr Metab Care 2009; 12(4): 366-71.
[http://dx.doi.org/10.1097/MCO.0b013e32832c5a12] [PMID: 19474714]

[97]    Yang Q, Zhong Y, Ritchey M, *et al.* Predicted 10-year risk of developing cardiovascular disease at the state level in the U.S. Am J Prev Med 2015; 48(1): 58-69.
[http://dx.doi.org/10.1016/j.amepre.2014.09.014] [PMID: 25450016]

[98]    Ference BA, Ginsberg HN, Graham I, *et al.* Low-density lipoproteins cause atherosclerotic cardiovascular disease. 1. Evidence from genetic, epidemiologic, and clinical studies. A consensus statement from the European Atherosclerosis Society Consensus Panel. Eur Heart J 2017; 38(32): 2459-72.
[http://dx.doi.org/10.1093/eurheartj/ehx144] [PMID: 28444290]

[99]    Goff DC Jr, Bertoni AG, Kramer H, *et al.* Dyslipidemia prevalence, treatment, and control in the Multi-Ethnic Study of Atherosclerosis (MESA): gender, ethnicity, and coronary artery calcium. Circulation 2006; 113(5): 647-56.
[http://dx.doi.org/10.1161/CIRCULATIONAHA.105.552737] [PMID: 16461837]

[100]   Go AS, Mozaffarian D, Roger VL, *et al.* Heart disease and stroke statistics--2013 update: a report from the American Heart Association. Circulation 2013; 127(1): e6-e245.
[http://dx.doi.org/10.1161/CIR.0b013e31828124ad] [PMID: 23239837]

[101]   Kelemework B, Woubshet K, Tadesse S, Eshetu B, Geleta D, Ketema W. The Burden of Dyslipidemia and Determinant Factors Among Type 2 Diabetes Mellitus Patients at Hawassa University Comprehensive Specialized Hospital, Hawassa, Ethiopia. Diabetes Metab Syndr Obes 2024; 17: 825-32.
[http://dx.doi.org/10.2147/DMSO.S448350] [PMID: 38380274]

[102]   Zamora A, Masana L, Comas-Cufí M, *et al.* Familial hypercholesterolemia in a European Mediterranean population-Prevalence and clinical data from 2.5 million primary care patients. J Clin Lipidol 2017; 11(4): 1013-22.
[http://dx.doi.org/10.1016/j.jacl.2017.05.012] [PMID: 28826564]

[103]   Masana L, Zamora A, Plana N, *et al.* Incidence of Cardiovascular Disease in Patients with Familial Hypercholesterolemia Phenotype: Analysis of 5 Years Follow-Up of Real-World Data from More than 1.5 Million Patients. J Clin Med 2019; 8(7): 1080.
[http://dx.doi.org/10.3390/jcm8071080] [PMID: 31340450]

[104]   Garg A, Garg V, Hegele RA, Lewis GF. Practical definitions of severe *versus* familial hypercholesterolaemia and hypertriglyceridaemia for adult clinical practice. Lancet Diabetes

Endocrinol 2019; 7(11): 880-6.
[http://dx.doi.org/10.1016/S2213-8587(19)30156-1] [PMID: 31445954]

[105] Boekholdt SM, Arsenault BJ, Mora S, *et al.* Association of LDL cholesterol, non-HDL cholesterol, and apolipoprotein B levels with risk of cardiovascular events among patients treated with statins: a meta-analysis. JAMA 2012; 307(12): 1302-9.
[http://dx.doi.org/10.1001/jama.2012.366] [PMID: 22453571]

[106] Robinson JG, Wang S, Jacobson TA. Meta-analysis of comparison of effectiveness of lowering apolipoprotein B *versus* low-density lipoprotein cholesterol and nonhigh-density lipoprotein cholesterol for cardiovascular risk reduction in randomized trials. Am J Cardiol 2012; 110(10): 1468-76.
[http://dx.doi.org/10.1016/j.amjcard.2012.07.007] [PMID: 22906895]

[107] Cannon CP, Blazing MA, Giugliano RP, *et al.* Ezetimibe Added to Statin Therapy after Acute Coronary Syndromes. N Engl J Med 2015; 372(25): 2387-97.
[http://dx.doi.org/10.1056/NEJMoa1410489] [PMID: 26039521]

[108] Sabatine MS, Giugliano RP, Keech AC, *et al.* Evolocumab and Clinical Outcomes in Patients with Cardiovascular Disease. N Engl J Med 2017; 376(18): 1713-22.
[http://dx.doi.org/10.1056/NEJMoa1615664] [PMID: 28304224]

[109] Schalkwijk CG, Stehouwer CDA. Vascular complications in diabetes mellitus: the role of endothelial dysfunction. Clin Sci (Lond) 2005; 109(2): 143-59.
[http://dx.doi.org/10.1042/CS20050025] [PMID: 16033329]

[110] Incalza MA, D'Oria R, Natalicchio A, Perrini S, Laviola L, Giorgino F. Oxidative stress and reactive oxygen species in endothelial dysfunction associated with cardiovascular and metabolic diseases. Vascul Pharmacol 2018; 100: 1-19.
[http://dx.doi.org/10.1016/j.vph.2017.05.005] [PMID: 28579545]

[111] Wang L, Cheng CK, Yi M, Lui KO, Huang Y. Targeting endothelial dysfunction and inflammation. J Mol Cell Cardiol 2022; 168: 58-67.
[http://dx.doi.org/10.1016/j.yjmcc.2022.04.011] [PMID: 35460762]

[112] Rosen ED. The transcriptional basis of adipocyte development. Prostaglandins Leukot Essent Fatty Acids 2005; 73(1): 31-4.
[http://dx.doi.org/10.1016/j.plefa.2005.04.004] [PMID: 15936931]

[113] Rösen P, Nawroth PP, King G, Möller W, Tritschler HJ, Packer L. The role of oxidative stress in the onset and progression of diabetes and its complications: a summary of a Congress Series sponsored by UNESCO-MCBN, the American Diabetes Association and the German Diabetes Society. Diabetes Metab Res Rev 2001; 17(3): 189-212.
[http://dx.doi.org/10.1002/dmrr.196] [PMID: 11424232]

[114] Lasselin J, Capuron L. Chronic low-grade inflammation in metabolic disorders: relevance for behavioral symptoms. Neuroimmunomodulation 2014; 21(2-3): 95-101.
[http://dx.doi.org/10.1159/000356535] [PMID: 24557041]

[115] Tylutka A, Morawin B, Walas Ł, Michałek M, Gwara A, Zembron-Lacny A. Assessment of metabolic syndrome predictors in relation to inflammation and visceral fat tissue in older adults. Sci Rep 2023; 13(1): 89.
[http://dx.doi.org/10.1038/s41598-022-27269-6] [PMID: 36596839]

[116] Hanley AJG, Williams K, Festa A, Wagenknecht LE, D'Agostino RB Jr, Haffner SM. Liver markers and development of the metabolic syndrome: the insulin resistance atherosclerosis study. Diabetes 2005; 54(11): 3140-7.
[http://dx.doi.org/10.2337/diabetes.54.11.3140] [PMID: 16249437]

[117] Nakanishi N, Suzuki K, Tatara K. Serum gamma-glutamyltransferase and risk of metabolic syndrome and type 2 diabetes in middle-aged Japanese men. Diabetes Care 2004; 27(6): 1427-32.
[http://dx.doi.org/10.2337/diacare.27.6.1427] [PMID: 15161799]

[118] Lonardo A, Ballestri S, Marchesini G, Angulo P, Loria P. Nonalcoholic fatty liver disease: A precursor of the metabolic syndrome. Dig Liver Dis 2015; 47(3): 181-90.
[http://dx.doi.org/10.1016/j.dld.2014.09.020] [PMID: 25739820]

[119] Ballestri S, Zona S, Targher G, *et al.* Nonalcoholic fatty liver disease is associated with an almost twofold increased risk of incident type 2 diabetes and metabolic syndrome. Evidence from a systematic review and meta-analysis. J Gastroenterol Hepatol 2016; 31(5): 936-44.
[http://dx.doi.org/10.1111/jgh.13264] [PMID: 26667191]

[120] Mantovani A, Byrne CD, Bonora E, Targher G. Nonalcoholic Fatty Liver Disease and Risk of Incident Type 2 Diabetes: A Meta-analysis. Diabetes Care 2018; 41(2): 372-82.
[http://dx.doi.org/10.2337/dc17-1902] [PMID: 29358469]

[121] Rinella ME, Lazarus JV, Ratziu V, *et al.* A multisociety Delphi consensus statement on new fatty liver disease nomenclature. Hepatology 2023; 78(6): 1966-86.
[http://dx.doi.org/10.1097/HEP.0000000000000520] [PMID: 37363821]

[122] Chan WK, Chuah KH, Rajaram RB, Lim LL, Ratnasingam J, Vethakkan SR. Metabolic Dysfunction-Associated Steatotic Liver Disease (MASLD): A State-of-the-Art Review. J Obes Metab Syndr 2023; 32(3): 197-213.
[http://dx.doi.org/10.7570/jomes23052] [PMID: 37700494]

[123] Chalasani N, Younossi Z, Lavine JE, *et al.* The diagnosis and management of nonalcoholic fatty liver disease: Practice guidance from the American Association for the Study of Liver Diseases. Hepatology 2018; 67(1): 328-57.
[http://dx.doi.org/10.1002/hep.29367] [PMID: 28714183]

[124] Jarvis H, Craig D, Barker R, *et al.* Metabolic risk factors and incident advanced liver disease in non-alcoholic fatty liver disease (NAFLD): A systematic review and meta-analysis of population-based observational studies. PLoS Med 2020; 17(4): e1003100.
[http://dx.doi.org/10.1371/journal.pmed.1003100] [PMID: 32353039]

[125] Byrne CD, Targher G. NAFLD: A multisystem disease. J Hepatol 2015; 62(1) (Suppl.): S47-64.
[http://dx.doi.org/10.1016/j.jhep.2014.12.012] [PMID: 25920090]

[126] Younossi ZM, Golabi P, de Avila L, *et al.* The global epidemiology of NAFLD and NASH in patients with type 2 diabetes: A systematic review and meta-analysis. J Hepatol 2019; 71(4): 793-801.
[http://dx.doi.org/10.1016/j.jhep.2019.06.021] [PMID: 31279902]

[127] Yilmaz Y, Zeybel M, Adali G, *et al.* TASL Practice Guidance on the Clinical Assessment and Management of Patients with Nonalcoholic Fatty Liver Disease. Hepatol Forum 2023; 4 (Suppl. 1): 1-32.
[http://dx.doi.org/10.14744/hf.2023.2023.0011] [PMID: 37920782]

[128] Christensen P, Meinert Larsen T, Westerterp-Plantenga M, *et al.* Men and women respond differently to rapid weight loss: Metabolic outcomes of a multi-centre intervention study after a low-energy diet in 2500 overweight, individuals with pre-diabetes (PREVIEW). Diabetes Obes Metab 2018; 20(12): 2840-51.
[http://dx.doi.org/10.1111/dom.13466] [PMID: 30088336]

[129] Riccardi G, Rivellese AA. Dietary treatment of the metabolic syndrome - the optimal diet. Br J Nutr 2000; 83(S1) (Suppl. 1): S143-8.
[http://dx.doi.org/10.1017/S0007114500001082] [PMID: 10889805]

[130] Van Gaal LF, Rissanen AM, Scheen AJ, Ziegler O, Rössner S. Effects of the cannabinoid-1 receptor blocker rimonabant on weight reduction and cardiovascular risk factors in overweight patients: 1-year experience from the RIO-Europe study. Lancet 2005; 365(9468): 1389-97.
[http://dx.doi.org/10.1016/S0140-6736(05)66374-X] [PMID: 15836887]

[131] Whelton PK, Appel LJ, Espeland MA, *et al.* Sodium reduction and weight loss in the treatment of hypertension in older persons: a randomized controlled trial of nonpharmacologic interventions in the

elderly (TONE). JAMA 1998; 279(11): 839-46.
[http://dx.doi.org/10.1001/jama.279.11.839] [PMID: 9515998]

[132]  Baxheinrich A, Stratmann B, Lee-Barkey YH, Tschoepe D, Wahrburg U. Effects of a rapeseed oil-enriched hypoenergetic diet with a high content of α-linolenic acid on body weight and cardiovascular risk profile in patients with the metabolic syndrome. Br J Nutr 2012; 108(4): 682-91.
[http://dx.doi.org/10.1017/S0007114512002875] [PMID: 22894911]

[133]  Ambroselli D, Masciulli F, Romano E, *et al.* New Advances in Metabolic Syndrome, from Prevention to Treatment: The Role of Diet and Food. Nutrients 2023; 15(3): 640.
[http://dx.doi.org/10.3390/nu15030640] [PMID: 36771347]

**CHAPTER 2**

# Functional Changes in Metabolic Syndrome

**Esra Bihter Gürler[1], Hülya Çevik ARAS[2] and Nagihan Bostanci[3,\*]**

[1] *Department of Physiology, Faculty of Dentistry, İstanbul Galata University, İstanbul, Turkey*

[2] *Department of Oral Medicine and Pathology, University of Gothenburg, Göteborg, Sweden*

[3] *Department of Dental Medicine, Karolinska Institutet, Stockholm, Sweden*

**Abstract:** Metabolic Syndrome (MetS) is a condition characterized by the co-occurrence of several cardiovascular risk factors, including insulin resistance, obesity, dyslipidemia, and hypertension. The development of MetS is closely linked to visceral adiposity, which refers to fat accumulation around critical vital organs in the abdominal cavity. Visceral fat is metabolically active and produces adipokines, proteins that regulate energy balance and play a role in inflammation and atherosclerosis. Some adipokines, such as leptin and adiponectin, have beneficial effects on glucose homeostasis and are considered protective against MetS. However, other adipokines, such as visfatin and resistin, contribute to glucose intolerance and have pro-atherogenic properties. Visceral obesity also contributes to the development of MetS through its effects on blood pressure. It activates the sympathetic nervous system, the renin-angiotensin-aldosterone system, and insulin resistance, leading to elevated blood pressure.

Another critical factor in the development of MetS is the activation of the lectin-like oxidized low-density lipoprotein receptor-1 (LOX-1). LOX-1 is a protein that acts as a receptor for oxidized LDL on the cell surface. Its activation leads to the production of reactive oxygen species, a decrease in nitric oxide, and increased expression of molecules contributing to hypertension and vascular damage. LOX-1 is also involved in the development of other complications associated with MetS, such as nephropathy and left ventricular hypertrophy.

The renin-angiotensin-aldosterone system (RAAS) regulates blood volume, electrolyte balance, and vascular resistance. In patients with MetS, the activation of RAAS leads to increased levels of angiotensin II (Ang II) and aldosterone, which have various effects on blood pressure and sodium and water retention. Ang II also contributes to oxidative stress and inflammation in the vasculature.

Insulin resistance, a key feature of MetS, disrupts the insulin signaling process in adipose tissue, leading to increased lipolysis and elevated levels of circulating free fatty acids. These fatty acids further worsen insulin resistance and contribute to impaired glucose metabolism.

---

\* **Corresponding author Nagihan Bostanci:** Department of Dental Medicine, Karolinska Institutet, Stockholm, Sweden; E-mail: nagihan.bostanci@ki.se

**Hafize Uzun & Seyma Dumur (Eds.)**

Oxidative stress, characterized by an imbalance between the production of reactive oxygen species and the body's antioxidant defenses, is closely associated with the development of MetS. Hyperlipidemia and hyperglycemia, standard features of MetS, are linked to increased oxidative stress and ROS production. Oxidative stress and the activation of RAAS and LOX-1 contribute to the progression of dyslipidemia, type 2 diabetes, hypertension, and cardiovascular diseases.

The oral-gut-liver axis is an emerging concept that suggests a relationship between oral infections, such as periodontitis, and metabolic dysfunction, including MetS and liver diseases. Periodontitis has been associated with chronic liver diseases, such as non-alcoholic fatty liver disease (NAFLD) and liver cirrhosis. The translocation of oral bacteria from the mouth to the gut may contribute to gut dysbiosis, increased intestinal permeability, and systemic inflammation, which can worsen liver functions.

Overall, the development of MetS involves the interplay of various factors, including visceral obesity, adipokines, LOX-1 activation, insulin resistance, oxidative stress, and the oral-gut-liver axis. Understanding these mechanisms is crucial for preventing and managing MetS and its associated complications. Further research is needed to fully elucidate the roles of individual factors and develop targeted interventions for MetS.

**Keywords:** Gut dysbiosis, Hyperglycemia, Liver diseases, MetS, Oxidative stress, Translocation.

## INTRODUCTION

Metabolic Syndrome (MetS) represents a complex constellation of interconnected physiological, biochemical, clinical, and metabolic factors that directly increase the risk of cardiovascular disease, type 2 diabetes, and all-cause mortality. This syndrome has emerged as a significant public health challenge worldwide, paralleling the rising epidemic of obesity and sedentary lifestyles. At its core, MetS is characterized by the co-occurrence of several cardiovascular risk factors, including insulin resistance, visceral obesity, atherogenic dyslipidemia, and hypertension [1].

The pathophysiology of MetS is multifaceted, involving an intricate interplay of various mechanisms. Central to this syndrome is visceral adiposity, which goes beyond mere fat accumulation to represent metabolically active tissue-producing adipokines—proteins that play crucial roles in energy homeostasis, inflammation, and atherosclerosis. The balance between protective adipokines (such as leptin and adiponectin) and those contributing to metabolic dysfunction (like visfatin and resistin) is critical in the progression of MetS [1, 2, 3].

Furthermore, the activation of the lectin-like oxidized low-density lipoprotein receptor-1 (LOX-1) and the renin-angiotensin-aldosterone system (RAAS) contributes significantly to the development of hypertension and vascular damage associated with MetS [1, 4]. Insulin resistance, a hallmark of MetS, disrupts normal metabolic processes, leading to a cascade of events that further exacerbate the syndrome.

Oxidative stress, resulting from an imbalance between reactive oxygen species production and the body's antioxidant defenses, is another key player in the pathogenesis of MetS. This oxidative imbalance is closely linked to the lipid and glucose abnormalities characteristic of the syndrome [5, 6].

Recent research has also highlighted the potential role of the oral-gut-liver axis in metabolic dysfunction [7-10]. This emerging concept suggests a relationship between oral infections, particularly periodontitis, and the development of MetS and liver diseases, adding another layer of complexity to our understanding of this syndrome.

This chapter sets the stage for a deeper exploration of these mechanisms, their interactions, and their collective impact on the development and progression of Metabolic Syndrome. Understanding these pathways is crucial for developing effective strategies for prevention, early diagnosis, and targeted treatment of this increasingly prevalent condition.

## Role of Visceral Fat and Adipokines (Adipocytes) in Metabolic Syndrome

Metabolic syndrome (MetS), also variously known as syndrome X, refers to the co-occurrence of several known cardiovascular risk factors, including insulin resistance, obesity, atherogenic dyslipidemia, and hypertension. The incidence of metabolic syndrome often parallels that of obesity. However, obesity does not always reflect MetS without other features such as insulin resistance, visceral obesity, atherogenic dyslipidemia, and endothelial dysfunction [14, 15]. Of these, the first two appear to be required for metabolic syndrome.

Visceral adiposity is crucial for the development of MetS. This type of fat is stored in the abdominal cavity around important internal organs such as the liver, pancreas, and intestines (Fig. **1**). The adipocytes of obese patients usually show increased sensitivity to the lipolytic action of catecholamines. This increased lipolytic response can lead to elevated levels of free fatty acids in the bloodstream, affecting lipid metabolism and contributing to dyslipidemia [1, 11-13].

Visceral obesity can also elevate blood pressure. This is due to a variety of factors, including the activation of the sympathetic nervous system, the renin-angiotensin-aldosterone system, and the effects of insulin resistance [1, 12, 14].

Visceral fat is metabolically active and produces adipokines and secretes proteins called "adipocytokines," which regulate the body's energy homeostasis and play an essential role in pathophysiological events such as inflammation and atherosclerosis [15-18]. They regulate lipolysis, lipogenesis, and lipid uptake in different tissues and contribute to the development of metabolic syndrome through various mechanisms. Adipokines, such as leptin, adiponectin, resistin, and visfatin, as well as pro-inflammatory and anti-inflammatory cytokines, such as TNF-α, IL-6, IL-1β, monocyte chemoattractant protein-1, and serum amyloid A, originate from visceral fat (Fig. **2**) [19, 20].

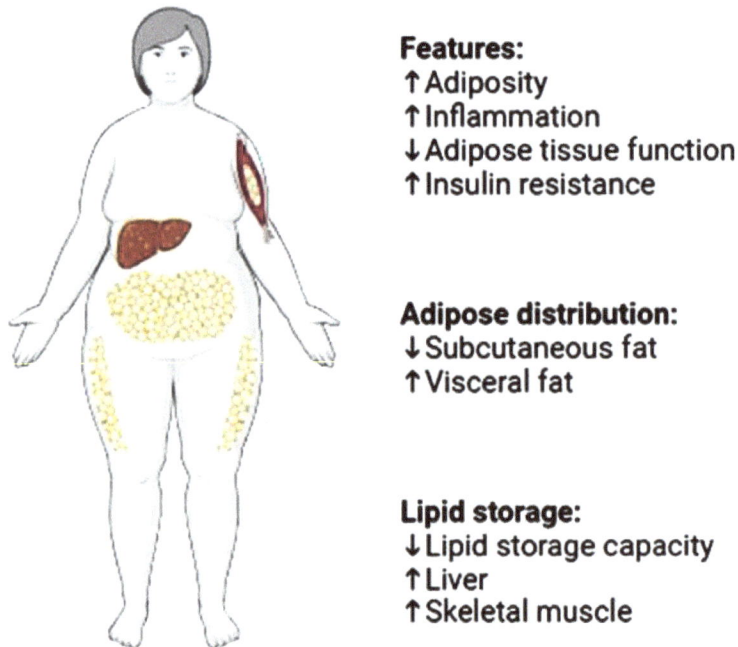

**Features:**
↑Adiposity
↑Inflammation
↓Adipose tissue function
↑Insulin resistance

**Adipose distribution:**
↓Subcutaneous fat
↑Visceral fat

**Lipid storage:**
↓Lipid storage capacity
↑Liver
↑Skeletal muscle

**Fig. (1).** Metabolically unhealthy obesity.

Adipokines such as leptin and adiponectin are involved in glucose homeostasis and lipid metabolism. Leptin and adiponectin improve insulin sensitivity, increase fatty acid oxidation, and prevent foam cell formation. These adipokines have beneficial effects on glucose homeostasis and are generally considered protective against metabolic syndrome [20].

On the other hand, adipokines like visfatin, fetuin-A, resistin, and plasminogen activator inhibitor-1 (PAI-1) are mentioned as contributors to the development of glucose intolerance and have pro-atherogenic properties [3, 21]. These adipokines may have harmful effects on metabolic syndrome.

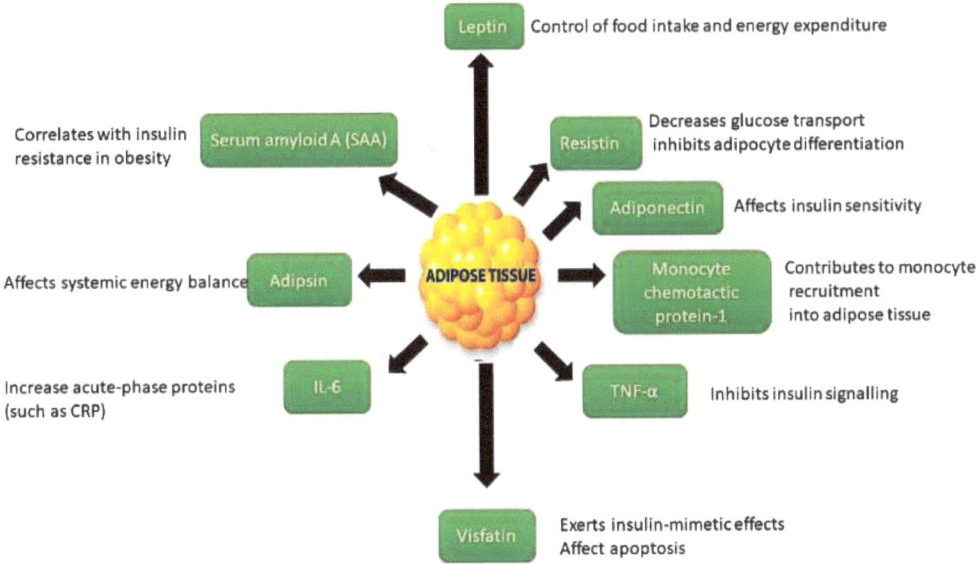

**Fig. (2).** Major adipokines and their functions.

Furthermore, chronic inflammation in adipose tissue, driven by elevated levels of cytokines and chemokines, recruits monocytes and produces vascular adhesion molecules. This process can result in hepatic fibroinflammatory injury, insulin resistance, and other complications associated with metabolic syndrome [17-23].

It is important to note that the contributions of individual adipokines to the pathophysiological features of metabolic syndrome are still a topic of debate, and further research is needed.

Obesity is a key feature of MetS, a state of chronic low-grade inflammation that contributes to insulin resistance and other metabolic abnormalities with increased levels of pro- and anti-inflammatory markers. These pro-inflammatory mediators trigger monocytes to differentiate macrophages in the adipose tissue, releasing cytokines.

However, the recruitment of monocytes into adipose tissue is not fully understood.

## Role of Lectin-Like Oxidized Low-Density Lipoprotein (LOX) Activation

Lectin-like oxidized low-density lipoprotein receptor-1 (LOX-1) is a membrane protein that acts as a receptor for oxidized LDL (ox-LDL) on the cell surface. LOX-1 activation produces reactive oxygen species, decreases nitric oxide from vascular endothelial cells, and increases the expression of endothelin-1, AT1R, and cell adhesion molecules [24, 25]. All of these factors contribute to both hypertension and vascular damage. In the case of high blood pressure, the expression of LOX-1 is increased in vascular smooth muscle cells [26]. Elevated concentrations of LOX-1 have been reported in adults with conditions such as hypertension, diabetes, and hyperlipidemia and cause oxLDL-induced apoptosis of endothelial cells. It can be down-regulated by Angiotensin I receptor blockers and statins [27, 28].

Moreover, LOX-1 is highly expressed in macrophages in human atherosclerotic lesions, and high glucose concentrations enhance LOX-1 expression in human macrophages. Endothelial dysfunction, in addition to disturbances in cholesterol metabolism, is associated with the development of atherosclerosis [26]. Endothelial cells, which form a single layer on the blood vessels' innermost surface, release molecules such as vasodilator nitric oxide, vasoconstrictor endothelin-1, adhesion molecules, and chemokines. Oxidized LDL (Low-Density Lipoprotein) causes the dysregulation of endothelial function, proinflammatory, prothrombotic, or proatherogenic through the LOX-1 receptor [29]. Urged by the endothelin-1, up-regulation of LOX-1 causes lipid accumulation in the coronary arteries of ApoE. By means of passivization through superoxide production and phosphorylation of endothelial synthase of endothelial nitric oxide, LOX-1 activation hinders nitric oxide discharge [30]. Depressed levels of NO also lead to increased endothelin-1 levels. In addition, LOX-1 stimulates various cellular signaling pathways such as rho and rac small GTPases, p38 MAP kinase, protein kinase C beta II, and NF-kB, thereby activating the expression of chemokines and molecules that facilitate the adhesion of leukocytes [31].

In addition to complications that are associated with diabetes and hypertension, LOX-1 is also associated with nephropathy and left ventricular hypertrophy. Depending on the extent of tubulointerstitial damage and urine protein concentrations, high LOX-1 expression is observed in tubulointerstitial regions in diabetic nephropathy [32]. Moreover, LOX-1 has been demonstrated to play a critical role in reforming cardiac myocytes as opposed to angiotensin II. Serum levels of soluble LOX-1 (sLOX-1) are elevated in the presence of ventricular hypertrophy in the pathophysiology of essential hypertension [27, 32].

The role of LOX-1 in visceral fat is thought to be associated with inflammation (Fig. **3**). It is suggested that elevated serum oxidized LDL (ox-LDL) levels in obesity demonstrate systemic oxidative stress due to escalating production of reactive oxygen species (ROS) by adipose tissue mitochondria [33].

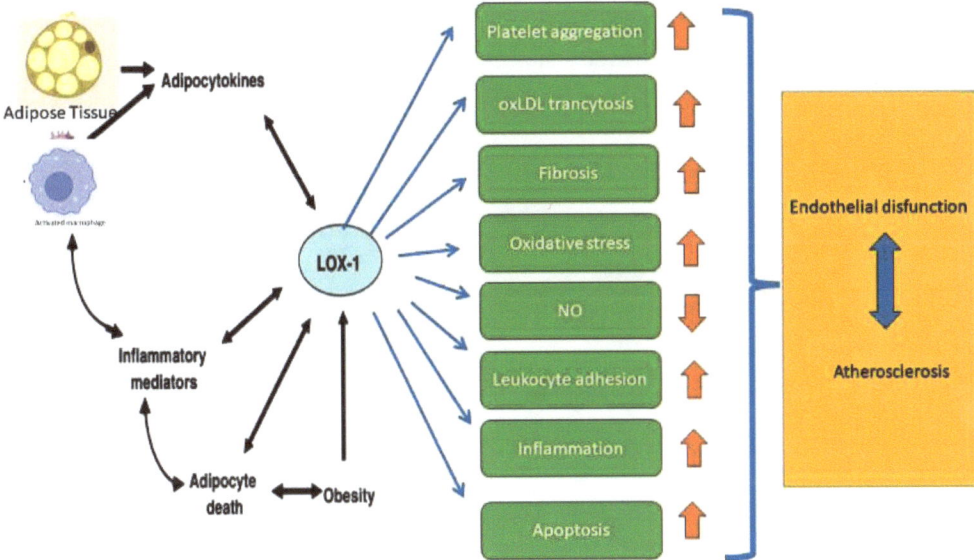

**Fig. (3).** Role of LOX-1 in MetS.

## Angiotensin II and Lox (lectin-like Oxidized low-density Lipoprotein) Activation

The renin-angiotensin-aldosterone system (RAAS) regulates blood volume, electrolyte balance, and systemic vascular resistance. In patients with over activated RAAS, pathological events promoting vascular disease are initiated. In type 2 diabetes, increased glucose levels initiate the activation of RAAS, which leads to increased levels of angiotensin II (Ang II) and aldosterone [34]. Ang II has various effects on blood pressure, including vasoconstriction, sympathetic nervous system stimulation, and sodium and water retention promotion through aldosterone release. Ang II's pathologic effects on the vasculature occur *via* oxidative stress by generating reactive oxygen species (ROS). The overproduction of Ang II, the activation of NAD(P)H oxidases, and the generation of ROS contribute to the pathophysiology of type 2 diabetes (Fig. **4**) [35].

The Angiotensin type 1 receptors (AT1R) are widely distributed in all organs and mediate most of the physiological effects of Ang II, such as blood pressure elevation, vasoconstriction, increased cardiac contractility, renal sodium retention, water reabsorption, and aldosterone release from the adrenal gland. AT1R expression in vascular smooth muscle cells is upregulated by LDL, insulin, progesterone, and erythropoietin and downregulated by epidermal growth factor, platelet-derived growth factor, thyroid hormone, nitric oxide, forskolin, angiotensin II, interferon-gamma, estrogen, vitamin A and HMG (3-hydroxy-

3-methyl-glutaryl) CoA reductase inhibitors. Both native LDL and oxidized LDL (ox-LDL) increase the expression of AT1R, which mediates most of the recognized cardiovascular effects of Ang II [29, 36].

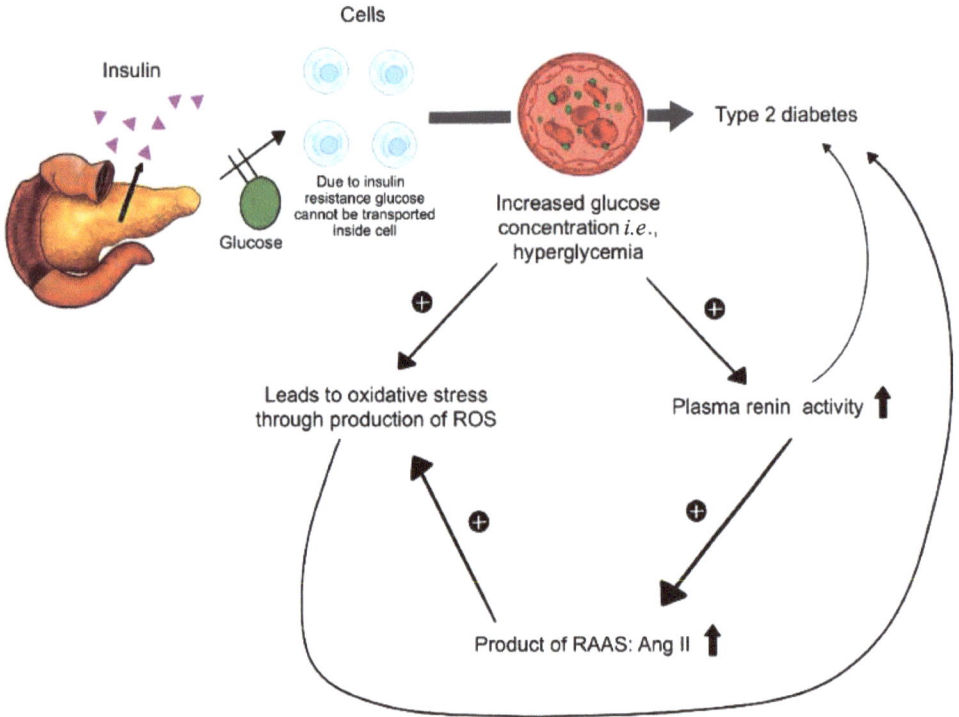

**Fig. (4).** The role of Ang-II and ROS generation in diabetes type 2 pathophysiology.

In obesity, increased body weight results in elevated cardiac output [33]. As a result, an increased metabolic rate due to functional vasodilatation causes greater tissue oxygen consumption. The exact mechanisms responsible for the harmful effects of obesity on the blood vessels have not been completely clarified. However, these effects likely result from complex interactions among various factors, including elevated blood pressure, inflammation, hyperglycemia, the accumulation of lipids leading to "lipotoxicity" through non-beta oxidative metabolism of fatty acids, oxidative stress, and the activation of various neurohumoral systems. Visceral obesity causes excessive secretion of pro-inflammatory and vasoactive adipokines such as angiotensinogen, Ang II, aldosterone, and resisting, along with increased plasma renin activity, which has been implicated in blood pressure control. RAAS activation occurs despite NaCl retention, volume expansion, and hypertension, which typically suppress renin secretion and Ang II formation [32, 34, 37]. Multiple mechanisms activate RAAS activation in obesity, including kidney compression and increased sympathetic nervous system activation. Although angiotensinogen is produced in adipocytes, the importance of adipose tissue as a source of Ang II formation remains unclear. An essential role for Ang II in stimulating renal NaCl reabsorption and in mediating obesity hypertension is supported by studies on experimental animals demonstrating that Ang II receptor blockade or ACE inhibition attenuates sodium retention, volume expansion, and increased BP. Activation of the RAAS may contribute to glomerular injury and nephron loss associated with obesity not only by increasing but also through intrarenal effects.

Many of these effects have been observed in experimental models of obesity-related hypertension that exhibit the characteristics of metabolic syndrome. Specific metabolic syndrome factors, such as high cholesterol levels, elevated blood sugar levels, and obesity, as indicated by an increased waist circumference, regulate the expression of components of the renin-angiotensin system (RAAS). This activation of the RAAS leads to the production of Ang II in specific tissues and cell types. The mechanisms mediated by Ang II contribute to the development of metabolic syndrome by exacerbating pathologies in various organs, including the vascular system (smooth muscle cells, endothelial cells), adipocytes, liver, pancreas, and kidney (Fig. **5**) [24, 26, 27, 32].

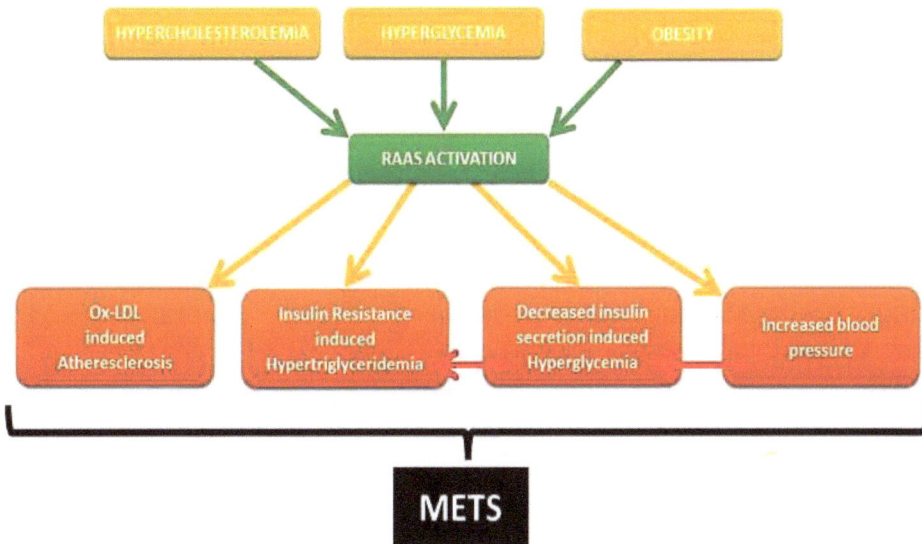

**Fig. (5).**   The interplay between RAAS components and other specific factors (hypercholesterolemia, hyperglycemia, obesity) regarding the development of metabolic syndrome.

## The Role of Insulin Resistance and Adipose Tissue

In healthy individuals, insulin signaling plays a crucial role in regulating the synthesis and storage of triacylglycerol in adipose tissue. However, insulin's ability to inhibit lipolysis in adipose tissue is impaired when insulin resistance develops. This leads to an increase in the levels of circulating free fatty acids, which further worsens insulin resistance by disrupting the insulin signaling process in various organs (Fig. **5**). The elevated levels of circulating fatty acids and triacylglycerol are strongly associated with impaired insulin signaling and glucose intolerance in obesity and type 2 diabetes [1, 31, 35, 37]. Dysfunctional lipid metabolism is considered the primary underlying cause of metabolic diseases. The accumulation of fat in non-adipose tissues, such as the liver and muscles, has been identified as a significant predictor of type 2 diabetes mellitus. In muscles, free fatty acids affect insulin receptor substrate (IRS-1), leading to reduced glucose uptake. In the liver, free fatty acids stimulate the production of glucose and fats. As a result, there is an increased demand for insulin to maintain normal blood glucose levels.

## Role of Oxidative Stress

Oxidative stress is a state of imbalance between the oxidative and anti-oxidative systems of cells and tissues, resulting in the overproduction of reactive oxygen species (ROS). Excessive oxidative stress is implicated in metabolic syndrome-related manifestations, including obesity, type 2 diabetes, hypertension, and cardiovascular diseases. In addition to increased oxidative activity, a reduced antioxidant state strongly correlates with MetS occurrence.

Hyperlipidemia and hyperglycemia are highly associated with oxidative stress and increased ROS production. ROS has multiple pleiotropic effects in the vascular system, including endothelial injury, LDL oxidation, and LOX-1 expression [32]. Increased ROS production, together with RAAS and LOX-1, contribute to the progression of dyslipidemia, type 2 diabetes, hypertension, and cardiovascular diseases. Total body fat and waist circumference are positively associated with oxidative stress-mediated endothelial dysfunction. Ang II is a principal NAD(P)H oxidase activator expressed in vascular smooth muscle cells and fibroblasts [35-39]. This oxidase system, similar to neutrophil oxidase, is a significant source of ROS in the vascular system. In hyperlipidemia and atherosclerosis, endothelial nitric oxide synthase may become dysfunctional and produce large amounts of superoxide.

Possible contributors to oxidative stress in obesity include hyperglycemia, hyperlipidemia, chronic inflammation, endothelial dysfunction, vitamin and mineral deficiencies, hyperleptinemia, increased muscle activity to carry excessive weight, impaired mitochondrial function, and diet. The relationship between oxidative stress and obesity is bidirectional and multifaceted. Oxidative stress can be a trigger and the outcome of obesity [35]. Obesity is highly associated with reduced antioxidant status due to continuous overeating, especially high-calorie, low-nutrient foods, which overwhelm the body's metabolic processes. This excess nutrient intake can lead to the production of ROS that the body's antioxidant defenses can neutralize, resulting in oxidative stress.

It is well documented that reducing visceral adiposity (waist circumference) through lifestyle modifications such as dietary changes and physical activity positively impacts overall health, specifically concerning metabolic syndrome and oxidative stress.

## Role of the Oral-Gut-Liver Axis in Metabolic Dysfunction

Obesity, metabolic syndrome, and oral infections are some of the most prevalent non-communicable diseases, and a substantial body of evidence from the published studies substantiates the correlation among these conditions. It is estimated that 3.5 billion people worldwide live with oral diseases [38]. Dental caries and periodontitis are the most prevalent oral infections, impacting approximately 35% and 11% of the worldwide population [39]. Extensive research has delineated plausible mechanisms elucidating how these conditions can detrimentally influence one another, indicating a mutually adverse relationship. The oral cavity hosts the second largest and most diverse microbiota, comprising more than 770 bacterial species engaging with diverse microbial populations at distinct anatomical sites within the human body, including the gut and liver. It is estimated that a person swallows up to 1.5 L of saliva each day, which can contain $10^8$–$10^{12}$ oral bacteria in the presence of periodontitis [40]. Although there is a growing body of knowledge regarding the dissemination of oral bacteria to distant organs *via* hematogenous and enteral routes, the functional impact of oral bacteria in the pathogenesis of intestinal and liver disorders remains relatively understudied.

Cross-sectional studies have found associations between periodontitis and the onset and progression of chronic liver diseases such as non-alcoholic fatty liver disease (NAFLD) and liver cirrhosis [8, 41, 42]. Common risk factors such as diabetes, smoking, and alcohol use partially explain the connections between these conditions. NAFLD is the most widespread chronic liver condition globally, with a notable rise in cases among individuals with metabolic syndrome. Population-based health examination surveys in the USA, Asia, and Europe indicated that advanced forms of periodontitis were linked to a heightened risk of developing NAFLD [9, 43, 44]. Salivary *P. gingivalis* is more frequently detected in saliva in patients with NAFLD than in controls [45]. Potentially, swallowed periodontal bacteria can translocate to the gut and cause gut dysbiosis, increased intestinal permeability, and subsequent systemic inflammation. Moreover, individuals with NAFLD showed elevated serum antibody levels against periodontitis-related bacteria such as *P. gingivalis and A. actinomycetemcomitans*. Periodontopathic bacteria may aggravate NAFLD by affecting lipid and glucose metabolism and altering the gut microbiota in experimental periodontitis models [10]. In a mouse model inducing NAFLD *via* a high-fat diet, intravenous *P. gingivalis* treatment led to notable increases in body and liver weight compared with NAFLD controls [45]. More interestingly, oral bacteria are overrepresented in the fecal microbiome of patients with liver cirrhosis [46]. Oral bacteria have been observed to infiltrate and persist within immune cells, suggesting that they may exploit host immune cells as Trojan horses for transportation from the oral mucosa to the gut mucosa [47]. The exact mechanism by which oral bacteria contribute to the pathogenesis of liver diseases remains elusive (Fig. **6**). Once periodontitis is established, oral bacteria can invade the gut, spreading adverse events to the intestinal microbiome and likely affecting liver functions. This may not be surprising as the liver has very close anatomical proximity and physiological interdependence with the intestine *via* metabolic exchange and translocation of bacteria. Ectopically colonized oral bacteria may contribute to the worsening of liver functions through the combined effects of two separate mechanisms: triggering mucosal inflammatory responses directly and acting as specific antigens for migrated oral T cells indirectly.

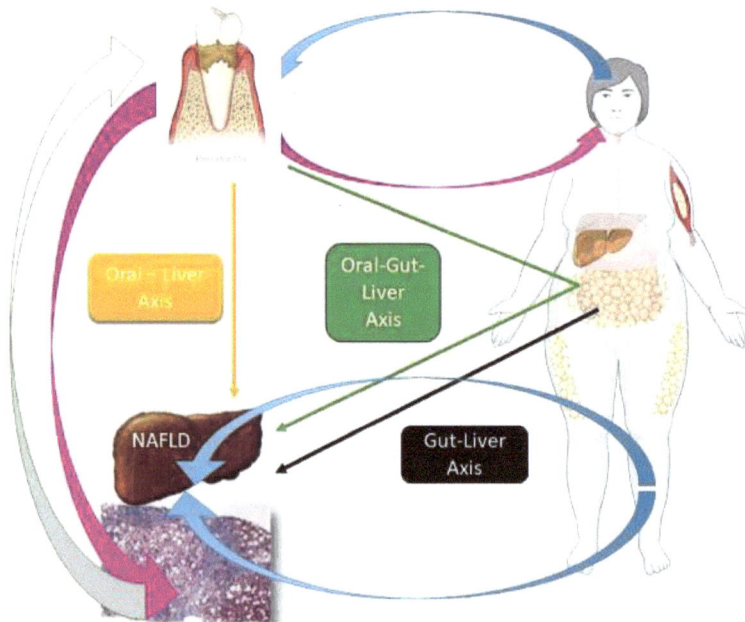

**Fig. (6).** The interplay between the gut, liver, and mouth.

Direct transfer occurs from mouth to gut due to impaired intestinal permeability. An imbalanced microbiota causes gut dysbiosis, and inflammatory mediators lead to systemic inflammation.

The blue arrow shows established links, the pink arrow shows possible links, and the white arrow shows indeterminate links.

Recent animal studies have revealed biologically plausible mechanisms by which experimental periodontitis can modify gut microbiota and impair gut tight junction integrity and insulin resistance [48, 49]. Periodontal pathogens impair glucose tolerance and insulin resistance in mice fed a standard or high-fat diet, leading to a significant accumulation of lipids in the liver. This is accompanied by elevated gene expression of acetyl-CoA carboxylase, a key enzyme in hepatic lipid metabolism, and glucokinase, a pivotal glucose sensor governing the regulation of insulin secretion. This body of evidence collectively supports a consensus between clinical and experimental research, indicating a distinct involvement of specific periodontal pathogens in modulating the oral-gut-liver axis. These observations have brought forward the hypothesis of an oral-gut-liver axis, justifying longitudinal studies to influence liver-related outcomes through periodontal interventions [50]. To date, periodontal treatment seems to alter the composition of the intestinal microbiota of liver diseases, modulate their systemic immune response, and potentially benefit liver health; clear evidence demonstrating that periodontitis treatment can arrest or reverse liver disease progression and improve outcomes is still lacking [51]. Given the existing evidence, offering education and guidance on oral examinations and self-care to all patients with liver disease is advisable. Employing an integrated care approach and fostering close collaboration between hepatologists and dentists is strongly recommended for managing patients dealing with liver disease and periodontitis.

## CONCLUSION

In conclusion, MetS's complex etiology necessitates a multifaceted approach to its prevention and treatment. Future research should focus on elucidating individual factors' precise roles and interactions to develop more targeted and effective interventions. A comprehensive understanding of these mechanisms is crucial for addressing the growing prevalence of MetS and associated complications.

As our knowledge of MetS continues to evolve, it becomes increasingly clear that effective management strategies must simultaneously address multiple aspects of the syndrome. This may involve lifestyle modifications, pharmacological interventions, and potentially novel approaches targeting specific pathways such as the oral-gut-liver axis.

# REFERENCES

[1]     Bernabe E, Marcenes W, Hernandez CR, *et al.* Global, Regional, and National Levels and Trends in Burden of Oral Conditions from 1990 to 2017: A Systematic Analysis for the Global Burden of Disease 2017 Study. J Dent Res 2020; 99(4): 362-73.
[http://dx.doi.org/10.1177/0022034520908533] [PMID: 32122215]

[2]     Kassebaum NJ, Bernabé E, Dahiya M, Bhandari B, Murray CJL, Marcenes W. Global burden of severe periodontitis in 1990-2010: a systematic review and meta-regression. J Dent Res 2014; 93(11): 1045-53.
[http://dx.doi.org/10.1177/0022034514552491] [PMID: 25261053]

[3]     Greenwood D, Afacan B, Emingil G, Bostanci N, Belibasakis GN. Salivary Microbiome Shifts in Response to Periodontal Treatment Outcome. Proteomics Clin Appl 2020; 14(3): 2000011.
[http://dx.doi.org/10.1002/prca.202000011] [PMID: 32223062]

[4]     Kobayashi T, Iwaki M, Nogami A, *et al.* Involvement of Periodontal Disease in the Pathogenesis and Exacerbation of Nonalcoholic Fatty Liver Disease/Nonalcoholic Steatohepatitis: A Review. Nutrients 2023; 15(5): 1269.
[http://dx.doi.org/10.3390/nu15051269] [PMID: 36904268]

[5]     Grønkjær LL, Holmstrup P, Schou S, Kongstad J, Jepsen P, Vilstrup H. Periodontitis in patients with cirrhosis: a cross-sectional study. BMC Oral Health 2018; 18(1): 22.
[http://dx.doi.org/10.1186/s12903-018-0487-5] [PMID: 29439734]

[6]     Sandler HC, Sigmund Stahl S. Prevalence of periodontal disease in a hospitalized population. J Dent Res 1960; 39(3): 439-49.
[http://dx.doi.org/10.1177/00220345600390030401] [PMID: 14441428]

[7]     Shin HS. Association between periodontal status and non-alcoholic fatty liver disease in a Korean adult population: A nationwide cross-sectional study. J Periodontol 2020; 91(4): 524-32.
[http://dx.doi.org/10.1002/JPER.19-0291] [PMID: 31484207]

[8]     Weintraub JA, Lopez Mitnik G, Dye BA. Oral Diseases Associated with Nonalcoholic Fatty Liver Disease in the United States. J Dent Res 2019; 98(11): 1219-26.
[http://dx.doi.org/10.1177/0022034519866442] [PMID: 31369716]

[9]     Helenius-Hietala J, Suominen AL, Ruokonen H, *et al.* Periodontitis is associated with incident chronic liver disease—A population-based cohort study. Liver Int 2019; 39(3): 583-91.
[http://dx.doi.org/10.1111/liv.13985] [PMID: 30300961]

[10]    Yoneda M, Naka S, Nakano K, *et al.* Involvement of a periodontal pathogen, Porphyromonas gingivalis on the pathogenesis of non-alcoholic fatty liver disease. BMC Gastroenterol 2012; 12(1): 16.
[http://dx.doi.org/10.1186/1471-230X-12-16] [PMID: 22340817]

[11]    Komazaki R, Katagiri S, Takahashi H, *et al.* Periodontal pathogenic bacteria, Aggregatibacter actinomycetemcomitans affect non-alcoholic fatty liver disease by altering gut microbiota and glucose metabolism. Sci Rep 2017; 7(1): 13950.
[http://dx.doi.org/10.1038/s41598-017-14260-9] [PMID: 29066788]

[12]    Qin N, Yang F, Li A, *et al.* Alterations of the human gut microbiome in liver cirrhosis. Nature 2014; 513(7516): 59-64.
[http://dx.doi.org/10.1038/nature13568] [PMID: 25079328]

[13]    Hajishengallis G. Periodontitis: from microbial immune subversion to systemic inflammation. Nat Rev Immunol 2015; 15(1): 30-44.
[http://dx.doi.org/10.1038/nri3785] [PMID: 25534621]

[14]    Blasco-Baque V, Garidou L, Pomié C, *et al.* Periodontitis induced by *Porphyromonas gingivalis* drives periodontal microbiota dysbiosis and insulin resistance *via* an impaired adaptive immune response. Gut 2017; 66(5): 872-85.

[http://dx.doi.org/10.1136/gutjnl-2015-309897] [PMID: 26838600]

[15]    Kitamoto S, Nagao-Kitamoto H, Jiao Y, *et al.* The Intermucosal Connection between the Mouth and Gut in Commensal Pathobiont-Driven Colitis. Cell 2020; 182(2): 447-462.e14.
[http://dx.doi.org/10.1016/j.cell.2020.05.048] [PMID: 32758418]

[16]    Nickenig G, Harrison DG. The AT(1)-type angiotensin receptor in oxidative stress and atherogenesis: part I: oxidative stress and atherogenesis. Circulation 2002; 105(3): 393-6.
[http://dx.doi.org/10.1161/hc0302.102618] [PMID: 11804998]

[17]    Li DY, Zhang YC, Philips MI, Sawamura T, Mehta JL. Upregulation of endothelial receptor for oxidized low-density lipoprotein (LOX-1) in cultured human coronary artery endothelial cells by activating angiotensin II type 1 receptor. Circ Res 1999; 84(9): 1043-9.
[http://dx.doi.org/10.1161/01.RES.84.9.1043] [PMID: 10325241]

[18]    Mehta PK, Griendling KK. Angiotensin II cell signaling: physiological and pathological effects in the cardiovascular system. Am J Physiol Cell Physiol 2007; 292(1): C82-97.
[http://dx.doi.org/10.1152/ajpcell.00287.2006] [PMID: 16870827]

[19]    Kataoka H, Kume N, Miyamoto S, *et al.* Expression of lectinlike oxidized low-density lipoprotein receptor-1 in human atherosclerotic lesions. Circulation 1999; 99(24): 3110-7.
[http://dx.doi.org/10.1161/01.CIR.99.24.3110] [PMID: 10377073]

[20]    Li L, Sawamura T, Renier G. Glucose enhances human macrophage LOX-1 expression: role for LOX-1 in glucose-induced macrophage foam cell formation. Circ Res 2004; 94(7): 892-901.
[http://dx.doi.org/10.1161/01.RES.0000124920.09738.26] [PMID: 15001526]

[21]    Nurun Nabi AHMEA. Diabetes and Renin-angiotensin-Aldosterone System: Pathophysiology and Genetics. Renin-Angiotensin Aldosterone System 2021.

[22]    Li D, Saldeen T, Romeo F, Mehta JL. Oxidized LDL upregulates angiotensin II type 1 receptor expression in cultured human coronary artery endothelial cells: the potential role of transcription factor NF-kappaB. Circulation 2000; 102(16): 1970-6.
[http://dx.doi.org/10.1161/01.CIR.102.16.1970] [PMID: 11034947]

[23]    Nickenig G, Sachinidis A, Michaelsen F, Bo¨hm M, Seewald S, Vetter H. Upregulation of vascular angiotensin II receptor gene expression by low-density lipoprotein in vascular smooth muscle cells. Circulation 1997; 95(2): 473-8.
[http://dx.doi.org/10.1161/01.CIR.95.2.473] [PMID: 9008466]

[24]    Putnam K, Shoemaker R, Yiannikouris F, Cassis LA. The renin-angiotensin system: a target of and contributor to dyslipidemias, altered glucose homeostasis, and hypertension of the metabolic syndrome. Am J Physiol Heart Circ Physiol 2012; 302(6): H1219-30.
[http://dx.doi.org/10.1152/ajpheart.00796.2011] [PMID: 22227126]

[25]    El Meouchy P, Wahoud M, Allam S, Chedid R, Karam W, Karam S. Hypertension Related to Obesity: Pathogenesis, Characteristics and Factors for Control. Int J Mol Sci 2022; 23(20): 12305.
[http://dx.doi.org/10.3390/ijms232012305] [PMID: 36293177]

[26]    Alicka M, Marycz K. The Effect of Chronic Inflammation and Oxidative and Endoplasmic Reticulum Stress in the Course of Metabolic Syndrome and Its Therapy. Stem Cells Int 2018; 2018: 1-13.
[http://dx.doi.org/10.1155/2018/4274361] [PMID: 30425746]

[27]    Rani V, Deep G, Singh RK, Palle K, Yadav UCS. Oxidative stress and metabolic disorders: Pathogenesis and therapeutic strategies. Life Sci 2016; 148: 183-93.
[http://dx.doi.org/10.1016/j.lfs.2016.02.002] [PMID: 26851532]

[28]    Kawashima S, Yokoyama M. Dysfunction of endothelial nitric oxide synthase and atherosclerosis. Arterioscler Thromb Vasc Biol 2004; 24(6): 998-1005.
[http://dx.doi.org/10.1161/01.ATV.0000125114.88079.96] [PMID: 15001455]

[29]    Manna P, Jain SK. Obesity, Oxidative Stress, Adipose Tissue Dysfunction, and the Associated Health Risks: Causes and Therapeutic Strategies. Metab Syndr Relat Disord 2015; 13(10): 423-44.

[http://dx.doi.org/10.1089/met.2015.0095] [PMID: 26569333]

[30]  Clemente-Suárez VJ, Redondo-Flórez L, Beltrán-Velasco AI, *et al.* The Role of Adipokines in Health and Disease. Biomedicines 2023; 11(5): 1290.
[http://dx.doi.org/10.3390/biomedicines11051290] [PMID: 37238961]

[31]  Deng Y, Scherer PE. Adipokines as novel biomarkers and regulators of the metabolic syndrome. Ann N Y Acad Sci 2010; 1212(1): E1-E19.
[http://dx.doi.org/10.1111/j.1749-6632.2010.05875.x] [PMID: 21276002]

[32]  Wajchenberg BL. Subcutaneous and visceral adipose tissue: their relation to the metabolic syndrome. Endocr Rev 2000; 21(6): 697-738.
[http://dx.doi.org/10.1210/edrv.21.6.0415] [PMID: 11133069]

[33]  Gade W, Schmit J, Collins M, Gade J. Beyond obesity: the diagnosis and pathophysiology of metabolic syndrome. Clin Lab Sci 2010; 23(1): 51-61.
[http://dx.doi.org/10.29074/ascls.23.1.51] [PMID: 20218095]

[34]  Chistiakov DA, Orekhov AN, Bobryshev YV. LOX-1-Mediated Effects on Vascular Cells in Atherosclerosis. Cell Physiol Biochem 2016; 38(5): 1851-9.
[http://dx.doi.org/10.1159/000443123] [PMID: 27160316]

[35]  Kim JE, Kim JS, Jo MJ, *et al.* The Roles and Associated Mechanisms of Adipokines in Development of Metabolic Syndrome. Molecules 2022; 27(2): 334.
[http://dx.doi.org/10.3390/molecules27020334] [PMID: 35056647]

[36]  McCracken E, Monaghan M, Sreenivasan S. Pathophysiology of the metabolic syndrome. Clin Dermatol 2018; 36(1): 14-20.
[http://dx.doi.org/10.1016/j.clindermatol.2017.09.004] [PMID: 29241747]

[37]  Francisqueti FV, Chiaverini LC, Santos KC, *et al.* The role of oxidative stress on the pathophysiology of metabolic syndrome. Rev Assoc Med Bras (1992) 1992; 1;63(1): 85-91.

[38]  Kahn CR, Wang G, Lee KY. Altered adipose tissue and adipocyte function in the pathogenesis of metabolic syndrome. J Clin Invest 2019; 129(10): 3990-4000.
[http://dx.doi.org/10.1172/JCI129187] [PMID: 31573548]

[39]  Yan M, Mehta JL, Hu C. LOX-1 and Obesity. Cardiovasc Drugs Ther 2011; 25(5): 469-76.
[http://dx.doi.org/10.1007/s10557-011-6335-3] [PMID: 21881850]

# CHAPTER 3

# New Approach to the Diagnosis of Metabolic Syndrome in Children

Omer Okuyan[1,*]

[1] *Istanbul Atlas University, Istanbul, Turkey*

**Abstract:** Metabolic syndrome (MetS) is a disorder with central obesity, essential hypertension (HT), glucose tolerance disorder, diabetes mellitus (DM), dyslipidaemia, and an increased risk of cardiovascular disease (CVD), which occurs under the influence of genetic predisposition and is based on insulin resistance (IR). MetS is well defined in adults, although MetS is a complex multifactorial disease with a not entirely recognized definition in childhood. Nevertheless, MetS is described as the presence of obesity, IR, dyslipidaemia, and HT. The increase in the rate of MetS in children is at alarming levels. The first step in the prevention and treatment of MetS is to recommend and implement healthy lifestyle changes from an early age. Healthy lifestyle changes should include not only children but also all family members and should be targeted to be maintained throughout life. One method of preventing CVD in adulthood should be the care of children with MetS. It is necessary to carry out studies to prevent MetS and to measure the effect of these studies on the frequency of MetS. In terms of preventive medicine, children with a family history of T2DM and/or MetS burden, body obesity on physical examination, and IR findings such as acanthosis nigricans should be monitored more closely and early treatment should be initiated in cases with IR at-risk for T2DM. In line with the objectives, continuous training on the evaluation of childhood obesity is necessary for paediatricians and general practitioners.

**Keywords:** Children, Diabetes mellitus, Dyslipidaemia, Glucose tolerance disorder, Metabolic Syndrome, Obesity.

## INTRODUCTION

Metabolic syndrome (MetS) is an important cause of morbidity and mortality with an increasing prevalence in the world, and while it was first known as an adult problem, it is now seen very frequently in childhood and adolescence and forms the basis of cardiovascular diseases which are the most common cause of death in adulthood. Genetic and environmental factors underlie MetS. There is a strong association between the physiopathology of MetS and insulin resistance (IR). In

---

* **Corresponding author Omer Okuyan:** Istanbul Atlas University, Istanbul, Turkey; E-mail: dmemhs@gmail.com

**Hafize Uzun & Seyma Dumur (Eds.)**

people with a genetic predisposition to IR, a sedentary lifestyle, unbalanced and excessive nutrition, and physical inactivity increase the risk of developing MetS [1 - 4].

MetS is a risk factor for type 2 diabetes (T2DM) and cardiovascular disease (CVD) in adults. In children, there are no studies directly describing the impact of MetS on these diseases, but autopsy studies in young people have shown that cardiovascular risk factors (obesity, high blood pressure (BP), elevated triglycerides (TG), and low high-density lipoprotein (HDL)) are associated with early coronary atherosclerosis [5, 6]. In recent years, the prevalence of MetS has increased in paediatric and adolescent age groups [7].

## THE DEFINITION OF THE METABOLIC SYNDROME

In the following years, the diagnostic criteria for MetS, which has been referred to by various names such as "syndrome X", "insulin resistance syndrome", "metabolic cardiovascular syndrome", "*the deadly* quartet*"*, "dysmetabolic syndrome" and "Reaven syndrome", were defined by the World Health Organization (WHO) in 1998 [8] and by the National Cholesterol Education Program's Adult Treatment Panel III (NCEP-ATP III) in 2001 [9]. Finally, it was reorganised by "The International Diabetes Federation (IDF)" in 2005 [10]. Although MetS is a complex multifactorial disease with a not entirely recognized definition in childhood, MetS is described as the presence of obesity, IR, dyslipidaemia, and HT [11, 12].

In addition to the abnormal glucose balance found in the patient for the diagnosis of MetS according to WHO criteria, at least two of the criteria given in Table **1** must be present [13].

According to NCEP-ATP III criteria, 3 of 5 criteria are sufficient (Table **2**) [14].

While MetS definitions specific to children and adolescents are adaptations of those used in adults, IDF published criteria that can be used in children in 2007 (Table **3**) [15, 16].

**Table 1. Definition of metabolic syndrome according to WHO criteria.**

| WHO Criteria | WHO Criteria Adjusted for Children |
|---|---|
| Hyperinsulinaemia or FBG ≥ 110 mg/dL or OGTT 2nd hour FBG > 200 mg/dL with two of the following; | Abnormal glucose balance. <br>• fasting hyperinsulinaemia. <br>• impaired fasting glucose. <br>• impaired glucose tolerance. |
| Abdominal obesity (BMI>30kg/m², waist/hip ratio female > 0.8, male > 0.9). | BMI > 95th percentile level. |

*(Table 1) cont.....*

| WHO Criteria | WHO Criteria Adjusted for Children |
|---|---|
| Dyslipidaemia (TG ≥ 150 mg/dL or HDL ≤ 35 mg/dL (male), HDL ≤ 39 mg/dL (female). | TG>105 mg/dL (<10 years), TG>136 mg/dL (>10 years) or.<br>• HDL<35 mg/dL or.<br>• TC > 95th percentile level. |
| Blood pressure ≥ 130/85 mmHg or use of anti-hypertensive drug. | Systolic blood pressure > 95th percentile level. |
| Microalbumiuria (≥20 mcg/min, albumin/creatinine > 30 mg/g). | Two of three criteria in addition to abnormal glucose balance. |

**OGTT**: oral glucose tolerance test; **FBG**: fasting blood glucose; **BMI**: body mass index; **TG**: triglyceride; **HDL**: high density lipoprotein; **TC**: total cholesterol.

**Table 2. Definition of metabolic syndrome according to NCEP ATP III criteria.**

| NCEP ATP III Criteria | WHO Criteria Adjusted for Children |
|---|---|
| FBG ≥100-125 mg/dL. | FBG >100 mg/dL. |
| Abdominal obesity.<br>>102 cm (male).<br>>88 cm (female). | Waist circumference > 75th percentile level. |
| TG ≥ 150 mg/dL.<br>HDL < 40 mg/dL (male).<br>HDL < 50 mg/dL (female). | TG ≥ 100 mg/dL.<br>15-19 years.<br>HDL < 45 mg/dL (male).<br>HDL < 50 mg/dL (female). |
| Blood pressure ≥ 130/85 mmHg. | Blood pressure ≥ 90th percentile level. |

**FBG**: fasting blood glucose; **TG**: triglyceride; **HDL**: high density lipoprotein.

**Table 3. Pediatrics definitions of metabolic syndrome according to IDF criteria.**

| Variables | IDF Definition Age <10 Years | IDF Definition Ages 10-16 Years | Cook *et al.* [17] |
|---|---|---|---|
| Defining criteria | Cannot be diagnosed in the age group. | Central obesity plus at least 2 out of 4 criteria. | ≥3 criteria. |
| Central obesity. | - | WC ≥90th percentile or adult cut-off if lower. | WC≥90th percentile. |
| Hypertension. | - | SBP ≥130 mmHg or DBP ≥85 mmHg or treatment with anti-hypertensive medication. | BP≥90th percentile. |
| Hypertriglyceridemia. | - | TG ≥150 mg/dL. | TG ≥110 mg/dL. |
| Low HDL. | - | HDL <40 mg/dL. | HDL ≤40 mg/dL. |
| Impaired glucose. | - | FPG ≥100 mg/dL or known T2DM. | FPG ≥110 mg/dL. |

**IDF**: International Diabetes Federation; **WC**: waist circumference; **SBP**: systolic blood pressure; **FBG**: fasting blood glucose; **TG**: triglyceride; **HDL**: high density lipoprotein; **T2DM**: Type 2 Diabetes Mellitus.

The first large study on children was conducted within the scope of the "Bogalusa Hearth Study" and in this study, body mass index (BMI), HT, TG, HDL and fasting insulin levels above the 75th percentile were used for the definition of MetS [18]. The diagnosis of MetS in children can be made with modified NCEP ATP III criteria [19, 20]. According to these criteria, at least 3 of the criteria of TG >95 percentile, HDL <5 percentile, and impaired glucose tolerance must be met [20].

The IDF criteria are not used in children under 6 years of age. It is not recommended for children under 10 years of age, but it is recommended for follow-up in those with a waist circumference (WC) over the 90th percentile and those with a family history of MetS, Type 2 DM, CVS diseases, HT, and obesity. In addition to BMI, WC measurement, which reflects excess abdominal fat accumulation, was also added to determine obesity and its risks. Other criteria are the same in the adult age group, except that the WC in children between the ages of 10 and 16 is above the 90th percentile for age. Children and adolescents who meet at least three criteria, regardless of age, are considered to have MetS. WHO MetS diagnostic criteria have been developed and modified [21, 22].

## EPIDEMIOLOGY OF THE METABOLIC SYNDROME

The increase in the rate of MetS in children is at alarming levels. Obesity plays an important role in increasing the prevalence of diseases such as T2DM, HT and dyslipidemia that accompany metabolic syndrome [23]. The prevalence of MetS in children and adolescents remains unclear [16]. The prevalence of MetS in children varies considerably in different studies. This variability is partly due to different measurement methods and partly due to different diagnostic criteria [17].

In the review examining 98 studies, the prevalence of MetS according to IDF criteria was reported as 1-7% in the whole population, the prevalence of MetS in overweight and obese children as 16-44% according to IDF criteria, and 23-42% according to WHO criteria. There is no difference between boys and girls. The prevalence of MetS in European and Asian studies (3.3-4.2%) was found to be lower than the prevalence in the Middle East and North America (4.2-10%) [24]. In a review of 85 articles published in recent years, the prevalence of MS was reported as 11.9% (2.8%-29.3%) in overweight children and 29.2% (10%-66%) in obese children. When looked at by region, the prevalence of MetS in obese children is reported as 21% in Europe, 34.2-37% in the Middle East, 24.3% in the Far East, and 9.6-21% in the USA. In studies conducted in different regions according to modified WHO criteria, the prevalence of MetS in obese children was reported to be 28.2% in Europe, 27.2-38.8% in the Middle East, 42.3% in the

Far East, and 38.7-38.9% in the USA. Additionally, in this study, the prevalence of MS was found to be higher in men and older children [25].

Although the prevalence of metabolic syndrome is not known exactly, a previous review revealed that it ranged from 0.2 to 38.9%, with a median of 3.3% (range, 0-19.2) in the general population and relatively higher in overweight (11.9%) and obese (29.2%) children [16, 25, 26]. In a study in which different definitions were used, it was shown that the frequency of MetS varied between 13.4% and 25.1% [27]. In another study, it was reported that the prevalence of MetS in obese adolescents varied according to diagnostic criteria and was 19.5% according to NCEP/ATPIII and 38.9% according to WHO criteria [28]. This study shows that the prevalence of MetS is low when fasting glucose is taken as a criterion instead of hyperinsulinaemia in childhood. However, some features related to the prevalence of MetS are similar. MetS is more common in boys than in girls. In addition, the prevalence of metabolic syndrome increases in puberty compared to pre-puberty. MetS has also been shown to be associated with the degree of obesity. According to the NHANES 2014 study, the prevalence of MetS was reported to be 6.8% in overweight boys, 34.5% in obese boys and 9.2% and 24.6% in girls, respectively [29, 30]. In a study conducted by Weiss *et al.* [20] in 2004, 490 obese individuals aged 4-20 years were analysed in terms of the frequency of metabolic syndrome and the rates were 38.7% in mildly obese and 49.7% in severely obese individuals metabolic syndrome was found.

In the systematic review and meta-analysis of Bitew *et al.* [31], 142,142 children and adolescents from 76 eligible articles were included to compute the pooled prevalence of MetS and its components in low and middle-income countries. In their study, MetS among overweight and obese populations was computed from 20 articles with the pooled prevalence of 24.09%, 36.5%, and 56.32% in IDF, ATP III and de Ferranti criteria, respectively [31]. Reisinger *et al.* [32] conducted a systematic literature review of the prevalence of paediatric MetS and included articles published in the last 5 years (2014-2019) using at least one of four predefined classifications (IDF, Cook *et al.*, Ford *et al.*, and de Ferranti *et al.*). The prevalence of MetS ranged between 0.3 and 26.4%, whereby the rising number of children and adolescents with MetS partly depended on the definition used. The IDF definition generally provided the lowest prevalences (0.3-9.5%), whereas the classification of de Ferranti *et al.* yielded the highest (4.0-26.4%) [32]. In a recent systematic review [33], the prevalence of MetS was underestimated at 2.8% in children (6 to 12 years) and 4.8% in adolescents (13 to 18 years).

In studies conducted in Korea, pediatric abdominal obesity is one of the primary diagnostic criteria for the prevalence of MetS [34, 35]. The prevalence of MetS in childhood and adolescence has been estimated to differ between 6 and 39%, depending on which diagnostic criteria are applied [36, 37].

## PATHOGENESIS OF THE METABOLIC SYNDROME

Studies indicate that MetS begins in the early period of life [38 - 40]. It has been determined that the main factor in the pathogenesis of MetS is IR and that there is a relationship between the degree of IR and the frequency of MetS [41, 42]. Although MetS is not fully understood, it is known that IR and inflammation play an important role in pathogenesis. It is thought that free fatty acids (FFAs) accumulated in the liver, adipose tissue, striated muscles and pancreas disrupt the insulin signalling pathway and cause IR. In response to IR in the liver, gluconeogenesis is suppressed. The resulting hyperinsulinaemia triggers lipogenic enzymes in the liver and increases triglyceride production. It is also thought that HT may occur as a result of sympathetic nervous system activity and renal sodium retention due to hyperinsulinaemia [43]. In addition, the vasodilator effect of insulin through nitric oxide production is suppressed in the presence of IR [44].

MetS is a cluster of findings, and the underlying pathophysiology of all the elements that make up this cluster paves the way for coronary artery disease (CAD) [45 - 48]. These metabolic risk factors are: High plasma glucose (T2DM, impaired glucose intolerance or impaired fasting glucose), IR, central obesity, high blood pressure and atherogenic dyslipidemia. IR, which is the most important factor in the pathogenesis of MetS, is the condition in which insulin in normal concentration in plasma cannot stimulate peripheral glucose uptake sufficiently and cannot suppress glucose and VLDL cholesterol production from the liver. IR causes the development of atherosclerosis and diabetes. The central distribution of body fat reflects visceral adipose tissue. Factors that increase IR include genetic predisposition, insulin receptor defects, drug use such as steroids, and disorders such as generalized lipodystrophy [49].

Although obesity and IR constitute the basis of the pathophysiology of MetS, chronic stress, disruption of the hypothalamic-pituitary adrenal axis and autonomic nervous system, increased cellular oxidative stress, renin-angiotensi- -aldosterone system activity and glucocorticoid effect in intrinsic tissues, and recently discovered molecules such as micro RNA (miRNA) are also play an important role [50].

Fat distribution is one of the most important factors affecting the formation of MetS. Central obesity is one of the indicators of fat in the organs (visceral obesity). The most important clinical indicator of organ fat is WC. In a study conducted in the 6-12 age group, an increase in WC was associated with high systolic and diastolic blood pressure, high LDL-cholesterol, and high triglyceride and insulin levels in children as well as in adults [51]. It has been shown that high BMI and high WC are separate risk factors for MetS [52].

In the aetiology, anthropometric measurements as well as family history should be questioned in addition to obesity. The heritability for obesity varies between 60-80%, for blood pressure changes between 11-37%, and for changes in lipid levels between 43-54% [53].

Some compounds produced in adipose tissue especially non-esterified FFAs are important in the pathogenesis of MetS. In the presence of IR, FFA formation from triglycerides of stored adipose tissue is accelerated. In the liver, a vicious cycle is formed with an increase in glucose, triglycerides and VLDL due to increased IR and an increase in FFA.

Increased FFA level inhibits insulin-related glucose uptake in muscle and decreases insulin sensitivity by increasing fibrinogen and plasminogen activator inhibitor (PAI)-1 production [54].

Visceral adipose tissue secretes bioactive substances called adipocytokines such as leptin, resistin, tumour necrosis factor-α (TNF-α), interleukin-6 (IL-6), and angiotensin 2, which stimulate insulin resistance, and plasminogen activator inhibitor-1, which is associated with thrombogenic vascular diseases. The level of the newly defined visvatin was found to be high in obese children with IR or hyperinsulinaemia. Visvatin has an insulin-like effect and regulates the proinflammatory response by increasing cytokine production [55].

Chronic hypersecretion of stress mediators, chronic hypercortisolism, low growth hormone secretion and hypogonadism lead to increased visceral adipose tissue. Prenatal, infancy, and adolescence are periods characterised by increased sensitivity to stressors. Hypercortisolism causes insulin resistance in peripheral tissues depending on glucocorticoid levels. These hormonal changes lead to reactive hyperinsulinaemia and an increase in visceral adipose tissue resulting in dyslipidaemia, HT, and T2DM [56].

The nutritional, metabolic, and hormonal status of the mother in the intrauterine period, as well as in the postnatal period, causes reprogramming of the physiological and structural characteristics of the fetus, leading to the development of metabolic diseases later in life. Birth weight and the uterine environment influence the MetS in childhood. In addition, it has been found that the likelihood of MetS in childhood increases in fetuses born larger than gestational age or whose mothers have obesity or gestational diabetes [57]. In addition, inadequate protein intake in the intrauterine period contributes to the development of MetS by causing the production of special epigenotypes and by having detrimental effects on the sleep-wake cycle and locomotor activity rhythm of the fetus in adulthood [58].

In a study, low vitamin D levels in adolescents were associated with MetS and cardiovascular risk factors such as HT, dyslipidaemia, and hyperglycaemia [59].

Omentin has anti-inflammatory, antiatherogenic, anti cardiovascular disease and anti-diabetic properties. The ability of omentin to reduce IR, together with its anti-inflammatory and anti-atherogenic properties, makes omentin a promising therapeutic target. Therefore, omentin may have beneficial effects on MetS and can be used as a potential pharmacological agent/target in this regard [60].

Adiponectin is an adipokine with a wide range of effects that fulfills its function inversely proportional to insulin, BMI, triglyceride, WC, IR values and directly proportional to HDL-cholesterol values [61]. The production of adiponectin, which increases insulin sensitivity, decreases in obese individuals despite the increase in adipose tissue. This decrease is an indication that adiponectin regulation is impaired in obesity. In addition, low serum adiponectin levels have been found to be strongly associated with T2DM, IR, and dyslipidaemia [62].

Intestinal microbiota (IM) has been associated with many features of MetS (especially obesity and T2DM). Metabolic bacteremia is the translocation of live bacteria into the host, similar to metabolic endotoxemia. This is thought to be a feature of diabetes. Endotoxaemia contributes to subclinical inflammation, IR, adipose tissue hyperplasia, and decreased β cell function, which are components of MetS [63]. Improvement in IR has been reported with the transfer of IM from lean healthy donors to individuals with MetS [64].

**Risk Factors**

Six components of the metabolic syndrome have been identified by ATP III [65].

• Abdominal obesity.
• Atherogenic dyslipidemia.
• High blood pressure.
• Insulin resistance ± glucose intolerance.
• Proinflammatory state.
• Prothrombotic state.

ATP III categorised these components into 3 different groups.

• Underlying risk factors (obesity, physical inactivity, atherogenic diet).
• Major risk factors (smoking, hypertension, high LDL cholesterol, low HDL cholesterol, family history of premature CAD - female <65 years, male <55

years, ageing).
• Emerging risk factors (increased TG and small LDL particles, IR, glucose intolerance, proinflammatory and prothrombotic state).

MetS is a risk factor for T2DM and cardiovascular disease in adults. In children, although there are no studies that directly explain the effect of MetS on these diseases, autopsy studies in young people have shown that cardiovascular risk factors (obesity, high blood pressure, elevated triglycerides and low HDL) are associated with early coronary atherosclerosis. T2DM and impaired fasting glucose tolerance have also recently emerged as a critical health problem in obese adolescents [5].

## CLINICAL FEATURES OF THE METABOLIC SYNDROME

Obesity, dyslipidemia, HT, glucose intolerance, and T2DM, are the most common clinical features in MetS. Although the clinical features of MetS in children resemble those of adults in many aspects, it also includes some additional findings specific to childhood. Clinical signs and symptoms of children with MetS are presented in Table **4**.

**Table 4. Clinical features of metabolic syndrome in childhood.**

| |
|---|
| • Family history of diabetes, obesity, HT, cardiovascular disease and/or history of stroke. |
| • Maternal history of gestational diabetes. |
| • Low or high birth weight. |
| • Asthma, allergic rhinitis, T2DM. |
| • Premature pubarche, hypertension. |
| • Old or new striae, early atherosclerosis. |
| • Development or progression of obesity with adrenarche decreased energy expenditure at rest. |
| • Low fat and carbohydrate oxidation rate at rest. |
| • Acanthosis nigricans, acute pancreatitis. |
| • Development of hirsutism or polycystic ovary syndrome with adrenarche. |
| • Gynaecomastia. |

## Obesity

Obesity is a combination of the effects of genetic and environmental factors on energy metabolism and adipose tissue. In an individual with a genetic predisposition, ongoing multifaceted environmental factors facilitate the formation of obesity. Obesity is one of the most important clinical findings of MetS. It has been reported that obesity is the main risk factor for T2DM and 1 kg increase in body weight increases the frequency of diabetes by 5% (5). One in three of obese children and 80% of obese adolescents remain obese when they reach adulthood. It is known that the onset of obesity in 30% of cases of obesity in adulthood dates back to childhood [66].

Waist/hip ratio is one of the criteria used to determine fat distribution. The thinnest part of the waist and the widest part of the hip should be determined during measurement [67]. There are standard values determined according to gender in adults. In children, no consensus has yet been reached on waist/hip ratio norms according to age and gender. However, in 2023, an increased waist-to-hip ratio > 0.89 in adolescents was associated with a higher risk of developing metabolic syndrome and can be proposed as a predictor for MetS in obese adolescents in Indonesia [68].

## Insulin resistance and hyperinsulinaemia

Insulin resistance is the fact that insulin at normal concentrations produces less biological response than normal, in other words, the effect of stimulating glucose utilisation is reduced. The development of IR is one of the most important causes in the pathogenesis of MetS.

The higher the IR in obese children and adolescents, the higher the likelihood of developing MetS. In addition to the relationship between increased visceral adipose tissue and IR, the relationship between fat accumulation in muscle cells and insulin sensitivity is known [69].

The causes of IR can be categorised into three groups [70];

1. Insulin resistance at the pre-receptor level.

- Abnormal beta cell secretion products.
- Presence of circulating insulin antagonists.
- Disturbance in skeletal muscle blood flow and endothelial cells.

2. Insulin resistance at the receptor level.

- Decreased number of receptors.
- Mutations in the receptor.

3. Postreceptor insulin resistance.

- Decreased insulin receptor tyrosine kinase activity.
- Defects in the receptor signal transduction system.
- Decreased glucose transport.
- Decrease in glucose phosphorylation.
- Impairment of glycogen synthetase activity.

• Defects in glycolysis/glucose oxidation.

MetS, more precisely IR and the associated increased insulin secretion leads to chronic changes in many tissues and organs. These include central obesity, acne, skin cracks and acanthosis nigricans, hirsutism, frontal hair loss, allergic problems such as asthma, HT, atherogenic dyslipidaemia, early atherosclerosis, hepatic steatosis, excessive androgen secretion in ovarian and adrenal glands [71].

Hyperinsulinaemia also affects lipid metabolism. It stimulates triglyceride synthesis by increasing gene transcription related to lipogenic enzymes in the liver. In the liver with IR, hepatic VLDL is produced in excessive amounts by increasing FoxO1 transcription factor activity, and the ground is prepared for hypertriglyceridemia [72]. Persistently high insulin levels in children and young people are strongly associated with the development of CAD [73, 74].

### Insulin measurement methods

The "hyperinsulinaemic euglycaemic index" and "modified minimal model (Frequently Sampled Intravenous Glucose Tolerance Test -FSIVGTT)" are the gold standard methods used to assess insulin sensitivity. However, since these clamping techniques are time-consuming, expensive, and invasive, it is difficult to use them in practice [75].

The oral glucose tolerance test (OGTT) is as reliable as these invasive techniques in detecting insulin sensitivity [76]. However, since OGTT is limited in population screening, fasting insulin level, fasting glucose/insulin ratio, and Homeostasis Model Assesment for Insulin Resistance (HOMA-IR) techniques are used for population screening. It has been shown that the HOMA-IR index correlates with the euglycaemic index and is more reliable than the fasting glucose/insulin ratio and quantitative insulin sensitivity check index (QUICKI) in demonstrating insulin sensitivity in obese children [77].

### HOMA-IR is calculated according to the following formulas:

HOMA-IR= Fasting plasma glucose (nmol/L) x fasting insulin level (microU/L)/22.5.

HOMA-IR= Fasting plasma glucose (mg/dl) x fasting insulin level (µU/ml) / 405.

In studies conducted in adults, the limit value was found to be between 2-2.5. However, studies conducted in children and adolescents have shown that temporary IR develops during puberty. In addition, the frequency of IR varies according to gender and race. Arellano-Ruiz *et al.* [78] reported the HOMA-IR test may be useful for early evaluations in children and adolescents with IR and presents a good diagnostic accuracy independently of the definition of MetS used. The HOMA-IR cut point to avoid MetS risk ranged from 2.30 to 3.59. In the study conducted by Reihner *et al.* [79] HOMA-IR>4 was defined as insulin resistance in adolescents. In a study conducted in Turkey, the cut-off value for obese adolescents was defined as 3.16 [77]. Kurtoğlu *et al.* [80] reported that HOMA-IR cut-off values were determined according to prepubertal/pubertal periods in boys and girls. Accordingly, a value above 2.16 in prepubertal boys, 2.22 in prepubertal girls, 5.2 in pubertal boys, and 3.82 in pubertal girls was defined as insulin resistance [80].

### The Fasting Insulin Sensitivity Index is Calculated According to the Formula [81] (Table 5):

Fasting insulin sensitivity index=fasting blood glucose (mg/dl) / fasting insulin (mIU/mL).

According to this formula, it is expected to be above 6.

Fasting insulin level;

prepubertal>15μU/mL,

postpubertal > 20μU/mL,

OGTT peak insulin level >150μU/mL, 120 minutes insulin level >75μU/mL

is defined as hyperinsulinaemia [80].

**Table 5. Main laboratory tests used in the diagnosis of insulin resistance and their evaluation.**

| |
|---|
| **Insulin sensitivity index:** <br> Fasting blood sugar (mg/dl)/fasting insulin (mU/L): <6 <br> **OGTT** <br> • Fasting (0.min) insulin level >15-20 mU/L. <br> • Peak insulin level >150 mU/L. <br> • 120th minute insulin level >75 mU/L. <br> **HOMA-IR** > 2.5 |

IR is an important risk factor in the development of T2DM. T2DM develops as a result of IR resulting from obesity and subsequent beta cell dysfunction [82, 83].

### Hypertension (HT)

Hyperinsulinaemia leads to increased vascular resistance and proliferation of vascular smooth muscle cells in the long term. Insulin affects ion transport mechanisms in cell membranes and causes HT by changing intracellular electrolyte density. Another effect of insulin leading to the development of HT is its growth factor property. Insulin itself is a powerful growth factor and directly or indirectly stimulates other growth factors such as insulin-like growth factor I deficiency (IGF-1). The resulting vascular hypertrophy may lead to the development of HT by narrowing the diameter of the vessels. Sympathetic nervous system activation, increased sodium reabsorption, and increased renin-angiotensin-aldosterone system (RAS) activation are other factors leading to HT in MetS [84].

The definition of HT in children, which is one of the components of MetS, is systolic and diastolic blood pressure above the 95th percentile for age and sex. Persistently high insulin levels in children and young people are strongly associated with the development of CAD. The effect of insulin on blood pressure may be explained by activation of the sympathetic nervous system and baroreceptor dysfunction, increased renal water retention and stimulation of vascular smooth muscle growth [72].

## Dyslipidaemia

The dyslipidaemia seen in obesity is explained by increased lipolysis of visceral fat cells and the resulting increase in FFAs. This has been reported to be related with peripheral IR, another change seen in obesity. In studies, it was found that there was a linear relationship between insulin level and triglyceride, total cholesterol and LDL-cholesterol levels, whereas there was an inverse relationship with HDL level [85].

The atherosclerosis-promoting effect of obesity increases with the combination of dyslipidaemia, insulin resistance and HT. The dyslipidaemia pattern associated with childhood obesity is defined as increased triglyceride level, decreased HDL-cholesterol and moderately elevated LDL-cholesterol level [86]. There are epidemiological studies related with normal lipid levels in childhood [87, 88].

## SCREENING OF THE METABOLIC SYNDROME

The American Diabetes Association (ADA) recommends screening every three years from the age of 10 years in asymptomatic children if the following criteria are present. Obese or overweight and two of the following risk factors:

- T2DM in the family or 2nd degree relative.
- High-risk ethnic group.
- If there are markers of insulin resistance or concomitant conditions (Acanthosis, Hypertension, Dyslipidaemia, PCOS, SGA birth history).

- Maternal diabetes or a history of gestational diabetes while pregnant with that child.

These criteria are for asymptomatic patients. If symptoms are present, test without waiting should be performed. Fasting blood glucose and HbA1C or OGTT can be used for screening [89].

According to the recommendation of the American Diabetes Association (ADA), screening tests should be performed in children at high risk of developing T2DM, as in adults [89]. Although there are insufficient data to make definite recommendations, according to the recommendation of the Consensus Panel, if a person is overweight (BMI above the 85th percentile for age, ideal weight for height greater than 120%) and has any two of the following risk factors, a test should be performed every two years from the age of 10 years or the onset of puberty. Testing should also be considered for other high-risk patients with any of the following risk factors:

- History of type 2 diabetes in first or second-degree relatives.
- Belonging to a distinct racial/ethnic group (American Indian, African descent Americans, Asians and South Pacific islanders).
- Those with signs of insulin resistance or conditions associated with insulin resistance (acanthosis nigricans, hypertension, dyslipidaemia, polycystic ovary disease).

As a screening test, fasting blood glucose (although the 2nd hour blood glucose value is more appropriate in OGTT, fasting blood glucose is preferred because it is a cheaper and less time-consuming method) is recognised. It is recommended to perform the test every 2 years [89 - 93].

Lee *et al.* [94] showed that the 2010 ADA recommendations would lead to increased uptake of HbA1c as a screening test for identifying adolescent patients for T2DM, which may impact detection rates and the cost-effectiveness of screening.

According to the report in which cardiovascular risk factors in children and adolescents were determined by the National Hearth, Lung, Blood Institute (NHLBI), screening is recommended in the presence of the following conditions [95];

1. Routine screening is not recommended for the first 2 years.

2. 2-8 years.

- History of myocardial infarction, stroke, coronary artery disease/bypass/stent/angioplasty in parents, grandparents, siblings (F<65 years, M<55 years if).
- Parental triglycerides >250mg/dl or unexplained dyslipidaemia.
- Diabetes, hypertension, BMI>95 p, smoking in the child.
- Disease status that creates risk in the child (T1DM or T2DM, CRF, Kawasaki, Renal transplantation, HIV, SLE, JIA).

3. Recommends screening in the 9-11 age range.

4. Recommends screening in the age range of 12-16 years in the presence of risk factors mentioned in the age range of 2-8 years (BMI>85p for this period, that is, it is also recommended if overweight).

## PREVENTION AND TREATMENT OF METABOLIC SYNDROME

The general approach in the treatment of MetS is to correct IR. There is no definitive treatment for IR. However, a healthy diet and regular exercise are the first steps to reduce IR. For this purpose, lifestyle changes such as exercising 30-40 minutes a day and increasing the consumption of fibrous foods should be initiated [96]. Metformin, which has been approved for the treatment of T2DM in children, is considered as an option in the treatment of children with MetS, especially in the high-risk group [97]. In adolescents and young people with MetS and polycystic ovary syndrome (PCOS), use of 850 mg metformin daily for 8 months-1 year has been shown to lead to a significant improvement in insulin sensitivity as well as a decrease in triglyceride and androgen levels [96].

It is recommended that blood pressure should be measured at baseline and at each follow-up visit and evaluated according to percentile curves adjusted for age, sex, and weight. Lifestyle change (weight loss, salt-free diet, increased activity) is prioritised as initial treatment for blood pressure values above 95 percentile in at least 3 measurements. However, if the blood pressure is still above the 95th percentile in the 6-month follow-up, pharmacotherapy, primarily angiotensin-converting-enzyme (ACE) inhibitors, is recommended [98].

In the SEARCH (Search for Diabetes in Youth Study Group) study, low HDL cholesterol levels were found in 61% and high triglyceride levels in 65% of patients with T2DM [99]. It is recommended that fasting lipid profile should be checked in all patients diagnosed with T2DM after glycaemic control is achieved at the first presentation and if baseline values are normal, fasting lipid profile should be checked every 2 years. If LDL-cholesterol is 130mg/dl, it is recommended that 25-30% of total calories should be fat (7% saturated fat, cholesterol intake >300mg/day) and lipid profile should be checked after 6 months and if it is still in the range of 130-160mg/dl, statins should be started. The goal is to keep the LDL-cholesterol level below 130 mg/dl, ideally 100 mg/dl. If the basal triglyceride level is between 150-600 mg/dl, weight loss is tried to be achieved by restricting simple carbohydrate and fat intake. If it is above 700 mg/dl, since there is a risk of pancreatitis at these values, fibrate or niacin treatment should be started over the age of 10 years.

In patients who develop glucose intolerance, diet and exercise therapy alone is recommended first, and if this is not sufficient, metformin therapy should be initiated to decrease insulin resistance. In cases in which diabetes occurs, insulin treatment should be initiated when adequate metabolic control cannot be achieved with diet, exercise, and oral anti-diabetic treatment [96].

Increasing physical activity, consuming healthy, balanced diets, and preventing obesity play a key role in the treatment of MetS in children. Studies related to MetS have shown that nutrients and dietary practices affect the components of MetS and the incidence of metS. Increasing physical activity, consumption of healthy, balanced diets, and prevention of obesity play a key role in the treatment of MetS in children [100].

The first step in the prevention and treatment of metS is to recommend and implement healthy lifestyle changes from an early age. Healthy lifestyle changes should include not only children but also all family members and should be aimed to be maintained throughout life. Many problems arise due to obesity in children. The condition defined as metabolic syndrome is characterised by obesity (obesity), insulin resistance, hyperlipidaemia (increase in bad cholesterol and decrease in good cholesterol) and hypertension (high blood pressure). Diabetes, fatty liver, gall bladder diseases, puberty disorders, orthopaedic problems, respiratory disorders, and psychosocial problems in children due to obesity may develop. Therefore, the factors that may cause obesity should be known and preventive measures should be taken. It is important to recognise and start treatment at an early stage [16, 100].

The first step in the prevention and treatment of metabolic syndrome is to recommend and implement healthy lifestyle changes from an early age. Healthy lifestyle changes should include not only children but also all family members and should be aimed to be maintained throughout life.

## CONCLUDING REMARKS

In conclusion, MetS has been a global pandemic affecting children and adults. MetS is a fatal endocrinopathy that begins with insulin resistance and is accompanied by systemic disorders such as abdominal obesity, glucose intolerance or DM, dyslipidemia, HT and CHD. The prevalence of MetS is increasing rapidly, especially in obese children and adolescents. As a result of clinical observations, various MetS criteria have been suggested for children and adolescents, but there is no consensus on any of them. Firstly, a common consensus on the diagnostic criteria for MetS in children and adults should be established. Although there is no consensus on the diagnostic criteria for MetS in childhood and adolescence, there is common agreement that the main features defining MetS include (i) disturbed glucose metabolism, (ii) arterial hypertension, (iii) dyslipidemia, and (iv) abdominal obesity.

## REFERENCES

[1]     Berenson GS, Srinivasan SR, Bao W, Newman WP III, Tracy RE, Wattigney WA. Association between multiple cardiovascular risk factors and atherosclerosis in children and young adults. The Bogalusa Heart Study. N Engl J Med 1998; 338(23): 1650-6.
        [http://dx.doi.org/10.1056/NEJM199806043382302] [PMID: 9614255]

[2]     Reaven GM. Banting lecture 1988. Role of insulin resistance in human disease. Diabetes 1988; 37(12): 1595-607.
        [http://dx.doi.org/10.2337/diab.37.12.1595] [PMID: 3056758]

[3]     Meigs JB. Epidemiology of the metabolic syndrome, 2002. Am J Manag Care 2002; 8(11) (Suppl.): S283-92.
        [PMID: 12240700]

[4]     DeBoer MD. Assessing and Managing the Metabolic Syndrome in Children and Adolescents. Nutrients 2019; 11(8): 1788.
        [http://dx.doi.org/10.3390/nu11081788] [PMID: 31382417]

[5]     Cruz ML, Goran MI. The metabolic syndrome in children and adolescents. Curr Diab Rep 2004; 4(1): 53-62.
        [http://dx.doi.org/10.1007/s11892-004-0012-x] [PMID: 14764281]

[6]     Cruz ML, Weigensberg MJ, Huang TTK, Ball G, Shaibi GQ, Goran MI. The metabolic syndrome in overweight Hispanic youth and the role of insulin sensitivity. J Clin Endocrinol Metab 2004; 89(1): 108-13.
        [http://dx.doi.org/10.1210/jc.2003-031188] [PMID: 14715836]

[7]     Abarca-Gómez L, Abdeen ZA, Hamid ZA, *et al.* Worldwide trends in body-mass index, underweight, overweight, and obesity from 1975 to 2016: a pooled analysis of 2416 population-based measurement studies in 128·9 million children, adolescents, and adults. Lancet 2017; 390(10113): 2627-42.
        [http://dx.doi.org/10.1016/S0140-6736(17)32129-3] [PMID: 29029897]

[8]     Alberti KG, Zimmet PZ. Definition, diagnosis and classification of diabetes mellitus and its complications. Part 1: diagnosis and classification of diabetes mellitus provisional report of a WHO consultation. Dia Med 1998; 15: 539e53.

[9]     Executive Summary of the Third Report of the National Cholesterol Education Program (NCEP) Expert Panel on Detection, Evaluation, and Treatment of High Blood Cholesterol in Adults (Adult Treatment Panel III). JAMA 2001; 285(19): 2486-97.
        [http://dx.doi.org/10.1001/jama.285.19.2486] [PMID: 11368702]

[10]    International Diabetes Federation . The IDF consensus worldwide definition of the metabolic syndrome      [article        online]        2005;        Available        from http://www.idf.org/webdata/docs/metac_syndrome_def.pdf

[11]    Christian Flemming GM, Bussler S, Körner A, Kiess W. Definition and early diagnosis of metabolic syndrome in children. J Pediatr Endocrinol Metab 2020; 33(7): 821-33.

[http://dx.doi.org/10.1515/jpem-2019-0552] [PMID: 32568734]

[12]   Sangun Ö, Dündar B, Köşker M, Köşker M, Pirgon Ö, Dündar N. Prevalence of metabolic syndrome in obese children and adolescents using three different criteria and evaluation of risk factors. J Clin Res Pediatr Endocrinol 2011; 3(2): 70-6.
[http://dx.doi.org/10.4274/jcrpe.v3i2.15] [PMID: 21750635]

[13]   Alberti KGMM, Zimmet PZ. Definition, diagnosis and classification of diabetes mellitus and its complications. Part 1: diagnosis and classification of diabetes mellitus. Provisional report of a WHO Consultation. Diabet Med 1998; 15(7): 539-53.
[http://dx.doi.org/10.1002/(SICI)1096-9136(199807)15:7<539::AID-DIA668>3.0.CO;2-S] [PMID: 9686693]

[14]   Ford ES, Giles WH, Dietz WH. Prevalence of the metabolic syndrome among US adults: findings from the third National Health and Nutrition Examination Survey. JAMA 2002; 287(3): 356-9.
[http://dx.doi.org/10.1001/jama.287.3.356] [PMID: 11790215]

[15]   Zimmet P, Alberti KGMM, Kaufman F, *et al.* The metabolic syndrome in children and adolescents? an IDF consensus report. Pediatr Diabetes 2007; 8(5): 299-306.
[http://dx.doi.org/10.1111/j.1399-5448.2007.00271.x] [PMID: 17850473]

[16]   Al-Hamad D, Raman V. Metabolic syndrome in children and adolescents. Transl Pediatr 2017; 6(4): 397-407.
[http://dx.doi.org/10.21037/tp.2017.10.02] [PMID: 29184820]

[17]   Cook S, Weitzman M, Auinger P, Nguyen M, Dietz WH. Prevalence of a metabolic syndrome phenotype in adolescents: findings from the third National Health and Nutrition Examination Survey, 1988-1994. Arch Pediatr Adolesc Med 2003; 157(8): 821-7.
[http://dx.doi.org/10.1001/archpedi.157.8.821] [PMID: 12912790]

[18]   Chen W, Bao W, Begum S, Elkasabany A, Srinivasan SR, Berenson GS. Age-related patterns of the clustering of cardiovascular risk variables of syndrome X from childhood to young adulthood in a population made up of black and white subjects: the Bogalusa Heart Study. Diabetes 2000; 49(6): 1042-8.
[http://dx.doi.org/10.2337/diabetes.49.6.1042] [PMID: 10866058]

[19]   Grundy SM, Cleeman JI, Daniels SR, *et al.* Diagnosis and Management of the Metabolic Syndrome. Circulation 2005; 112(17): 2735-52.
[http://dx.doi.org/10.1161/CIRCULATIONAHA.105.169404] [PMID: 16157765]

[20]   Weiss R, Dziura J, Burgert TS, *et al.* Obesity and the metabolic syndrome in children and adolescents. N Engl J Med 2004; 350(23): 2362-74.
[http://dx.doi.org/10.1056/NEJMoa031049] [PMID: 15175438]

[21]   Balkau B, Charles MA. Comment on the provisional report from the WHO consultation. Diabet Med 1999; 16(5): 442-3.
[http://dx.doi.org/10.1046/j.1464-5491.1999.00059.x] [PMID: 10342346]

[22]   Silveira LS, Buonani C, Monteiro PA, Mello Antunes BM, Freitas Júnior IF. Metabolic Syndrome: Criteria for Diagnosing in Children and Adolescents. Endocrinol Metab Syndr 2013; 2(3): 118.
[http://dx.doi.org/10.4172/2161-1017.1000118]

[23]   Mallare JT, Karabell AH, Velasquez-Mieyer P, Stender SRS, Christensen ML. Current and future treatment of metabolic syndrome and type 2 diabetes in children and adolescents. Diabetes Spectr 2005; 18(4): 220-8.
[http://dx.doi.org/10.2337/diaspect.18.4.220]

[24]   Friend A, Craig L. Turner SThe prevalence of metabolic syndrome in children - a systematic reviewArchives of Disease in Childhood 2012; 97: A116-7.

[25]   Friend A, Craig L, Turner S. The prevalence of metabolic syndrome in children: a systematic review of the literature. Metab Syndr Relat Disord 2013; 11(2): 71-80.

[http://dx.doi.org/10.1089/met.2012.0122] [PMID: 23249214]

[26]   Agudelo GM, Bedoya G, Estrada A, Patiño FA, Muñoz AM, Velásquez CM. Variations in the prevalence of metabolic syndrome in adolescents according to different criteria used for diagnosis: which definition should be chosen for this age group? Metab Syndr Relat Disord 2014; 12(4): 202-9.
[http://dx.doi.org/10.1089/met.2013.0127] [PMID: 24564686]

[27]   Lee S, Bacha F, Gungor N, Arslanian S. Comparison of different definitions of pediatric metabolic syndrome: relation to abdominal adiposity, insulin resistance, adiponectin, and inflammatory biomarkers. J Pediatr 2008; 152(2): 177-184.e3.
[http://dx.doi.org/10.1016/j.jpeds.2007.07.053] [PMID: 18206686]

[28]   Goodman E, Daniels SR, Morrison JA, Huang B, Dolan LM. Contrasting prevalence of and demographic disparities in the World Health Organization and National Cholesterol Education Program Adult Treatment Panel III definitions of metabolic syndrome among adolescents. J Pediatr 2004; 145(4): 445-51.
[http://dx.doi.org/10.1016/j.jpeds.2004.04.059] [PMID: 15480365]

[29]   Laurson KR, Welk GJ, Eisenmann JC. Diagnostic performance of BMI percentiles to identify adolescents with metabolic syndrome. Pediatrics 2014; 133(2): e330-8.
[http://dx.doi.org/10.1542/peds.2013-1308] [PMID: 24470650]

[30]   Kassi E, Pervanidou P, Kaltsas G, Chrousos G. Metabolic syndrome: definitions and controversies. BMC Med 2011; 9(1): 48.
[http://dx.doi.org/10.1186/1741-7015-9-48] [PMID: 21542944]

[31]   Bitew ZW, Alemu A, Ayele EG, Tenaw Z, Alebel A, Worku T. Metabolic syndrome among children and adolescents in low and middle income countries: a systematic review and meta-analysis. Diabetol Metab Syndr 2020; 12(1): 93.
[http://dx.doi.org/10.1186/s13098-020-00601-8] [PMID: 33117455]

[32]   Reisinger C, Nkeh-Chungag BN, Fredriksen PM, Goswami N. The prevalence of pediatric metabolic syndrome—a critical look on the discrepancies between definitions and its clinical importance. Int J Obes 2021; 45(1): 12-24.
[http://dx.doi.org/10.1038/s41366-020-00713-1] [PMID: 33208861]

[33]   Noubiap JJ, Nansseu JR, Lontchi-Yimagou E, *et al.* Global, regional, and country estimates of metabolic syndrome burden in children and adolescents in 2020: a systematic review and modelling analysis. Lancet Child Adolesc Health 2022; 6(3): 158-70.
[http://dx.doi.org/10.1016/S2352-4642(21)00374-6] [PMID: 35051409]

[34]   Lee J, Kang SC, Kwon O, *et al.* Temporal Trends of the Prevalence of Abdominal Obesity and Metabolic Syndrome in Korean Children and Adolescents between 2007 and 2020. J Obes Metab Syndr 2023; 32(2): 170-8.
[http://dx.doi.org/10.7570/jomes22059] [PMID: 37073728]

[35]   Cho JH. The Prevalence of Abdominal Obesity and Metabolic Syndrome in Korean Children and Adolescents. J Obes Metab Syndr 2023; 32(2): 103-5.
[http://dx.doi.org/10.7570/jomes23025] [PMID: 37311703]

[36]   Reinehr T, de Sousa G, Toschke AM, Andler W. Comparison of metabolic syndrome prevalence using eight different definitions: a critical approach. Arch Dis Child 2007; 92(12): 1067-72.
[http://dx.doi.org/10.1136/adc.2006.104588] [PMID: 17301109]

[37]   Weihe P, Weihrauch-Blüher S. Metabolic Syndrome in Children and Adolescents: Diagnostic Criteria, Therapeutic Options and Perspectives. Curr Obes Rep 2019; 8(4): 472-9.
[http://dx.doi.org/10.1007/s13679-019-00357-x] [PMID: 31691175]

[38]   Ozanne S, Hales C. Early programming of glucose-insulin metabolism. Trends Endocrinol Metab 2002; 13(9): 368-73.
[http://dx.doi.org/10.1016/S1043-2760(02)00666-5] [PMID: 12367817]

[39] Caprio S. Insulin resistance in childhood obesity. J Pediatr Endocrinol Metab 2002; 15 (Suppl. 1): 487-92.
[PMID: 12017221]

[40] Bao W, Srinivasan SR, Berenson GS. Persistent elevation of plasma insulin levels is associated with increased cardiovascular risk in children and young adults. The Bogalusa Heart Study. Circulation 1996; 93(1): 54-9.
[http://dx.doi.org/10.1161/01.CIR.93.1.54] [PMID: 8616941]

[41] Reaven GM. Banting lecture 1988. Role of insulin resistance in human disease. Diabetes 1988; 37(12): 1595-607.
[http://dx.doi.org/10.2337/diab.37.12.1595] [PMID: 3056758]

[42] Son DH, Lee HS, Lee YJ, Lee JH, Han JH. Comparison of triglyceride-glucose index and HOMA-IR for predicting prevalence and incidence of metabolic syndrome. Nutr Metab Cardiovasc Dis 2022; 32(3): 596-604.
[http://dx.doi.org/10.1016/j.numecd.2021.11.017]

[43] Wittcopp C, Conroy R. Metabolic Syndrome in Children and Adolescents. Pediatr Rev 2016; 37(5): 193-202.
[http://dx.doi.org/10.1542/pir.2014-0095] [PMID: 27139327]

[44] Natali A, Ferrannini E. Hypertension, insulin resistance, and the metabolic syndrome. Endocrinol Metab Clin North Am 2004; 33(2): 417-29.
[http://dx.doi.org/10.1016/j.ecl.2004.03.007] [PMID: 15158527]

[45] Dunger DB. Obesity and the insulin resistance syndrome. Arch Dis Child 2005; 90(1): 1.
[http://dx.doi.org/10.1136/adc.2003.046854] [PMID: 15613499]

[46] Lobstein TJ, James WPT, Cole TJ. Increasing levels of excess weight among children in England. Int J Obes 2003; 27(9): 1136-8.
[http://dx.doi.org/10.1038/sj.ijo.0802324] [PMID: 12917722]

[47] Reilly JJ, Dorosty AR, Emmett PM. Prevalence of overweight and obesity in British children: cohort study. BMJ 1999; 319(7216): 1039.
[http://dx.doi.org/10.1136/bmj.319.7216.1039] [PMID: 10521196]

[48] Fagot-Campagna A, Pettitt DJ, Engelgau MM, *et al.* Type 2 diabetes among North American children and adolescents: an epidemiologic review and a public health perspective. J Pediatr 2000; 136(5): 664-72.
[http://dx.doi.org/10.1067/mpd.2000.105141] [PMID: 10802501]

[49] Ten S, Maclaren N. Insulin resistance syndrome in children. J Clin Endocrinol Metab 2004; 89(6): 2526-39.
[http://dx.doi.org/10.1210/jc.2004-0276] [PMID: 15181020]

[50] Kassi E. Pervanidou, Kaltas G, Churousos G. Metabolic syndrome: definition and controversies. BMC Med 2011; 9: 48.
[http://dx.doi.org/10.1186/1741-7015-9-48] [PMID: 21542944]

[51] Maffeis C, Pietrobelli A, Grezzani A, Provera S, Tatò L. Waist circumference and cardiovascular risk factors in prepubertal children. Obes Res 2001; 9(3): 179-87.
[http://dx.doi.org/10.1038/oby.2001.19] [PMID: 11323443]

[52] Barzin M, Hosseinpanah F, Fekri S, Azizi F. Predictive value of body mass index and waist circumference for metabolic syndrome in 6-12-year-olds. Acta Paediatr 2011; 100(5): 722-7.
[http://dx.doi.org/10.1111/j.1651-2227.2011.02162.x] [PMID: 21244485]

[53] Kraja AT, Hunt Sc, Pankow JS, Myers RH, Heiss G. Lewis Ce, Rao D, Province MA. An evalution of the metabolic syndrome in the hypergen study. Nutr Metab 2005; 18: 2:2.

[54] Cornier MA, Dabelea D, Hernandez TL, *et al.* The metabolic syndrome. Endocr Rev 2008; 29(7):

777-822.
[http://dx.doi.org/10.1210/er.2008-0024] [PMID: 18971485]

[55]   Stofkova A. Resistin and visvatin: regulators of insülin sensitivity, inflammation and immunity. Endocr Regul 2010; 44-25-36.

[56]   Charmandari E, Tsigos C, Chrousos G. Endocrinology of the stress response. Annu Rev Physiol 2005; 67(1): 259-84.
[http://dx.doi.org/10.1146/annurev.physiol.67.040403.120816] [PMID: 15709959]

[57]   Boney CM, Verma A, Tucker R, Vohr BR. Metabolic syndrome in childhood: association with birth weight, maternal obesity, and gestational diabetes mellitus. Pediatrics 2005; 115(3): e290-6.
[http://dx.doi.org/10.1542/peds.2004-1808] [PMID: 15741354]

[58]   Bruce KD, Cagampang FR. Epigenetic priming of the metabolic syndrome. Toxicol Mech Methods 2011; 21(4): 353-61.
[http://dx.doi.org/10.3109/15376516.2011.559370] [PMID: 21495873]

[59]   Reis JP, von Mühlen D, Miller ER III, Michos ED, Appel LJ. Vitamin D status and cardiometabolic risk factors in the United States adolescent population. Pediatrics 2009; 124(3): e371-9.
[http://dx.doi.org/10.1542/peds.2009-0213] [PMID: 19661053]

[60]   Zengi S, Zengi O, Kirankaya A, Kucuk SH, Kutanis EE, Yigit O. Serum omentin-1 levels in obese children. J Pediatr Endocrinol Metab 2019; 32(3): 247-51.
[http://dx.doi.org/10.1515/jpem-2018-0231] [PMID: 30817300]

[61]   Chakraborti CK. Role of adiponectin and some other factors linking type 2 diabetes mellitus and obesity. World J Diabetes 2015; 6(15): 1296-308.
[http://dx.doi.org/10.4239/wjd.v6.i15.1296] [PMID: 26557957]

[62]   Ganesh V, M M, Palem SP. Adiponectin Can Be an Early Predictable Marker for Type 2 Diabetes Mellitus and Nephropathy. Cureus 2022; 14(7): e27308.
[http://dx.doi.org/10.7759/cureus.27308] [PMID: 36039271]

[63]   Brun P, Castagliuolo I, Leo VD, *et al.* Increased intestinal permeability in obese mice: new evidence in the pathogenesis of nonalcoholic steatohepatitis. Am J Physiol Gastrointest Liver Physiol 2007; 292(2): G518-25.
[http://dx.doi.org/10.1152/ajpgi.00024.2006] [PMID: 17023554]

[64]   Vrieze A, Van Nood E, Holleman F, *et al.* Transfer of intestinal microbiota from lean donors increases insulin sensitivity in individuals with metabolic syndrome. Gastroenterology 2012; 143(4): 913-916.e7.
[http://dx.doi.org/10.1053/j.gastro.2012.06.031] [PMID: 22728514]

[65]   Type 2 diabetes in children and adolescents. Diabetes Care 2000; 23(3): 381-9.
[http://dx.doi.org/10.2337/diacare.23.3.381] [PMID: 10868870]

[66]   Lobstein T, Baur L, Uauy R. Obesity in children and young people: a crisis in public health. Obes Rev 2004; 5(s1) (Suppl. 1): 4-85.
[http://dx.doi.org/10.1111/j.1467-789X.2004.00133.x] [PMID: 15096099]

[67]   Chiarelli F, Mohn A. Early diagnosis of metabolic syndrome in children. Lancet Child Adolesc Health 2017; 1(2): 86-8.
[http://dx.doi.org/10.1016/S2352-4642(17)30043-3] [PMID: 30169210]

[68]   Widjaja NA, Arifani R, Irawan R. Value of waist-to-hip ratio as a predictor of metabolic syndrome in adolescents with obesity. Acta Biomed 2023; 94(3): e2023076.
[PMID: 37326280]

[69]   Lee SH, Park SY, Choi CS. Insulin Resistance: From Mechanisms to Therapeutic Strategies. Diabetes Metab J 2022; 46(1): 15-37.
[http://dx.doi.org/10.4093/dmj.2021.0280] [PMID: 34965646]

[70]　Shulman GI. Cellular mechanisms of insulin resistance. J Clin Invest 2000; 106(2): 171-6.
[http://dx.doi.org/10.1172/JCI10583] [PMID: 10903330]

[71]　Bovolini A, Garcia J, Andrade MA, Duarte JA. Metabolic Syndrome Pathophysiology and Predisposing Factors. Int J Sports Med 2021; 42(3): 199-214.
[http://dx.doi.org/10.1055/a-1263-0898]

[72]　Biddinger SB, Hernandez-Ono A, Rask-Madsen C, *et al.* Hepatic insulin resistance is sufficient to produce dyslipidemia and susceptibility to atherosclerosis. Cell Metab 2008; 7(2): 125-34.
[http://dx.doi.org/10.1016/j.cmet.2007.11.013] [PMID: 18249172]

[73]　Khalil A, Prakash V, Bhattacharjee J. Insulin resistance and lipid profile in the children of young ischemic parents. Indian Pediatr 2003; 40(10): 946-50.
[PMID: 14581731]

[74]　Tagi VM, Mainieri F, Chiarelli F. Hypertension in Patients with Insulin Resistance: Etiopathogenesis and Management in Children. Int J Mol Sci 2022; 23(10): 5814.
[http://dx.doi.org/10.3390/ijms23105814] [PMID: 35628624]

[75]　Henderson M, Rabasa-Lhoret R, Bastard JP, *et al.* Measuring insulin sensitivity in youth: How do the different indices compare with the gold-standard method? Diabetes Metab 2011; 37(1): 72-8.
[http://dx.doi.org/10.1016/j.diabet.2010.06.008] [PMID: 21126900]

[76]　Matsuda M, DeFronzo RA. Insulin sensitivity indices obtained from oral glucose tolerance testing: comparison with the euglycemic insulin clamp. Diabetes Care 1999; 22(9): 1462-70.
[http://dx.doi.org/10.2337/diacare.22.9.1462] [PMID: 10480510]

[77]　Keskin M, Kurtoğlu S, Kendirci M, Atabek ME, Yazici C. Homeostasis model assesment is more reliable than the fasting glucose/insülin ratio and quantitative insülin sensitivity check index for assesing insülin resistancce among obese children and adolescents. Pediatrics 2005; 115: 500-503.

[78]　Arellano-Ruiz P, García-Hermoso A, Cavero-Redondo I, Pozuelo-Carrascosa D, Martínez-Vizcaíno V, Solera-Martinez M. Homeostasis Model Assessment cut-off points related to metabolic syndrome in children and adolescents: a systematic review and meta-analysis. Eur J Pediatr 2019; 178(12): 1813-22.
[http://dx.doi.org/10.1007/s00431-019-03464-y] [PMID: 31522316]

[79]　Reinehr T, Andler W. Changes in the atherogenic risk factor profile according to degree of weight loss. Arch Dis Child 2004; 89(5): 419-22.
[http://dx.doi.org/10.1136/adc.2003.028803] [PMID: 15102630]

[80]　Kurtoğlu S, Hatipoğlu N, Mazıcıoğlu M, Kendirci M, Keskin M, Kondolot M. Insulin resistance in obese children and adolescents: HOMA-IR cut-off levels in the prepubertal and pubertal periods. J Clin Res Pediatr Endocrinol 2010; 2(3): 100-6.
[http://dx.doi.org/10.4274/jcrpe.v2i3.100] [PMID: 21274322]

[81]　Tura A, Sbrignadello S, Succurro E, Groop L, Sesti G, Pacini G. An empirical index of insulin sensitivity from short IVGTT: validation against the minimal model and glucose clamp indices in patients with different clinical characteristics. Diabetologia 2010; 53(1): 144-52.
[http://dx.doi.org/10.1007/s00125-009-1547-9] [PMID: 19876614]

[82]　Wang T, Lu J, Shi L, *et al.* Association of insulin resistance and β-cell dysfunction with incident diabetes among adults in China: a nationwide, population-based, prospective cohort study. Lancet Diabetes Endocrinol 2020; 8(2): 115-24.
[http://dx.doi.org/10.1016/S2213-8587(19)30425-5] [PMID: 31879247]

[83]　Inaishi J, Saisho Y. Beta-Cell Mass in Obesity and Type 2 Diabetes, and Its Relation to Pancreas Fat: A Mini-Review. Nutrients 2020; 12(12): 3846.
[http://dx.doi.org/10.3390/nu12123846] [PMID: 33339276]

[84]　Francischetti EA, Genelhu VA. Obesity-hypertension: an ongoing pandemic. Int J Clin Pract 2007; 61(2): 269-80.

[http://dx.doi.org/10.1111/j.1742-1241.2006.01262.x] [PMID: 17263714]

[85]    Daniels SR, Morrison JA, Sprecher DL, Khoury P, Kimball TR. Association of body fat distribution and cardiovascular risk factors in children and adolescents. Circulation 1999; 99(4): 541-5.
[http://dx.doi.org/10.1161/01.CIR.99.4.541] [PMID: 9927401]

[86]    Cook S, Kavey REW. Dyslipidemia and pediatric obesity. Pediatr Clin North Am 2011; 58(6): 1363-1373, ix.
[http://dx.doi.org/10.1016/j.pcl.2011.09.003] [PMID: 22093856]

[87]    National Cholesterol Education Program (NCEP): Highlights of the Report of the Expert Panel on Blood Cholesterol Levels in Children and Adolescents. Pediatrics 1992; 89(3): 495-501.
[http://dx.doi.org/10.1542/peds.89.3.495] [PMID: 1741227]

[88]    Kwiterovich PO Jr. Recognition and management of dyslipidemia in children and adolescents. J Clin Endocrinol Metab 2008; 93(11): 4200-9.
[http://dx.doi.org/10.1210/jc.2008-1270] [PMID: 18697860]

[89]    *Standards of Medical Care in Diabetes—2017* : Summary of Revisions. Diabetes Care 2017; 40 (Suppl. 1): S4-5.
[http://dx.doi.org/10.2337/dc17-S003] [PMID: 27979887]

[90]    Type 2 diabetes in children and adolescents. Pediatrics 2000; 105(3 Pt 1): 671-80.
[PMID: 10699131]

[91]    Nesmith JD. Type 2 diabetes mellitus in children and adolescents. Pediatr Rev 2001; 22(5): 147-52.
[http://dx.doi.org/10.1542/pir.22.5.147] [PMID: 11331736]

[92]    Kapadia CR. Kapadia CR. Are the ADA hemoglobin A(1c) criteria relevant for the diagnosis of type 2 diabetes in youth? Curr Diab Rep 2013; 13(1): 51-.
[http://dx.doi.org/10.1007/s11892-012-0343-y] [PMID: 23109000]

[93]    Lee JM, Eason A, Nelson C, Kazzi NG, Cowan AE, Tarini BA. Screening practices for identifying type 2 diabetes in adolescents. J Adolesc Health 2014; 54(2): 139-43.
[http://dx.doi.org/10.1016/j.jadohealth.2013.07.003] [PMID: 23968881]

[94]    Lee JM, Wu EL, Tarini B, Herman WH, Yoon E. Diagnosis of diabetes using hemoglobin A1c: should recommendations in adults be extrapolated to adolescents? J Pediatr 2011; 158(6): 947-952. e1-3.
[http://dx.doi.org/10.1016/j.jpeds.2010.11.026] [PMID: 21195416] [PMCID: 3210198]

[95]    Expert Panel on Integrated Guidlines for Cardiovasculer Health and Risk Reduction in Children and Adolescent: Full Report. National Institutes of Health. National Heart, Lung and Blood Institute. 2012 Oct NIH Publication No.12-7486.

[96]    Kent SC, Legro RS. Polycystic ovary syndrome in adolescents. Adolesc Med 2002; 13(1): 73-88, vi.
[PMID: 11841956]

[97]    Al Dubayee MS, Alayed H, Almansour R, *et al.* Differential Expression of Human Peripheral Mononuclear Cells Phenotype Markers in Type 2 Diabetic Patients and Type 2 Diabetic Patients on Metformin. Front Endocrinol (Lausanne) 2018; 9: 537.
[http://dx.doi.org/10.3389/fendo.2018.00537]

[98]    Springer SC, Silverstein J, Copeland K, *et al.* Management of type 2 diabetes mellitus in children and adolescents. Pediatrics 2013; 131(2): e648-64.
[http://dx.doi.org/10.1542/peds.2012-3496] [PMID: 23359584]

[99]    Search for Diabetes in Youth Study Group. Cardiovascular disease risk factors in youth with type 1 and 2 diabetes: implications of a factor analysis of clustering. Metab Syndr Relat Disord 2009; 7(2): 89-95.
[http://dx.doi.org/10.1089/met.2008.0046] [PMID: 18847385]

[100]  Halpern A, Mancini MC, Magalhães MEC, *et al.* Metabolic syndrome, dyslipidemia, hypertension and type 2 diabetes in youth: from diagnosis to treatment. Diabetol Metab Syndr 2010; 2(1): 55.
[http://dx.doi.org/10.1186/1758-5996-2-55] [PMID: 20718958]

**CHAPTER 4**

# Association of Metabolic Syndrome with Gastrointestinal Disorders

**Berrin Papila[1,\*]**

[1] *Istanbul University-Cerrahpasa, Cerrahpasa Medical Faculty, Istanbul, Turkey*

**Abstract:** Metabolic syndrome (MetS) is a collection of risk factors that should be evaluated for cardiovascular diseases, which are increasing in frequency worldwide. It is a prothrombotic and proinflammatory condition in which insulin resistance plays a central role and manifests itself with abdominal obesity, high triglyceride levels, atherogenic dyslipidemia, high blood pressure and high blood glucose. The intestinal-blood barrier, also known as the intestinal barrier, plays an important role in maintaining the homeostasis of the organism. The intestinal barrier ensures nutrient uptake through the lumen and at the same time restricts the passage of harmful substances. Increasing evidence suggests a relationship between intestinal barrier function and other body systems. Many studies have identified insulin resistance and metabolic syndrome as risk factors for reflux oesophagitis. Insulin resistance is also associated with metabolic syndrome and is known as a fundamental factor in its development. Abdominal obesity in particular is an independent risk factor for erosive esophagitis and increases the symptoms of gastroesophageal reflux. Subcutaneous and visceral adipose tissues, the main feature of MetS, secrete a variety of bioactive substances known as adipocytokines. Activation of inflammatory signaling pathways in the metabolic syndrome results in altered circulating and tissue levels of proinflammatory and anti-inflammatory cytokines, leading to systemic inflammation and tissue damage. The process of microbial dysbiosis, in which the ratio of beneficial to harmful bacteria is disrupted, is associated with many diseases such as inflammatory bowel disease, cancer, obesity, diabetes and cardiovascular disease. There is a relationship between the human gut microbiome and obesity.

**Keywords:** Abdominal obesity, Gastrointestinal disorders, Microbiota, Metabolic syndrome, Visceral fat.

## INTRODUCTION

Metabolic syndrome (MetS) is generally described as a cluster/complex of factors that are risk factors for cardiovascular disease (CVD) and type 2 diabetes, including hyperglycemia, insulin resistance, hypertension, hypertriglyceridemia,

---

[\*] **Corresponding author Berrin Papila:** Istanbul University-Cerrahpasa, Cerrahpasa Medical Faculty, Istanbul, Turkey; E-mail: papilaberrin@yahoo.com

**Hafize Uzun & Seyma Dumur (Eds.)**

decreased HDL-cholesterol concentration and central obesity [1]. MetS is also defined by different terms such as insulin resistance syndrome, syndrome X, polymetabolic syndrome, fatal quartet and civilization syndrome [2]. For the first time in 1988, Reaven drew attention to the frequent coexistence of various risk factors and stated that this association, which he called syndrome X, increased the risk of developing cardiovascular diseases (CVD) [3].

## Synonyms of MetS

- Syndrome X.
- Insulin resistance syndrome.
- Obesity dyslipidemia syndrome.

## Epidemiology of Metabolic Syndrome

When countries are analysed in terms of the prevalence of MetS, different results are obtained from each country. The most important factor affecting the incidence of metabolic syndrome in a country is the percentage of obesity and abdominal obesity in that country. Although obesity and physical activity have an effect on the incidence of MetS, it is an undeniable fact that genetic factors also have an important effect [4]. In the development of obesity, ready-to-eat food, appetitive diet, decrease in physical activity, age, gender and genetic factors are effective [5].

A steady increase in the prevalence of MetS in the US since 2011 has shown a rising trend in hyperglycemia, thus increasing the urgent need for measures to prevent diabetes. Today, factors such as fast pace of life, irregular eating habits and sedentary lifestyle facilitate the occurrence of MetS. However, it is possible to reduce the risk of MetS by making simple lifestyle changes such as healthy eating, regular exercise and stress management [6].

## Diagnostic Criteria for Metabolic Syndrome

The definition of MetS is based on the current NCEP (ATP III)= National Cholesterol Education Program (Adult Treatment Panel III) criteria [7].

### *National Cholesterol Education Programme 3rd Adult Treatment Panel (NCEP ATP III) Description*

The existence, effects and improvement of high blood cholesterol in adults are discussed in the report prepared by the NCEP on the criteria to be determined in the diagnosis of metabolic syndrome and called ATP III. In this report, MetS is diagnosed in the presence of hypertriglyceridemia, low HDL-C, HT, serum glucose $\geq$ 100 mg/dl and three of the criteria of abdominal obesity. Table **1** shows the National Cholesterol Education Programme 3rd Adult Treatment Panel (NCEP ATP III) Definition for diagnosing MetS [7].

**Table 1. NCEP ATP III diagnostic criteria for metabolic syndrome.**

| Measure | Presence of any Three or More of the Five Features Below: |
|---|---|
| **Fasting blood glucose** | >100 mg/dL (5.6 mmol/L). |
| **Blood pressure** | ≥130/85 mmHg or hypertension. |
| **Waist circumference** | Women≥ 88 cm, Men ≥ 102 cm. |
| **Triglyceride** | ≥ 150 m g/dL (1.7 mmol/L). |
| **High density lipoprotein cholesterol (HDL-C)** | Women≤ 50 mg/dL (1.29 mmol/L), Men ≤ 40 mg/dL (1.03 mmol/ L). |
| **Others** | Type 2 diabetes mellitus (T2DM). |

## *Pathogenesis of Metabolic Syndrome*

MetS is a chronic inflammatory condition resulting from the interaction of genetic and environmental factors. Several factors include insulin resistance, visceral adiposity, atherogenic dyslipidemia, endothelial dysfunction, inherited gene susceptibility, hypertension, hypercoagulable state and chronic stress syndrome [8]. No single factor, such as genetic, infectious or environmental, has yet been described to explain the etiopathogenesis of all MetS components.

Although there is a polygenic predisposition, a sedentary lifestyle and a high-calorie diet aggravate the course of the syndrome. It is still debated whether the separate components of MetS represent separate pathologies or a common pathogenetic mechanism. There are several hypotheses for the underlying pathophysiology of MetS, the most common being fatty acid flux and insulin resistance. Visceral adiposity is also thought to be the main trigger of the abnormalities involved in MetS [9, 10].

## *Components of Metabolic Syndrome*

The components of metabolic syndrome are analysed under 4 main headings. These are: insulin resistance, visceral obesity, atherogenic dyslipidaemia, and endothelial dysfunction. The first two of these are considered absolutely necessary for the diagnosis of metabolic syndrome. Most individuals with metabolic syndrome are obese, with a body mass index above 30 kg/m$^2$. It is believed that obesity provides excess fat to various organs or tissues, especially muscle and liver. Excess fat in tissues is defined as ectopic fat. Ectopic fat in muscle is closely associated with insulin resistance. In the liver, excess fatty acids can be completely burned or partially broken down into ketone bodies. The remaining fatty acids are re-esterified to triglycerides, which are incorporated into very low-density lipoproteins (VLDL) and secreted into the circulation [11].

## Gastrointestinal System

The digestive system, consisting of oesophagus, stomach, liver, pancreas and intestine, fulfills many functions such as digestion, absorption, and absorption of wastes, which are the digestive products of food and nutrients, and provides a barrier function against ingested pathogens, while also providing a healthy microbiota. The liver and pancreas, which are connected to the gastrointestinal system (GI) by the hepatopancreatic duct system, perform a number of metabolic functions, including the secretion of exocrine, endocrine enzymes and bile necessary for digestion, regulation of blood glucose homeostasis and blood detoxification [12].

The digestive system, which ensures that nutrients are broken down into their smallest building blocks after ingestion into the body, is regulated by neural, hormonal and paracrine factors. The central nervous system and the gastrointestinal system are in constant bidirectional communication with neural pathways such as the vagus nerve, the immune system including humoral and cellular mediators, and the hypothalamic-pituitary-adrenal (HPA) axis. The gut is colonised by a complex bacterial community (microbiota) that helps shape the immune system, metabolic functions, and health and disease behaviour throughout life [13].

Digestive system problems and diseases are among the most common health problems today. MetS, a major public health problem, is considered to be a combination of metabolic abnormalities such as abdominal obesity, hypertension, hyperglycaemia, low-density lipoprotein cholesterol (HDL-C) and high triglycerides (TG) [14]. In addition to the increased intra-abdominal pressure caused by visceral adiposity, metabolically active visceral adipose tissue has a proinflammatory effect and leads to an insulin-resistant state. Obesity-related hypertension, hyperglycaemia, dyslipidaemia and other metabolic abnormalities are important risk factors for reflux oesophagitis [15]. Both subcutaneous and visceral fats are considered to be the main feature of the metabolic syndrome, and in particular excessive visceral fat accumulation releases several bioactive substances known as adipocytokines, including tumour necrosis factor-$\alpha$ (TNF-$\alpha$), interleukin-6 (IL-6), leptin and adiponectin [16]. These cytokines are proinflammatory and have been shown in many studies to be overexpressed in patients with erosive oesophagitis.

Humoral factors such as insulin and leptin as well as hormonal factors such as growth factors or estrogen may influence the development of gastroesophageal reflux disease (GERD) [17, 18]. There are many studies demonstrating that MetS is associated with erosive oesophagitis [19, 20]. Some studies have shown that abdominal obesity, which is the main component of MetS, may be a stronger predictor of erosive oesophagitis than obesity.

In a study conducted by Fujikawa *et al.* [21] serum total cholesterol and triglyceride levels were found to be risk factors associated with GERD symptoms in patients with non-alcoholic fatty liver disease (NAFLD).

In a study conducted in Taiwan in 2019, Hsieh *et al.* [22] examined the effect of MetS components on reflux oesophagitis and found that there was a linear relationship between the number of MetS components and the severity of erosive oesophagitis. Hypertension has been reported to be significantly associated with erosive oesophagitis [23 - 25]. Chung *et al.* [26] found that smoking, alcohol and MetS were associated with increased risk of reflux oesophagitis. Gunji *et al.* [27] found erosive oesophagitis in 1831 patients in a study of 9840 asymptomatic Japanese male patients. They found that factors such as alcohol, smoking, metabolic changes and hiatal hernia increased the risk of erosive oesophagitis. Insulin resistance and MetS have been identified as risk factors for reflux oesophagitis [28]. Insulin resistance is also known as a major factor in the development of MetS.

Sogabe *et al.* [16], in a study conducted on 265 Japanese male individuals with MetS, found that the risk of erosive oesophagitis was higher in individuals with more visceral adiposity than in those with more subcutaneous adipose tissue. Sogabe *et al.* [16] performed ultrasonography (USG) to determine visceral and subcutaneous adipose tissues and then performed upper gastrointestinal endoscopy in individuals with MetS without reflux or dyspepsia symptoms.

They reported that the frequency of erosive oesophagitis was higher in individuals with MetS in accordance with the literature [28, 29]. There are many studies showing that visceral adiposity increases the risk of erosive oesophagitis. These studies have evaluated visceral fat ratios with expensive examinations such as magnetic resonance imaging (MRI), USG, and computerised tomographies (CT). Ze *et al.* [24] studied 728 patients over 40 years of age between 2007 and 2012 to evaluate the visceral-subcutaneous fat ratio in patients with erosive oesophagitis. These patients underwent endoscopy, blood tests for metabolic parameters, waist circumference measurement, and CT to analyse fat distribution. They reported that the frequency of erosive oesophagitis was higher in individuals with MetS in accordance with the literature. There are many studies showing that visceral adiposity increases the risk of erosive oesophagitis. They found the visceral subcutaneous fat ratio of patients with erosive oesophagitis was significantly higher. These studies have evaluated visceral fat ratios with expensive examinations such as magnetic resonance imaging (MRI), USG, and computerised tomographies (CT).

Nurleili *et al.* [30], in their study conducted in 2019 to reveal the difference in visceral fat between erosive and non-erosive reflux patients, first applied gastroesophageal reflux disease questionnaire (GERDQ) to the patients. In this study, upper gastrointestinal endoscopy was performed in 56 patients diagnosed with reflux as a result of the questionnaire and visceral fat ratios were evaluated by USG. Erosive oesophagitis was found in 54% of the subjects and 64% of the group with erosive oesophagitis was male. As a result of the study, no significant difference was found between non-erosive reflux disease (NERD) and ERD subjects in visceral fat thickness measurements. However, it was reported that there was a tendency to increase in oesophagitis severity with an increase in visceral fat thickness. Visceral adipose tissue is a source of inflammatory cytokines and is associated with systemic inflammation in obese individuals.

Both subcutaneous fat and visceral fat are considered to be the main feature of MetS, and in particular, excessive visceral fat deposition releases several bioactive substances known as adipocytokines, including tumour necrosis factor-α, resistin, leptin, and adiponectin. These mediators can affect the stomach and/or oesophagogastric junction. Proinflammatory cytokines IL-1 and TNF-α have been reported to stimulate gastrin release in the gastric antrum [31]. Thus, proinflammatory mediators such as adipocytokines may exacerbate or perpetuate local inflammation at the oesophagogastric junction after local damage resulting from the pathological levels of oesophageal acid exposure [16]. It is also known that obesity is associated with transient lower oesophageal sphincter relaxation and increased frequency of acid exposure [32]. However, it remains unclear what the underlying metabolic mechanisms are and whether other factors play a role in the pathogenesis of obesity-related erosive oesophagitis.

## *Zonulin*

Zonulin is considered a biomarker of increased intestinal permeability. Intestinal permeability is regulated to a significant extent by tight junctions in the intestinal epithelium. The role of zonulin protein is very important in regulating the function of tight junctions. Zonulin binds to special receptors in the intestinal epithelium and is involved in the structure of intercellular tight junctions. Separation of this protein from the tight junction causes an increase in intestinal permeability. The first barrier or brake system in the mucosal immune system is the epithelial barrier. In the gastrointestinal system, the epithelial cover and the tight junctions between them restrict the access of immunogenic material in the intestinal lumen to immunologically active sites [33, 34].

Zonulin is the best-known physiological modulator of intercellular tight junctions involved in the permeability of macromolecules and thus in the balance of tolerance/immunity response. When the precisely regulated zonulin mechanism is damaged in genetically susceptible individuals, it may cause intestinal and extraintestinal autoimmune, inflammatory, and neoplastic disorders [35].

Serum zonulin level was significantly higher in patients with MetS compared to those without MetS in renal transplant patients. Serum zonulin level correlated with the presence of MetS, abdominal obesity, fasting glucose level, presence of fasting glucose/diabetes criterion of MetS, presence of low HDL criterion of MetS, and body mass index (BMI). A zonulin-mediated increase in intestinal permeability may play a role in the pathogenesis of MetS [36].

Increased intestinal permeability is associated with intestinal dysbiosis, chronic systemic inflammation, insulin resistance, metabolic syndrome and nonalcoholic fatty liver disease (NAFLD). Zonulin levels increase in the blood when there are problems in the intestinal barrier and increased intestinal permeability [37]. High zonulin levels are associated with higher waist circumference, diastolic blood pressure, fasting glucose, and increased risk of metabolic disease [38, 39]. In recent studies conducted with zonulin, insulin resistance and metabolic effects of zonulin on obesity have been investigated. Moreno-Navarrete *et al.* [40] showed that increased zonulin levels were associated with obesity-related insulin resistance. It has been shown that zonulin levels are increased by 50% in type 1 diabetic patients and this is related to increased intestinal permeability [41]. Furthermore, a recent study by Mokkala *et al.* [42] showed that increased zonulin levels were associated with increased insulin resistance, inflammation, and metabolic toxicity in overweight pregnant women.

The relationship between intestinal permeability and obesity is known [43]. The relationship between hypertension and zonulin protein was investigated and zonulin was found to be significantly higher in hypertensive patients [44, 45]. High zonulin levels are associated with higher waist circumference, diastolic blood pressure, fasting glucose and increased risk of metabolic disease. At the same time, there is increasing evidence that intestinal wall permeability plays a role in the development of MetS [36].

Recently, great interest has been shown in the role of intestinal wall permeability and gut microbiota in the pathogenesis of obesity and its complications [46, 47]. Loss of intestinal barrier function or alterations in intestinal microbiota appear to be key mechanisms involved in the pathogenesis of metabolic disorders [40, 42].

# Microbiota

Each organ has a microbiota, also known as flora. Although the gastrointestinal system comes to mind first when microbiota is mentioned, it is also found in the oral cavity, skin, lungs, genitourinary system and amniotic fluid [48]. The microbes in these tissues are defined as "organs" and are actively involved in shaping and maintaining human physiology and homeostasis [49]. Among these, the gut microbiota is called the second brain because it contains the highest number of bacteria and nerve cells and is associated with chronic diseases [50].

## *Gut Microbiota*

All microorganisms found in humans are called "microbiota" and the genome of microorganisms is called "microbiome". The human being is a superorganism consisting of roughly 10% human cells and 90% microbial cells settled in this macroscopic host [51]. The flora contains a certain ratio of beneficial and harmful bacteria. When the ratio of beneficial to harmful bacteria decreases, a pathological process called "microbial dysbiosis" begins [52]. It matures and remains stable during the first years of life [52, 53].

The gut microbiota is like a fingerprint and each person has a unique content and distribution. The microbiota varies depending on endogenous and exogenous factors such as geographical origin, genetics, mode of birth, age, lifestyle, nutrition, antibiotic use, and illnesses throughout a person's life. For example, from infancy to old age, Firmicutes bacteria increase and Bacteriodetes decrease. The use of antibiotics can cause temporary or permanent microbial dysbiosis, depending on the type and age of use [54].

With the understanding of its role in pathophysiology, the use of microbiota-targeted agents in the treatment of metabolic diseases, especially diabetes and obesity, has come to the fore. For this purpose, treatments such as prebiotics, probiotics, synbiotics in which prebiotics and probiotics are given together, and fecal transplantation have been considered as new treatment options [55, 56].

## Gut Microbiota and Metabolic Syndrome

MetS includes risk factors for T2DM and cardiovascular diseases. These include overweight, obesity, hypertension, hyperglycaemia, and impaired lipid and carbohydrate metabolism. A diet rich in fat is a dietary pattern that plays a role in the emergence of MetS, leading to chronic inflammation and increased intestinal permeability. Low levels of inflammation are derived from adipose tissue and gut microbiota. and in the MetS is gradually increasing. Some studies have reported that changes in gut microbiota are associated with metabolic disorders. Based on these findings, pharmacological and nutritional treatment options for the control of gut microbiota should be considered in the management of MetS and obesity-related diseases, among other treatments [57]. Mice lacking Toll-Like Receptor 5 (TLR5) receptor, which is released from the intestinal mucosa, has anti-inflammatory properties and plays an important role in resistance to the components of MetS, have increased MetS. In the study of Gregor *et al.* [58] the intestinal microbiota of mice lacking TLR5 receptor was transferred to mice with natural microbiota and metabolic syndrome components were observed in the recipient mice.

The relationship between adipose tissue, liver and hematopoietic system plays an important role in the development of MetS. The primary treatment approach for MetS has focussed on reducing morbidity related to coronary artery disease by lowering blood glucose levels, serum cholesterol, and blood pressure [59]. Other therapeutic approaches focus on weight control and daily regular physical activities. Health professionals agree that lifestyle changes consisting of following a healthy diet, reducing calorie intake, and engaging in physical activity are the basis for long-term weight loss [60]. At least 3-5 days a week, 150 minutes of moderate-intensity or 75 minutes of vigorous physical activity reduces all-cause mortality and cardiovascular risk factors, including the incidence of MetS [61]. The fact that the level of physical activity is inversely correlated with the incidence of MetS has made physical activity a key component of treatment [62]. However, the long duration of weight loss and weight management strategies and patient compliance problems with the treatment protocol have led to the need for more effective medical interventions [63].

Bariatric surgery is one of the surgical methods used in the treatment of obesity, which is indicated for adult patients with BMI >40 kg/m$^2$ or with a BMI value between 35-40 kg/m$^2$ with obesity-related comorbidities in clinical evaluation and when other treatment options are not sufficient [64]. When surgical procedures were analysed, it was observed that many methods were used but laparoscopic transit bipartition and sleeve gastrectomy (SG) techniques were relatively superior to others [65].

C-reactive protein (CRP) is a marker of inflammatory and metabolic syndrome [66]. Increased CRP levels are also seen in T2DM [67]. Recent studies have reported that CRP can be used as a marker to determine the risk of developing coronary artery disease in metabolically healthy individuals with abdominal obesity [68]. In light of recent studies on obesity, it has been shown that obesity is associated with a chronic low-grade inflammatory state. Obesity-induced chronic inflammation is associated with diabetes, insulin resistance, and cancer [69].

Surgically induced weight loss and anatomical changes may play an important role in the improvement of chronic inflammation.

## CONCLUSION

As a result, there is no effective treatment for MetS and its components, which is a serious public health problem. The incidence of MetS is increasing parallel to time. People do not pay attention to their lifestyles, do not eat a regular and balanced diet, and do not spare time for physical exercise due to busy lives. However, MetS is a difficult and expensive disease to treat. This places heavy burdens on national economies. Therefore, the methods to be developed for the prevention of MetS should be new treatment strategies designed with the least cost. Increased zonulin levels are associated with obesity-related insulin resistance. By determining the individual gut microbiota, personalised advice and treatment approaches are possible.

## REFERENCES

[1]     Third Report of the National Cholesterol Education Program (NCEP) Expert Panel on Detection, Evaluation, and Treatment of High Blood Cholesterol in Adults (Adult Treatment Panel III) Final Report. Circulation 2002; 106(25): 3143-421.
[http://dx.doi.org/10.1161/circ.106.25.3143] [PMID: 12485966]

[2]     Alberti KGMM, Zimmet PZ. Definition, diagnosis and classification of diabetes mellitus and its complications. Part 1: diagnosis and classification of diabetes mellitus. Provisional report of a WHO Consultation. Diabet Med 1998; 15(7): 539-53.
[http://dx.doi.org/10.1002/(SICI)1096-9136(199807)15:7<539::AID-DIA668>3.0.CO;2-S] [PMID: 9686693]

[3]     Reaven GM. Banting lecture 1988. Role of insulin resistance in human disease. Diabetes 1988; 37(12): 1595-607.
[http://dx.doi.org/10.2337/diab.37.12.1595] [PMID: 3056758]

[4]     Roberts CK, Hevener AL, Barnard RJ. Metabolic syndrome and insulin resistance: underlying causes and modification by exercise training. Compr Physiol 2013; 3(1): 1-58. 22.
[http://dx.doi.org/10.1002/cphy.c110062]

[5]     Moore JX, Chaudhary N, Akinyemiju T. Metabolic syndrome prevalence by race/ethnicity and sex in the united states, national health and nutrition examination survey, 1988-2012. Prev Chronic Dis 2017; 14: 160287.
[http://dx.doi.org/10.5888/pcd14.160287] [PMID: 28301314]

[6]     Liang X, Or B, Tsoi MF, Cheung CL, Cheung BMY. Prevalence of metabolic syndrome in the United States National Health and Nutrition Examination Survey 2011–18. Postgrad Med J 2023; 99(1175): 985-92.
[http://dx.doi.org/10.1093/postmj/qgad008] [PMID: 36906842]

[7]     Nwankwo M, Okamkpa CJ, Danborno B. Comparison of diagnostic criteria and prevalence of metabolic syndrome using WHO, NCEP-ATP III, IDF and harmonized criteria: A case study from urban southeast Nigeria. Diabetes Metab Syndr 2022; 16(12): 102665.
[http://dx.doi.org/10.1016/j.dsx.2022.102665] [PMID: 36417829]

[8]     Alkhulaifi F, Darkoh C. Meal Timing, Meal Frequency and Metabolic Syndrome. Nutrients 2022; 14(9): 1719.
[http://dx.doi.org/10.3390/nu14091719] [PMID: 35565686]

[9]　Park YW, Zhu S, Palaniappan L, Heshka S, Carnethon MR, Heymsfield SB. The metabolic syndrome: prevalence and associated risk factor findings in the US population from the Third National Health and Nutrition Examination Survey, 1988-1994. Arch Intern Med 2003; 163(4): 427-36.
[http://dx.doi.org/10.1001/archinte.163.4.427] [PMID: 12588201]

[10]　Rochlani Y, Pothineni NV, Kovelamudi S, Mehta JL. Metabolic syndrome: pathophysiology, management, and modulation by natural compounds. Ther Adv Cardiovasc Dis 2017; 11(8): 215-25.
[http://dx.doi.org/10.1177/1753944717711379] [PMID: 28639538]

[11]　Aromolaran AS, Boutjdir M. Cardiac ion channel regulation in obesity and the metabolic syndrome: relevance to long qt syndrome and atrial fibrillation. Front Physiol 2017; 8: 431.
[http://dx.doi.org/10.3389/fphys.2017.00431] [PMID: 28680407]

[12]　Zorn AM. Development of the digestive system. Semin Cell Dev Biol 2017; 66: 1-2.
[http://dx.doi.org/10.1016/j.semcdb.2017.05.015] [PMID: 28624076]

[13]　De Palma G, Collins SM, Bercik P, Verdu EF. The microbiota–gut–brain axis in gastrointestinal disorders: stressed bugs, stressed brain or both? J Physiol 2014; 592(14): 2989-97.
[http://dx.doi.org/10.1113/jphysiol.2014.273995] [PMID: 24756641]

[14]　Mokhsin A, Mokhtar SS, Mohd Ismail A, *et al.* Observational study of the status of coronary risk biomarkers among Negritos with metabolic syndrome in the east coast of Malaysia. BMJ Open 2018; 8(12): e021580.
[http://dx.doi.org/10.1136/bmjopen-2018-021580] [PMID: 30518581]

[15]　Kim TJ, Lee H, Baek SY, *et al.* Metabolically Healthy Obesity and the Risk of Erosive Esophagitis: A Cohort Study. Clin Transl Gastroenterol 2019; 10(9): e00077.
[http://dx.doi.org/10.14309/ctg.0000000000000077] [PMID: 31498243]

[16]　Sogabe M, Okahisa T, Kimura Y, Hibino S, Yamanoi A. Visceral fat predominance is associated with erosive esophagitis in Japanese men with metabolic syndrome. Eur J Gastroenterol Hepatol 2012; 24(8): 910-6.
[http://dx.doi.org/10.1097/MEG.0b013e328354a354] [PMID: 22617364]

[17]　Weinsier RL, Hunter GR, Gower BA, Schutz Y, Darnell BE, Zuckerman PA. Body fat distribution in white and black women: different patterns of intraabdominal and subcutaneous abdominal adipose tissue utilization with weight loss. Am J Clin Nutr 2001; 74(5): 631-6.
[http://dx.doi.org/10.1093/ajcn/74.5.631] [PMID: 11684531]

[18]　Ha NR, Lee HL, Lee OY, *et al.* Differences in clinical characteristics between patients with non-erosive reflux disease and erosive esophagitis in Korea. J Korean Med Sci 2010; 25(9): 1318-22.
[http://dx.doi.org/10.3346/jkms.2010.25.9.1318] [PMID: 20808675]

[19]　Park JH, Park DIL, Kim HJ, *et al.* Metabolic syndrome is associated with erosive esophagitis. World J Gastroenterol 2008; 14(35): 5442-7.
[http://dx.doi.org/10.3748/wjg.14.5442] [PMID: 18803357]

[20]　Ierardi E, Rosania R, Zotti M, *et al.* Metabolic syndrome and gastro-esophageal reflux: A link towards a growing interest in developed countries. World J Gastrointest Pathophysiol 2010; 1(3): 91-6.
[http://dx.doi.org/10.4291/wjgp.v1.i3.91] [PMID: 21607146]

[21]　Fujikawa Y, Tominaga K, Fujii H, *et al.* High prevalence of gastroesophageal reflux symptoms in patients with non-alcoholic fatty liver disease associated with serum levels of triglyceride and cholesterol but not simple visceral obesity. Digestion 2012; 86(3): 228-37.
[http://dx.doi.org/10.1159/000341418] [PMID: 22964626]

[22]　Hsieh YH, Wu MF, Yang PY, *et al.* What is the impact of metabolic syndrome and its components on reflux esophagitis? A cross-sectional study. BMC Gastroenterol 2019; 19(1): 33.
[http://dx.doi.org/10.1186/s12876-019-0950-z] [PMID: 30782138]

[23]　Moki F, Kusano M, Mizuide M, *et al.* Association between reflux oesophagitis and features of the metabolic syndrome in Japan. Aliment Pharmacol Ther 2007; 26(7): 1069-75.

[http://dx.doi.org/10.1111/j.1365-2036.2007.03454.x] [PMID: 17877514]

[24]    Ze EY, Kim BJ, Kang H, Kim JG. Abdominal Visceral to Subcutaneous Adipose Tissue Ratio Is Associated with Increased Risk of Erosive Esophagitis. Dig Dis Sci 2017; 62(5): 1265-71.
[http://dx.doi.org/10.1007/s10620-017-4467-4] [PMID: 28281164]

[25]    Niigaki M, Adachi K, Hirakawa K, Furuta K, Kinoshita Y. Association between metabolic syndrome and prevalence of gastroesophageal reflux disease in a health screening facility in Japan. J Gastroenterol 2013; 48(4): 463-72.
[http://dx.doi.org/10.1007/s00535-012-0671-3] [PMID: 22976934]

[26]    Chung SJ, Kim D, Park MJ, *et al.* Metabolic syndrome and visceral obesity as risk factors for reflux oesophagitis: a cross-sectional case-control study of 7078 Koreans undergoing health check-ups. Gut 2008; 57(10): 1360-5.
[http://dx.doi.org/10.1136/gut.2007.147090] [PMID: 18441006]

[27]    Gunji T, Sato H, Iijima K, *et al.* Risk factors for erosive esophagitis: a cross-sectional study of a large number of Japanese males. J Gastroenterol 2011; 46(4): 448-55.
[http://dx.doi.org/10.1007/s00535-010-0359-5] [PMID: 21229366]

[28]    Mohammadi M, Ramezani Jolfaie N, Alipour R, Zarrati M. Is Metabolic Syndrome Considered to Be a Risk Factor for Gastroesophageal Reflux Disease (Non-Erosive or Erosive Esophagitis)?: A Systematic Review of the Evidence. Iran Red Crescent Med J 2016; 18(11): e30363.
[http://dx.doi.org/10.5812/ircmj.30363]

[29]    Mohammadi M, Ramezani Jolfaie N, Alipour R, Zarrati M. Is Metabolic Syndrome Considered to Be a Risk Factor for Gastroesophageal Reflux Disease (Non-Erosive or Erosive Esophagitis)?: A Systematic Review of the Evidence. Iran Red Crescent Med J 2016; 18(11): e30363.
[http://dx.doi.org/10.5812/ircmj.30363] [PMID: 28191340]

[30]    Nurleili RA, Purnamasari D, Simadibrata M, Rachman A, Tahapary DL, Gani RA. Visceral fat thickness of erosive and non-erosive reflux disease subjects in Indonesia's tertiary referral hospital. Diabetes Metab Syndr 2019; 13(3): 1929-33.
[http://dx.doi.org/10.1016/j.dsx.2019.04.025] [PMID: 31235117]

[31]    Endo Y, Kumagai K. Induction by interleukin-1, tumor necrosis factor and lipopolysaccharides of histidine decarboxylase in the stomach and prolonged accumulation of gastric acid. Br J Pharmacol 1998; 125(4): 842-8.
[http://dx.doi.org/10.1038/sj.bjp.0702108] [PMID: 9831923]

[32]    Wu JCY, Mui LM, Cheung CMY, Chan Y, Sung JJY. Obesity is associated with increased transient lower esophageal sphincter relaxation. Gastroenterology 2007; 132(3): 883-9.
[http://dx.doi.org/10.1053/j.gastro.2006.12.032] [PMID: 17324403]

[33]    Vanuytsel T, Vermeire S, Cleynen I. The role of Haptoglobin and its related protein, Zonulin, in inflammatory bowel disease. Tissue Barriers 2013; 1(5): e27321.
[http://dx.doi.org/10.4161/tisb.27321] [PMID: 24868498]

[34]    Sapone A, de Magistris L, Pietzak M, *et al.* Zonulin upregulation is associated with increased gut permeability in subjects with type 1 diabetes and their relatives. Diabetes 2006; 55(5): 1443-9.
[http://dx.doi.org/10.2337/db05-1593] [PMID: 16644703]

[35]    Fasano A. Zonulin and its regulation of intestinal barrier function: the biological door to inflammation, autoimmunity, and cancer. Physiol Rev 2011; 91(1): 151-75.
[http://dx.doi.org/10.1152/physrev.00003.2008] [PMID: 21248165]

[36]    Erkan G, Sumnu A, Ertugrul G, *et al.* The Relationship between Zonulin and Metabolic Syndrome in Renal Transplant Patients. Clin Lab 2023; 69(1)
[http://dx.doi.org/10.7754/Clin.Lab.2022.220341] [PMID: 36649519]

[37]    Teixeira TFS, Souza NCS, Chiarello PG, *et al.* Intestinal permeability parameters in obese patients are correlated with metabolic syndrome risk factors. Clin Nutr 2012; 31(5): 735-40.

[http://dx.doi.org/10.1016/j.clnu.2012.02.009] [PMID: 22444236]

[38]   Gami AS, Witt BJ, Howard DE, *et al.* Metabolic syndrome and risk of incident cardiovascular events and death: a systematic review and meta-analysis of longitudinal studies. J Am Coll Cardiol 2007; 49(4): 403-14.
[http://dx.doi.org/10.1016/j.jacc.2006.09.032] [PMID: 17258085]

[39]   Grundy SM, Cleeman JI, Daniels SR, *et al.* Diagnosis and Management of the Metabolic Syndrome. Circulation 2005; 112(17): 2735-52.
[http://dx.doi.org/10.1161/CIRCULATIONAHA.105.169404] [PMID: 16157765]

[40]   Moreno-Navarrete JM, Sabater M, Ortega F, Ricart W, Fernández-Real JM. Circulating zonulin, a marker of intestinal permeability, is increased in association with obesity-associated insulin resistance. PLoS One 2012; 7(5): e37160.
[http://dx.doi.org/10.1371/journal.pone.0037160] [PMID: 22629362]

[41]   Meddings JB, Jarand J, Urbanski SJ, Hardin J, Gall DG. Increased gastrointestinal permeability is an early lesion in the spontaneously diabetic BB rat. Am J Physiol 1999; 276(4): G951-7.
[PMID: 10198339]

[42]   Mokkala K, Pellonperä O, Röytiö H, Pussinen P, Rönnemaa T, Laitinen K. Increased intestinal permeability, measured by serum zonulin, is associated with metabolic risk markers in overweight pregnant women. Metabolism 2017; 69: 43-50.
[http://dx.doi.org/10.1016/j.metabol.2016.12.015] [PMID: 28285651]

[43]   Camilleri M. Is intestinal permeability increased in obesity? A review including the effects of dietary, pharmacological and surgical interventions on permeability and the microbiome. Diabetes Obes Metab 2023; 25(2): 325-30.
[http://dx.doi.org/10.1111/dom.14899] [PMID: 36263962]

[44]   E Ntlahla E, MO Mfengu M, A Engwa G, N Nkeh-Chungag B, R Sewani-Rusike C. Gut permeability is associated with hypertension and measures of obesity but not with Endothelial Dysfunction in South African youth. Afr Health Sci 2021; 21(3): 1172-84.
[http://dx.doi.org/10.4314/ahs.v21i3.26] [PMID: 35222580]

[45]   Bawah AT, Tornyi H, Seini MM, Ngambire LT, Yeboah FA. Zonulin as marker of pregnancy induced hypertension: a case control study. Clin Hypertens 2020; 26(1): 7.
[http://dx.doi.org/10.1186/s40885-020-00139-x] [PMID: 32313692]

[46]   Sekirov I, Russell SL, Antunes LCM, Finlay BB. Gut microbiota in health and disease. Physiol Rev 2010; 90(3): 859-904.
[http://dx.doi.org/10.1152/physrev.00045.2009] [PMID: 20664075]

[47]   Vajro P, Paolella G, Fasano A. Microbiota and gut-liver axis: their influences on obesity and obesity-related liver disease. J Pediatr Gastroenterol Nutr 2013; 56(5): 461-8.
[http://dx.doi.org/10.1097/MPG.0b013e318284abb5] [PMID: 23287807]

[48]   Pelzer E, Gomez-Arango LF, Barrett HL, Nitert MD. Review: Maternal health and the placental microbiome. Placenta 2017; 54: 30-7.
[http://dx.doi.org/10.1016/j.placenta.2016.12.003] [PMID: 28034467]

[49]   Yang NJ, Chiu IM. Bacterial Signaling to the Nervous System through Toxins and Metabolites. J Mol Biol 2017; 429(5): 587-605.
[http://dx.doi.org/10.1016/j.jmb.2016.12.023] [PMID: 28065740]

[50]   Sonnenburg J, Sonnenburg E. Gut Feelings. The Second Brain. in Our Gastrointestinal Systems.'' Scientific American, May 1, 2015. From The Good Gur: Taking Control of Your Weight, Your Mood and Your Long-Term. Health New York: Penguin Books 2015.

[51]   Belkaid Y, Hand TW. Role of the microbiota in immunity and inflammation. Cell 2014; 157(1): 121-41.
[http://dx.doi.org/10.1016/j.cell.2014.03.011] [PMID: 24679531]

[52]  Sun J, Kato I. Gut microbiota, inflammation and colorectal cancer. Genes Dis 2016; 3(2): 130-43.
[http://dx.doi.org/10.1016/j.gendis.2016.03.004] [PMID: 28078319]

[53]  Sommer F, Bäckhed F. Know your neighbor: Microbiota and host epithelial cells interact locally to control intestinal function and physiology. BioEssays 2016; 38(5): 455-64.
[http://dx.doi.org/10.1002/bies.201500151] [PMID: 26990415]

[54]  Ottman N, Smidt H, de Vos WM, Belzer C. The function of our microbiota: who is out there and what do they do? Front Cell Infect Microbiol 2012; 2: 104.
[http://dx.doi.org/10.3389/fcimb.2012.00104] [PMID: 22919693]

[55]  Li C, Li X, Han H, *et al.* Effect of probiotics on metabolic profiles in type 2 diabetes mellitus. Medicine (Baltimore) 2016; 95(26): e4088.
[http://dx.doi.org/10.1097/MD.0000000000004088] [PMID: 27368052]

[56]  Yoo SR, Kim YJ, Park DY, *et al.* Probiotics L. plantarum and L. curvatus in combination alter hepatic lipid metabolism and suppress diet-induced obesity. Obesity (Silver Spring) 2013; 21(12): 2571-8.
[http://dx.doi.org/10.1002/oby.20428] [PMID: 23512789]

[57]  de Cossío LF, Fourrier C, Sauvant J, *et al.* Impact of prebiotics on metabolic and behavioral alterations in a mouse model of metabolic syndrome. Brain Behav Immun 2017; 64: 33-49.
[http://dx.doi.org/10.1016/j.bbi.2016.12.022] [PMID: 28027925]

[58]  Gregor MF, Hotamisligil GS. Inflammatory mechanisms in obesity. Annu Rev Immunol 2011; 29(1): 415-45.
[http://dx.doi.org/10.1146/annurev-immunol-031210-101322] [PMID: 21219177]

[59]  Martin KA, Mani MV, Mani A. New targets to treat obesity and the metabolic syndrome. Eur J Pharmacol 2015; 763(Pt A): 64-74.
[http://dx.doi.org/10.1016/j.ejphar.2015.03.093] [PMID: 26001373]

[60]  Pittler MH, Ernst E. Dietary supplements for body-weight reduction: a systematic review. Am J Clin Nutr 2004; 79(4): 529-36.
[http://dx.doi.org/10.1093/ajcn/79.4.529] [PMID: 15051593]

[61]  Khatoon R, Sinnathuray AR. A case of metabolic syndrome. Malays Fam Physician 2006; 1(2-3): 58-61.
[PMID: 27570588]

[62]  Zota IM, Statescu C, Sascau R, *et al.* Exercise-based rehabilitation for metabolic syndrome-case report. Med Surg J 2018; 122(1): 82-6.

[63]  Liu LY, Zhou L, Liu XZ, Zou DJ. Effect of Hedan Tablets on Body Weight and Insulin Resistance in Patients with Metabolic Syndrome. Obes Facts 2022; 15(2): 180-5.
[http://dx.doi.org/10.1159/000520711]

[64]  Sauerland S, Angrisani L, Belachew M, *et al.* Obesity surgery: evidence-based guidelines of the European Association for Endoscopic Surgery (EAES). Surg Endosc 2005; 19(2): 200-21.
[http://dx.doi.org/10.1007/s00464-004-9194-1] [PMID: 15580436]

[65]  Yormaz S, Yılmaz H, Ece I, Sahin M. Laparoscopic ileal interposition with diverted sleeve gastrectomy *versus* laparoscopic transit bipartition with sleeve gastrectomy for better glycemic outcomes in T2DM patients. Obes Surg 2018; 28(1): 77-86.
[http://dx.doi.org/10.1007/s11695-017-2803-6] [PMID: 28681261]

[66]  Chiappetta S, Schaack HM, Wölnerhannsen B, Stier C, Squillante S, Weiner RA. The Impact of Obesity and Metabolic Surgery on Chronic Inflammation. Obes Surg 2018; 28(10): 3028-40.
[http://dx.doi.org/10.1007/s11695-018-3320-y] [PMID: 29876839]

[67]  Schmidt MI, Duncan BB, Sharrett AR, *et al.* Markers of inflammation and prediction of diabetes mellitus in adults (Atherosclerosis Risk in Communities study): a cohort study. Lancet 1999; 353(9165): 1649-52.

[http://dx.doi.org/10.1016/S0140-6736(99)01046-6] [PMID: 10335783]

[68]    De Luca M, Angrisani L, Himpens J, *et al.* Indications for surgery for obesity and weight-related diseases: position statements from the International Federation for the Surgery of Obesity and metabolic disorders (IFSO). Obes Surg 2016; 26(8): 1659-96.
[http://dx.doi.org/10.1007/s11695-016-2271-4] [PMID: 27412673]

[69]    Hotamisligil GS. Inflammation and metabolic disorders. Nature 2006; 444(7121): 860-7.
[http://dx.doi.org/10.1038/nature05485] [PMID: 17167474]

# CHAPTER 5

# Related Anatomy of Gastrointestinal, Endocrine, Urinary, Nervous System and Morphometric Evaluation in Metabolic Syndrome

Hurriyet Cetinok[1,*]

[1] *Faculty of Medicine, Istanbul Atlas University, Istanbul, Turkey*

**Abstract:** Being overweight, hyperlipidemia, hypertension, type II diabetes mellitus(DM) or high blood sugar, and glucose intolerances are all clinical disorders collectively referred to as the metabolic syndrome (MetS). MetS affects multiple systems in the body, including cardiovascular, endocrine, urinary, nervous, and gastrointestinal systems. Atherosclerosis risk is increased by chronic inflammation and vascular endothelial dysfunction, which are both closely related to MetS. The risk of cardiovascular illnesses, the world's leading cause of mortality, is also increased by metabolic syndrome. Cancers such as the endometrium, breast, colon, liver, gallbladder, oesophageal, pancreas, kidney, and prostate, also chronic kidney disease, IBD (idiopathic inflammatory bowel disease), chronic gastritis, and dysplasia, are all caused by MetS enhanced by abdominal obesity, dyslipidemia, and poor glucose control. Besides, those with normal glucose metabolism are more likely to develop various peripheral nerve issues related to MetS. There is a connection between MetS and a number of cognitive deficiencies. Endocrine-disrupting substances (EDS) also have a detrimental effect on human health, which includes their influence on metabolic procedures. The gold standard for non-invasive pancreatic fat quantification is magnetic resonance spectroscopy (MRS). Anthropometry is quickly and accurately assessed on a wide scale by three-dimensional (3D) body surface scanners (BS). Indicators of waist circumference, sagittal diameter, and body weight are strongly correlated with areas of deep abdominal adipose tissue in both sexes. Each system listed above is examined in this chapter in relation to MetS, new diagnostic insights are presented, and pathogenesis and consequences that were not identified and treated as early on are summarized.

**Keywords:** Abdominal obesity, BMI, Metabolic syndrome, Neuropathy.

## INTRODUCTION

Due to its high occurrence rate and the detrimental effects of lifestyle choices on overall quality of life, metabolic syndrome is an important public health issue. It

* **Corresponding author Hurriyet Cetinok:** Faculty of Medicine, Istanbul Atlas University, Istanbul, Turkey; E-mail: hurriyet.cetinok@atlas.edu.tr

**Hafize Uzun & Seyma Dumur (Eds.)**

is estimated that over 30% of adults and an increasing number of children suffer from this condition [1]. Various factors such as demographics (gender, age, living status, education, income), lifestyle, physical performance, mechanical factors, genetics, inflammation, environment (EDC- endocrine disrupting chemicals. *etc.*), microorganisms, adipokines, eating behaviors, and growth factors may contribute to the development of MetS. Three or more of the following symptoms are necessary for the diagnosis of metabolic syndrome; abdominal obesity, hyperglycemia, dyslipidemia, diabetes mellitus or prediabetes, and hypertension. An inflammatory and thrombotic condition brought on by abdominal obesity and insulin resistance raises the risk of cardiovascular pathologies and DM type II [1]. MetS has an impact on the neurological, gastrointestinal, endocrine, cardiovascular, and urinary systems in the body. There is a higher chance of developing hypertension, Diabetes mellitus (Type II), stroke, coronary artery disease, fatty liver disease, and osteoarthritis. Obesity is a problem that is spreading around the world and raises the risk of several gastrointestinal (GI) illnesses, including non-neoplastic ones such as gastro-oesophageal reflux disease (GORD), gallstones, and Barret's esophagus. Additionally, it raises the chance of neoplastic illnesses including gallbladder cancer, esophageal adenocarcinoma, and colorectal carcinoma. Metabolic syndrome is also associated with fatty pancreatic and liver diseases. Radiological imaging should be used for early diagnosis, treatment, and prevention of both neoplastic and non-neoplastic conditions and anatomical changes associated with metabolic syndrome. Magnetic Resonance Spectroscopy (MRS) is widely acknowledged as the gold standard for non-invasive quantification of pancreatic fat. In addition to being frequently brought on by metabolic syndrome, visceral obesity raises the risk of developing and worsening chronic kidney disease (CKD). CKD development could be linked to adipokines due to metabolic syndrome's effects on the prostate, detrusor enlargement may be a factor in poor bladder function. Gut hormones and afferent neurons play a significant part in communication between the brain and the gut, as well as in metabolism. The communication involves the hypothalamus, nucleus tractus solitarius (NTS), prefrontal cortex (PFC), ventral tegmental area (VTA), and nucleus accumbens (NAc). Recent research has demonstrated a link between sympathetic dysfunction and obesity, which affects the cardiovascular system and results in issues. There is a link between microvascular damage and high blood glucose levels, which can lead to neuropathy. Patients with MetS are more likely to get radiculopathy, entrapment neuropathy, and peripheral neuropathy even if their blood glucose levels are normal. Numerous factors, such as glucose-mediated endothelial damage, oxidative stress, and advanced glycation end products, can cause neuronal injury. There is a link between microvascular damage and high blood glucose levels, which can lead to neuropathy. There are several mechanisms for neuron damage, including oxidative stress, advanced glycation end products, and damage to endothelial cells caused by glucose. When it comes to more severe brain and cognitive abnormalities, including those shown by DTI and MRI in different regions of both white and gray matter in people with bipolar disorder, obesity, and associated cardiovascular risk factors play a significant role. Predicting risk is crucial because GI illness and obesity are so common. Although the BMI is useful, other measurements, such as visceral fat and central (abdominal) obesity buildup, may be more accurate [2]. Researchers have demonstrated a relationship between waist circumference assessed by hand and the metabolic syndrome's characteristics and abdominal volume as evaluated by body surface scanner. BMI, sagittal diameter, and waist circumference are anthropometric measurements used in metabolic syndrome. The elements of the MetS were determined using the Adult Treatment Panel III of the National Cholesterol Education Program [3]. Participants were deemed to have metabolic syndrome if at least three of the following five symptoms were present [4]: abdominal obesity (waist circumference >102 cm in men or >88 cm in women), high triglycerides ($\geq$1.7 mmol/L), low high-density lipoprotein (HDL) (<1.0 mmol/L in men or <1.3 mmol/L in women), high serum fructosamine ($\geq$247 $\mu$mol/L or use of antidiabetic medication), and high blood pressure ($\geq$160/90 mmHg or use of antihypertensive medication). At the Department of Clinical Chemistry at the VU University Medical Center (VUmc) in Amsterdam, fructosamine, HDL, and triglycerides were measured using an enzymatic colorimetric assay (Roche Diagnostics, Mannheim, Germany). Following a typical expiration, abdominal obesity was measured to the nearest 0.1 cm at the midpoint between the lower rib edge and the iliac crest. A regular mercury sphygmomanometer (Omron HEM 706) was used to take blood pressure readings in the upper arm while the subject was seated.

## Pathoanatomical Approach of the Gastrointestinal System in Metabolic Syndrome

Obesity is a growing problem globally. It increases the risk of various gastrointestinal (GI) diseases, including non-neoplastic conditions such as gastroesophageal reflux and Barrett's esophagus, as well as neoplastic conditions like esophageal adenocarcinoma, pancreatic carcinoma, gallbladder carcinoma and, CRC. In addition, obesity has been linked to poorer outcomes for GI cancer. BMI is frequently used to quantify fat, however, certain patterns, such as visceral fat and abdominal obesity, better indicate the risk of developing disease. Overweight individuals are more likely to develop cancer-related conditions such as Barrett's esophagus, colorectal adenoma, gallstones, pancreatic intraepithelial neoplasia, and colorectal serrated lesions. Carcinogens including adipokines, vascular endothelial growth factors, and insulin-like growth factors can be released by adipocytes at the cellular level. Additionally, in obese individuals, the number of inflammatory cells that can be a potential source of carcinogens is increased both systemically and in adipose tissue [2].

Obesity is associated with a higher risk of GORD, Barrett's esophagus. Due to higher intra-abdominal pressure, reduced esophageal sphincter relaxation, and hiatus hernia, GORD is linked to a high BMI [5, 6]. A more acid-sensitive mucosa [7], elevated bile acid and pancreatic enzyme levels in the refluxate [8], and changed hormone levels are possible additional contributory causes.

Gallstones are more likely to form when a person has metabolic syndrome and a high body mass index, which may help to explain why these conditions consistently carry a high risk of developing gallbladder cancer [9, 10].

Although neuroendocrine or squamous types of adenocarcinoma might occasionally be seen, the most prevalent kind of that is gallbladder cancer.

The likelihood of developing both intrahepatic and extrahepatic cholangiocarcinoma may be greater in people with diabetes mellitus.

The association between obesity/MetS and cancer may be influenced by known risk factors including GORD, gallstones, preneoplastic lesions, growth factors, adipokines, inflammation, microorganisms, and mechanical factors.

Dysplasia and cancer risk are elevated in chronic inflammatory disorders including IBD and chronic gastritis. Additionally, there are strong connections between ongoing colonic inflammation and CRC development in test animals [11]. Inflammatory cells release a variety of chemicals that could eventually cause cancer. Chronic inflammation underlies obesity [12], which is frequently brought on by elevated cytokine levels. Visceral fat is intimately associated with both insulin resistance and systemic inflammation. Reduced anti-tumor activity in T cells brought on by systemic inflammation may encourage carcinogenesis. Adipose tissue's inflammatory cells release substances that raise the likelihood of neoplasia [13].

It is well established that obesity and insulin resistance are linked to the onset and development of non-alcoholic fatty liver disease (NAFLD). Notably, NAFLD patients typically experience a mild form of the disease and rarely progress to cirrhosis. However, non-alcoholic steatohepatitis (NASH), a more serious condition that can result in cirrhosis and end-stage liver disease, can develop in up to 20% of patients with steatosis [1]. It has been observed that lipid build up also occurs in the pancreas in cases of this condition, although it has not been studied as extensively. When a person is obese, their pancreas can become infiltrated with adipocytes, which is why terms such as NAFPD and nonalcoholic fatty steatopancreatitis (NASP) have been suggested when there are accompanying inflammatory changes [14, 15]. Studies on animals have shown that pancreatic steatosis leads to abnormal pancreatic islet cells and elevated blood sugar levels. A dangerous liver condition called NAFLD is brought on by metabolic syndrome. It is critical to understand that hepatocellular carcinoma and intrahepatic cholangiocarcinoma are both greatly increased by both metabolic syndrome and NAFLD. In Western countries, NAFLD has emerged as the leading reason for liver transplants. Patients with MetS and/or NAFLD must receive specialized evaluation and perioperative management because they are at increased operative risk during liver resection and transplantation. The most reliable approach to calculating pancreatic fat and its correlation with pancreatic cancer is through MRI-PDFF (Magnetic Resonance Imaging- Proton Density Fat Fraction). In contrast, the accuracy of PI (Pancreatic Index) in predicting the likelihood of developing pancreatic cancer falls short of this imaging biomarker. Therefore, it is essential to prioritize MRI-PDFF when assessing pancreatic well-being. MRI-PDFF is a good non-invasive tool to evaluate fatty pancreas and potentially predict pancreatic cancer more accurately than PI, as it correlates well with histologic pancreatic fat fraction [16].

## Clinical Anatomy of Endocrine & Urinary System in Metabolic Syndrome

Endocrine disruptors (EDCs) are substances that are released into the environment from a variety of sources, such as the food industry, pesticide manufacturers, and the packaging industry. EDCs can target a variety of bodily organs and systems, including the reproductive system, breast tissue, pancreas, adipose tissue, and more, according to clinical evidence, experimental models, and epidemiological research. Given that parabens, bisphenol A, and phthalates are commonly present in human environments, the most recent research are on their impacts during key exposure times, such as during pregnancy, infancy, and children. It is important to thoroughly investigate the ways that Endocrine Disrupting Chemicals (EDCs) affect human health, including their impact on metabolic processes, in addition to their known effects on the endocrine system. Examining how they relate to conditions like infertility, breast, testicular, and ovarian cancers as well as metabolic conditions like diabetes and obesity is part of this [17]. Through the direct activation or inactivation of endocrine target receptors, interference with the production of hormones, or the inhibition/activation of metabolizing enzymes, EDCs have the power to disrupt endocrine functioning. Nuclear receptors such as glucocorticoid, mineralocorticoid, androgen, progesterone, estrogen, thyroid, and peroxisome proliferator-activated receptors (PPAR) are among the classical targets of EDCs [18, 19]. Additionally, studies have shown that these substances have an impact on the hormone-metabolizing enzymes aromatase [20], 5-reductase [21], 3-hydroxysteroid dehydrogenase (3-HSD) [22], and 11- [21]

hydroxysteroid dehydrogenases (11-HSDs) [23, 24]. By altering the availability of active hormones, they can also affect nuclear receptor responses. Depending on the individual endocrine pathway that is impacted, endocrine system disruption can have an impact on a variety of body functions. The body's naturally occurring effects of estrogen and androgen hormones can be interfered with by a class of chemicals known as EDCs. This may be accomplished by preventing the formation of sex steroids or by obstructing their breakdown [25]. EDCs that have negative effects on reproduction can bind to either androgen receptors (ARs) or estrogen receptors (ERs), which can then either activate or suppress certain genetic mechanisms [19]. Breast health (cancer) and reproductive systems may be impacted by EDC exposure [2].

As previously mentioned, MetS is a collection of clinical conditions, including overweight, hyperglycemia or DM Type II, hypertension, and hyperlipidemia [26]. Atherosclerosis risk is increased by chronic inflammation and vascular endothelial dysfunction, which are both closely related to metabolic syndrome. Cardiovascular illnesses, the main cause of death globally, are also made more likely by MetS [27]. People with MetS, including children, adolescents, and young women with polycystic ovarian syndrome, are becoming more common as a result of sedentary lifestyles [28].

According to recent evidence, hyperinsulinemia occurs before the beginning of (pre)diabetes. These include eating a "modern" Western diet, being overweight, having less hepatic insulin clearance, having a genetic predisposition, and having fetal/metabolic programming that might enhance insulin secretion and result in persistent hyperinsulinemia. MetS, DM type II, cardiovascular disease, Alzheimer's disease, and polycystic ovarian syndrome are all significantly influenced by hyperinsulinemia. The hypothalamic-adrenal-pituitary (HPA) axis becomes more activated in individuals with the MetS, resulting in "functional hypercortisolism" in these individuals. Abdominal obesity, insulin resistance, and the MetS are all caused by the interaction of elevated insulin levels and "functional hypercortisolism". It is believed that the overproduction of insulin, known as hyperinsulinemia, can lead to the development of MetS and its associated health problems by activating the HPA axis. Many studies have shown that hyperinsulinemia can be managed and even reversed through lifestyle changes, surgery, and medication. To determine if reducing hyperinsulinemia in its early stages can prevent the HPA axis from becoming overactive and causing MetS, further long-term research is needed [29].

Previous research has indicated that individuals with obesity and metabolic syndrome tend to have a higher rate of daily cortisol production [30, 31]. This is reinforced by evidence that shows increased responsiveness in the HPA axis among those with obesity, especially those with visceral obesity when exposed to stimuli such as hypoglycemia, CRH/arginine vasopressin, acute stress, or a standard meal [32 - 34]. Furthermore, it appears that hyperinsulinemia may be linked to hyper-responsiveness to ACTH following CRH/AVP stimulation, although the specific mechanism behind this relationship remains unclear [34]. In the abdominal adipose tissue of obese people, 11b-HSD-1 expression and activity are both elevated. Contrary to people with Cushing syndrome, those with central obesity frequently have basal plasma cortisol levels that are normal [32].

Males were more likely than females to experience MetS in general. Men's metabolism was greatly impacted by overt hyperthyroidism and subclinical hypothyroidism. Males in the overt hyperthyroidism group had considerably lower BMI, systolic blood pressure (SBP), waist circumference, and triglycerides (TGs) than males in the subclinical hypothyroidism group, who had significantly greater TGs. Women's metabolic components were significantly impacted by both overt and subclinical hypothyroidism. In comparison to the euthyroid group, women with subclinical and overt hypothyroidism had significantly greater SBP&DBP(diastolic blood pressure), BMI, TGs, and waist circumference. The relative risk of abdominal obesity and hypertriglyceridemia rose in hypothyroid women. There was no impact of subclinical hyperthyroidism on the MetS or any of its elements. Before and after menopause, thyroid impairment has varied impacts on the MetS and its constituent parts. Compared to men, postmenopausal women with hypothyroidism had a higher prevalence of MetS [35]. Men and postmenopausal women are more likely to quickly accumulate abdominal fat, leading to central obesity, while peripheral obesity, which is accompanied by hypodermic and adipose accumulation, is more common in premenopausal women. The likelihood of developing DM type II, dying from cardiovascular disease, and having abdominal obesity all rise [36]. Having hypothyroidism results in weight gain. BMI and obesity are positively associated with TSH.

The most prevalent circulating adipokine, adiponectin, possesses anti-inflammatory and insulin-sensitizing effects. Even though it has been hypothesized that decreased renal clearance and compensatory responses related to adiponectin resistance are to blame for kidney function decline associated with elevated adiponectin [37], it is still unknown how elevated adiponectin affects clinical outcomes in people with chronic kidney disease (CKD) and whether these effects are similar to those in the general population.

Adiponectin, the most prevalent adipokine made by adipocytes, is under expressed in obese persons and circulates in the blood as various multimers. Adiponectin has insulin-sensitizing, anti-atherogenic anti-inflammatory, anti-oxidative stress, and, cardioprotective actions in contrast to the pro-inflammatory features of most adipokines [38 - 42]. Body composition heavily influences adiponectin levels, which are mostly negatively related to total body and visceral fat, waist circumference, and BMI [43 - 47].

Adipokines that circulate throughout the body may contribute to the development of chronic kidney disease (CKD) since visceral obesity, which frequently coexists with metabolic syndrome, increases the risk of its initiation and progression. Lower adiponectin levels have been associated with coronary artery disease (CAD), DM type II and, insulin resistance in the general population, according to studies [48 - 50]. These diseases may facilitate the development of CKD.

The consequences of protein-energy wasting (PEW) or chronic inflammation as well as decreased renal excretion may all contribute to the population with CKD, there is a dysregulated metabolism of adipokines. Despite substantial cardiovascular (CV) risks and mortality, adiponectin levels are noticeably increased with diminishing renal function [51] and have a significantly negative connection with eGFR [52 - 55]. In fact, because CKD patients have a variety of illness conditions and several metabolic pathways, adiponectin's clinical function is more nuanced. Higher rather than lower adiponectin levels are linked with a higher progression of renal disease, which is in contrast to the beneficial benefits of adiponectin in the general population [56, 57]. Studies in the CKD population have produced varying conclusions about the impact of adiponectin on mortality and CV outcomes. The clinical importance of MetS in CKD has been outlined; specifically, MetS has been linked to insulin resistance, eGFR decrease, and hypoadiponectinemia [47, 58]. Additionally, clustering the elements of the metabolic syndrome increased the chance of a fast drop in eGFR rather than a gradual one [59].

MetS causes detrusor enlargement and may be a factor in decreased bladder function. This is probably connected to how the prostate is affected by the disorder [60]. Bothersome Lower Urinary Tract Symptoms (LUTS) and BPH have been associated with MetS, a set of conditions that cause ongoing, low-grade inflammation. The accumulation of collagen and prostate fibrosis, which restrict the bladder outlet and increase prostate volume, is likely caused by persistent prostate inflammation [61 - 72].

An innovative technique for assessing crucial aspects of the lower urinary tract(LUT) is the manual and semi-automated segmentation of pelvic magnetic resonance imaging (MRI) with 3D anatomical representations [73 - 75]. This technology might make it possible to measure the modifications in people with MetS's lower urinary tract.

Males with MetS showed increased prostate volume (PV), raised postvoid residual (PVR), and increased bladder wall volume (BWV). Additionally, men with BPE had a higher risk of developing MetS, while men with MetS had higher PV [60]. The lower urinary tract's clinically important anatomical and functional aspects can be measured with the help of MRI.

Renin-angiotensin-aldosterone(RAA) system activation is linked to obesity [76]. Animal investigations have shown that angiotensin II can increase sympathetic nervous system activity centrally [77]. Additionally, it has been demonstrated in humans that angiotensin-converting enzyme inhibitor decreases sympathetic nerve traffic whereas angiotensin II infusion increases it [78]. In addition, visceral adipocytes express angiotensinogen more than subcutaneous adipocytes do, and certain renin-angiotensin system components are present in adipose tissue [79]. As a result, elevated levels of circulating angiotensin II may assist in triggering the sympathetic nervous system in cases of visceral obesity. This is corroborated by the discovery that in obese hypertension patients, angiotensin II receptor blockade reduces sympathetic nerve activity [80].

Nitric oxide synthases are downregulated and the renin-angiotensin system is upregulated as a result of the persistent visceral fat hypoxia [81]. Increased peripheral chemoreflex sensitivity and direct effects on sites of central control are two of the mechanisms, that may cause sympathoexcitation in response to hypoxia. Hypoxia increases oxidative stress (The increase in several of these genes' protein products, such as erythropoietin, endothelin-1, and vascular endothelial growth factor, suggests that reduction-oxidation-sensitive gene expression has been activated.), blood pressure, sympathetic activity, inflammatory mediators (Pentraxin, interleukin 6, tumor necrosis factor-α, and T lymphocyte), and antifibrinolytic activity (plasminogen activator inhibition type 1).

**Clinical Anatomy of Nervous System in Metabolic Syndrome**

Even when their blood glucose levels are normal, patients with MetS are more likely to develop entrapment neuropathy, peripheral neuropathy and radiculopathy. The complexity of their symptoms and overlapping illnesses in this population typically necessitates electrodiagnostic testing. If the nerve disease in patients with metabolic syndrome is not treated, they run the danger of functional deterioration [82].

It is generally known that the microvascular damage and hyperglycemia that causes neuropathy are related. Among the neuropathies connected to hyperglycemia are proximal, autonomic, focal and, small fiber neuropathies, and also distal symmetric sensorimotor polyneuropathy (DPN). Neurons are susceptible to damage from hyperglycemia through a variety of pathways, including oxidative stress, advanced glycation end products, and glucose-mediated endothelium damage [83]. Waist circumference and the presence of DPN appear to be specifically correlated.

Additionally, entrapment neuropathies and lumbar radiculopathy are risk factors for obesity [84, 85].

Although the association between dyslipidemia and neuropathy is not entirely certain, there are numerous factors, including mitochondrial dysregulation, oxidative stress, and the function of free fatty acids, that are probably at play. While some studies have not shown these connections, the exact relationship and underlying mechanisms are still unclear, high triglycerides have been linked to the development of neuropathy [86]. Several sizable observational studies have discovered that people who have an aberrant lipid profile and DM Type II are more likely than people with normal lipid profiles to develop DPN. Sensorimotor polyneuropathy, which is symmetric and length-dependent, is the classic polyneuropathy linked to MetS.

Foot discomfort, paresthesias, and numbness are typical symptoms. However, a diagnosis of neuropathy cannot be made only on the basis of symptoms. For instance, the symptom of daily numbness in the feet had only 22% sensitivity and 92% specificity in patients older than age 68 and 28% sensitivity and 93% specificity in younger patients for the presence of neuropathy in a study of 588 patients with type 2 DM where the diagnostic standard was an abnormal clinical neurologic examination [87]. Even worse diagnosis accuracy resulted from the inclusion of additional symptoms, such as foot discomfort, which had a minimal predictive value for neuropathy. A battery of questions about neuropathic symptoms is used to evaluate patients, which improves sensitivity but reduces specificity.

A lack of Achilles reflexes, poor great toe proprioception, and diminished feeling, including cold, vibratory, pinprick, and two-point discrimination, are common physical examination symptoms in patients with neuropathy. Physical examination findings of severe illness include distal weakness. The absence of the Achilles reflex and proprioception are two isolated physical examination indicators that have a high specificity but a reduced sensitivity [88].

Electrodiagnosis is used to gauge the degree of neuropathy. Action potentials of the sensory nerve are determined to assess severity. The first objective sign of neuropathy in typical DPN is anomalies in the sensory nerve action potential, which makes the diagnosis more accurate.

Patients with metabolic syndrome are more likely to develop spine problems. The risk factor for metabolic syndrome that has received the most research is obesity. Patients who are obese are more susceptible to sciatica and low back pain.

Additionally, clinically and radiologically detected spinal stenosis is more common in them.

The most prevalent and most researched entrapment neuropathy in MetS is carpal tunnel syndrome (CTS), which involves entrapment of the median nerve at the wrist. Among individuals with CTS who were part of a case series, MetS was present in 75% of the patients. Additionally, those with MetS had more aberrant electrophysiological parameters than those without [89].

In other instances, the link between the MetS and CTS appears to be unique. It indicates that having more body mass poses a particularly high danger. They discovered a dose-dependent relationship between weight and CTS in overweight and obese people in a meta-analysis of 58 trials with more than 1.3 million participants. The risk of CTS rose by more than 7.4% for every unit higher body mass index. Obesity doubled the risk compared to participants who were of normal weight. Waist-to-hip ratios and larger waist circumferences seem to be particularly dangerous, as they are in some other medical problems [85].

Prediabetes, which is commonly overlooked in this circumstance, is another risk factor for CTS. An Italian research study, for instance, found that 14% of 117 people with chronic idiopathic CTS had undiagnosed diabetes and that 45% of those people had abnormal results from a 2-hour glucose tolerance test. Even after accounting for obesity and waist size, the number of people with CTS remained considerable. The authors suggested that every patient with idiopathic CTS is tested for glucose tolerance to see whether they have a greater prevalence of incorrect glucose metabolism. This implies that CTS might be a separate risk factor for MetS [90]. DM is another well-known risk element for CTS. The symptoms of diabetic individuals with entrapment neuropathies may be misinterpreted for length-dependent polyneuropathy rather than a treatable entrapment, leading to a misdiagnosis.

The second-most frequent entrapment neuropathy is ulnar neuropathy at the elbow, which is more common among diabetics [91].

Even those with normal glucose metabolism are more likely to develop various peripheral nerve issues if they have metabolic syndrome. It can be difficult to diagnose nerve illness in this population. Because metabolic syndrome has an effect on many different disorders, the symptoms' differential diagnosis could be complex. An electrodiagnostic evaluation that has been adequately planned and carried out can contribute important information that alters patient management. Additional ways in which electrodiagnosis offers benefits include determining individuals who pose a high danger for functional problems, gauging the extent of nerve damage, and giving patients important health information. It also often reveals more than one diagnosis [82].

When compared to the general population, patients with bipolar disorder (BD) have greater rates of obesity and related cardiovascular risk factors such as DM and hypertension [92].

Numerous research works [93 - 96] have shown that obesity, MetS, and its components are significant risk factors for incidences of dementia and cognitive impairment in the general population. The brain's structural integrity is also adversely affected by obesity and elements of MetS [97, 98].

In comparison to individuals with normal weight, overweight/obese BD showed decreased fractional anisotropy (FA) in the occipital, temporal, frontal, and right parietal regions, according to the DTI study by Kuswanto *et al.* [99]. Only obese individuals, in comparison to healthy controls, have thinner cortical layers in the left and right inferior frontal cortex of BD, according to Soares *et al.* [100]. Patients with obesity or overweight have a more serious neurochemical impairment in the hippocampus than patients who are of normal weight, according to the findings of the Stop-EM experiment [101 - 103], although no such finding was reported for the volume of the cortical regions [104]. BMI was examined as a dimensional variable in six more brain-imaging studies [104 - 108]. Increased BMI was associated with disrupted white matter volume and microstructure [108], reduced gray matter volume in the temporal lobe) [104, 108], decreased cortical thickness in the frontal lobe [107], and neurochemical abnormality [100, 104], but not with decreased hippocampal volume) [106].

Three studies [108 - 110] examined the connection between DM (or glucose levels) and MRI findings [109]. In the frontoparietal, subcortical, and hippocampal regions, patients with poor glucose metabolism exhibit more extensive gray matter abnormalities than other patients. Using DTI, the other study [108] discovered elevated glucose levels and disturbed white matter integrity. The body of the corpus callosum, the left external capsule, and the fornix showed the strongest associations. Last but not least, another study [109] compared BD patients with euglycemia, and BD patients with diabetes and prediabetes had altered neurochemical processes.

With the help of DTI [108], the authors looked into the connection between white matter integrity and serum triglyceride/cholesterol levels. They discovered a substantial link between compromised white matter integrity and elevated blood levels of both variables.

Serum cholesterol had a negative correlation with FA and signal peaks in the corpus callosum, fasciculus right superior longitudinal fasciculus, the left inferior frontal-occipital fasciculus, and right posterior thalamic radiation [108].

According to some studies [93 - 96], significant risk factors for dementia and cognitive decline include MetS and its components. Cognitive impairment is a hallmark of schizophrenia, which adds to the functional deficit in this condition [111, 112]. Cognitive impairment in schizophrenia is significantly influenced by neurodevelopmental disorders [113]. According to other writers [114], schizophrenia can be distinguished from other mental illnesses by a neurodegenerative process and progressive cognitive impairment.

Since the use of antipsychotics is one of the key factors contributing to weight gain and a rise in the prevalence of MetS in schizophrenia, it is also crucial to estimate the effect size of cognitive abnormalities associated with MetS in schizophrenia [115].

There is reason to believe that cutting-edge precision drugs with the capacity to imitate, augment, and/or alter gut-brain transmission could put an end to the pandemics of DM type II and obesity. Recent research has uncovered the high-risk molecular signaling pathways that connect the brain and gastrointestinal system to control energy. Homeostasis and newly discovered molecular processes underlie effective bariatric surgery [116].

Afferent neurons and gut hormones are important messengers in human energy metabolism and gut-brain communication. In order to influence feeding behavior, homeostatic (hypothalamus and NTS) and hedonistic (VTA-Nac) brain regions, which are ordinarily divided, produce signals in conjunction with cognitive processes and data collected from visual, gustatory, and olfactory inputs. The brain is represented by the abbreviations nucleus accumbens, hypothalamus, prefrontal cortex, ventral tegmental region, hypothalamus, and nucleus tractus solitarius [116].

Tremendous brain enlargement was accompanied by equivalent changes in gut size in order to keep the metabolic rate essentially constant. This gut-brain coevolution may have been largely influenced by the expansion of energy-producing, easily digested, and nutrient-rich food sources [117]. This coevolution was mirrored by an analogous expansion of metabolic cues that were reciprocally coordinated between peripheral tissues and the central nervous system.

Intake and content of nutrients are promptly detected and transformed into humoral and neurological signals obtained from the gut. The CNS receives and processes this information, combining it with internal cues like adiposity, stress, prior experience, and a variety of other cues to produce the necessary behavioral, autonomic, and endocrine output to close the energy homeostatic loop. Ironically, modern humans have (mis)used the inheritance of superior intelligence to engineer a dietary environment that outweighs peripherally derived satiation and adiposity signals, takes advantage of the limbic system, is "unnaturally" energy-dense and hyper-palatable, and is available in practically unlimited quantities. This is despite our knowledge of systems biology and the molecular regulation of metabolism exponentially expanding.

Surgery to reorganize the gastrointestinal (GI) system is the most efficient treatment for severe obesity and DM. A majority of patients who undergo bariatric procedures, such as gastric bypass, experience a remission of their lifestyle-related comorbidities, such as DM type II, obesity, and cardiovascular disease [118, 119]. The physiological and molecular mechanisms behind the metabolic benefits of bariatric surgery are only now beginning to become known, which is significant [120], providing clues for developing more potent pharmacotherapies that might take the place of these invasive and irreversible surgical operations.

In the middle of the 20th century, a series of elegant brain-lesion studies led to the discovery of distinct hypothalamic regions that, respectively, encourage increased food intake and weight gain (lateral hypothalamic area [LHA]) and decreased food intake and weight loss (ventromedial hypothalamic nucleus [VMH]) [121]. Parallel to this, it was hypothesized that a component originating from adipose tissue alerts the same brain regions to the availability of externally stored energy [122, 123]. Even while the identification of leptin did not immediately lead to the treatment of human obesity, it sparked significant interest among researchers everywhere in identifying other signals and circuits controlling metabolic processes in both health and disease. As a result of insights from bariatric surgery, ground-breaking advancements in research on molecular metabolism, technological revolutions transforming neuroscience, and a wealth of information generated by Genome-Wide Association Studies (GWAS), gut-brain communication is now being positioned as a primary target for developing better therapeutics for metabolic diseases. The critical role of the CNS in the etiology of obesity has been established by each of these findings.

Because of its location, circulating hormones and nutrients directly send signals to the hypothalamic arcuate nucleus (ARC). ARC cells express a variety of hormone receptors and nutrition sensors as a result. The ARC is in a unique position to act as a sensing and orchestrating conduit because of its proximity to the neighboring median eminence, a circumventricular organ that is not completely shielded by a functional blood-brain barrier [124].

One area where significant progress has been made over the past two decades is the physiological and molecular functions of sub-populations of ARC neurons that express different neuropeptides and, as a result, have different functional profiles, such as those that express the anorexigenic pro-opiomelanocortin (POMC) and the orexigenic Agouti-related protein (Agrp). The typical regulators of energy metabolism are these neuropeptides. These neurons are highly responsive to metabolic conditions and regulate energy intake through bimodal modulation of the melanocortin-4 receptor (MC4R). Co-expressing with AGRP is the potent orexigenic peptide Neuropeptide Y (NPY). Inhibitory Y1 and GABA receptors are employed by AGRP/NPY neurons to directly project to POMC neurons and, upon stimulation, decrease POMC firing, among presumably countless further layers of intercellular communication [125].

The coordinated activity of the POMC in connection to the AGRP and NPY is a crucial element in the control of eating habits and body weight. The importance of MC4Rs found in the nearby hypothalamic paraventricular nucleus (PVN) to integrate this knowledge into a larger neural feeding circuitry represents a hallmark success of modern obesity research. Loss-of-function mutations in the MC4R gene cause severe obesity in humans and rodents [126, 127]. In order to advance effective MC4R agonists, a number of pharmacological research activities have been started [128].

Another significant integrative gut-brain connection is the caudal brainstem. This area of the brain receives a lot of afferent information about the type and amount of nutrients being consumed during a meal [129]. The area postrema (AP), a circumventricular organ analogous to the hypothalamic ARC, is located on the caudal brainstem and ideally situated to receive and integrate circulating metabolic signals including cholecystokinin (CCK), amylin, leptin, peptide YY (PYY), glucagon-like peptide-1 (GLP-1), ghrelin, and others, each of which can influence satiation, or how much food will be consumed in the ongoing meal. The AP transmits signals to the neighboring nucleus tractus solitarius (NTS), which subsequently delivers signals *via* monoamine-expressing neuronal projections to several hypothalamic nuclei and other parts of the brain [129].

The NTS receives a continuous stream of information from the gut *via* the vagal afferent fibers, which innervate significant portions of the intestinal wall and gastric mucosa and transmit data about the volume and composition of food being consumed by secreting peptide hormones like CCK and GLP-1. By acting in a paracrine manner on their receptors found on the surface of local vagal afferent fibers in the intestine that project to the NTS, these vagal neurons then translate nutrient-dependent changes in the gut-hormonal milieu into electro-chemical information that is transmitted to the NTS [130]. Neurons in the NTS integrate the incoming vagal information with other neuroendocrine signals, such as locally synthesized CCK and GLP- 1, to alter the magnitude of the incoming responses to the gut-derived signals before relaying them from the NTS to other brain areas [131 - 134].

The sympathetic nervous system is triggered by a variety of metabolic and cardiovascular issues, many of which are more frequent in obese people. Obesity amplifies sympathetic nervous system activation in people with hypertension, and increased sympathetic nervous system activity is connected to worse clinical outcomes [135].

The sympathetic nervous system plays a major role in maintaining the physiological homeostasis of the cardiovascular system. The sympathetic nervous system is influenced to carry out this function by a number of processes, including hormones (cortisol, vasopressin, renin-angiotensin-aldosterone system, growth hormone, gonadic hormones, asymmetric dimethylarginine), reflex (cardiopulmonary receptors, baroreceptors, chemoreceptors), metabolic (insulin, leptin, free fatty acids), inflammatory (ROS system, cytokines), endothelial and hematologic are the other categories [76].

The results of microneurographic studies evaluating abdominal and peripheral obesity show that the degree of sympathetic activation (and the magnitude of the insulin resistance state) is clearly higher in patients with visceral body fat deposits compared to those with peripheral distribution of adipose tissue [136]. Research results showing that subcutaneous body fat growth is unrelated to an adrenergic overdrive have further strengthened this conclusion [137]. The metabolic syndrome is also associated with an independent hyperadrenergic state, which may make treating hyperadrenergic illnesses like congestive heart failure more challenging.

Short sleepers, both in children and adults, consistently have a higher risk of becoming obese, according to cross-sectional research conducted worldwide [138]. Leptin levels are thought to decrease, ghrelin levels to rise, and insulin sensitivity to decline as a result of sleep loss [139].

According to human research, insulin triggers a variety of sympathetic responses. Acute hyperinsulinemia increases muscular sympathetic nerve activity, but renal norepinephrine spillover is unaffected [140, 141], and in obese individuals, there is no association between acute hyperinsulinemia and the frequency of renal norepinephrine spill over to plasma [142]. Given that norepinephrine spill over from the kidneys is frequently associated with obesity and hypertension [142, 143], it appears that factors other than hyperinsulinemia are responsible for the enhanced sympathetic nerve output in obesity and metabolic syndrome. Emphasizing the detrimental effects of sympathetic activation on the cell's capacity to transport glucose across its membrane, which is a marker of insulin resistance, increased norepinephrine release in the human forearm reduces forearm blood flow and is connected to decreased forearm glucose uptake which decreases forearm blood flow [144].

Numerous studies [139, 145, 146] suggest that sympathetic activation in obesity may be caused by high plasma leptin concentrations. Recent studies further reveal that leptin's effects on renal and brown adipose tissue thermal sympathetic nerve activity are mediated through the brain's renin-angiotensin system (RAS), irrespective of the hormone's effects on food intake. These findings imply that changes in the brain RAS's activity could modify leptin's effects on blood pressure and energy expenditure without affecting leptin's ability to make people eat less. There is evidence that genetic differences in the leptin receptor affect sympathetic activity and blood pressure in humans, despite studies failing to show a rise in blood pressure with leptin administration [147].

Similar to those documented in the metabolic syndrome and each of its constituent components, the observed changes in sympathetic drive are likely the outcome of a number of pathological mechanisms. One of the hypotheses advanced is that the neurogenic alterations are brought on by a baroreflex malfunction (*i.e.*, a considerable inhibition of sympathetic tone) [139, 148]. This has been confirmed by studies demonstrating that the sympatho-inhibitory and sympatho-excitatory baroreflex components are both involved in the plainly impaired modulation of sympathetic nerve traffic by arterial baroreceptors in people with metabolic syndrome [139]. Other reflexogenic regions, like the chemoreceptors and the cardiopulmonary receptors, may also be affected by reflex dysfunction [139].

## New Insights of Morphometric Evaluation in Metabolic Syndrome

One study comparing manually measured WC with BS-based abdominal volume found that the relationship with MetS features appeared to be much greater and that the goodness-of-fit likely to be marginally better for abdominal volume than for waist circumference (WC). Differences, though, were negligible. For both abdominal volume and WC, the ability to distinguish between the existence of MetS components was comparable. In terms of metabolic health, an ideal cut-off for abdominal volume is 12.8 L for men and 9.5 L for women. The outcomes demonstrate that abdominal volume is at least as suitable for metabolic characterisation as the conventional manually measured WC as a result [149].

We explore abdominal volume as an anthropometric indicator of MetS and compare its components to manually measure WC. Three-dimensional (3D) body surface scanners (BS) quickly and thoroughly evaluated anthropometry on a broad scale. These gadgets, which were first created for the textile industry, automatically take a 3D image of the human body and enable the determination of more than 150 anthropometric measurements. Some research has indicated that BS can be used to accurately and consistently quantify WC and total body volume [150, 151].

The BS allows for the volumetric determination of overall volume as well as the volume of the lower/upper arms, hands, legs, feet, head, and, torso, in addition to many other anthropometric measurements.

According to the World Health Organization requirements, all anthropometric studies must be conducted manually by skilled staff [152]. Compared to WC, which is merely a 2-dimensional horizontal measure, or related indices, directly measured abdominal volume as a 3D measure was anticipated to better capture visceral fat accumulation and, consequently, metabolic status.

The accumulation of central body fat was the primary contributor to cardiovascular disease (CVD), according to a sequential examination of the risk factors for the condition, starting with overweight and continuing to obesity, BMI, and anatomical distribution of body fat. Initial research revealed a substantial relationship between mortality from CVD and the distribution of body fat [153 - 155]. Regional body fat, however, dispersal became the key factor [156, 157,]. Hyperlipidemia, hypertension, DM type II, and the newly emerging MetS were all found to be strongly correlated with abdominal obesity [158 - 165].

Using more precise measures of the regional fat distribution from Computed Tomography (CT) scans, it was discovered that the deep abdominal adipose tissue (DAAT) areas were the main CVD risk markers [166 - 170]. The difficulty is quantifying these adipose tissue (AT) locations in the general population after a long history of pinpointing specific risk factors. Although CT scanners have a lot of potential for body composition study, practical issues including radiation exposure, cost, and technological challenges prevent them from being widely used. Simple anthropometric data were used to build predictive models to calculate the deep abdominal fat depots. While Despres *et al.* [171] provided the earliest predictive equations. Koester *et al.* [172]. provided the best equations that best explain 70-80% of the variance in visceral AT regions. Later, Lemieux *et al.* determined the cut-off dimensions for waist and waist-to-hip ratios (WHR). There are limitations on the general applicability of these currently available equations because there is solid evidence of the variations in the DAAT areas among populations [173 - 175]. Worldwide, population-specific predictive algorithms for measuring the DAAT regions are being created [176]. The predictive power of all anthropometric variables was only boosted by the absolute body fat indices of circumferences, skinfolds, and sagittal diameters; however, the relative body fat indices of WHR, the sum of skinfolds, the sum of trunk skinfolds, and trunk extremity ratio did not. In step-up regression analysis, it was discovered that there was a gender-specific association between anthropometric indices and DAAT regions.

In women, waist and arm measurements (central and upper peripheral circumference measures) and waist and thigh measurements (central and lower peripheral circumference measures) boosted the predictive power. Skinfold measurements added somewhat to the model's robustness, and women were more likely to notice the relationships. Sagittal diameters played a substantial role, and this was particularly pronounced in men. BMI and body weight have been found to be of exceptional value; this confirms the usefulness of these factors in addition to the measurement of the deep abdomen adipose tissue areas [176].

## CONCLUSION

According to the information that has been proven to date, the development of metabolic syndrome may be influenced by a number of variables, including demographics (gender, age, living situation, education, and income), lifestyle, physical performance, mechanical factors, genetics, environment (endocrine disrupting chemicals, *etc.*), eating habits, adipokines, inflammation, growth factors, and microorganisms. However, there are still mechanisms that need to be elucidated in the fields of genetics, inflammation, ethnic diversity, oncogenesis, and immunology related to MetS. In addition to existing diagnostic modalities, studies on new diagnostic and treatment methods that can be effective in individual diagnosis and treatment will be effective in minimizing morbidity and mortality caused by MetS and its components. Anthropometric measurements and new diagnostic approaches developed manually or in parallel with technology are very important in the diagnosis of MetS. It should not be forgotten that complications may develop in MetS even in individuals with normal blood glucose levels. Further long-term studies are required to evaluate whether decreasing hyperinsulinemia in its early stages can stop the HPA axis from becoming overactive and producing metabolic syndrome. Both overt and subclinical hypothyroidism have a considerable impact on women's metabolic components. A separate hyperadrenergic state that is present in conjunction with metabolic syndrome may make the treatment of hyperadrenergic conditions like congestive heart failure more challenging. Although leptin treatment has not been shown to raise blood pressure, there is proof that human sympathetic activity and blood pressure are impacted by leptin receptor gene variants. In primary care, a higher BMI is already acknowledged as a significant risk factor for age-related disease, but it should also be utilized to identify older persons at risk of developing MetS. It is challenging to estimate how obesity affects GI disease. 'Dose-response' relationships are frequent. There are occasionally distinctions based on gender and ethnicity. The risk of disease and excess body fat can be inversely correlated, and connections with specific anatomical patterns of fat deposition rather than high BMI may exist. It is undeniable that gaining weight raises the chance of certain GI conditions that may or may not be cancerous such as oesophageal adenocarcinoma, colorectal cancer, and gallbladder cancer. Lower adiponectin levels are related to insulin resistance, type 2 diabetes mellitus (DM), and coronary artery disease (CAD). These conditions could result in CKD being more likely to develop. Due to MetS's effects on the prostate, detrusor enlargement and possible contributions to reduced bladder function are likely associated.

In fact, metabolic syndrome has an impact on many disorders, and there may be a wide range of differential diagnoses for symptoms. Electrodiagnosis adds value in additional ways, such as assessing the degree of nerve damage, identifying patients at high risk for functional issues, and giving patients important health information. It also often reveals more than one diagnosis. Body weight was shown to be the most significant indicator for measuring DAAT regions. The BMI, sagittal diameters, and waist circumferences are the next anthropometric measurements. Despite the limitations of estimating DAAT using anthropometry, useful predictive models have been created. Different distributions of DAAT regions of different ethnic communities around the world, mapping them according to age and gender will be important in the diagnosis and treatment of metabolic syndrome. Significantly more severe cognitive and brain imaging impairments in BD are correlated with obesity and related cardiovascular risk factors. Medical co-morbidities may have an impact on the functional deterioration that some patients experience during BD. MetS is significantly linked to cognitive impairment in schizophrenia and may be a factor in some patients' functional decline during the course of their illness. Recently, there has been a lot of attention on the connections between sympathetic dysfunction, obesity, particularly complex obesity, and the risk of cardiovascular disease. As a result, therapeutic approaches are heavily targeted at lowering global cardiovascular, diabetic, and cancer risks.

# REFERENCES

[1]     Ballester-Vallés C, Flores-Méndez J, Delgado-Moraleda J, *et al.* Hepatic and pancreatic fat as imaging biomarkers of metabolic syndrome. Radiología (English Edition) 2020; 62(2): 122-30.
[http://dx.doi.org/10.1016/j.rxeng.2019.10.005] [PMID: 31447050]

[2]     Feakins RM. Obesity and metabolic syndrome: pathological effects on the gastrointestinal tract. Histopathology 2016; 68(5): 630-40.
[http://dx.doi.org/10.1111/his.12907] [PMID: 26599607]

[3]     Third Report of the National Cholesterol Education Program (NCEP) Expert Panel on Detection, Evaluation, and Treatment of High Blood Cholesterol in Adults (Adult Treatment Panel III) Final Report. Circulation 2002; 106(25): 3143-421.
[http://dx.doi.org/10.1161/circ.106.25.3143] [PMID: 12485966]

[4]     Van Ancum JM, Jonkman NH, van Schoor NM, *et al.* Predictors of metabolic syndrome in community-dwelling older adults. PLoS One 2018; 13(10): e0206424.
[http://dx.doi.org/10.1371/journal.pone.0206424] [PMID: 30379967]

[5]     Ashburn DD, Reed MJ. Gastrointestinal system and obesity. Crit Care Clin 2010; 26(4): 625-7.
[http://dx.doi.org/10.1016/j.ccc.2010.06.006] [PMID: 20970047]

[6]     Singh S, Sharma AN, Murad MH, *et al.* Central adiposity is associated with increased risk of esophageal inflammation, metaplasia, and adenocarcinoma: a systematic review and meta-analysis. Clin Gastroenterol Hepatol 2013; 11(11): 1399-1412.e7.
[http://dx.doi.org/10.1016/j.cgh.2013.05.009] [PMID: 23707461]

[7]     Ryan AM, Duong M, Healy L, *et al.* Obesity, metabolic syndrome and esophageal adenocarcinoma: Epidemiology, etiology and new targets. Cancer Epidemiol 2011; 35(4): 309-19.
[http://dx.doi.org/10.1016/j.canep.2011.03.001] [PMID: 21470937]

[8]     Barak N, Ehrenpreis ED, Harrison JR, Sitrin MD. Gastro-oesophageal reflux disease in obesity: pathophysiological and therapeutic considerations. Obes Rev 2002; 3(1): 9-15.
[http://dx.doi.org/10.1046/j.1467-789X.2002.00049.x] [PMID: 12119661]

[9]     Donohoe CL, Pidgeon GP, Lysaght J, Reynolds JV. Obesity and gastrointestinal cancer. Br J Surg 2010; 97(5): 628-42.
[http://dx.doi.org/10.1002/bjs.7079] [PMID: 20306531]

[10]    Borena W, Stocks T, Jonsson H, *et al.* Serum triglycerides and cancer risk in the metabolic syndrome and cancer (Me-Can) collaborative study. Cancer Causes Control 2011; 22(2): 291-9.
[http://dx.doi.org/10.1007/s10552-010-9697-0] [PMID: 21140204]

[11]    Liu Z, Brooks RS, Ciappio ED, *et al.* Diet-induced obesity elevates colonic TNF-α in mice and is accompanied by an activation of Wnt signaling: a mechanism for obesity-associated colorectal cancer. J Nutr Biochem 2012; 23(10): 1207-13.
[http://dx.doi.org/10.1016/j.jnutbio.2011.07.002] [PMID: 22209007]

[12]    Donohoe CL, O'Farrell NJ, Doyle SL, Reynolds JV. The role of obesity in gastrointestinal cancer: evidence and opinion. Therap Adv Gastroenterol 2014; 7(1): 38-50.
[http://dx.doi.org/10.1177/1756283X13501786] [PMID: 24381646]

[13]    Howe LR, Subbaramaiah K, Hudis CA, Dannenberg AJ. Molecular pathways: adipose inflammation as a mediator of obesity-associated cancer. Clin Cancer Res 2013; 19(22): 6074-83.
[http://dx.doi.org/10.1158/1078-0432.CCR-12-2603] [PMID: 23958744]

[14]    Dong Z, Luo Y, Cai H, *et al.* Noninvasive fat quantification of the liver and pancreas may provide potential biomarkers of impaired glucose tolerance and type 2 diabetes. Medicine (Baltimore) 2016; 95(23): e3858.
[http://dx.doi.org/10.1097/MD.0000000000003858] [PMID: 27281097]

[15]    Begovatz P, Koliaki C, Weber K, *et al.* Pancreatic adipose tissue infiltration, parenchymal steatosis and beta cell function in humans. Diabetologia 2015; 58(7): 1646-55.

[http://dx.doi.org/10.1007/s00125-015-3544-5] [PMID: 25740696]

[16]   Fukui H, Hori M, Fukuda Y, *et al.* Evaluation of fatty pancreas by proton density fat fraction using 3-T magnetic resonance imaging and its association with pancreatic cancer. Eur J Radiol 2019; 118: 25-31.
[http://dx.doi.org/10.1016/j.ejrad.2019.06.024] [PMID: 31439250]

[17]   Giulivo M, Lopez de Alda M, Capri E, Barceló D. Human exposure to endocrine disrupting compounds: Their role in reproductive systems, metabolic syndrome and breast cancer. A review. Environ Res 2016; 151: 251-64.
[http://dx.doi.org/10.1016/j.envres.2016.07.011] [PMID: 27504873]

[18]   Yang O, Kim HL, Il Weon J, Seo YR. Endocrine-disrupting Chemicals: Review of Toxicological Mechanisms Using Molecular Pathway Analysis. Journal of cancer prevention 2015; 20(2): 12.
[http://dx.doi.org/10.15430/JCP.2015.20.1.12]

[19]   Wuttke W, Jarry H, Seidlova-Wuttke D. Definition, classification and mechanism of action of endocrine disrupting chemicals. Hormones (Athens) 2010; 9(1): 9-15.
[http://dx.doi.org/10.1007/BF03401276] [PMID: 20363717]

[20]   Sanderson JT. The steroid hormone biosynthesis pathway as a target for endocrine-disrupting chemicals. Toxicol Sci 2006; 94(1): 3-21.
[http://dx.doi.org/10.1093/toxsci/kfl051] [PMID: 16807284]

[21]   Kalfa N, Philibert P, Sultan C. Is hypospadias a genetic, endocrine or environmental disease, or still an unexplained malformation? Int J Androl 2008.
[PMID: 18637150]

[22]   Ye L, Su ZJ, Ge RS. Inhibitors of testosterone biosynthetic and metabolic activation enzymes. Molecules 2011; 16(12): 9983-10001.
[http://dx.doi.org/10.3390/molecules16129983] [PMID: 22138857]

[23]   Odermatt A, Gumy C, Atanasov AG, Dzyakanchuk AA. Disruption of glucocorticoid action by environmental chemicals: Potential mechanisms and relevance. J Steroid Biochem Mol Biol 2006; 102(1-5): 222-31.
[http://dx.doi.org/10.1016/j.jsbmb.2006.09.010] [PMID: 17045799]

[24]   Guo Y, Kannan K. A survey of phthalates and parabens in personal care products from the United States and its implications for human exposure. Environ Sci Technol 2013; 47(24): 14442-9.
[http://dx.doi.org/10.1021/es4042034] [PMID: 24261694]

[25]   Lee CC, Jiang LY, Kuo YL, Hsieh CY, Chen CS, Tien CJ. The potential role of water quality parameters on occurrence of nonylphenol and bisphenol A and identification of their discharge sources in the river ecosystems. Chemosphere 2013; 91(7): 904-11.
[http://dx.doi.org/10.1016/j.chemosphere.2013.02.006] [PMID: 23473432]

[26]   Chen G, Li H, Zhao Y, *et al.* Saponins from stems and leaves of Panax ginseng prevent obesity *via* regulating thermogenesis, lipogenesis and lipolysis in high-fat diet-induced obese C57BL/6 mice. Food Chem Toxicol 2017; 106(Pt A): 393-403.
[http://dx.doi.org/10.1016/j.fct.2017.06.012] [PMID: 28599882]

[27]   Kang JG, Park CY. Anti-obesity drugs: A review about their effects and safety. Diabetes Metab J 2012; 36(1): 13-25.
[http://dx.doi.org/10.4093/dmj.2012.36.1.13] [PMID: 22363917]

[28]   Vassallo P, Driver SL, Stone NJ. Metabolic syndrome: An evolving clinical construct. Prog Cardiovasc Dis 2016; 59(2): 172-7.
[http://dx.doi.org/10.1016/j.pcad.2016.07.012] [PMID: 27497505]

[29]   Janssen JAMJL. New Insights into the Role of Insulin and Hypothalamic-Pituitary-Adrenal (HPA) Axis in the Metabolic Syndrome. Int J Mol Sci 2022; 23(15): 8178.
[http://dx.doi.org/10.3390/ijms23158178] [PMID: 35897752]

[30]   Andrew R, Phillips DIW, Walker BR. Obesity and gender influence cortisol secretion and metabolism

in man. J Clin Endocrinol Metab 1998; 83(5): 1806-9.
[http://dx.doi.org/10.1210/jcem.83.5.4951] [PMID: 9589697]

[31]  Vicennati V, Pasquali R. Abnormalities of the hypothalamic-pituitary-adrenal axis in nondepressed women with abdominal obesity and relations with insulin resistance: evidence for a central and a peripheral alteration. J Clin Endocrinol Metab 2000; 85(11): 4093-8.
[http://dx.doi.org/10.1210/jcem.85.11.6946] [PMID: 11095438]

[32]  Asensio C, Muzzin P, Rohner-Jeanrenaud F. Role of glucocorticoids in the physiopathology of excessive fat deposition and insulin resistance. Int J Obes 2004; 28(S4) (Suppl. 4): S45-52.
[http://dx.doi.org/10.1038/sj.ijo.0802856] [PMID: 15592486]

[33]  Stewart PM, Boulton A, Kumar S, Clark PM, Shackleton CH. Cortisol metabolism in human obesity: impaired cortisone-->cortisol conversion in subjects with central adiposity. J Clin Endocrinol Metab 1999; 84(3): 1022-7.
[http://dx.doi.org/10.1210/jc.84.3.1022] [PMID: 10084590]

[34]  Pasquali R, Gagliardi L, Vicennati V, *et al.* ACTH and cortisol response to combined corticotropin releasing hormone-arginine vasopressin stimulation in obese males and its relationship to body weight, fat distribution and parameters of the metabolic syndrome. Int J Obes 1999; 23(4): 419-24.
[http://dx.doi.org/10.1038/sj.ijo.0800838] [PMID: 10340821]

[35]  He J, Lai Y, Yang J, *et al.* The Relationship Between Thyroid Function and Metabolic Syndrome and Its Components: A Cross-Sectional Study in a Chinese Population. Front Endocrinol (Lausanne) 2021; 12: 661160.
[http://dx.doi.org/10.3389/fendo.2021.661160] [PMID: 33868183]

[36]  Pellegrini M, Pallottini V, Marin R, Marino M. Role of the sex hormone estrogen in the prevention of lipid disorder. Curr Med Chem 2014; 21(24): 2734-42.
[http://dx.doi.org/10.2174/0929867321666140303123602] [PMID: 24606523]

[37]  Kuo IC, Wu PH, Lin HYH, *et al.* The association of adiponectin with metabolic syndrome and clinical outcome in patients with non-diabetic chronic kidney disease. PLoS One 2019; 14(7): e0220158.
[http://dx.doi.org/10.1371/journal.pone.0220158] [PMID: 31323071]

[38]  Ohashi K, Ouchi N, Matsuzawa Y. Anti-inflammatory and anti-atherogenic properties of adiponectin. Biochimie 2012; 94(10): 2137-42.
[http://dx.doi.org/10.1016/j.biochi.2012.06.008] [PMID: 22713764]

[39]  Ebrahimi-Mamaeghani M, Mohammadi S, Arefhosseini SR, Fallah P, Bazi Z. Adiponectin as a potential biomarker of vascular disease. Vasc Health Risk Manag 2015; 11: 55-70.
[PMID: 25653535]

[40]  Nigro E, Scudiero O, Monaco ML, *et al.* New insight into adiponectin role in obesity and obesity-related diseases. BioMed Res Int 2014; 2014: 1-14.
[http://dx.doi.org/10.1155/2014/658913] [PMID: 25110685]

[41]  Matsuda M, Shimomura I. Roles of adiponectin and oxidative stress in obesity-associated metabolic and cardiovascular diseases. Rev Endocr Metab Disord 2014; 15(1): 1-10.
[http://dx.doi.org/10.1007/s11154-013-9271-7] [PMID: 24026768]

[42]  Tao L, Gao E, Jiao X, *et al.* Adiponectin cardioprotection after myocardial ischemia/reperfusion involves the reduction of oxidative/nitrative stress. Circulation 2007; 115(11): 1408-16.
[http://dx.doi.org/10.1161/CIRCULATIONAHA.106.666941] [PMID: 17339545]

[43]  Rhee CM, Nguyen DV, Moradi H, *et al.* Association of Adiponectin With Body Composition and Mortality in Hemodialysis Patients. Am J Kidney Dis 2015; 66(2): 313-21.
[http://dx.doi.org/10.1053/j.ajkd.2015.02.325] [PMID: 25824125]

[44]  Zoccali C, Postorino M, Marino C, Pizzini P, Cutrupi S, Tripepi G. Waist circumference modifies the relationship between the adipose tissue cytokines leptin and adiponectin and all-cause and cardiovascular mortality in haemodialysis patients. J Intern Med 2011; 269(2): 172-81.

[http://dx.doi.org/10.1111/j.1365-2796.2010.02288.x] [PMID: 21138492]

[45]   Delgado C, Chertow GM, Kaysen GA, *et al.* Associations of Body Mass Index and Body Fat With Markers of Inflammation and Nutrition Among Patients Receiving Hemodialysis. Am J Kidney Dis 2017; 70(6): 817-25.
[http://dx.doi.org/10.1053/j.ajkd.2017.06.028] [PMID: 28870376]

[46]   Hyun YY, Lee KB, Oh KH, *et al.* Serum adiponectin and protein–energy wasting in predialysis chronic kidney disease. Nutrition 2017; 33: 254-60.
[http://dx.doi.org/10.1016/j.nut.2016.06.014] [PMID: 27692989]

[47]   Yoon CY, Kim YL, Han SH, *et al.* Hypoadiponectinemia and the presence of metabolic syndrome in patients with chronic kidney disease: results from the KNOW-CKD study. Diabetol Metab Syndr 2016; 8(1): 75.
[http://dx.doi.org/10.1186/s13098-016-0191-z] [PMID: 27895721]

[48]   Spranger J, Kroke A, Möhlig M, *et al.* Adiponectin and protection against type 2 diabetes mellitus. Lancet 2003; 361(9353): 226-8.
[http://dx.doi.org/10.1016/S0140-6736(03)12255-6] [PMID: 12547549]

[49]   Shand BI, Scott RS, Elder PA, George PM. Plasma adiponectin in overweight, nondiabetic individuals with or without insulin resistance. Diabetes Obes Metab 2003; 5(5): 349-53.
[http://dx.doi.org/10.1046/j.1463-1326.2003.00279.x] [PMID: 12940874]

[50]   Mohan V, Deepa R, Pradeepa R, *et al.* Association of low adiponectin levels with the metabolic syndrome—the Chennai Urban Rural Epidemiology Study (CURES-4). Metabolism 2005; 54(4): 476-81.
[http://dx.doi.org/10.1016/j.metabol.2004.10.016] [PMID: 15798954]

[51]   Huang JW, Yen CJ, Chiang HW, Hung KY, Tsai TJ, Wu KD. Adiponectin in peritoneal dialysis patients: a comparison with hemodialysis patients and subjects with normal renal function. Am J Kidney Dis 2004; 43(6): 1047-55.
[http://dx.doi.org/10.1053/j.ajkd.2004.02.017] [PMID: 15168385]

[52]   Becker B, Kronenberg F, Kielstein JT, *et al.* Renal insulin resistance syndrome, adiponectin and cardiovascular events in patients with kidney disease: the mild and moderate kidney disease study. J Am Soc Nephrol 2005; 16(4): 1091-8.
[http://dx.doi.org/10.1681/ASN.2004090742] [PMID: 15743998]

[53]   Nanayakkara PWB, Poole CYL, Fouque D, *et al.* Plasma adiponectin concentration has an inverse and a non linear association with estimated glomerular filtration rate in patients with K/DOQI 3 – 5 chronic kidney disease. Clin Nephrol 2009; 72(7): 21-30.
[http://dx.doi.org/10.5414/CNP72021] [PMID: 19640384]

[54]   Mills KT, Hamm LL, Alper AB, *et al.* Circulating adipocytokines and chronic kidney disease. PLoS One 2013; 8(10): e76902.
[http://dx.doi.org/10.1371/journal.pone.0076902] [PMID: 24116180]

[55]   Ortega Moreno L, Lamacchia O, Copetti M, *et al.* Serum Adiponectin and Glomerular Filtration Rate in Patients with Type 2 Diabetes. PLoS One 2015; 10(10): e0140631.
[http://dx.doi.org/10.1371/journal.pone.0140631] [PMID: 26465607]

[56]   Kollerits B, Fliser D, Heid IM, Ritz E, Kronenberg F. Gender-specific association of adiponectin as a predictor of progression of chronic kidney disease: The Mild to Moderate Kidney Disease Study. Kidney Int 2007; 71(12): 1279-86.
[http://dx.doi.org/10.1038/sj.ki.5002191] [PMID: 17457380]

[57]   Jorsal A, Tarnow L, Frystyk J, *et al.* Serum adiponectin predicts all-cause mortality and end stage renal disease in patients with type I diabetes and diabetic nephropathy. Kidney Int 2008; 74(5): 649-54.
[http://dx.doi.org/10.1038/ki.2008.201] [PMID: 18496510]

[58]    Yun HR, Kim H, Park JT, *et al.* Obesity, Metabolic Abnormality, and Progression of CKD. Am J Kidney Dis 2018; 72(3): 400-10.
[http://dx.doi.org/10.1053/j.ajkd.2018.02.362] [PMID: 29728317]

[59]    Huh JH, Yadav D, Kim JS, *et al.* An association of metabolic syndrome and chronic kidney disease from a 10-year prospective cohort study. Metabolism 2017; 67: 54-61.
[http://dx.doi.org/10.1016/j.metabol.2016.11.003] [PMID: 28081778]

[60]    Tannenbaum AP, Grimes MD, Brace CL, *et al.* Effect of Metabolic Syndrome on Anatomy and Function of the Lower Urinary Tract Assessed on MRI. Urology 2022; 159: 176-81.
[http://dx.doi.org/10.1016/j.urology.2021.09.006]

[61]    McConnell JD, Roehrborn CG, Bautista OM, *et al.* The long-term effect of doxazosin, finasteride, and combination therapy on the clinical progression of benign prostatic hyperplasia. N Engl J Med 2003; 349(25): 2387-98.
[http://dx.doi.org/10.1056/NEJMoa030656] [PMID: 14681504]

[62]    Robert G, Descazeaud A, Nicolaïew N, *et al.* Inflammation in benign prostatic hyperplasia: A 282 patients' immunohistochemical analysis. Prostate 2009; 69(16): 1774-80.
[http://dx.doi.org/10.1002/pros.21027] [PMID: 19670242]

[63]    Delongchamps NB, de la Roza G, Chandan V, *et al.* Evaluation of prostatitis in autopsied prostates--is chronic inflammation more associated with benign prostatic hyperplasia or cancer? J Urol 2008; 179(5): 1736-40.
[http://dx.doi.org/10.1016/j.juro.2008.01.034] [PMID: 18343414]

[64]    Begley LA, Kasina S, MacDonald J, Macoska JA. The inflammatory microenvironment of the aging prostate facilitates cellular proliferation and hypertrophy. Cytokine 2008; 43(2): 194-9.
[http://dx.doi.org/10.1016/j.cyto.2008.05.012] [PMID: 18572414]

[65]    Penna G, Fibbi B, Amuchastegui S, *et al.* Human benign prostatic hyperplasia stromal cells as inducers and targets of chronic immuno-mediated inflammation. J Immunol 2009; 182(7): 4056-64.
[http://dx.doi.org/10.4049/jimmunol.0801875] [PMID: 19299703]

[66]    Fujita K, Ewing CM, Getzenberg RH, Parsons JK, Isaacs WB, Pavlovich CP. Monocyte chemotactic protein-1 (MCP-1/CCL2) is associated with prostatic growth dysregulation and benign prostatic hyperplasia. Prostate 2010; 70(5): 473-81.
[http://dx.doi.org/10.1002/pros.21081] [PMID: 19902472]

[67]    Schauer IG, Ressler SJ, Tuxhorn JA, Dang TD, Rowley DR. Elevated epithelial expression of interleukin-8 correlates with myofibroblast reactive stroma in benign prostatic hyperplasia. Urology 2008; 72(1): 205-13.
[http://dx.doi.org/10.1016/j.urology.2007.11.083] [PMID: 18314176]

[68]    Gacci M, Corona G, Vignozzi L, *et al.* Metabolic syndrome and benign prostatic enlargement: a systematic review and meta-analysis. BJU Int 2015; 115(1): 24-31.
[http://dx.doi.org/10.1111/bju.12728] [PMID: 24602293]

[69]    Yim SJ, Cho YS, Joo KJ. Relationship between metabolic syndrome and prostate volume in Korean men under 50 years of age. Korean J Urol 2011; 52(6): 390-5.
[http://dx.doi.org/10.4111/kju.2011.52.6.390] [PMID: 21750749]

[70]    De Nunzio C, Cindolo L, Gacci M, *et al.* Metabolic syndrome and lower urinary tract symptoms in patients with benign prostatic enlargement: a possible link to storage symptoms. Urology 2014; 84(5): 1181-7.
[http://dx.doi.org/10.1016/j.urology.2014.07.018] [PMID: 25443931]

[71]    Russo GI, Regis F, Spatafora P, *et al.* Association between metabolic syndrome and intravesical prostatic protrusion in patients with benign prostatic enlargement and lower urinary tract symptoms ( MIPS Study). BJU Int 2018; 121(5): 799-804.
[http://dx.doi.org/10.1111/bju.14007] [PMID: 28872764]

[72] Gacci M, Corona G, Sebastianelli A, *et al.* Male lower urinary tract symptoms and cardiovascular events: A systematic review and meta-analysis. Eur Urol 2016; 70(5): 788-96.
[http://dx.doi.org/10.1016/j.eururo.2016.07.007] [PMID: 27451136]

[73] Anzia LE, Johnson CJ, Mao L, *et al.* Comprehensive non-invasive analysis of lower urinary tract anatomy using MRI. Abdom Radiol (NY) 2021; 46(4): 1670-6.
[http://dx.doi.org/10.1007/s00261-020-02808-9] [PMID: 33040167]

[74] Turkbey B, Fotin SV, Huang RJ, *et al.* Fully automated prostate segmentation on MRI: comparison with manual segmentation methods and specimen volumes. AJR Am J Roentgenol 2013; 201(5): W720-9.
[http://dx.doi.org/10.2214/AJR.12.9712] [PMID: 24147502]

[75] Tian Z, Liu L, Zhang Z, Xue J, Fei B. A supervoxel-based segmentation method for prostate MR images. Med Phys 2017; 44(2): 558-69.
[http://dx.doi.org/10.1002/mp.12048] [PMID: 27991675]

[76] Seravalle G, Grassi G. Sympathetic Nervous System, Hypertension, Obesity and Metabolic Syndrome. High Blood Press Cardiovasc Prev 2016; 23(3): 175-9.
[http://dx.doi.org/10.1007/s40292-016-0137-4] [PMID: 26942609]

[77] Reid IA. Interactions between ANG II, sympathetic nervous system, and baroreceptor reflexes in regulation of blood pressure. Am J Physiol 1992; 262(6 Pt 1): E763-78.
[PMID: 1616014]

[78] Miyajima EIJI, Shigemasa TOMOHIKO, Yamada YUTAKA, Tochikubo OSAMU, Ishii MASAO. Angiotensin II blunts, while an angiotensin-converting enzyme inhibitor augments, reflex sympathetic inhibition in humans. Clin Exp Pharmacol Physiol 1999; 26(10): 797-802.
[http://dx.doi.org/10.1046/j.1440-1681.1999.03122.x] [PMID: 10549404]

[79] Engeli S, Negrel R, Sharma AM. Physiology and pathophysiology of the adipose tissue renin-angiotensin system. Hypertension 2000; 35(6): 1270-7.
[http://dx.doi.org/10.1161/01.HYP.35.6.1270] [PMID: 10856276]

[80] Prabhakar NR, Fields RD, Baker T, Fletcher EC. Intermittent hypoxia: cell to system. Am J Physiol Lung Cell Mol Physiol 2001; 281(3): L524-8.
[http://dx.doi.org/10.1152/ajplung.2001.281.3.L524] [PMID: 11504675]

[81] Belaidi E, Joyeux-Faure M, Ribuot C, Launois SH, Levy P, Godin-Ribuot D. Major role for hypoxia inducible factor-1 and the endothelin system in promoting myocardial infarction and hypertension in an animal model of obstructive sleep apnea. J Am Coll Cardiol 2009; 53(15): 1309-17.
[http://dx.doi.org/10.1016/j.jacc.2008.12.050] [PMID: 19358946]

[82] Phillips BG, Kato M, Narkiewicz K, Choe I, Somers VK. Increases in leptin levels, sympathetic drive, and weight gain in obstructive sleep apnea. Am J Physiol Heart Circ Physiol 2000; 279(1): H234-7.
[http://dx.doi.org/10.1152/ajpheart.2000.279.1.H234] [PMID: 10899061]

[83] Peppard PE, Young T, Palta M, Skatrud J. Prospective study of the association between sleep-disordered breathing and hypertension. N Engl J Med 2000; 342(19): 1378-84.
[http://dx.doi.org/10.1056/NEJM200005113421901] [PMID: 10805822]

[84] Hla KM, Young TB, Bidwell T, Palta M, Skatrud JB, Dempsey J. Sleep apnea and hypertension. A population-based study. Ann Intern Med 1994; 120(5): 382-8.
[http://dx.doi.org/10.7326/0003-4819-120-5-199403010-00005] [PMID: 8304655]

[85] Mills PJ, Kennedy BP, Loredo JS, Dimsdale JE, Ziegler MG. Effects of nasal continuous positive airway pressure and oxygen supplementation on norepinephrine kinetics and cardiovascular responses in obstructive sleep apnea. J Appl Physiol 2006; 100(1): 343-8.
[http://dx.doi.org/10.1152/japplphysiol.00494.2005] [PMID: 16357087]

[86] Krieger J, Pépin JL, Kurtz D, *et al.* Blood pressure and heart rate variability in the European Sleep Apnea Database (ESADA) subjects. Physiol Meas 2016; 37: 1284-96.

[http://dx.doi.org/10.1088/0967-3334/37/8/1284]

[87]   Sforza E, Roche F, Thomas-Anterion C, *et al.* Cognitive function and sleep related breathing disorders in a healthy elderly population: the SYNAPSE study. Sleep 2010; 33(4): 515-21.
[http://dx.doi.org/10.1093/sleep/33.4.515] [PMID: 20394321]

[88]   Karamanli H, Kizilirmak D, Akgedik R, *et al.* The effects of continuous positive airway pressure therapy on blood pressure and renal function in obstructive sleep apnea patients with hypertension and diabetic nephropathy. Ren Fail 2012; 34: 1170-4.
[http://dx.doi.org/10.3109/0886022X.2012.715750]

[89]   Pépin JL, Tamisier R, Hwang D, *et al.* Does obstructive sleep apnea favor cancer? Sleep Med Rev 2018; 41: 28-36.
[http://dx.doi.org/10.1016/j.smrv.2017.12.007]

[90]   Huang T, Lin BM, Markt SC, *et al.* Associations of Untreated Sleep Duration and Snoring with Incident Excessive Daytime Sleepiness: The Framingham Heart Study. BMC Pulm Med 2017; 17: 63.
[http://dx.doi.org/10.1186/s12890-017-0411-7]

[91]   Zhang W, si L. Obstructive sleep apnea syndrome (OSAS) and hypertension: Pathogenic mechanisms and possible therapeutic approaches. Ups J Med Sci 2012; 117(4): 370-82.
[http://dx.doi.org/10.3109/03009734.2012.707253] [PMID: 23009224]

[92]   Bagai K. The Relationship Between Sleep-Disordered Breathing and Hypertension: A Review. Cardiol Ther 2015; 4: 43-52.
[http://dx.doi.org/10.1007/s40119-015-0033-z]

[93]   Ong CW, O'Driscoll DM, Truby H, Naughton MT, Hamilton GS. The reciprocal interaction between obesity and obstructive sleep apnoea. J Thorac Dis 2015; 7: 543-51.
[http://dx.doi.org/10.3978/j.issn.2072-1439.2015.02.05]

[94]   Liu L, Cao Q, Guan X, Li R, Yang Y, Yao Y. Obstructive sleep apnea is associated with 4-hydroxynonenal-related atherosclerosis. Mol Med Rep 2016; 13: 5203-8.
[http://dx.doi.org/10.3892/mmr.2016.5174]

[95]   Steiropoulos P, Papanas N, Nena E, *et al.* Inflammatory markers in middle-aged obese subjects: does obstructive sleep apnea syndrome play a role? Mediators Inflamm 2010; 2010: 1-6.
[http://dx.doi.org/10.1155/2010/675320] [PMID: 20628509]

[96]   Leproult R, Van Cauter E. Effect of 1 week of sleep restriction on testosterone levels in young healthy men. JAMA 2011; 305(21): 2173-4.
[http://dx.doi.org/10.1001/jama.2011.710] [PMID: 21632481]

[97]   Luboshitzky R, Zabari Z, Shen-Orr Z, Herer P, Lavie P. Disruption of the nocturnal testosterone rhythm by sleep fragmentation in normal men. J Clin Endocrinol Metab 2001; 86(3): 1134-9.
[http://dx.doi.org/10.1210/jcem.86.3.7296] [PMID: 11238497]

[98]   Penev PD. Association between sleep and morning testosterone levels in older men. Sleep 2007; 30(4): 427-32.
[http://dx.doi.org/10.1093/sleep/30.4.427] [PMID: 17520786]

[99]   Axelsson J, Ingre M, Åkerstedt T, Holmbäck U. POINT Group. Effects of Acute Sleep Loss on Diurnal Plasma Dynamics of CNS Health Biomarkers in Young Men. Neurology 2018; 91(10): e1177-85.
[http://dx.doi.org/10.1212/WNL.0000000000006125]

[100]  Pilz LK, Keller LK, Lenssen D, Roenneberg T. Time to rethink sleep quality: PSQI scores reflect sleep quality on workdays. Sleep 2018; 41(5): zsy029.
[http://dx.doi.org/10.1093/sleep/zsy029] [PMID: 29420828]

[101]  Vgontzas AN, Zoumakis E, Bixler EO, *et al.* Adverse effects of modest sleep restriction on sleepiness, performance, and inflammatory cytokines. J Clin Endocrinol Metab 2004; 89(5): 2119-26.
[http://dx.doi.org/10.1210/jc.2003-031562] [PMID: 15126529]

[102]   Kim JH, Chang JH, Kim DY, Kang JW. Effects of Sleep Duration on Blood Pressure and Arterial Stiffness in Healthy College Students. Korean Circ J 2021; 51(9): 840-50.
        [http://dx.doi.org/10.4070/kcj.2020.0456] [PMID: 34227268]

[103]   Nabe-Nielsen J, Rod NH, Hansen AM, *et al.* The Job-Demand-Control-Support model and circadian blood pressure variation in Danish nurses: a cross-sectional study. Scand J Work Environ Health 2010; 36(2): 127-35.
        [http://dx.doi.org/10.5271/sjweh.2892]

[104]   Brindle RC, Yu L, Buysse DJ, Hall MH. Empirical derivation of cutoff values for the sleep health metric and its relationship to cardiometabolic morbidity: results from the Midlife in the United States (MIDUS) study. Sleep 2019; 42(9): zsz116.
        [http://dx.doi.org/10.1093/sleep/zsz116] [PMID: 31083710]

[105]   Shea SA, Hilton MF, Hu K, Scheer FAJL. Existence of an endogenous circadian blood pressure rhythm in humans that peaks in the evening. Circ Res 2011; 108(8): 980-4.
        [http://dx.doi.org/10.1161/CIRCRESAHA.110.233668] [PMID: 21474818]

[106]   Shinozaki N, Murata M, Maruyama T, *et al.* Relationship between lifestyle factors and defecatory dysfunction. Biomed Rep 2016; 4(6): 747-51.
        [http://dx.doi.org/10.3892/br.2016.642]

[107]   Shimizu S, Hirose Y, Yamamoto T, Tatsuoka H, Okuyama T, Abe T. Long-term lifestyle and attitude of the defecation in middle-aged and elderly Japanese people. J Phys Ther Sci 2019; 31(5): 423-8.
        [http://dx.doi.org/10.1589/jpts.31.423]

[108]   Kim JW, Kim BC, Hong KS, *et al.* The relationship between dietary habits and defecation. Korean J Intern Med (Korean Assoc Intern Med) 2009; 24(3): 303-9.
        [http://dx.doi.org/10.3904/kjim.2022.338]

[109]   Singh RK, Chang HW, Yan D, *et al.* Influence of diet on the gut microbiome and implications for human health. J Transl Med 2017; 15(1): 73.
        [http://dx.doi.org/10.1186/s12967-017-1175-y] [PMID: 28388917]

[110]   Sanz Y, Santacruz A, De Palma G. Insights into the roles of gut microbes in obesity. Interdiscip Perspect Infect Dis 2008; 2008: 1-9.
        [http://dx.doi.org/10.1155/2008/829101] [PMID: 19259329]

[111]   Duncan SH, Lobley GE, Holtrop G, *et al.* Human colonic microbiota associated with diet, obesity and weight loss. Int J Obes 2008; 32(11): 1720-4.
        [http://dx.doi.org/10.1038/ijo.2008.155] [PMID: 18779823]

[112]   Turnbaugh PJ, Hamady M, Yatsunenko T, *et al.* A core gut microbiome in obese and lean twins. Nature 2009; 457(7228): 480-4.
        [http://dx.doi.org/10.1038/nature07540] [PMID: 19043404]

[113]   Eckburg PB, Bik EM, Bernstein CN, *et al.* Diversity of the human intestinal microbial flora. Science 2005; 308(5728): 1635-8.
        [http://dx.doi.org/10.1126/science.1110591] [PMID: 15831718]

[114]   Ley RE, Bäckhed F, Turnbaugh P, Lozupone CA, Knight RD, Gordon JI. Obesity alters gut microbial ecology. Proc Natl Acad Sci USA 2005; 102(31): 11070-5.
        [http://dx.doi.org/10.1073/pnas.0504978102] [PMID: 16033867]

[115]   Jumpertz R, Le DS, Turnbaugh PJ, *et al.* Energy-balance studies reveal associations between gut microbes, caloric load, and nutrient absorption in humans. Am J Clin Nutr 2011; 94(1): 58-65.
        [http://dx.doi.org/10.3945/ajcn.110.010132] [PMID: 21543530]

[116]   Cani PD, Amar J, Iglesias MA, *et al.* Metabolic endotoxemia initiates obesity and insulin resistance. Diabetes 2007; 56(7): 1761-72.
        [http://dx.doi.org/10.2337/db06-1491] [PMID: 17456850]

[117]   Muccioli GG, Naslain D, Bäckhed F, *et al.* The endocannabinoid system links gut microbiota to adipogenesis. Mol Syst Biol 2010; 6(1): 392.
[http://dx.doi.org/10.1038/msb.2010.46] [PMID: 20664638]

[118]   Diamant M, Blaak EE, de Vos WM. Do nutrient–gut–microbiota interactions play a role in human obesity, insulin resistance and type 2 diabetes? Obes Rev 2011; 12(4): 272-81.
[http://dx.doi.org/10.1111/j.1467-789X.2010.00797.x] [PMID: 20804522]

[119]   Geurts L, Neyrinck AM, Delzenne NM, Knauf C, Cani PD. Gut microbiota controls adipose tissue expansion, gut barrier and glucose metabolism: novel insights into molecular targets and interventions using prebiotics. Benef Microbes 2014; 5(1): 3-18.
[http://dx.doi.org/10.3920/BM2012.0065] [PMID: 23886976]

[120]   Tilg H, Kaser A. Gut microbiome, obesity, and metabolic dysfunction. J Clin Invest 2011; 121(6): 2126-32.
[http://dx.doi.org/10.1172/JCI58109] [PMID: 21633181]

[121]   Cani PD, Bibiloni R, Knauf C, *et al.* Changes in gut microbiota control metabolic endotoxemia-induced inflammation in high-fat diet-induced obesity and diabetes in mice. Diabetes 2008; 57(6): 1470-81.
[http://dx.doi.org/10.2337/db07-1403] [PMID: 18305141]

[122]   Ley RE, Turnbaugh PJ, Klein S, Gordon JI. Human gut microbes associated with obesity. Nature 2006; 444(7122): 1022-3.
[http://dx.doi.org/10.1038/4441022a] [PMID: 17183309]

[123]   Cani PD, Possemiers S, Van de Wiele T, *et al.* Changes in gut microbiota control inflammation in obese mice through a mechanism involving GLP-2-driven improvement of gut permeability. Gut 2009; 58(8): 1091-103.
[http://dx.doi.org/10.1136/gut.2008.165886] [PMID: 19240062]

[124]   Jais A, Brüning JC. Arcuate Nucleus-Dependent Regulation of Metabolism-Pathways to Obesity and Diabetes Mellitus. Endocr Rev 2022; 43(2): 314-28.
[http://dx.doi.org/10.1210/endrev/bnab025]

[125]   Ziętek M, Kaczmarczyk M, Król M, Skała J, Stojko J, Folwarski M. The significant impact of long-term lifestyle education on metabolic syndrome components in postmenopausal obese women. Climacteric 2019; 22(6): 592-9.
[http://dx.doi.org/10.1080/13697137.2019.1598425]

[126]   Valdes AM, Walter J, Segal E, Spector TD. Role of the gut microbiota in nutrition and health. BMJ 2018; 361: k2179.
[http://dx.doi.org/10.1136/bmj.k2179] [PMID: 29899036]

[127]   Kim BS, Jeon YD, Hong SB, Kim JW. Association between circadian preference and academic achievement: A systematic review and meta-analysis. Chronobiol Int 2020; 37(6): 905-22.
[http://dx.doi.org/10.1080/07420528.2020.1755900]

[128]   Roenneberg T, Kuehnle T, Pramstaller PP, *et al.* A marker for the end of adolescence. Curr Biol 2004; 14(24): R1038-9.
[http://dx.doi.org/10.1016/j.cub.2004.11.039] [PMID: 15620633]

[129]   Wittmann M, Dinich J, Merrow M, Roenneberg T. Social jetlag: misalignment of biological and social time. Chronobiol Int 2006; 23(1-2): 497-509.
[http://dx.doi.org/10.1080/07420520500545979] [PMID: 16687322]

[130]   Paruthi S, Brooks LJ, D'Ambrosio C, *et al.* Recommended Amount of Sleep for Pediatric Populations: A Consensus Statement of the American Academy of Sleep Medicine. J Clin Sleep Med 2016; 12(6): 785-6.
[http://dx.doi.org/10.5664/jcsm.5866] [PMID: 27250809]

[131]   Watson NF, Badr MS, Belenky G, *et al.* Recommended Amount of Sleep for a Healthy Adult: A Joint

Consensus Statement of the American Academy of Sleep Medicine and Sleep Research Society. J Clin Sleep Med 2015; 11(6): 591-2.
[http://dx.doi.org/10.5664/jcsm.4758] [PMID: 25979105]

[132]  Suzuki E, Yorifuji T, Ueshima K, *et al.* Sleep duration, sleep quality and cardiovascular disease mortality among the elderly: A population-based cohort study. Prev Med 2009; 49(2-3): 135-41.
[http://dx.doi.org/10.1016/j.ypmed.2009.06.016] [PMID: 19573557]

[133]  Gallicchio L, Kalesan B. Sleep duration and mortality: a systematic review and meta-analysis. J Sleep Res 2009; 18(2): 148-58.
[http://dx.doi.org/10.1111/j.1365-2869.2008.00732.x] [PMID: 19645960]

[134]  Knutson KL, Turek FW. The U-shaped association between sleep and health: the 2 peaks do not mean the same thing. Sleep 2006; 29(7): 878-9.
[http://dx.doi.org/10.1093/sleep/29.7.878] [PMID: 16895253]

[135]  Cappuccio FP, D'Elia L, Strazzullo P, Miller MA. Quantity and quality of sleep and incidence of type 2 diabetes: a systematic review and meta-analysis. Diabetes Care 2010; 33(2): 414-20.
[http://dx.doi.org/10.2337/dc09-1124] [PMID: 19910503]

[136]  Kripke DF, Garfinkel L, Wingard DL, Klauber MR, Marler MR. Mortality associated with sleep duration and insomnia. Arch Gen Psychiatry 2002; 59(2): 131-6.
[http://dx.doi.org/10.1001/archpsyc.59.2.131] [PMID: 11825133]

[137]  Cappuccio FP, Cooper D, D'Elia L, Strazzullo P, Miller MA. Sleep duration predicts cardiovascular outcomes: a systematic review and meta-analysis of prospective studies. Eur Heart J 2011; 32(12): 1484-92.
[http://dx.doi.org/10.1093/eurheartj/ehr007] [PMID: 21300732]

[138]  Cappuccio FP, Taggart FM, Kandala NB, *et al.* Meta-analysis of short sleep duration and obesity in children and adults. Sleep 2008; 31(5): 619-26.
[http://dx.doi.org/10.1093/sleep/31.5.619] [PMID: 18517032]

[139]  Gangwisch JE, Malaspina D, Boden-Albala B, Heymsfield SB. Inadequate sleep as a risk factor for obesity: analyses of the NHANES I. Sleep 2005; 28(10): 1289-96.
[http://dx.doi.org/10.1093/sleep/28.10.1289] [PMID: 16295214]

[140]  Stranges S, Cappuccio FP, Kandala NB, *et al.* Cross-sectional *versus* prospective associations of sleep duration with changes in relative weight and body fat distribution: the Whitehall II Study. Am J Epidemiol 2008; 167(3): 321-9.
[http://dx.doi.org/10.1093/aje/kwm302] [PMID: 18006903]

[141]  Patel SR, Hu FB. Short sleep duration and weight gain: a systematic review. Obesity (Silver Spring) 2008; 16(3): 643-53.
[http://dx.doi.org/10.1038/oby.2007.118] [PMID: 18239586]

[142]  Vorona RD, Winn MP, Babineau TW, Eng BP, Feldman HR, Ware JC. Overweight and obese patients in a primary care population report less sleep than patients with a normal body mass index. Arch Intern Med 2005; 165(1): 25-30.
[http://dx.doi.org/10.1001/archinte.165.1.25] [PMID: 15642870]

[143]  Kim CW, Yun KE, Jung HS, *et al.* Sleep duration and quality in relation to non-alcoholic fatty liver disease in middle-aged workers and their spouses. J Hepatol 2013; 59(2): 351-7.
[http://dx.doi.org/10.1016/j.jhep.2013.03.035] [PMID: 23578884]

[144]  Kastorini CM, Panagiotakos DB, Chrysohoou C, *et al.* Metabolic syndrome, adherence to the Mediterranean diet and 10-year cardiovascular disease incidence: The ATTICA study. Atherosclerosis 2016; 246: 87-93.
[http://dx.doi.org/10.1016/j.atherosclerosis.2015.12.025] [PMID: 26761772]

[145]  Bibiloni MD, Julibert A, Argelich E, *et al.* Nut intake is associated with better nutrient adequacy and diet quality in Spanish children and adolescents: The ANIBES study. Nutrients 2017; 9(3): 269.

[http://dx.doi.org/10.3390/nu9030269] [PMID: 28287486]

[146]  St-Onge MP, Mikic A, Pietrolungo CE. Effects of diet on sleep quality. Adv Nutr 2016; 7(5): 938-49.
[http://dx.doi.org/10.3945/an.116.012336] [PMID: 27633109]

[147]  Hirota N, Sone Y, Tokura H. Relative effectiveness of a rich-flavoured tea and a non-caloric tea in suppressing the caloric intake from food. Food Qual Prefer 2000; 11(1-2): 163-8.
[http://dx.doi.org/10.1016/S0950-3293(99)00040-4]

[148]  Veerman JL, Sacks G, Antonopoulos N, Martin J. The impact of a tax on sugar-sweetened beverages on health and health care costs: a modelling study. PLoS One 2016; 11(4): e0151460.
[http://dx.doi.org/10.1371/journal.pone.0151460] [PMID: 27073855]

[149]  Jaeschke L, Steinbrecher A, Hansen G, *et al.* Association of body surface scanner-based abdominal volume with parameters of the Metabolic Syndrome and comparison with manually measured waist circumference. Sci Rep 2020; 10(1): 9324.
[http://dx.doi.org/10.1038/s41598-020-66095-6] [PMID: 32518262]

[150]  Jaeschke L, Steinbrecher A, Pischon T. Measurement of waist and hip circumference with a body surface scanner: feasibility, validity, reliability, and correlations with markers of the metabolic syndrome. PLoS One 2015; 10(3): e0119430.
[http://dx.doi.org/10.1371/journal.pone.0119430] [PMID: 25749283]

[151]  Adler C, Steinbrecher A, Jaeschke L, *et al.* Validity and reliability of total body volume and relative body fat mass from a 3-dimensional photonic body surface scanner. PLoS One 2017; 12(7): e0180201.
[http://dx.doi.org/10.1371/journal.pone.0180201] [PMID: 28672039]

[152]  2011. World Health Organization. Waist Circumference and Waist–Hip Ratio. Report of a WHO Expert Consultation. Geneva, World Health Organization, Geneva, 2008; 8–11. Available from: http://www.who.int/nutrition/publications/obesity/WHO_report_waistcircumference_and_waisthip_rat io/en/

[153]  Lapidus L, Bengtsson C, Larsson B, Pennert K, Rybo E, Sjöström L. Distribution of adipose tissue and risk of cardiovascular disease and death: a 12 year follow up of participants in the population study of women in Gothenburg, Sweden. BMJ 1984; 289(6454): 1257-61.
[http://dx.doi.org/10.1136/bmj.289.6454.1257] [PMID: 6437507]

[154]  Larsson B, Svärdsudd K, Welin L, Wilhelmsen L, Björntorp P, Tibblin G. Abdominal adipose tissue distribution, obesity, and risk of cardiovascular disease and death: 13 year follow up of participants in the study of men born in 1913. BMJ 1984; 288(6428): 1401-4.
[http://dx.doi.org/10.1136/bmj.288.6428.1401] [PMID: 6426576]

[155]  Ducimetiere P, Richard J, Cambien F. The pattern of subcutaneous fat distribution in middle-aged men and the risk of coronary heart disease: the Paris Prospective Study. Int J Obes 1986; 10(3): 229-40.
[PMID: 3759330]

[156]  Kissebah AH, Vydelingum N, Murray R, *et al.* Relation of body fat distribution to metabolic complications of obesity. J Clin Endocrinol Metab 1982; 54(2): 254-60.
[http://dx.doi.org/10.1210/jcem-54-2-254] [PMID: 7033275]

[157]  Krotkiewski M, Björntorp P, Sjöström L, Smith U. Impact of obesity on metabolism in men and women. Importance of regional adipose tissue distribution. J Clin Invest 1983; 72(3): 1150-62.
[http://dx.doi.org/10.1172/JCI111040] [PMID: 6350364]

[158]  Després JP, Allard C, Tremblay A, Talbot J, Bouchard C. Evidence for a regional component of body fatness in the association with serum lipids in men and women. Metabolism 1985; 34(10): 967-73.
[http://dx.doi.org/10.1016/0026-0495(85)90147-7] [PMID: 4046840]

[159]  Baumgartner RN, Roche AF, Chumlea WC, Siervogel RM, Glueck CJ. Fatness and fat patterns: associations with plasma lipids and blood pressures in adults, 18 to 57 years of age. Am J Epidemiol 1987; 126(4): 614-28.
[http://dx.doi.org/10.1093/oxfordjournals.aje.a114701] [PMID: 3498363]

[160]  Fujioka S, Matsuzawa Y, Tokunaga K, Tarui S. Contribution of intra-abdominal fat accumulation to the impairment of glucose and lipid metabolism in human obesity. Metabolism 1987; 36(1): 54-9.
[http://dx.doi.org/10.1016/0026-0495(87)90063-1] [PMID: 3796297]

[161]  Després JP, Nadeau A, Tremblay A, *et al.* Role of deep abdominal fat in the association between regional adipose tissue distribution and glucose tolerance in obese women. Diabetes 1989; 38(3): 304-9.
[http://dx.doi.org/10.2337/diab.38.3.304] [PMID: 2645187]

[162]  Peiris AN, Sothmann MS, Hoffmann RG, *et al.* Adiposity, fat distribution, and cardiovascular risk. Ann Intern Med 1989; 110(11): 867-72.
[http://dx.doi.org/10.7326/0003-4819-110-11-867] [PMID: 2655520]

[163]  Pouliot MC, Després JP, Nadeau A, *et al.* Visceral obesity in men. Associations with glucose tolerance, plasma insulin, and lipoprotein levels. Diabetes 1992; 41(7): 826-34.
[http://dx.doi.org/10.2337/diab.41.7.826] [PMID: 1612197]

[164]  Després JP, Lamarche B. Effects of diet and physical activity on adiposity and body fat distribution: implications for the prevention of cardiovascular disease. Nutr Res Rev 1993; 6(1): 137-59.
[http://dx.doi.org/10.1079/NRR19930010] [PMID: 19094306]

[165]  Poirier P, Despres JP. Obesity and cardiovascular disease 2003; 19: 943-9.

[166]  Leenen R, Kooy K, Seidell JC, Deurenberg P. Visceral fat accumulation measured by magnetic resonance imaging in relation to serum lipids in obese men and women. Atherosclerosis 1992; 94(2-3): 171-81.
[http://dx.doi.org/10.1016/0021-9150(92)90242-9] [PMID: 1632871]

[167]  Hunter GR, Snyder SW, Kekes-Szabo T, Nicholson C, Berland L. Intra-abdominal adipose tissue values associated with risk of possessing elevated blood lipids and blood pressure. Obes Res 1994; 2(6): 563-8.
[http://dx.doi.org/10.1002/j.1550-8528.1994.tb00106.x] [PMID: 16355516]

[168]  Pouliot MC, Després JP, Lemieux S, *et al.* Waist circumference and abdominal sagittal diameter: Best simple anthropometric indexes of abdominal visceral adipose tissue accumulation and related cardiovascular risk in men and women. Am J Cardiol 1994; 73(7): 460-8.
[http://dx.doi.org/10.1016/0002-9149(94)90676-9] [PMID: 8141087]

[169]  Lemieux S, Prud'homme D, Bouchard C, Tremblay A, Després JP. A single threshold value of waist girth identifies normal-weight and overweight subjects with excess visceral adipose tissue. Am J Clin Nutr 1996; 64(5): 685-93.
[http://dx.doi.org/10.1093/ajcn/64.5.685] [PMID: 8901786]

[170]  Williams MJ, Hunter GR, Kekes-Szabo T, Snyder S, Treuth MS. Regional fat distribution in women and risk of cardiovascular disease. Am J Clin Nutr 1997; 65(3): 855-60.
[http://dx.doi.org/10.1093/ajcn/65.3.855] [PMID: 9062540]

[171]  Després JP, Prud'homme D, Pouliot MC, Tremblay A, Bouchard C. Estimation of deep abdominal adipose-tissue accumulation from simple anthropometric measurements in men. Am J Clin Nutr 1991; 54(3): 471-7.
[http://dx.doi.org/10.1093/ajcn/54.3.471] [PMID: 1877502]

[172]  Koester RS, Hunter GR, Snyder S, Khaled MA, Berland LL. Estimation of computerized tomography derived abdominal fat distribution. Int J Obes 1992; 16(8): 543-54.
[PMID: 1326484]

[173]  Schwartz RS, Shuman WP, Bradbury VL, *et al.* Body fat distribution in healthy young and older men. J Gerontol 1990; 45(6): M181-5.
[http://dx.doi.org/10.1093/geronj/45.6.M181] [PMID: 2229940]

[174]  Conway JM, Yanovski SZ, Avila NA, Hubbard VS. Visceral adipose tissue differences in black and white women. Am J Clin Nutr 1995; 61(4): 765-71.

[http://dx.doi.org/10.1093/ajcn/61.4.765] [PMID: 7702017]

[175]  Lovejoy JC, de la Bretonne JA, Klemperer M, Tulley R. Abdominal fat distribution and metabolic risk factors: Effects of race. Metabolism 1996; 45(9): 1119-24.
[http://dx.doi.org/10.1016/S0026-0495(96)90011-6] [PMID: 8781299]

[176]  Brundavani V, Murthy SR, Kurpad AV. Estimation of deep-abdominal-adipose-tissue (DAAT) accumulation from simple anthropometric measurements in Indian men and women. Eur J Clin Nutr 2006; 60(5): 658-66.
[http://dx.doi.org/10.1038/sj.ejcn.1602366] [PMID: 16391572]

# CHAPTER 6

# Novel Metabolic Panel in Metabolic Syndrome

**Dahlia Badran**[1,2,*]

[1] *Medical Biochemistry & Molecular Biology department, Medicine faculty, Suez Canal University, Egypt*

[2] *Medical Biochemistry & Molecular Biology department, Medicine faculty, Badr University in Cairo, Egypt*

**Abstract:** MetS is a multifaceted disease that embraces multiple disorders such as obesity, hyperlipidemia, hyperglycemia, insulin resistance, and hypertension. These disorders are characterized by specific metabolic aberrations presenting at different stages, which can be detected and monitored through a wide panel of serum biomarkers. Providing a minimally invasive technique thus can help greatly in the prediction, early screening and management of metabolic syndrome in high-risk communities and minimize its complications.

However, no sole biomarker is sensitive nor distinct for the diagnosis of metabolic syndrome, arousing the necessity of performing a panel that includes related biomarkers.

Metabolic biomarkers associated with metabolic syndrome are released primarily due to lipid accumulation and the dysregulated production of adipokines (ex. leptin, adiponectin) or oxidative stress brought on by obesity (ex. malondialdehyde, F-2 isoprostanes, paraoxonase, and oxidized LDL) or the associated inflammatory reaction (ex.IL-6, IL-10, tumor necrosis factor (TNFα), uric acid as well as heparanase).

Since obesity and insulin resistance are the cornerstones in metabolic syndrome pathogenesis, Leptin, an adipokine whose function is to reduce appetite and increase energy expenditure, and adiponectin represent striking biomarkers for metabolic syndrome.

In addition, the importance of uric acid, the product of purine metabolism, as a pro-oxidant inflammatory marker that contributes to metabolic syndrome pathogenesis has also been elucidated in multiple studies.

Recently, a newly discovered metabolic syndrome biomarker, ''Heparanase (HPA)'' is closely related to the degradation of heparan sulfate proteoglycan (HSPG) and is associated with inflammatory responses as it could be secreted by various immune cells including macrophages.

---

[*] **Corresponding author Dahlia Badran:** Medical Biochemistry & Molecular Biology department, Medicine faculty, Suez Canal University, Egypt; Medical Biochemistry & Molecular Biology department, Medicine faculty, Badr University in Cairo, Egypt; E-mail: dalia_badran@med.suez.edu.eg

**Hafize Uzun & Seyma Dumur (Eds.)**

Since many studies have denoted the role of many biomarkers related to metabolic syndrome, this chapter will highlight the newly discovered ones that will help in the construction of a metabolic panel that could pave the way to precision medicine and help personalize the treatment given to metabolic syndrome patients.

**Keywords:** Asprosin, Adipokines, GGT, Leptin, Metabolic syndrome, Oxidative stress, Obesity, Subfatin, Visfatin.

## INTRODUCTION

MetS is a progressive metabolic disease that includes multiple disorders as abdominal obesity, dyslipidemia, glucose intolerance, insulin resistance and high blood pressure causing a worldwide health problem [1]. Although its pathogenesis is very complex, the core of the disease involves a significant metabolic disturbance combined with imbalanced oxidant/ antioxidant activities resulting in cellular damage. Early diagnosis of metabolic syndrome helps prevent further progression of the disease and minimize its complications [2].

However, the design of a non-invasive new biomarker panel for the diagnosis of MetS will help relieve the burden caused by the disease on the patients and assist in targeting molecules involved in the pathogenesis of the disease.

Since many studies have denoted the role of many biomarkers related to MetS, this chapter will focus on the promising biomarkers that will aid in the early diagnosis and treatment of MetS I in high-risk communities.

### MetS biomarkers

Metabolic biomarkers associated with MetS are released primarily due to lipid accumulation and the dysregulated production of adipokines (ex. leptin, adiponectin, ghrelin) or the oxidative stress brought on by obesity (ex. malondialdehyde, F-2 isoprostanes, paraoxonase and oxidized LDL) or the associated inflammatory reaction (ex.IL-6, tumor necrosis factor (TNFα), uric acid and heparanase) Fig. (**1**).

### *Adipokines*

Since obesity and insulin resistance are the cornerstones in MetS pathogenesis, leptin, and adiponectin represent striking biomarkers for MetS.

Leptin is an adipokine whose function is to reduce appetite by affecting the satiety center, increase energy utilization, and improve insulin sensitivity [3]. High levels of leptin, which denote leptin resistance, are positively correlated with the risk of MetS [4, 5].

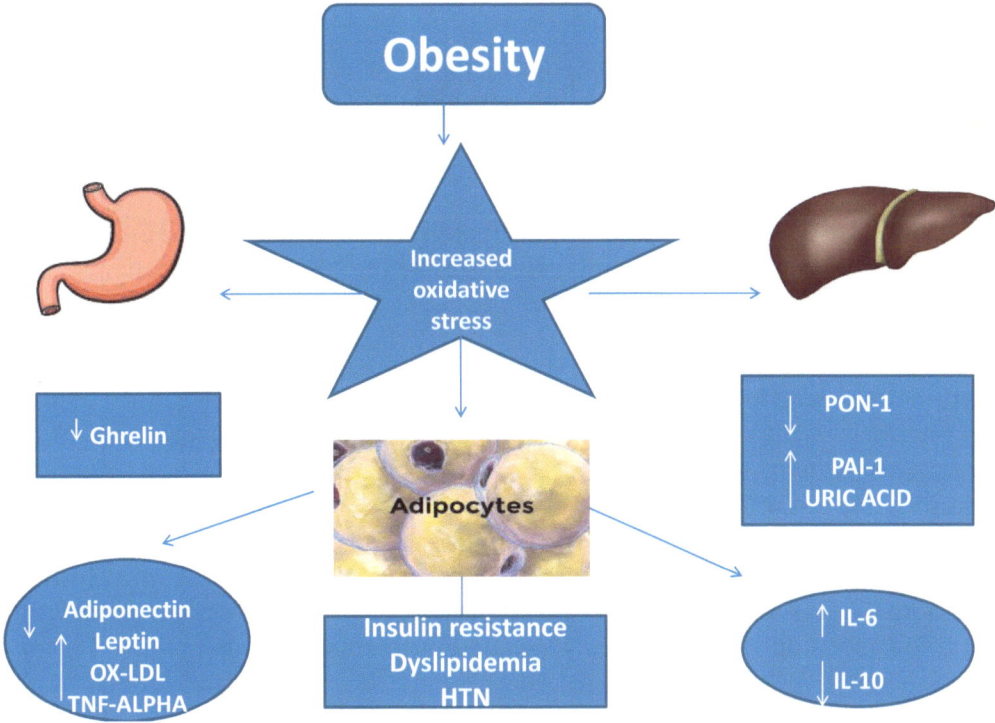

**Fig. (1).** Biomarkers panel of MetS (Srikanthan *et al.*, 2016).

Adiponectin enhances glucose metabolism and adjusts energy expenditure; its level correlates indirectly with MetS risk [6]. However, the active form of adiponectin: High-molecular-weight (HMW) adiponectin, is more potent than total adiponectin for prognosticating the development of MetS [7].

In addition, a newly conducted prospective study demonstrated that the leptin to adiponectin (LA) ratio is supposed to be a recommended marker for predicting newly diagnosed cases of MetS [8].

METRNL (Meteorin-like protein) or Subfatin, is a recently detected adipokine secreted by the adipose tissue as well as by skeletal muscle reversing insulin resistance through two signaling transduction pathways either: the AMP-activated protein kinase (AMPK) pathway or the peroxisome proliferator-activated receptor δ (PPAR-δ) [9], having an anti-inflammatory effect by inhibiting the release of inflammatory mediators [10]. It induces the browning of white adipose tissue (BWT) during exercise and cold exposure increasing energy expenditure, and glucose tolerance and upregulating the transcription of genes involved in fat thermogenesis [11].

Obesity is associated with depressed serum levels of subfatin. which induce fat proliferation and consequently adipocyte hypertrophy [12]. However, a recent study demonstrated that regular exercises greatly increased the circulatory level of subfatin and reversed the disturbance in glucose and lipid metabolism [13].

Visfatin named nicotinamide phosphoribosyl transferase (NAMPT), is another adipokine whose plasma levels increased greatly in obese diabetic patients [14] as well as in patients with MetS [15–17].

Fibrillin -1 and Asprosin: As a key component of extracellular microfibrils, fibrillin-1 encoded by *FBN1*, controls the bioavailability of TGF family members and interacts with the adjacent extracellular matrix (ECM) proteins to give connective tissues flexibility. Asprosin is a recently discovered glucogenic hormone that stimulates the liver to elucidate its role in maintaining glucose homeostasis in a fasting state by releasing glucose to the blood, it is a peptide chain made up of the 140 amino acids at the C-terminus of profibrillin-1. Additionally, it is a crucial part of the adipose ECM during development playing a key role in sending signals to the hypothalamus to augment appetite [18] Fig. (**2**).

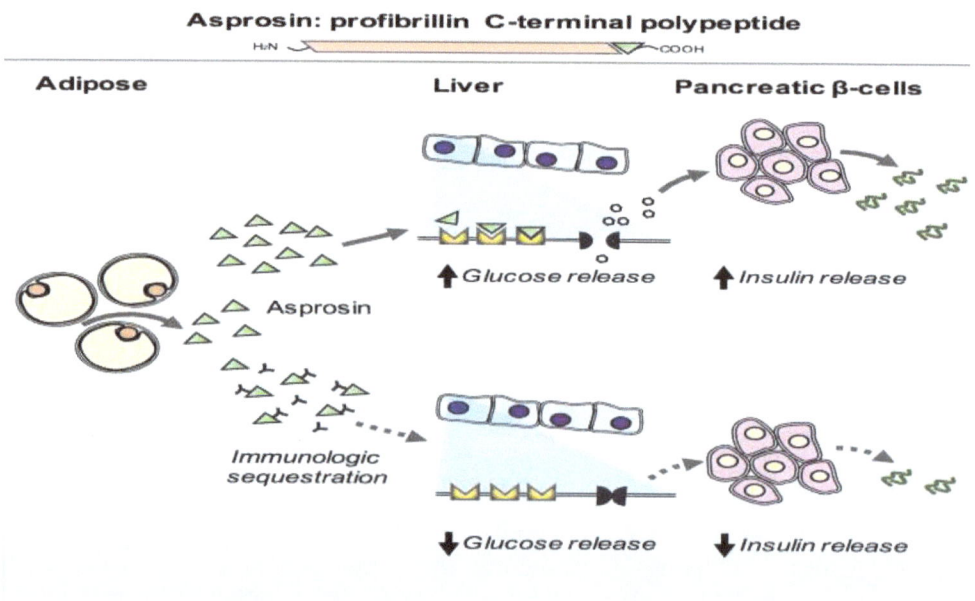

**Fig (2).** Asprosin role in glucose homeostasis.

The high plasma level of asprosin has been shown to be directly proportional to insulin resistance, both in human and mouse models, and is strongly associated with type 2 DM, obesity, and MetS considering it a plausible target in the treatment of these disorders by opposing its activity [19, 20].

Asprosin is a glucogenic hormone released in fasting state and involved in MetS pathogenesis (Romere *et al.* 2016)

## Oxidative Stress Biomarkers

MetS is a multifactorial disease characterized by the imbalance between reactive oxygen species production and antioxidants systems scavenging with the subsequent exoneration of glycation end products, proinflammatory mediators and cytokines resulting in mitochondrial dysfunction and protein damage induced by the increased adiposity [21]. Fig. (3).

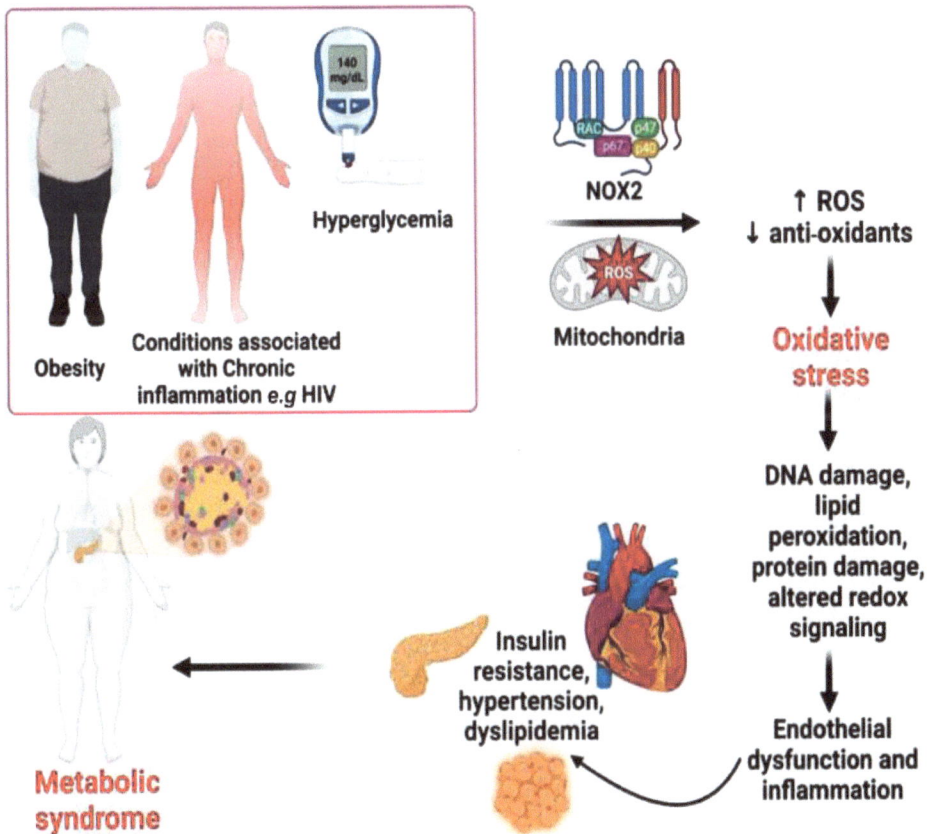

**Fig (3).** Mechanism of oxidative stress in MetS.

Numerous researches have proved that compared to healthy people, patients with metabolic syndrome exhibited higher levels of oxidative damage biomarkers and decreased plasma antioxidant enzyme activity, which may be a cause of oxidative stress [22].

Excessive ROS formation can take place under pathological situations such as obesity, ongoing inflammation, and hyperglycemia. The activation of enzymes in the cytosol, membrane, and mitochondria results in the formation of ROS. Oxidative stress is brought on by an increase in ROS production and a reduction in antioxidant capacity. The resultant oxidative stress causes intracellular cell damage and altered redox, which in turn causes an irreversible buildup of oxidation products and encourages endothelial dysfunction. Insulin resistance, hypertension, dyslipidemia, and metabolic syndrome are the results of these conditions. Reactive oxygen species (ROS) and nicotinamide adenine dinucleotide oxidase (NOX) enzymes are both examples of NOX2. (Masenga *et al.*, 2023).

The most precise technique to gauge the level of oxidative stress existing *in vivo* is by the quantification of its biomarkers. The biomarkers of lipid peroxidation, protein and amino acid oxidation, and DNA oxidation are all examples of oxidative stress [23].

Lipid peroxidation biomarkers include malondialdehyde (MDA), thiobarbituric acid-reactive substances (TBARS), and F2-isoproteins. Protein oxidation is indicated by protein carbonyls, AGEs and oxidized LDL (ox-LDL) while 8-oxo-2 deoxyguanosine (8-0xo-Dg), 5-chlorouracil, and 5-chlorocytosine are examples of DNA oxidation biomarkers [24].

Paraoxonase-1 (PON-1): On the other hand, the antioxidant and anti-inflammatory protective characteristics of HDL are thought to be contributed to by the multifunctional enzyme PON-1, which has anti-toxic and antioxidant capabilities through protecting LDL from oxidation and prohibits the progression of MetS complications notably the vascular dysfunction. It may be a valuable indicator for determining antioxidant capability. Hyperlipidaemia, insulin resistance, hyperglycaemia with impaired glucose metabolism, and elevated oxidative stress biomarkers were all linked to reduced levels of PON-1 [25].

Xanthine oxidase, myeloperoxidase (MPO), and nitric oxide synthase (NOS) as well as gamma-glutamyl transferase (GGT), are all the markers linked to ROS production [26].

However, the non-specific inflammatory markers: C-reactive protein (CRP), ferritin, and uric acid are examples of non-enzymatic indicators.

According to previous research, liver damage and insulin resistance, two signs of oxidative stress, were strongly linked with serum ferritin [27].

Uric acid, the product of purine metabolism, scavenges free radicals extracellularly in contrast to its intracellular effect acting as a pro-oxidant inflammatory marker that oxidizes lipid, decreases the effectiveness of NO and promotes the release of TNF-α, which leads to an aggravation of inflammation in a vicious circle and contributes to MetS pathogenesis [28].

Heparanase (HPA) is a newly discovered MetS biomarker, 'closely related to the breakdown of heparan sulphate proteoglycan (HSPG) and is strongly linked to inflammatory responses as it could be secreted by various immune cells including macrophages [29].

According to Shafat *et al.*, patients with T2DM had serum HPA levels that were significantly greater than those of healthy individuals as it positively iinteracts with CRP and IL-6 [30].

### *Inflammatory Markers*

MetS patients have activated pro-inflammatory transcription factors in their adipocytes, counting NF-B and activator protein-1 (AP-1), which are redox-sensitive and cause the release of pro-inflammatory cytokines like tumor necrosis factor-alpha (TNFα) and interleukin-6 (IL-6), which in turn aggravates the generation of oxidants [31].

TNFα is secreted by visceral adipocytes and is considered as a hallmark feature of MetS secreted by the dysregulated fat cells. Due to the abnormal stimulation of the mTOR and PKC signaling pathways by increased TNFα, insulin resistance is linked to this protein [32]. Multiple studies had noticed significant elevated levels of TNFα with MetS [33–35].

The anti-inflammatory cytokine biomarker IL-10 secreted from macrophages helps to modulate normal tissue after inflammation induced by oxidative stress by inhibiting NADPH oxidase. In MetS patients, low levels of IL-10 had been observed indicating a decreased protective action of IL-10 exerted on IL-6 and TNFα activities denoting a failure of antagonizing their destructive effects.

## CONCLUSION

MetS is a multifactorial disease with multiple etiologies that causes significant morbidity and mortality worldwide with a consequent economic burden on the health care systems. To identify those at risk and design an effective management plan, an updated panel of biomarkers with a known and predictable association with MetS should be developed.

# REFERENCES

[1]     Spahis S, Delvin E, Borys JM, Levy E. Oxidative Stress as a Critical Factor in Nonalcoholic Fatty Liver Disease Pathogenesis. Antioxid Redox Signal 2017; 26(10): 519-41.
[http://dx.doi.org/10.1089/ars.2016.6776] [PMID: 27452109]

[2]     Monserrat-Mesquida M, Quetglas-Llabrés M, Capó X, *et al.* Metabolic Syndrome Is Associated with Oxidative Stress and Proinflammatory State. Antioxidants 2020; 9(3): 236.
[http://dx.doi.org/10.3390/antiox9030236] [PMID: 32178436]

[3]     Tawfik MK, Mohamed MI. Exenatide suppresses 1,2-dimethylhydrazine-induced colon cancer in diabetic mice: Effect on tumor angiogenesis and cell proliferation. Biomed Pharmacother 2016; 82: 106-16.
[http://dx.doi.org/10.1016/j.biopha.2016.05.005] [PMID: 27470345]

[4]     Esteghamati A, Noshad S, Khalilzadeh O, *et al.* Contribution of serum leptin to metabolic syndrome in obese and nonobese subjects. Arch Med Res 2011; 42(3): 244-51.
[http://dx.doi.org/10.1016/j.arcmed.2011.05.005] [PMID: 21722822]

[5]     Madeira I, Bordallo MA, Rodrigues NC, *et al.* Leptin as a predictor of metabolic syndrome in prepubertal children. Arch Endocrinol Metab 2017; 61(1): 7-13.
[http://dx.doi.org/10.1590/2359-3997000000199] [PMID: 27598976]

[6]     Lindberg S, Jensen JS, Bjerre M, *et al.* Low adiponectin levels at baseline and decreasing adiponectin levels over 10 years of follow-up predict risk of the metabolic syndrome. Diabetes Metab 2017; 43(2): 134-9.
[http://dx.doi.org/10.1016/j.diabet.2016.07.027] [PMID: 27639310]

[7]     Seino Y, Hirose H, Saito I, Itoh H. High-molecular-weight adiponectin is a predictor of progression to metabolic syndrome: a population-based 6-year follow-up study in Japanese men. Metabolism 2009; 58(3): 355-60.
[http://dx.doi.org/10.1016/j.metabol.2008.10.008] [PMID: 19217451]

[8]     Lee KW, Shin D. Prospective Associations of Serum Adiponectin, Leptin, and Leptin-Adiponectin Ratio with Incidence of Metabolic Syndrome: The Korean Genome and Epidemiology Study. Int J Environ Res Public Health 2020; 17(9): 3287.
[http://dx.doi.org/10.3390/ijerph17093287] [PMID: 32397260]

[9]     Zheng S, Li Z, Song J, Liu J, Miao C. Metrnl: a secreted protein with new emerging functions. Acta Pharmacol Sin 2016; 37(5): 571-9.
[http://dx.doi.org/10.1038/aps.2016.9] [PMID: 27063217]

[10]    Huang S, Cao L, Cheng H, Li D, Li Y, Wu Z. The blooming intersection of subfatin and metabolic syndrome. Rev Cardiovasc Med 2021; 22(3): 799-805.
[http://dx.doi.org/10.31083/j.rcm2203086] [PMID: 34565078]

[11]    Rao RR, Long JZ, White JP, *et al.* Meteorin-like is a hormone that regulates immune-adipose interactions to increase beige fat thermogenesis. Cell 2014; 157(6): 1279-91.
[http://dx.doi.org/10.1016/j.cell.2014.03.065] [PMID: 24906147]

[12]    Du Y, Ye X, Lu A, *et al.* Inverse relationship between serum Metrnl levels and visceral fat obesity (VFO) in patients with type 2 diabetes. Diabetes Res Clin Pract 2020; 161: 108068.
[http://dx.doi.org/10.1016/j.diabres.2020.108068] [PMID: 32044349]

[13]    Patterson CM, Levin BE. Role of exercise in the central regulation of energy homeostasis and in the prevention of obesity. Neuroendocrinology 2008; 87(2): 65-70.
[http://dx.doi.org/10.1159/000100982] [PMID: 17374946]

[14] Garten A, Schuster S, Penke M, Gorski T, de Giorgis T, Kiess W. Physiological and pathophysiological roles of NAMPT and NAD metabolism. Nat Rev Endocrinol 2015; 11(9): 535-46.
[http://dx.doi.org/10.1038/nrendo.2015.117] [PMID: 26215259]

[15] Choi KM, Kim JH, Cho GJ, Baik SH, Park HS, Kim SM. Effect of exercise training on plasma visfatin and eotaxin levels. Eur J Endocrinol 2007; 157(4): 437-42.
[http://dx.doi.org/10.1530/EJE-07-0127] [PMID: 17893257]

[16] Zahorska-Markiewicz B, Olszanecka-Glinianowicz M, Janowska J, *et al.* Serum concentration of visfatin in obese women. Metabolism 2007; 56(8): 1131-4.
[http://dx.doi.org/10.1016/j.metabol.2007.04.007] [PMID: 17618961]

[17] Filippatosm TD, Derdemezis CS, Kiortsis DN, Tselepis AD, Elisaf MS. Increased plasma levels of visfatin/pre-B cell colony-enhancing factor in obese and overweight patients with metabolic syndrome. J Endocrinol Invest 2007; 30(4): 323-6.
[http://dx.doi.org/10.1007/BF03346300] [PMID: 17556870]

[18] Summers KM, Bush SJ, Davis MR, Hume DA, Keshvari S, West JA. Fibrillin-1 and asprosin, novel players in metabolic syndrome. Mol Genet Metab 2023; 138(1): 106979.
[http://dx.doi.org/10.1016/j.ymgme.2022.106979] [PMID: 36630758]

[19] Romere C, Duerrschmid C, Bournat J, *et al.* Asprosin, a Fasting-Induced Glucogenic Protein Hormone. Cell 2016; 165(3): 566-79.
[http://dx.doi.org/10.1016/j.cell.2016.02.063] [PMID: 27087445]

[20] Zhang L, Chen C, Zhou N, Fu Y, Cheng X. Circulating asprosin concentrations are increased in type 2 diabetes mellitus and independently associated with fasting glucose and triglyceride. Clin Chim Acta 2019; 489: 183-8.
[http://dx.doi.org/10.1016/j.cca.2017.10.034] [PMID: 29104036]

[21] Roy I, Jover E, Matilla L, *et al.* Soluble ST2 as a New Oxidative Stress and Inflammation Marker in Metabolic Syndrome. Int J Environ Res Public Health 2023; 20(3): 2579.
[http://dx.doi.org/10.3390/ijerph20032579] [PMID: 36767947]

[22] Bekkouche L, Bouchenak M, Malaisse W, Yahia D. The Mediterranean diet adoption improves metabolic, oxidative, and inflammatory abnormalities in Algerian metabolic syndrome patients. Horm Metab Res 2014; 46(4): 274-82.
[http://dx.doi.org/10.1055/s-0033-1363657] [PMID: 24446153]

[23] Ho E, Karimi Galougahi K, Liu CC, Bhindi R, Figtree GA. Biological markers of oxidative stress: Applications to cardiovascular research and practice. Redox Biol 2013; 1(1): 483-91.
[http://dx.doi.org/10.1016/j.redox.2013.07.006] [PMID: 24251116]

[24] Masenga SK, Kabwe LS, Chakulya M, Kirabo A. Mechanisms of Oxidative Stress in Metabolic Syndrome. Int J Mol Sci 2023; 24(9): 7898.
[http://dx.doi.org/10.3390/ijms24097898] [PMID: 37175603]

[25] Srikanthan K, Feyh A, Visweshwar H, Shapiro JI, Sodhi K. Systematic Review of Metabolic Syndrome Biomarkers: A Panel for Early Detection, Management, and Risk Stratification in the West Virginian Population. Int J Med Sci 2016; 13(1): 25-38.
[http://dx.doi.org/10.7150/ijms.13800] [PMID: 26816492]

[26] Marrocco I, Altieri F, Peluso I. Measurement and Clinical Significance of Biomarkers of Oxidative Stress in Humans. Oxid Med Cell Longev 2017; 2017(1): 6501046.
[http://dx.doi.org/10.1155/2017/6501046] [PMID: 28698768]

[27] Avila F, Echeverría G, Pérez D, *et al.* Serum Ferritin Is Associated with Metabolic Syndrome and Red Meat Consumption. Oxid Med Cell Longev 2015; 2015: 769739.
[PMID: 26451235]

[28] Billiet L, Doaty S, Katz JD, Velasquez MT. Review of hyperuricemia as new marker for metabolic syndrome. ISRN Rheumatol 2014; 2014: 1-7.

[http://dx.doi.org/10.1155/2014/852954] [PMID: 24693449]

[29]     Zhou X, Wang Q, Mei G, *et al.* Serum Heparanase: A New Clinical Biomarker Involved in Senile Metabolic Inflammatory Syndrome. Diabetes Metab Syndr Obes 2021; 14: 3221-8.
[http://dx.doi.org/10.2147/DMSO.S291612] [PMID: 34285529]

[30]     Shafat I, Ilan N, Zoabi S, Vlodavsky I, Nakhoul F. Heparanase Levels Are Elevated in the Urine and Plasma of Type 2 Diabetes Patients and Associate with Blood Glucose Levels. Vella A, editor. PLoS ONE. 2011 Feb 22; 6(2): e17312.

[31]     Čolak E, Pap D. The role of oxidative stress in the development of obesity and obesity-related metabolic disorders. J Med Biochem 2021; 40(1): 1-9.
[http://dx.doi.org/10.5937/jomb0-24652] [PMID: 33584134]

[32]     Aroor AR, McKarns S, DeMarco VG, Jia G, Sowers JR. Maladaptive immune and inflammatory pathways lead to cardiovascular insulin resistance. Metabolism 2013; 62(11): 1543-52.
[http://dx.doi.org/10.1016/j.metabol.2013.07.001] [PMID: 23932846]

[33]     Gormez S, Demirkan A, Atalar F, *et al.* Adipose tissue gene expression of adiponectin, tumor necrosis factor-α and leptin in metabolic syndrome patients with coronary artery disease. Intern Med 2011; 50(8): 805-10.
[http://dx.doi.org/10.2169/internalmedicine.50.4753] [PMID: 21498926]

[34]     Indulekha K, Surendar J, Mohan V. High sensitivity C-reactive protein, tumor necrosis factor-α, interleukin-6, and vascular cell adhesion molecule-1 levels in Asian Indians with metabolic syndrome and insulin resistance (CURES-105). J Diabetes Sci Technol 2011; 5(4): 982-8.
[http://dx.doi.org/10.1177/193229681100500421] [PMID: 21880241]

[35]     Musialik K. The influence of chosen adipocytokines on blood pressure values in patients with metabolic syndrome. Kardiol Pol 2012; 70(12): 1237-42.
[PMID: 23264241]

# CHAPTER 7

# How Would Metabolic Syndrome Disturb the Normal Endothelial Function?

**Eman Mamdouh Kolieb**[1] and **Dina A Ali**[2,*]

[1] *Physiology Department, Faculty of Medicine, Suez Canal University, Ismailia, 41522, Egypt*

[2] *Clinical pharmacology Department, Faculty of Medicine, Suez Canal University, Ismailia, 41522, Egypt*

**Abstract:** Metabolic syndrome (MetS) is an escalating epidemic that could influence more than one billion people worldwide. It is expressed as the presence of visceral obesity, hyperglycemia, dyslipidemia, and elevated blood pressure. MetS is a multifactorial disorder affecting all features of the community and extensively affects morbidity and mortality. Independently, the constituents of metabolic syndrome have the potential to influence the endothelium causing vascular dysfunction and interrupt vascular homeostasis. Since all components of MetS have unfavorable effects on the endothelium, endothelial dysfunction is more prevalent in MetS patients. Endothelial dysfunction could be a part of the pathogenesis of atherosclerosis in MetS. The nominated mechanisms of endothelial dysfunction linked with MetS are reduced NO production, upraised reactive oxygen species and high production of vasoconstrictors. All the elements of MetS especially the compromised endothelial function could participate in increasing the risks of cardiovascular disease, stroke, myocardial infarction and type 2 DM. Endothelial dysfunction, moreover, stimulates pro-inflammatory and oxidative stress pathways *via* endothelial mitochondrial reactive oxygen species (ROS) forcing vascular growth and remodeling. Because MetS is a multifactorial disorder, numerous signaling pathways manipulate the succeeding endothelial dysfunction. In the current review, we will discuss the incidence and pathogenesis of altered endothelial function in MetS. We will also discuss the impending effects of lifestyle measures and pharmacological interventions on endothelial function in patients with MetS .

**Keywords:** Atherosclerosis, Endothelial dysfunction, Insulin resistance, Metabolic syndrome, Reactive oxygen species (ROS) .

## INTRODUCTION

Metabolic syndrome (MetS) is a series of metabolic changes concomitant with cardiovascular disease (CVD). Metabolic syndrome, also called insulin resis-

---

* **Corresponding author Dina A Ali:** Clinical pharmacology Department, Faculty of Medicine, Suez Canal University, Ismailia, 41522, Egypt; E-mail: dina_abdel-karim@med.suez.edu.eg

**Hafize Uzun & Seyma Dumur (Eds.)**

tance syndrome, includes high blood glucose, central obesity, hypertension, high triglyceride levels, and low HDL-cholesterol. The main pathogenesis of MetS is insulin resistance (IR) with other factors that increase the risk of IR such as an unhealthy diet, sedentary lifestyle, and genetic and epigenetic factors. MetS includes a combination of major and modifiable CVD risk factors [1].

## Vascular Endothelium and its Physiological Function

Vascular endothelium consists of a single cell layer, completely lining the blood vessels. It has a fundamental role in hemostasis, muscle tone control, angiogenesis, vascular repair, and transportation of important metabolites from blood to tissues and *vice versa* [2]. Endothelial dysfunction results in arterial stiffness and remodeling. Many studies have shown that endothelial dysfunction represents the cornerstone to the onset and progression of CVD. Moreover, endothelial dysfunction is a crucial therapeutic target for CVD [3]. Normally, the endothelium regulates the homeostasis of the blood vessels by modulation of vascular permeability, vasomotor tone, coagulation, inflammation, immunity, and cell growth. These factors are mediated through mainly nitric oxide (NO).

Formation and liberation of endothelial NO can be accelerated by many neuroendocrine mediators (*e.g.* bradykinin, acetylcholine, substance P), and by some mechanical factors (*e.g.* shear stress) [4]. After the release of NO, it activates the guanylate cyclase enzyme and the intracellular increase of 4 guanosine 3,5 monophosphate, causing relaxation of endothelial smooth muscle cells causing endothelium-dependant/ NO-dependent vasodilatation. The inorganic nitrates, such as sodium nitroprusside or nitroglycerin, can activate the same pathway as external NO donors resulting in endothelium-independent/NO-independent vasodilation.

NO inhibits NF-kB resulting in an anti-inflammatory effect. Furthermore, NO down-regulates the receptors of angiotensin II and endothelin I leading to an antithrombotic effect [5]. NO also plays an important role in the cardiac tissue. NO causes coronary vasodilation and regulates cardiac function regarding the ventricular systolic and diastolic properties. There are 3 main types of NO synthase; the cardiac cells contain at least one of the forms of NO synthase (NOS): nNOS, eNOS, and iNOS [6].

The sympathetic nervous endings express the nNOS, which is responsible for regulating catecholamine release at the cardiac level causing stimulation of beta-adrenergic receptors. While the cardiomyocytes contain eNOS causing inhibition of platelet aggregation and an inhibition of the positive inotropic action induced by catecholamine release.

iNOS expression is accelerated by proinflammatory cytokine. NO regulates the stretching of cardiac muscle fibers, so it increases diastolic cardiac function [7].

## Disturbed Endothelial Function

Endothelial dysfunction is known as the decline of vasodilators, mainly NO, and the increase of vasoconstrictor substances. Arterial remodeling and stiffness, represent the connection between CVD risk factors and the initiation of atherosclerosis [8]. The reduction in the NO can be due to a decrease or inhibition in eNOS production, and degradation of NO by reactive oxygen species (ROS) [9].

Increased oxidative stress synthesis occurring with cardiovascular risk factors could lead to increase in the permeability of abnormal endothelial cells for LDL-cholesterol particles, followed by oxidation of the arterial intima. Subsequently, cellular growth and release of profibrotic factors, stimulate smooth muscle cell proliferation and excessive collagen production, followed by the formation of the atheroma plaque. This leads to arterial remodeling in addition to an increase in the intima-media thickness resulting in early arterial stiffening [9].

Cardiovascular risk factors such as smoking, aging, dyslipidemia, high blood pressure, high blood glucose, and a family history of atherosclerosis are all combined with endothelial dysfunction [8]. This leads to chronic inflammation associated with thrombosis and vasoconstriction leading to an elevation of the risk of CVD [10]. Currently, disrupted endothelial function has also been found to be associated with obesity, high C-reactive protein, and recurrent infections [11].

## Insulin Resistance in METS and Endothelial Dysfunction

Most of the metabolic dysfunctions found in MetS patients result from insulin resistance. IR leads to an increase in insulin levels, which activates the sympathetic-adrenergic system and renin-angiotensin system leading to multiple metabolic and vascular alterations, such as endothelial dysfunction.

Insulin stimulates endothelial cells to produce NO leading to vasodilatation, which is decreased in the case of IR by decreased synthesis or response to NO. Additionally, IR increases endothelin-1-vasoconstrictor, which may lead to increased arterial pressure [12].

Insulin activates two main pathways: PI3 kinase pathway and MAP kinase pathway. The PI3 kinase pathway activation causes increased glucose consumption in muscles and an increase in NO synthesis in endothelial cells [13]. Moreover, the activation of MAP kinase pathway increases proinflammatory mediators. Therefore, the imbalance related to these pathways that occur in IR may explain the endothelial dysfunction associated with IR [14].

## Hyperglycemia in MetS and Endothelial Dysfunction

Hyperglycemia causes oxidative stress, inflammation, and activation of tissue factors, which is the most important factor in initiating the coagulation cascade. The mechanisms produced by hyperglycemia causing endothelial dysfunction in MetS are protein kinase C activation, which causes an immediate decrease of endothelial NO, and an increase in endothelin-1- 1 that causes vasoconstriction. This is associated with the production of many growth factors as vascular endothelial growth factor (VEGF), epidermal growth factor (EGF), and growth factor (TGF-ß), causing vascular remodeling [15].

## CONCLUSION

Lastly, the activation of the protein kinase C pathway seems to be the most important factor responsible for the creation of several prothrombotic factors, such as von Willebrand factor, plasminogen activator inhibitor 1 (PAI 1), factor X, and fibrinogen. The second pathway is the activation of the proinflammatory nuclear transcription factor, nuclear factor kappa B leading to an increase of TNF alpha and IL-1 b [16]. The third pathway is the activation of the polyol pathway; this leads to the depletion of NADPH, which is essential for the regeneration of antioxidant enzymes such as glutathione and ascorbic acid as well as NADPH, which is a co-factor of endothelial nitric oxide synthesis [17].

## REFERENCES

[1]     Dobrowolski P, Prejbisz A, Kuryłowicz A, *et al.* Metabolic syndrome – a new definition and management guidelines. Arch Med Sci 2022; 18(5): 1133-56.
        [http://dx.doi.org/10.5114/aoms/152921] [PMID: 36160355]

[2]     Krüger-Genge A, Blocki A, Franke RP, Jung F. Vascular Endothelial Cell Biology: An Update. Int J Mol Sci 2019; 20(18): 4411.
        [http://dx.doi.org/10.3390/ijms20184411] [PMID: 31500313]

[3]     Ahmad A, Dempsey SK, Daneva Z, *et al.* Role of Nitric Oxide in the Cardiovascular and Renal Systems. Int J Mol Sci 2018; 19(9): 2605.
        [http://dx.doi.org/10.3390/ijms19092605] [PMID: 30177600]

[4]     Förstermann U, Sessa WC. Nitric oxide synthases: regulation and function. Eur Heart J 2012; 33(7): 829-837, 837a-837d.
        [http://dx.doi.org/10.1093/eurheartj/ehr304] [PMID: 21890489]

[5]     Wierońska JM, Cieślik P, Kalinowski L. Nitric Oxide-Dependent Pathways as Critical Factors in the Consequences and Recovery after Brain Ischemic Hypoxia. Biomolecules 2021; 11(8): 1097.
        [http://dx.doi.org/10.3390/biom11081097] [PMID: 34439764]

[6]     Loscalzo J, Welch G. Nitric oxide and its role in the cardiovascular system. Prog Cardiovasc Dis 1995; 38(2): 87-104.
        [http://dx.doi.org/10.1016/S0033-0620(05)80001-5] [PMID: 7568906]

[7]     Ye Y, Martinez JD, Perez-Polo RJ, Lin Y, Uretsky BF, Birnbaum Y. The role of eNOS, iNOS, and NF-κB in upregulation and activation of cyclooxygenase-2 and infarct size reduction by atorvastatin. Am J Physiol Heart Circ Physiol 2008; 295(1): H343-51.
[http://dx.doi.org/10.1152/ajpheart.01350.2007] [PMID: 18469150]

[8]     Libby P, Ridker PM, Maseri A. Inflammation and Atherosclerosis. Circulation 2002; 105(9): 1135-43.
[http://dx.doi.org/10.1161/hc0902.104353] [PMID: 11877368]

[9]     Bonetti PO, Lerman LO, Lerman A. Endothelial Dysfunction. Arterioscler Thromb Vasc Biol 2003; 23(2): 168-75.
[http://dx.doi.org/10.1161/01.ATV.0000051384.43104.FC] [PMID: 12588755]

[10]    Hadi HA, Carr CS, Al Suwaidi J. Endothelial dysfunction: cardiovascular risk factors, therapy, and outcome. Vasc Health Risk Manag 2005; 1(3): 183-98.
[PMID: 17319104]

[11]    Prasad A, Zhu J, Halcox JPJ, Waclawiw MA, Epstein SE, Quyyumi AA. Predisposition to atherosclerosis by infections: role of endothelial dysfunction. Circulation 2002; 106(2): 184-90.
[http://dx.doi.org/10.1161/01.CIR.0000021125.83697.21] [PMID: 12105156]

[12]    Muniyappa R, Sowers JR. Role of insulin resistance in endothelial dysfunction. Rev Endocr Metab Disord 2013; 14(1): 5-12.
[http://dx.doi.org/10.1007/s11154-012-9229-1] [PMID: 23306778]

[13]    Potenza MA, Marasciulo FL, Chieppa DM, *et al.* Insulin resistance in spontaneously hypertensive rats is associated with endothelial dysfunction characterized by imbalance between NO and ET-1 production. Am J Physiol Heart Circ Physiol 2005; 289(2): H813-22.
[http://dx.doi.org/10.1152/ajpheart.00092.2005] [PMID: 15792994]

[14]    Montagnani M, Golovchenko I, Kim I, *et al.* Inhibition of phosphatidylinositol 3-kinase enhances mitogenic actions of insulin in endothelial cells. J Biol Chem 2002; 277(3): 1794-9.
[http://dx.doi.org/10.1074/jbc.M103728200] [PMID: 11707433]

[15]    Hadi HA, Suwaidi JA. Endothelial dysfunction in diabetes mellitus. Vasc Health Risk Manag 2007; 3(6): 853-76.
[PMID: 18200806]

[16]    Funk SD, Yurdagul A Jr, Orr AW. Hyperglycemia and endothelial dysfunction in atherosclerosis: lessons from type 1 diabetes. Int J Vasc Med 2012; 2012: 1-19.
[http://dx.doi.org/10.1155/2012/569654] [PMID: 22489274]

[17]    Meza CA, La Favor JD, Kim DH, Hickner RC. Endothelial Dysfunction: Is There a Hyperglycemia-Induced Imbalance of NOX and NOS? Int J Mol Sci 2019; 20(15): 3775.
[http://dx.doi.org/10.3390/ijms20153775] [PMID: 31382355]

# CHAPTER 8

# Molecular Mechanisms Underlying Metabolic Syndrome

**Marwa Mohamed Hosny[1,2,*], Nora Hosny[3] and Ahmed Saber Shams[4]**

[1] *Medical Biochemistry and Molecular Biology Department, Faculty of Medicine, Suez Canal University, Ismailia, Egypt*

[2] *Oncology Diagnostic Unit, Faculty of Medicine, Suez Canal University, Ismailia, Egypt*

[3] *Medical Biochemistry and Molecular Biology Department, Faculty of Medicine, Suez Canal University, Ismailia, Egypt*

[4] *Human Anatomy and Embryology Department, Faculty of Medicine, Suez Canal University, Ismailia, Egypt*

**Abstract:** Metabolic syndrome (MetS) has become a worldwide health problem, affecting children and adults globally. The prevalence of MetS is rising all over the world due to increasing obesity and sedentary lifestyles. MetS is caused by the interaction of both genetic and environmental factors.

MetS is characterized by complicated, multidimensional, and sophisticated molecular pathways that involve insulin resistance, inflammatory processes, and hereditary predispositions.

Here we are trying to focus on common molecular mechanisms that underlie MetS occurrence, aiming to offer a better understanding of their role in MetS and helping in developing prognostic/diagnostic tools and targeting novel therapeutic options.

**Keyword:** Cancer, Cardiovascular disease, Diagnostic tools, HDL, Insulin resistance, MetS.

## INTRODUCTION

### The Convergence of Genetic, Environmental Factors and Molecular Pathways in Metabolic Syndrome

Metabolic syndrome (MetS) is characterized by the occurrence of several cardiovascular risk factors as abnormal glucose metabolism, obesity, dyslipidemia, and hypertension [1]. The prevalence shows difference among ethnic groups, with the highest rates in Mexican American women. Other factors affecting the metabolic syndrome occurrence are age, smoking, alcohol, diet, and physical inactivity [2].

---
[*] **Corresponding author Marwa Mohamed Hosny:** Medical Biochemistry and Molecular Biology Department, Faculty of Medicine, Suez Canal University, Ismailia, Egypt and Oncology Diagnostic Unit, Faculty of Medicine, Suez Canal University, Ismailia, Egypt; E-mail: marwahosny@med.suez.edu.eg

**Hafize Uzun & Seyma Dumur (Eds.)**

The prevalence of MetS is rising worldwide due to increasing obesity and sedentary lifestyles [3]. About 12.5-31.4% population globally have MetS [3]. MetS is associated with an increased risk of occurrence of type 2 diabetes mellitus (T2DM), cardiovascular disease, and cancer [4]. Metabolic syndrome is the presence of at least three of the following five: abdominal obesity, increased blood pressure, hyperglycemia, raised serum triglycerides, and deceased serum high-density lipoprotein (HDL) [5].

Crosstalk among genetic predisposition, environmental factors, and molecular pathways regulating metabolism and inflammation, underlies the molecular basis for MetS. Insulin resistance has a very obvious role in disturbed glucose [6] and lipid metabolism [7]. Moreover, the chronic inflammatory process is supposed to be one of the molecular mechanisms for MetS. In adipose tissue, there is obesity-induced chronic inflammation [8] that is associated with disturbed composition and abnormal metabolic role of abdominal subcutaneous adipose tissue (aSAT) [9]. Chronic inflammation is aggravated by exposure to adipose tissue stresses that are associated with the activation of stress-responsive signaling pathways [10].

This chapter will shed light on molecular mechanisms that are considered as a basis for MetS development. It will show the crosstalk among insulin resistance, chronic inflammation, autophagy, adipose tissue dysfunction, disturbed adipokines secretion, mitochondrial dysfunction, oxidative stress, and epigenetics as micro-RNA in addition to the genetic and environmental factors.

## Insulin Resistance

A pathophysiological condition known as insulin resistance occurs when normal insulin levels are unable to trigger the proper insulin response in target tissues such the liver, muscle, and adipose tissue. Insulin resistance is thought to have a major role in initiating and maintaining the detrimental consequences associated with metabolic syndrome.

Under normal circumstances, elevated glucose levels cause the pancreatic β cells to produce insulin and decrease the synthesis of glucagon. As a result, this prevents the liver from producing glucose and improves the absorption of glucose in the muscle, liver, and adipose tissues.

Insulin resistance is characterized by malfunction of the β cell, which leads to either a reduced initial secretion of insulin or no release of insulin in response to a glucose load [11]. Postprandial hyperglycemia is the outcome of this inadequate rapid insulin release. In the next phase, an increased insulin response takes place to counteract this excess glucose. Insulin's efficacy is reduced when high levels of insulin are sustained over time because fewer insulin receptors are present [12, 13]. Indeed, this phenomenon has been demonstrated in genetically engineered mouse trials [14]. The blood levels of insulin in transgenic mice that have additional copies of the human insulin gene increase two to four times. Even with the extra insulin, the mice's blood sugar remains elevated. According to this study, a prolonged elevation in insulin levels causes a decrease in the number of insulin receptors, which in turn causes insulin resistance. Therefore, depending on the circumstances, lower glucose uptake and elevated blood sugar levels due to insulin resistance can result from hyperinsulinemia as well as be a cause of it.

The two α-subunits of the insulin receptor (IR) complex are in charge of binding insulin, whereas the other two β-subunits have built-in tyrosine kinase activity. Insulin binding causes IR to become autophosphorylated, which activates kinase activity. Tyrosine residues on downstream signaling substrates such as Src homology (Shc) and insulin receptor substrates (IRS-1, IRS-2) can be phosphorylated as a result of this activation. As a result, two important pathways are activated: the metabolic regulation-related phosphatidylinositol 3-kinase (PI3K) pathway and mitogen-activated protein kinase (MAPK) pathway, which is in charge of both mitogenesis and growth. These pathways promote cellular development and differentiation, as well as metabolic activities involving glucose and lipids [15].

Mutations in the genes encoding the insulin receptor (IR) and its downstream components can result in impaired insulin signaling, suggesting a genetic foundation for insulin resistance. A family with a known autosomal dominant deficiency in the Akt2 gene, a crucial protein in the insulin receptor signaling pathway, leading to severe insulin resistance, serves as an instructive example [16]. Even though they are not fat, the affected members of this family have significant insulin resistance and frequently have diabetes early in life.

The subtypes of the IRS family of signaling molecules appear to have distinct functions in modulating the activities of insulin in different tissues. For example, IRS-1 is mostly involved in skeletal muscle function, whereas IRS-2 is predominantly involved in liver function. Knockout mice display skeletal muscle insulin resistance due to mutations in IRS-1 [17], hepatic insulin resistance, and failure of β-cell secretion [10] due to mutations in IRS-2 [18] (Fig. **1**).

In instances of insulin resistance, defective tyrosine phosphorylation of the insulin receptor (IR) and IRS-1 is observed, accompanied by increased inhibitory serine phosphorylation (pS) and a significant reduction in IRS-1 protein levels compared to those in normal subjects. The heightened serine phosphorylation of IRS-1 may be linked to the enhanced activation of the mTOR-p70S6 pathway. Notably, mTOR, p70S6K1, and AMPK function as nutrient and energy sensors within the cell. The elevation in basal serine IRS-1 phosphorylation and the degradation of IRS-1 can be attributed to inflammatory mediators, cytokines, and reactive oxygen species (ROS). Consequently, the impaired PI3K activation resulting from increased serine phosphorylation of IRS-1 leads to diminished translocation of GLUT4 to the plasma membrane, culminating in reduced insulin-stimulated glucose uptake [6, 19].

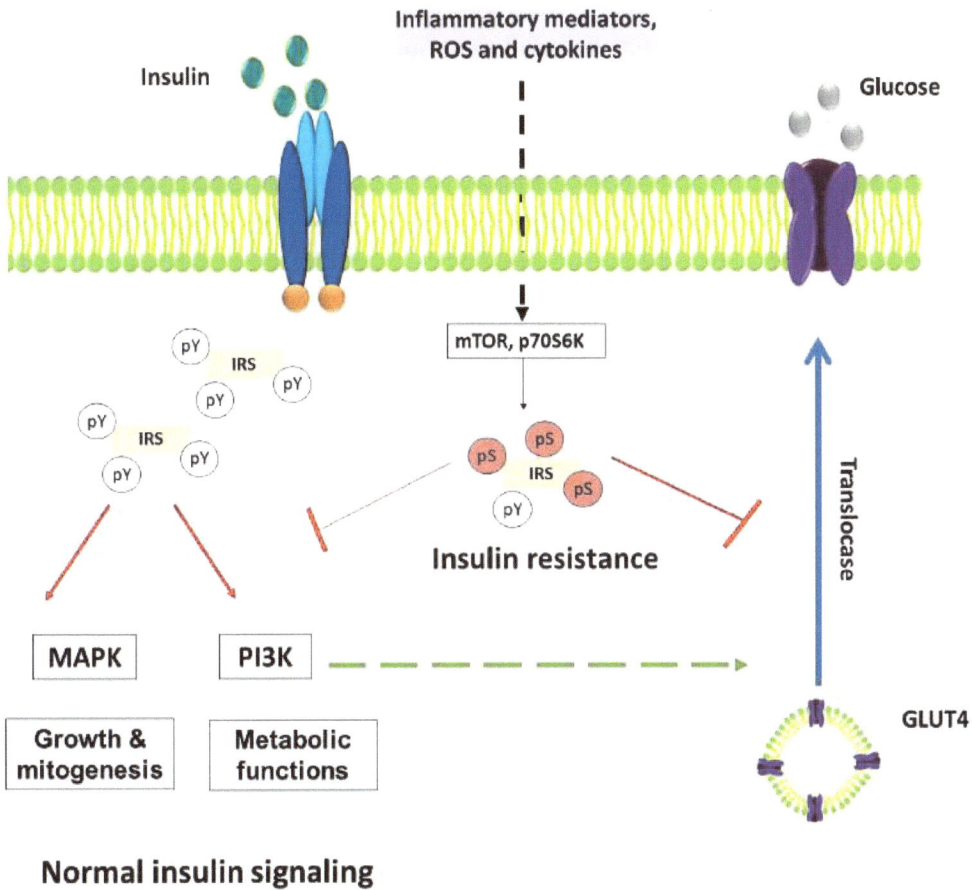

**Fig. (1). Potential mechanisms underlying insulin resistance involve the pathway for insulin-stimulated glucose transport.** This process entails the activation of the insulin receptor protein, which then associates with IRS-1 and IRS-2, phosphorylating these proteins at tyrosine residues (pY). Subsequently, IRS-1 recruits the p85 regulatory subunit of PI 3-kinase (p85-p110), leading to the phosphorylation of membrane-bound phospholipids at the 3 position, generating phosphoinositol-3,4,5-phosphate (PIP3). PIP3 production is essential for the activation of Akt and signaling for GLUT4 translocation.

Post-translational modifications that modify the activity of insulin signaling molecules represent a second proposed mechanism for inhibiting the insulin pathway and hence insulin resistance. Several kinases, including stress-activated protein kinase, c-Jun N-terminal kinase (JNK), and PKC can phosphorylate specific serine and threonine residues on IRS-1 and IRS-2, leading to the inhibition of insulin signaling [20]. Another underlying mechanism is linked to the induction of inhibitory factors, such as suppressors of cytokine signaling (SOCS-1,3). SOCS proteins hinder insulin signaling by competing with IRS-1 for binding to the insulin receptor and by promoting the proteasomal degradation of IRS-1 [21]. Additionally, increased activity of phosphatases, which dephosphorylates intermediate signaling molecules, can impede the insulin pathway [22].

While several phosphatases have been implicated as inhibitors of insulin action, in vivo studies in mice strongly support protein tyrosine phosphatase 1B (PTP1B) as the primary regulator of insulin signaling [23]. Remarkably, mice lacking PTP1B exhibited resistance to weight gain, enhanced insulin sensitivity, and maintained insulin sensitivity even when exposed to a high-fat diet [24]. Individuals who are obese, insulin resistant, and have type 2 diabetes display elevated PTP1B expression in their muscle and liver tissues [25]. Liver-specific overexpression of PTP1B has also demonstrated both hepatic and systemic insulin resistance [26]. Moreover, genetic variations within the promoter and untranslated regions of the PTP1B gene have been linked to insulin resistance and type 2 diabetes in the Iranian population [27, 28]. Other phosphatases, such as phosphatase and tensin homologue (PTEN), which inactivate PI3-K, and SH2-containing inositol 5′ phosphatase-2 (SHIP2), have been shown to exert a negative influence on insulin signaling [29, 30].

Hepatic insulin resistance and its associated metabolic disorders are pivotal factors in maintaining overall energy balance and metabolism since the liver is an insulin-sensitive organ. Impaired insulin signaling and the onset of insulin resistance in the liver can significantly disrupt energy regulation and metabolic processes. This dysfunction in insulin action within the liver is proposed as a fundamental contributor to Metabolic Syndrome (MetS) and its associated issues, encompassing elevated blood sugar levels, abnormal lipid profiles, and heightened inflammatory markers. The subsequent sections will delve into the role of hepatic insulin resistance in the development of MetS, elucidating the suggested molecular mechanisms involved.

## Insulin Resistance and Increased Blood Glucose Level

The liver holds a central position in gluconeogenesis, a process vital for glucose production, and insulin plays a crucial role in inhibiting gluconeogenic enzymes. However, hepatic insulin resistance disrupts this inhibition, leading to an incapacity to suppress these enzymes [31]. Consequently, insulin resistance is associated with an augmented production of glucose within the body. Studies on animals have shown that genetic disruption of the PI3K pathway results in decreased phosphorylation of Akt, causing increased gluconeogenesis, impaired glucose metabolism, and hyperinsulinemia [32]. The transcription factor forkhead box O1 (FoxO1) significantly influences hepatic gluconeogenesis. When insulin is present, FoxO1 undergoes phosphorylation through the PI3K pathway and is sequestered in the cytoplasm. This action inhibits FoxO1 from activating gluconeogenic genes through transcription [33]. Animal studies have distinctly indicated that the knockout of FoxO1 leads to an improvement in insulin resistance and provides protection against diabetes [34].

## Insulin Resistance and Disrupted Lipid Metabolism

Hepatic insulin resistance contributes to altered lipid metabolism, resulting in increased triglyceride (TG) synthesis and decreased free fatty acid (FFA) oxidation [35, 36]. In individuals with metabolic syndrome, elevated serum levels of triacylglycerols are observed due to hypertriglyceridemia, which is influenced by dysregulated transport mechanisms involving chylomicrons and very low-density lipoproteins (VLDLs) [35, 36]. Insulin's role in lipid metabolism is modulated through various mechanisms.

Normally, chylomicrons and TG acquire apoliprotein C (ApoC) during circulation, affecting lipolysis. ApoC-II activates lipoprotein lipase (LpL), facilitating TG breakdown in chylomicrons, whereas ApoC-III inhibits LpL. In insulin-resistant states, ApoC-III production increases, likely mediated by insulin and the transcription factor FoxO1, leading to reduced LpL levels [37]. Consequently, insulin resistance elevates VLDL production, competing with chylomicrons for LpL-mediated lipolysis [38]. There are three sources contributing to elevated VLDL levels in insulin resistance: increased serum fatty acid (FA) levels from adipose tissue lipolysis, inhibited lipolysis of TG, chylomicrons and VLDL due to reduced LpL, and heightened hepatic de novo TG synthesis due to insulin resistance [39].

Insulin plays a significant role in cardioprotective processes through high-density lipoprotein (HDL) and ApoA-I, primarily *via* reverse cholesterol transport (RCT). Insulin acts on the ApoA-1 promoter through the activation of the transcription factor Sp-1 *via* both MAPK and PI3K pathways. However, insulin resistance reduces HDL and ApoA-I levels, primarily due to increased fractional clearance and catabolism of HDL [40, 41]. In clinical practice, treating insulin-resistant dyslipidemia typically involves fibrates (PPARα agonists) and niacin. Fibrates increase LpL and ApoA-I levels and enhance hepatic FFA oxidation. Niacin, when appropriately monitored for glycemic control, has been shown to have minimal effects on insulin sensitivity [42]. Additionally, the PPARγ agonist pioglitazone (TZD) lowers TG levels by enhancing VLDL and TG lipolysis [43].

## Insulin Resistance and Pro-inflammatory State

Disrupted lipid metabolism is closely tied to chronic inflammation in conditions like insulin resistance, obesity, and type 2 diabetes (T2D). This inflammation arises from irregular cytokine production, activation of inflammatory signaling pathways, and heightened acute phase proteins that is often associated with the increased synthesis of C-reactive protein (CRP) in hepatocytes triggered by inflammatory stimuli [44]. Among cytokines, IL-6 is a notable inducer of CRP production, acting at the transcriptional level in human hepatocytes and hepatoma cells. This effect can be amplified by interleukin-1β (IL-1β) [45]. IL-6, along with IL-1β, is also produced by various other cell types, influencing acute phase protein gene expression through specific transcription factors like STAT3, C/EBP family members, and Rel proteins. C/EBP family members are particularly significant in inducing CRP [46]. It is important to mention that CRP can be produced by various cell types apart from hepatocytes, including neurons, atherosclerotic plaques, monocytes, and lymphocytes [47, 48].

Studies have established a correlation between serum CRP levels and components of metabolic syndrome (MetS), encompassing abdominal obesity, elevated triglycerides, reduced HDL cholesterol levels, high blood pressure, and high fasting glucose [49, 50]. Moreover, CRP has emerged as an independent predictor for both diabetes and cardiovascular disease (CVD) [51 - 54]. It is noteworthy that CRP levels also correlate with various other MetS components such as fasting insulin, microalbuminuria, and impaired fibrinolysis, although it is not included in the MetS definitions [50, 55, 56]. In numerous studies, CRP levels have shown a correlation with direct indicators of insulin resistance and endothelial dysfunction [57]. Collectively, evidence from human, animal, and in vitro studies strongly supports the hypothesis that CRP might be a crucial element in the syndrome, significantly elevating the risk of CVD in individuals with MetS.

## Adipose Tissue Dysfunction and Stresses

Adipose tissue dysfunction is an early occurrence in obesity development, characterized by visceral fat accumulation, alterations in cellular and intracellular matrix composition, increased infiltration of immune cells, enlarged adipocytes, heightened autophagy and apoptosis, and changes in mRNA and protein expression patterns. These changes may lead to a fibrotic state in adipose tissue mediated by mast cells. Besides, adipose tissue exhibits altered adipokine secretion patterns toward a proinflammatory, atherogenic, and diabetogenic profile, linking it to insulin resistance, cardiovascular disease, and MetS [58 - 62].

Adipose tissue dysfunction can develop due to continuous positive energy balance, especially in individuals with impaired subcutaneous adipose tissue expandability. Subcutaneous adipose tissue has a higher capacity to expand its capillary network compared to visceral tissue. As fat accumulation increases, this capacity decreases, correlating with insulin resistance. The inability to store excess calories in healthy subcutaneous fat may lead to subsequent ectopic fat deposition in visceral depots and other cell types. These initiate various mechanisms including adipocyte hypertrophy, hypoxia, adipose tissue stresses, autophagy, and inflammation, ultimately resulting in adipose tissue dysfunction and hence MetS [63, 64].

## Adipocyte Hypertrophy

Recent evidence indicates that the enlargement of adipocytes due to increased storage of triglycerides is a key factor driving the development of obesity. Adipose tissue enlargement without a proportional increase in the number of adipocytes (hypertrophy) is linked to the worsening of low-grade chronic inflammation and dyslipidemia, contributing to obesity-related diseases [65]. Conversely, the growth of adipose tissue by generating new adipocytes (hyperplasia) may provide some protection against lipid and glucose/insulin abnormalities in obesity [64]. Studies comparing insulin-sensitive and insulin-resistant individuals with healthy obesity demonstrate that larger average and maximal adipocyte volumes are associated with reduced whole-body insulin sensitivity, heightened levels of inflammation and oxidative stress markers, and increased macrophage presence in adipose tissue. Additionally, adipocyte size plays a role in determining the profile of secreted adipokines, shifting towards a predominantly proinflammatory pattern [64, 66]. These distinctions between hypertrophic and hyperplastic obesity are reflected in the levels of circulating inflammatory markers, such as elevated C-reactive protein (CRP), interleukin-6 (IL-6), monocyte chemoattractant protein-1 (MCP-1), progranulin, and chemerin, seen in obese individuals with hypertrophic adipose tissue expansion compared to those with smaller fat cells [65, 66].

## Hypoxia and its Role in Adipose Tissue Dysfunction

Adipose tissue dysfunction is suggested to be a response to relative hypoxia, occurring in clusters of adipocytes distant from vasculature as adipose tissue mass expands. Hypoxia may induce oxidative and endoplasmic reticulum stress, contributing to adipose tissue dysfunction [66].

## Adipose Tissue Stresses and Stress-Responsive Signaling Pathways

Adipose tissue, especially when subjected to overfeeding and obesity, experiences various stresses including metabolic, oxidative, and endoplasmic reticulum stress. These stressors activate stress-sensing pathways like p38MAPK and Jun N-terminal kinase (JNK) [10, 67, 68]. Increased activation of p38MAPK and JNK, especially in visceral adipose tissue, correlates with metabolic parameters and obesity-associated morbidity. JNK activation is linked to a shift towards a pro-inflammatory and diabetogenic adipokine secretion pattern. The activation of stress signaling pathways in adipose tissue leads to increased immune cell infiltration, particularly macrophages [69].

## Immune Cell Infiltration and Inflammation in Adipose Tissue

Obesity is associated with the infiltration of proinflammatory immune cells into adipose tissue, causing chronic, low-grade inflammation. This infiltration involves changes in T-cell phenotype, recruitment of B and T cells, and macrophage infiltration [70].

The accumulation of macrophages in visceral adipose tissue, possibly due to antigens absorbed from the gut, is thought to play a significant role in the development of visceral obesity and inflammation related to obesity. Various studies have consistently shown higher levels of macrophage infiltration in omental fat, compared to subcutaneous fat, across different research settings and diverse groups of participants.

Another crucial finding comes from research that compared extremely obese individuals who were either insulin-sensitive or insulin-resistant. By meticulously matching individuals for age, gender, BMI, and total body fat mass, it was discovered that increased infiltration of macrophages into omental adipose tissue strongly predicted the insulin-resistant phenotype in obese individuals. These findings underscore the importance of macrophages in the link between obesity and metabolic diseases [70, 71].

Moreover, differences in the composition of macrophage subtypes were observed in subcutaneous adipose tissue between lean and overweight individuals. Higher fat mass was associated with the accumulation of an M2 remodeling subtype of macrophages, characterized by reduced expression of proinflammatory markers such as IL-8 and cyclooxygenase-2, and increased expression of lymphatic vessel endothelial hyaluronan receptor-1. As secretory cells, these macrophages in human adipose tissue may contribute to the low-grade chronic inflammation often seen in obesity. The increased presence of macrophages in adipose tissue could result in higher systemic concentrations of pro-inflammatory cytokines, creating a molecular link between adipose tissue and the metabolic, cardiovascular, and hepatic complications of obesity. Notably, the higher levels of pro-inflammatory cytokines such as TNF-a, IL-6, and resistin, produced by activated macrophages, may directly contribute to changes in insulin sensitivity in various adipose depots [72, 73].

In accordance with these findings, studies on animal models have shown that lower immune cell infiltration is associated with improved glucose tolerance and increased insulin sensitivity. All of these data collectively support the notion that inflammation within adipose tissue is a significant contributor to insulin resistance in obesity, making macrophage infiltration a potential mechanistic link between adipose tissue dysfunction and systemic insulin resistance [73, 74].

## ER Stress and Unfolded Protein Response (UPR) in Obesity

Obesity is linked to endoplasmic reticulum (ER) stress and activation of the unfolded protein response (UPR) in adipose tissue. ER stress occurs due to an overload of the ER from increased protein synthesis or reduced elimination of misfolded proteins. Activation of UPR leads to transcriptional induction of genes involved in protein assembly, folding, and degradation to alleviate ER stress. Obesity, with increased nutrient flux, exposes adipose tissue to multidimensional stresses, possibly inducing a proinflammatory state and adipose tissue dysfunction. Additionally, oxidative stress, characterized by an imbalance between oxidant generation and antioxidant defense mechanisms, is a feature of obesity, with evidence of increased levels of oxidized proteins in adipose tissue [67, 75, 76].

## Autophagy and its Role in Obesity

Autophagy, a cellular process responsible for the breakdown and recycling of cellular components, has been recognized as playing a role in the development of obesity and its related metabolic complications. Studies on mice with a specific genetic deletion of the autophagy gene Atg7 in their adipose tissue have shown that autophagy contributes to the regulation of fat mass and the balance between white and brown adipocytes. These Atg7 knockout mice tend to be lean, insulin-sensitive, and have an increased metabolic rate, making them resistant to obesity development [77].

Human studies have also indicated that autophagy is up-regulated in the adipose tissue of obese and type 2 diabetic individuals, especially in the omental fat depot.

When researchers examined paired omental and subcutaneous adipose tissue samples from over 250 individuals with varying body mass index (BMI), glucose tolerance, and fat distribution, they found that markers of autophagy were elevated in the adipose tissue of obese individuals, particularly in visceral fat. These findings revealed a correlation between increased expression of autophagy genes and the degree of obesity, visceral fat distribution, and adipocyte hypertrophy [78, 79].

This suggests that autophagy activation may coincide with the development of insulin resistance and could precede the onset of obesity-related health issues. Therefore, autophagy might serve as an undiscovered mechanism that could either protect against dysfunction in adipose tissue associated with obesity or serve as an early indicator of impaired adipose tissue function.

## Adipokines as Mediators of Adipose Tissue Dysfunction in Obesity

Adipokines are the term used to describe the various substances that are released by adipose tissue [80, 81]. They exert their effects *via* auto/paracrine and endocrine pathways modulating glucose metabolism, adipogenesis, immune cell migration, adipocyte metabolism, influencing fat distribution, appetite, satiety, insulin sensitivity, insulin secretion, and inflammation.

Various cell types present in adipose tissue are responsible for producing pro-inflammatory molecules known as cytokines or adipocytokines. These include TNFα, TGFβ, interferon-ɤ, CRP, interleukins (IL-1, IL-6, IL-8, IL-10), PAI-1, RBP4, vaspin, endocannabinoids, fetuin-A, omentin, BMPs, clusterin, fractalkine, orosomucoid, fatty acid binding protein 4 (FABP4), fibrinogen, haptoglobin, angiopoietin-related proteins, metallothionein, complement factor 3, serum amyloid A (SAA) protein, anandamide, and chemoattractant cytokines like MCP-1, progranulin, and macrophage inflammatory protein-1α. Most of these adipokines are elevated in obesity and can induce insulin resistance. Interestingly, molecules known for their anti-inflammatory properties, including adiponectin, apelin, and IL-10, are reduced in obese individuals [58 - 60, 70, 82, 83].

Adipokines influence fat distribution, particularly intraabdominal fat accumulation. For example, adipokines like RBP4, chemerin, vaspin, and fetuin-A are linked to intraabdominal fat distribution. Additionally, adipokines have significant systemic effects on various target organs, linking fat accumulation and adipose tissue dysfunction to metabolic disorders associated with obesity, including effects on the brain, liver, muscle, vasculature, heart, and pancreatic β-cells. It is worth noting that the pattern of adipokine secretion mirrors the functionality of adipose tissue. This pattern is crucial in assessing an individual's susceptibility to developing metabolic and cardiovascular complications associated with obesity [58 - 60, 83, 84].

## Genetic Factors

Genetic factors can influence MetS through different perspectives [85]. Each of the fundamental components of this syndrome, including obesity, dyslipidemia, dysglycemia, and high blood pressure, has a genetic underpinning, with specific candidate genes that have been identified. These genetic associations may contribute to, or even enable, the manifestation of the syndrome. For instance, variations in the ADIPOQ gene, responsible for encoding adiponectin, have been linked to visceral obesity [86]. Similarly, variations in the AGT gene, which encode angiotensinogen, have been associated with blood pressure regulation [87], while plasma lipid concentrations have been tied to variations in the APOE and APOC3 genes, responsible for encoding apolipoproteins E and C-III, respectively [88, 89]. Consequently, genetic variants linked to individual components of the metabolic syndrome may also underlie associations with the entire syndrome.

Furthermore, certain products of candidate genes may operate within a common pathway that impacts more than one component of the syndrome. This suggests the possibility of single-gene associations. For example, the NR3C1 gene, which codes for the glucocorticoid receptor, has been implicated in obesity, hypertension, and insulin resistance [90]. ADIPOQ, in addition to its association with obesity, has also been linked to diabetes, hypertension, and dyslipidemia [91, 92]. Similarly, GNB3, encoding the β3 subunit of G protein, has demonstrated associations with both hypertension and obesity [93]. Variations in genes responsible for specific transcription factors, such as FOXC2 and SREBP1, have been linked to insulin sensitivity and plasma triglyceride concentrations [94, 95]. Hence, these genes present potential candidates for association studies investigating the complete metabolic syndrome phenotype.

## Heritability of the Metabolic Syndrome

The heritability of the metabolic syndrome is supported by findings from twin and family studies [89, 96 - 99]. These investigations suggest that there is a genetic contribution to the clustering of metabolic syndrome components. For instance, in a study involving 2,508 male twin pairs in the US, it was observed that the clustering of hypertension, diabetes, and obesity occurred in 31.6% of monozygotic (identical) twin pairs but only in 6.3% of dizygotic (fraternal) twin pairs [96]. Similar evidence for heritable factors was found in a study of female twin pairs [97]. Furthermore, in a study of 432 individuals from several Japanese American families, significant genetic influences were noted on all components of the metabolic syndrome, with dyslipidemia, in particular, showing that about 50% of the variance was attributable to genetic influences [98]. The suggestion of causative genes underlying the metabolic syndrome has prompted researchers to investigate both the rare monogenic forms of the syndrome and the more common trait using various approaches, including genetic linkage and association analysis.

## Single-gene Human Models

Studying the monogenic forms of the metabolic syndrome, which manifests in a small number of patients with specific single-gene disorders, may provide more insights into the genetic basis of this syndrome. For example, individuals with familial partial lipodystrophy, resulting from mutations in genes like LMNA (encoding lamin A/C) and PPARG (encoding peroxisome proliferative activated receptor γ), exhibit the hallmark features of the metabolic syndrome, including insulin resistance, dyslipidemia, and hypertension [100]. Moreover, these individuals, particularly women, face a significantly heightened risk of cardiovascular disease [101].

An in-depth examination of these patients has revealed distinct stages in the progression of the disease. In familial partial lipodystrophy, insulin resistance is the initial metabolic abnormality, followed by the development of dyslipidemia, with hypertension and diabetes emerging later in the course of the disease, and cardiovascular disease occurring even further along [100]. Understanding the sequence of abnormal phenotypes in familial partial lipodystrophy has suggested a logical, stepwise treatment approach that may help shape the natural history and the molecular basis of the disease and its development towards cardiovascular disease endpoints. This comprehension of disease progression stages in those patients could hold value not only for this rare condition but potentially also for patients with the common metabolic syndrome phenotype.

## Genome-wide Linkage Scanning

The approach of genome-wide linkage scanning, which involves a comprehensive exploration of the entire human genome to identify chromosomal regions linked to complex traits, has been employed in the study of metabolic syndrome.

A study, involving 2,209 individuals from 507 US families, revealed associations between the metabolic syndrome and specific chromosome loci, namely 3q27 and 17p12. The locus 3q27 displayed strong links to six pertinent traits, including weight, waist circumference, leptin, insulin, insulin-to-glucose ratio, and hip circumference, which encompass possibly relevant genes such as the solute carrier family 2 of the facilitated glucose transporter (GLUT2) and the catalytic α polypeptide of phosphoinositide 3-kinase, known to influence glucose-insulin homeostasis [98, 102]. On the other hand, the 17p12 locus was primarily linked to plasma leptin levels.

Another study, comprising 261 individuals without diabetes from 27 Mexican American families, identified a significant linkage between the metabolic syndrome and two distinct regions on chromosome 6 (D6S403 and D6S264) and one region on chromosome 7 (D7S479–D7S471) [103].

An additional study conducted in US families, which included 456 white and 217 black participants from 204 families in the HERITAGE Family Study, detected evidence for linkage on several chromosomal regions, including 1p34.1, 1q41, 2p22.3, 7q31.3, 9p13.1, 9q21.1, 10p11.2, and 19q13.4, emphasizing on strong evidence for linkage of two principal components in whites (comprising % body fat, abdominal visceral fat, HDL cholesterol, TG, glucose, insulin, and mean arterial BP) on 10p11.2 (2 markers) and on 19q13.4 [104]. It is worth mentioning that this study observed ethnic-group-specific linkages. Besides, a study of Hispanic families pinpointed the q23–q31 region of chromosome 1 as housing at least one gene related to the metabolic syndrome [89, 105].

In yet another linkage study encompassing 2,467 subjects from 387 families and 1,082 subjects from 256 sibships, evidence for linkage on chromosome 2 was found. This evidence was associated with a factor comprising BMI, waist-to-hip ratio, subscapular skinfold, TG, HDL cholesterol, homeostasis model assessment index, plasminogen activator inhibitor-1 antigen, and serum uric acid. These findings suggest the potential existence of a pleiotropic locus contributing to the clustering of metabolic syndrome-related phenotypes on chromosome 2 [99].

Furthermore, a genome-wide linkage study (the GENNID study) identified strong evidence for linkage related to metabolic syndrome phenotypes on chromosome 2 (2q12.1–2q13 in whites) and on chromosome 3 (3q26.1–3q29 in Mexican-Americans). This study included families from four different ethnic groups [106].

It is important to note that none of these studies have identified specific genes or mutations as a direct result. However, some of these chromosomal regions have previously been linked to cardiovascular disease and risk factors for diabetes, suggesting that they may harbor potential candidate genes for the metabolic syndrome. Nevertheless, these results must be interpreted with caution, as they are subject to the limitations inherent in all gene linkage studies focused on complex traits [100].

## Genetic Association Studies

Candidate gene association studies have explored various biologically plausible candidate genes involved in processes relevant to the metabolic syndrome, such as energy intake, energy expenditure, body weight, lipid and carbohydrate metabolism, inflammation, insulin signaling, and blood pressure regulation. These studies have examined the potential genetic basis of the metabolic syndrome, aiming to identify genetic variants associated with its components. Some candidate gene studies have reported associations between specific gene variants and metabolic syndrome. However, these associations are often weak and may not be consistently replicated in other populations due to limited statistical power.

For instance, APOC3 and PPARG are two genes that have shown positive associations with metabolic syndrome in multiple studies. The APOC3 gene, which encodes apolipoprotein C-III, has been linked to elevated plasma triglycerides and associated with metabolic syndrome in South Asian men and women [107] and Aboriginal Canadian women [108]. The PPARG gene, encoding a ligand-activated transcription factor with various roles in metabolism, has also demonstrated positive associations. Studies have reported associations between SNPs in PPARG and metabolic syndrome, with some findings showing a decreased risk of developing the syndrome in individuals with specific SNP genotypes [109, 110]. Furthermore, some gene variants, such as those in ACE, FABP2, and GNB3, have shown conflicting associations with the metabolic syndrome in different studies. In contrast, associations of the metabolic syndrome with APOC3 and PPARG have been replicated in more than one study sample [89, 109, 110].

In addition to candidate gene association studies, genome-wide association (GWA) studies have been conducted to identify genetic determinants of the metabolic syndrome. However, these studies have yielded mixed results. One GWA study in Indian Asian men failed to identify strong associations between specific single nucleotide polymorphisms (SNPs) and metabolic syndrome. Although some SNPs were associated with individual metabolic traits, no SNP exhibited a strong association with the syndrome as a whole [111]. Another GWA study involving participants of European ancestry identified five SNPs associated with the metabolic syndrome, with the APOA5 cluster, LPL, and CETP genes among the key genetic loci involved [101, 112].

A study on Finnish populations focused on the metabolic syndrome as defined by the IDF 2005 criteria and found a single SNP significantly associated with the syndrome, located within the APOA1/C3/A4/A5 genetic cluster. However, this study did not uncover evidence of pleiotropy linking dyslipidemia and obesity to other metabolic syndrome components [112 - 114]. Further study adopted a different strategy by clustering quantitative traits into six metabolic syndrome-related phenotype domains. This study identified new pleiotropic loci associated with multiple phenotype domains, such as APOC1, BRAP, and PLCG1 [112, 115]. Other GWA studies have unveiled specific genetic loci with pleiotropic effects on two or more components of the MetS. For example, the rs2943634 variant near IRS1, primarily associated with reduced adiposity, has also been linked to an increased visceral to subcutaneous fat ratio, insulin resistance, dyslipidemia (higher triglycerides and lower HDL cholesterol levels), risk of diabetes, coronary artery disease, and decreased adiponectin levels. Genetic variants in glucokinase regulator (GCKR) have been associated with fasting and 2-hour glucose levels, triglycerides, lipoprotein particles, and histological non-alcoholic fatty liver disease [116 - 122].

Variants in the fat mass and obesity-associated gene (FTO) and melanocortin-4 receptor (MC4R) genes, which primarily regulate body weight, have shown associations with various measures of adiposity, including waist circumference (WC), HDL cholesterol levels, insulin resistance, and the risk of type 2 diabetes. Growth factor receptor-bound protein 14 (GRB14) variants have been linked to BMI-adjusted waist-to-hip ratio, type 2 diabetes, and fasting insulin levels. CDK5 Regulatory Subunit Associated Protein 1 Like 1 (CDKAL1) and A disintegrin and metalloproteinase with thrombospondin motifs 9 ADAMTS9 variants have associations with type 2 diabetes, BMI-adjusted waist-to-hip ratio, BMI, and 2-hour glucose levels, while variants near gastric inhibitory polypeptide receptor (GIPR) have been linked to 2-hour glucose and BMI [123, 124].

Several candidate gene association studies have reported associations between these "pleiotropic" genetic loci and the MetS. These findings suggest that genetic regulation of adiposity and insulin resistance plays a role in the development of the MetS. Out of the various susceptibility loci associated with multiple MetS-related traits, FTO and MC4R appear to have primary effects on body weight regulation, while IRS1 is a key player in insulin resistance [112, 123, 124].

In summary, candidate gene association studies and GWA studies have provided insights into the potential genetic basis of the metabolic syndrome. While some gene variants have shown associations with the syndrome or its individual components, the overall genetic landscape of the metabolic syndrome remains complex and multifactorial. Many of the identified associations are related to genes involved in lipid metabolism, reflecting the importance of lipid parameters in defining the metabolic syndrome.

It is worth noting that genetic association studies between the metabolic syndrome and single nucleotide polymorphisms (SNPs) in human samples have their advantages and limitations. These studies offer several strengths [89] like simplicity, reliability, uncomplicated statistical analysis together with the potentiality of clear interpretation and direct relevance to human health and disease. However, there are several factors that can hinder the validity and application of genetic association studies. For instance, lack of replication, limited clinical use as in spite of extensive research, few DNA markers, typically SNPs, are currently incorporated into routine clinical practice beside some technological limitations represented in the limited ability of the current genotyping technologies to comprehensively investigate the vast amount of genetic variation in the human genome. In attempts to address these limitations and enhance the clinical utility of genetic associations, newer technologies like high-density SNP genotyping microarrays have been developed. These technologies will enable the simultaneous examination of thousands of polymorphisms, potentially leading to the identification of DNA markers that can be more useful for diagnostic and risk assessment purposes in conditions like the metabolic syndrome. However, these advancements are still a work in progress and validation to become standard practice in clinical settings.

## Epigenetics and Regulatory RNAs in the Pathogenesis of Metabolic Syndrome

Emerging evidence highlights the significance of epigenetic mechanisms in the development of Metabolic Syndrome (MetS). Epigenetic changes, which include DNA methylation and histone modifications, can lead to alterations in gene expression and cellular phenotypes, and these changes are passed on through cell divisions without affecting the DNA sequence itself. These epigenetic mechanisms potentially mediate the effects of environmental exposures on metabolism [125]. For example, there is growing support for the long-term impact of adverse intrauterine nutrition or gestational hyperglycemia on the metabolic health of offspring [126].

Studies examining the epigenetics of type 2 diabetes have revealed differences in DNA methylation between individuals with diabetes and those without, with specific loci, such as IRS1 and FTO, showing epigenetic changes. However, investigations into the epigenetics of the MetS are relatively limited. One study involving families discovered that DNA methylation of fatty acid binding protein 3, a key regulator of lipid homeostasis, was associated with various MetS-related phenotypes. Furthermore, methylation patterns of three clock genes, which play a role in regulating circadian rhythms (CLOCK, BMAL1, and PER2), were linked to MetS scores and anthropometric parameters such as body mass index and adiposity in a group of 60 women [112, 127 - 131].

In addition to epigenetic changes, small non-coding RNAs, specifically microRNAs, have gained attention for their potential roles in MetS pathogenesis. MicroRNAs regulate gene expression at both the transcriptional and post-transcriptional levels, influencing mRNA translation to proteins. Many microRNAs have been identified as regulators of MetS-related pathways, including those involved in insulin and glucose homeostasis (e.g., glucose uptake, insulin signaling, and insulin secretion), cholesterol and lipid regulation, adipogenesis, and inflammatory responses. These findings suggest that epigenetic mechanisms and microRNAs play pivotal roles in the complex pathogenesis of the MetS [132, 133].

## Mitochondrial Dysfunction and Oxidative Stress

Mitochondria are central players in the pathogenesis of the Metabolic Syndrome (MetS), insulin resistance, and type 2 diabetes (T2DM). Dysfunctional mitochondria contribute to oxidative stress, which plays a critical role in these conditions. It can result from factors such as nutrient overload, sedentary lifestyles, mitochondrial DNA polymorphisms, and environmental risk factors, including dietary habits, physical inactivity, exposure to chemicals, and certain drugs [134, 135].

The mitochondrial respiratory chain is a significant source of reactive oxygen species (ROS) in cells. When ROS levels exceed the antioxidant capacity of the cell, this leads to oxidative stress. Excessive nutrient intake in adipocytes can lead to increased mitochondrial fatty acid oxidation, resulting in excessive production of acetyl coenzyme A, NADH, and $FADH_2$ from the tricarboxylic acid cycle. This increased electron supply to the electron transport chain (ETC) generates excessive amounts of ROS [136, 137].

Accumulation of excessive free fatty acids (FFAs) in adipocytes can activate the NADPH oxidase enzyme, leading to further ROS production [134, 138], and consequently an escalated oxidative stress. Oxidative stress in adipocytes triggers a shift in adipose tissue macrophages from an anti-inflammatory state (M2) to a pro-inflammatory state (M1), initiating inflammation [139]. The increased oxidative stress can further damage ETC components and other mitochondrial constituents, leading to mitochondrial fragmentation and a decline in oxidative phosphorylation. This sets off a vicious cycle that ultimately leads to adipocyte apoptosis. Apoptosis of adipocytes triggers the proliferation of M1 macrophages, the release of inflammatory mediators, and the progression of local and systemic inflammation, exacerbating insulin resistance [134].

Mitochondrial Dysfunction in skeletal muscles and pancreatic beta cells are two main examples that can propagate the disease progression. For example, mitochondrial dysfunction in skeletal muscles is a significant contributor to insulin resistance. Initially, an increase in FFA availability leads to increased mitochondrial biogenesis and fatty acid oxidation *via* the activation of the PGC1α pathway. However, an overload of substrates in myocyte mitochondria contributes to oxidative stress and mitochondrial dysfunction. The accumulation of toxic lipids like diacylglycerol (DAG) and ceramide contributes to insulin resistance when FFAs are in relative excess beyond their utilization by oxidation or storage as neutral lipids [140]. Regarding the pancreatic beta cells, excessive and persistent ROS generation causes oxidative stress and mitochondrial dysfunction, leading to apoptosis of beta cells and a reduction in beta cell mass, which is a key event in the progression from insulin resistance to T2DM [141].

Additionally, mitochondrial dysfunction and oxidative stress can impact cellular signaling and metabolic reprogramming. Excessive ROS generation affects intracellular signaling by inhibiting tricarboxylic cycle enzyme aconitase, leading to citrate accumulation that is redirected to fat synthesis. Excessive hydrogen peroxide can inhibit beta fatty acid oxidation, resulting in increased fat storage and further insulin resistance. Insulin-resistant cells often have reduced mitochondrial energy production and increased susceptibility to oxidative stress that leads to a vicious cycle [142].

Genetic studies indicated a decrease in mitochondrial DNA (mtDNA) density in peripheral blood cells, which preceded the development of T2DM in a prospective cohort study. This mtDNA density was also associated with other components of metabolic syndrome, such as abdominal circumference and blood pressure before the onset of T2DM. These findings suggested a strong link between mitochondrial dysfunction and metabolic syndrome, indicating that changes in mtDNA density could serve as a biomarker for mitochondrial dysfunction and the risk of developing these conditions [135, 143 - 145]. Additionally, common mtDNA haplogroups have been associated with susceptibility to T2DM, with some haplogroups considered protective while others are associated with higher risk. Moreover, variants within the mtDNA control region have been linked to insulin resistance and T2DM risk in different populations, although the associations may vary among ethnic groups. This discrepancy could be due to the influence of nuclear genetic backgrounds and environmental factors [135, 146 - 148].

The interactions between mitochondrial dysfunction, insulin resistance, and the development of metabolic syndrome and T2DM are complex and multifaceted. With the fact that mitochondrial dysfunction can be both a cause and a consequence of insulin resistance and is associated with MetS [134, 135, 142].

Ongoing studies and further investigations are necessary to unravel the precise mechanisms and determinants that underlie these relationships.

## Brown Adipose Tissue (BAT)

Brown adipose tissue (BAT) has emerged as a key player in the development of metabolic syndrome (MetS), a cluster of conditions associated with heart disease and diabetes. While traditionally known for its role in thermoregulation and energy expenditure, BAT's recent prominence in metabolic health stems from several factors. BAT primarily functions in thermogenesis by generating heat through mitochondria, which helps burn stored fat and increase energy expenditure. This not only maintains body temperature but also aids in preventing obesity, a central feature of MetS. Furthermore, BAT's activation appears to improve insulin sensitivity, glucose homeostasis, and lipid metabolism, addressing key elements of MetS. It may also possess anti-inflammatory properties, impact appetite regulation, and secrete adipokines with potentially favourable effects. Nevertheless, understanding BAT's full role in MetS requires further research, considering that not everyone has substantial active BAT, and its levels can diminish with age and obesity [149 - 152].

## Dyslipidemia

Dyslipidemia, characterized by abnormal lipid levels in the blood, significantly influences the development of Metabolic Syndrome (MetS), a condition associated with an increased risk of cardiovascular disease and type 2 diabetes. It can result from multiple factors, including genetic factors, excessive calorie intake, obesity, chronic inflammation and insulin resistance. Dyslipidemia contributes to multiple aspects of MetS, including elevated triglycerides, low HDL cholesterol, the presence of small, dense LDL particles, and an unfavorable total cholesterol to HDL cholesterol ratio, all of which increase the risk of cardiovascular disease. Dyslipidemia is interconnected with other features of MetS, such as insulin resistance, obesity, inflammation, and genetics, making its management an essential component of the overall treatment and prevention strategies for MetS [153 - 155].

## SUMMARY

To summarize, an illustrative model to describe the outlines of complex interplay of those various factors in the pathogenesis of metabolic syndrome (MetS) has been described by Pankaj Prasun in 2020 [134]. This model is adapted and summarized below (Fig. **2**).

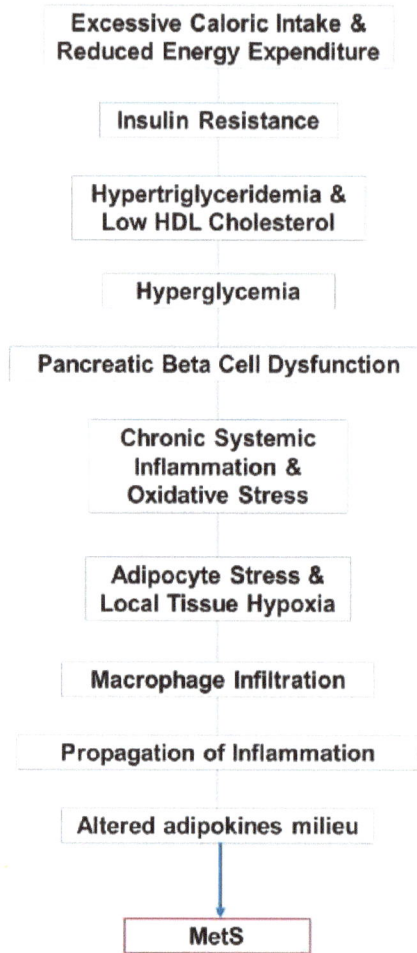

```
Excessive Caloric Intake &
Reduced Energy Expenditure

Insulin Resistance

Hypertriglyceridemia &
Low HDL Cholesterol

Hyperglycemia

Pancreatic Beta Cell Dysfunction

Chronic Systemic
Inflammation &
Oxidative Stress

Adipocyte Stress &
Local Tissue Hypoxia

Macrophage Infiltration

Propagation of Inflammation

Altered adipokines milieu

MetS
```

**Fig. (2).** Illustrative model to describe the outlines of complex interplay of those various factors in the pathogenesis of metabolic syndrome (MetS) [134].

## Excessive Caloric Intake and Reduced Energy Expenditure

These lead to lipid accumulation and obesity. The accumulated toxic lipids, particularly diacylglycerol (DAG) and ceramide, inhibit insulin signaling in the liver and skeletal muscle, resulting in insulin resistance.

## Insulin Resistance

As a consequence of lipid-induced insulin resistance, there is a state of relative hypoinsulinemia. This leads to increased hormone-sensitive lipase activity and lipolysis in adipose tissue, resulting in elevated plasma free fatty acids (FFA).

# Hypertriglyceridemia

The excessive FFA is shunted to the liver, causing the synthesis of excessive very-low-density lipoprotein (VLDL). This, in turn, results in hypertriglyceridemia.

# Low HDL Cholesterol

Excessive triglycerides in VLDL are exchanged for cholesterol in high-density lipoprotein (HDL), leading to low HDL cholesterol levels.

# Hyperglycemia

Insulin resistance leads to hyperglycemia due to decreased glucose uptake in skeletal muscles and enhanced gluconeogenesis in the liver.

# Pancreatic Beta Cell Dysfunction

Persistent hyperglycemia overstimulates pancreatic beta cells, leading to their eventual decompensation and failure. This progression results in the development of T2DM.

# Chronic Systemic Inflammation and Oxidative Stress

These are associated with MetS and are considered to mediate insulin resistance. They contribute to the pathogenesis of MetS and T2DM.

# Adipocyte Stress and Local Tissue Hypoxia

Progressive lipid accumulation in adipocytes leads to hypertrophy and the enlargement of adipose tissue, causing adipocyte stress and local tissue hypoxia. This sets the stage for tissue dysfunction.

# Macrophage Infiltration

Adipocyte necrosis and infiltration by macrophages are consequences of adipocyte stress. Macrophages secrete proinflammatory mediators such as interleukin-6 (IL-6), tumor necrosis factor-alpha (TNF-α), and prothrombotic mediator plasminogen activator inhibitor-1 (PAI-1).

# Propagation of Inflammation

The local inflammation initiated by these proinflammatory mediators propagates to systemic inflammation. This systemic inflammation contributes to the development of insulin resistance and other MetS components.

## Adipokines

Adipose tissue acts as an endocrine organ and secretes adipokines. Hypertrophied and stressed adipocytes have an altered adipokine secretory pattern. There is an increase in proinflammatory adipokines such as leptin and resistin, along with a decrease in the anti-inflammatory adipokine adiponectin.

## Effects of Altered Adipokine Milieu and Inflammation

The imbalance between pro- and anti-inflammatory adipokines exacerbates local and systemic inflammation. The overall effects of this altered adipokine milieu and chronic systemic inflammatory and prothrombotic status include insulin resistance, hepatic steatosis (fatty liver), endothelial dysfunction, hypertension, and atherosclerosis.

This model underscores the intricate relationships between metabolic factors, inflammation, and the progression of MetS and T2DM together with highlighting the importance of addressing both lifestyle and therapeutic interventions to prevent and manage these conditions effectively.

## REFERENCES

[1]     Duc Nguyen H, Ardeshir A, Fonseca VA, Kim WK. Cluster of differentiation molecules in the metabolic syndrome. Clin Chim Acta 2024; 561: 119819.
[http://dx.doi.org/10.1016/j.cca.2024.119819] [PMID: 38901629]

[2]     Coordinators NR. Database resources of the National Center for Biotechnology Information. Nucleic Acids Res 2016; 44(D1): D7-D19.
[http://dx.doi.org/10.1093/nar/gkv1290] [PMID: 26615191]

[3]     Wang J-S, Xia P-F, Ma M-N, Li Y, Geng T-T, Zhang Y-B, *et al.* Trends in the Prevalence of Metabolically Healthy Obesity Among US Adults, 1999-2018. JAMA Network Open. 2023; 6(3): e232145-e.

[4]     Shen X, Yang H, Yang Y, Zhu X, Sun Q. The cellular and molecular targets of natural products against metabolic disorders: a translational approach to reach the bedside. MedComm 2024; 5(8): e664.
[http://dx.doi.org/10.1002/mco2.664] [PMID: 39049964]

[5]     Huang PL. A comprehensive definition for metabolic syndrome. Dis Model Mech 2009; 2(5-6): 231-7.
[http://dx.doi.org/10.1242/dmm.001180] [PMID: 19407331]

[6]     Lann D, LeRoith D. Insulin resistance as the underlying cause for the metabolic syndrome. Med Clin North Am 2007; 91(6): 1063-1077, viii.
[http://dx.doi.org/10.1016/j.mcna.2007.06.012] [PMID: 17964909]

[7]     Schwarz JM, Linfoot P, Dare D, Aghajanian K. Hepatic de novo lipogenesis in normoinsulinemic and hyperinsulinemic subjects consuming high-fat, low-carbohydrate and low-fat, high-carbohydrate isoenergetic diets. Am J Clin Nutr 2003; 77(1): 43-50.
[http://dx.doi.org/10.1093/ajcn/77.1.43] [PMID: 12499321]

[8]     Hachiya R, Tanaka M, Itoh M, Suganami T. Molecular mechanism of crosstalk between immune and metabolic systems in metabolic syndrome. Inflamm Regen 2022; 42(1): 13.
[http://dx.doi.org/10.1186/s41232-022-00198-7] [PMID: 35490239]

[9]     Ahn C, Zhang T, Yang G, *et al.* Years of endurance exercise training remodel abdominal subcutaneous adipose tissue in adults with overweight or obesity. Nat Metab 2024; 6(9): 1819-36.
[http://dx.doi.org/10.1038/s42255-024-01103-x] [PMID: 39256590]

[10]    Sabio G, Das M, Mora A, *et al.* A stress signaling pathway in adipose tissue regulates hepatic insulin resistance. Science 2008; 322(5907): 1539-43.
[http://dx.doi.org/10.1126/science.1160794] [PMID: 19056984]

[11]    LeRoith D. β-cell dysfunction and insulin resistance in type 2 diabetes: role of metabolic and genetic abnormalities. Am J Med 2002; 113(6) (Suppl. 6A): 3-11.
[http://dx.doi.org/10.1016/S0002-9343(02)01276-7] [PMID: 12431757]

[12]    Del Prato S, Leonetti F, Simonson DC, Sheehan P, Matsuda M, DeFronzo RA. Effect of sustained physiologic hyperinsulinaemia and hyperglycaemia on insulin secretion and insulin sensitivity in man. Diabetologia 1994; 37(10): 1025-35.
[http://dx.doi.org/10.1007/BF00400466] [PMID: 7851681]

[13]    Roth J, Qiang X, Marbán SL, Redelt H, Lowell BC. The obesity pandemic: where have we been and where are we going? Obes Res 2004; 12(S11) (Suppl. 2): 88S-101S.
[http://dx.doi.org/10.1038/oby.2004.273] [PMID: 15601956]

[14]    Marbán SL, Roth J. Transgenic hyperinsulinemia: a mouse model of insulin resistance and glucose intolerance without obesity. Lessons from Animal Diabetes VI: 75th Anniversary of the Insulin Discovery. 1996: 201-24.
[http://dx.doi.org/10.1007/978-1-4612-4112-6_13]

[15]    Biddinger SB, Kahn CR. From mice to men: insights into the insulin resistance syndromes. Annu Rev Physiol 2006; 68(1): 123-58.
[http://dx.doi.org/10.1146/annurev.physiol.68.040104.124723] [PMID: 16460269]

[16]    George S, Rochford JJ, Wolfrum C, *et al.* A family with severe insulin resistance and diabetes due to a mutation in AKT2. Science 2004; 304(5675): 1325-8.
[http://dx.doi.org/10.1126/science.1096706] [PMID: 15166380]

[17]    Tamemoto H, Kadowaki T, Tobe K, *et al.* Insulin resistance and growth retardation in mice lacking insulin receptor substrate-1. Nature 1994; 372(6502): 182-6.
[http://dx.doi.org/10.1038/372182a0] [PMID: 7969452]

[18]    Withers DJ, Gutierrez JS, Towery H, *et al.* Disruption of IRS-2 causes type 2 diabetes in mice. Nature 1998; 391(6670): 900-4.
[http://dx.doi.org/10.1038/36116] [PMID: 9495343]

[19]    Barbour LA, McCurdy CE, Hernandez TL, Kirwan JP, Catalano PM, Friedman JE. Cellular mechanisms for insulin resistance in normal pregnancy and gestational diabetes. Diabetes Care 2007; 30 (Suppl. 2): S112-9.
[http://dx.doi.org/10.2337/dc07-s202] [PMID: 17596458]

[20]    Weickert MO, Pfeiffer AFH. Signalling mechanisms linking hepatic glucose and lipid metabolism. Diabetologia 2006; 49(8): 1732-41.
[http://dx.doi.org/10.1007/s00125-006-0295-3] [PMID: 16718463]

[21]    Kile BT, Schulman BA, Alexander WS, Nicola NA, Martin HME, Hilton DJ. The SOCS box: a tale of destruction and degradation. Trends Biochem Sci 2002; 27(5): 235-41.
[http://dx.doi.org/10.1016/S0968-0004(02)02085-6] [PMID: 12076535]

[22]    Schinner S, Scherbaum WA, Bornstein SR, Barthel A. Molecular mechanisms of insulin resistance. Diabet Med 2005; 22(6): 674-82.
[http://dx.doi.org/10.1111/j.1464-5491.2005.01566.x] [PMID: 15910615]

[23]    Kaszubska W, Falls HD, Schaefer VG, *et al.* Protein tyrosine phosphatase 1B negatively regulates leptin signaling in a hypothalamic cell line. Mol Cell Endocrinol 2002; 195(1-2): 109-18.
[http://dx.doi.org/10.1016/S0303-7207(02)00178-8] [PMID: 12354677]

[24]    Elchebly M, Payette P, Michaliszyn E, *et al.* Increased insulin sensitivity and obesity resistance in mice lacking the protein tyrosine phosphatase-1B gene. Science 1999; 283(5407): 1544-8. [http://dx.doi.org/10.1126/science.283.5407.1544] [PMID: 10066179]

[25]    Ahmad F, Azevedo JL, Cortright R, Dohm GL, Goldstein BJ. Alterations in skeletal muscle protein-tyrosine phosphatase activity and expression in insulin-resistant human obesity and diabetes. J Clin Invest 1997; 100(2): 449-58. [http://dx.doi.org/10.1172/JCI119552] [PMID: 9218523]

[26]    Haj FG, Zabolotny JM, Kim YB, Kahn BB, Neel BG. Liver-specific protein-tyrosine phosphatase 1B (PTP1B) re-expression alters glucose homeostasis of PTP1B-/-mice. J Biol Chem 2005; 280(15): 15038-46. [http://dx.doi.org/10.1074/jbc.M413240200] [PMID: 15699041]

[27]    Meshkani R, Taghikhani M, Al-Kateb H, *et al.* Polymorphisms within the protein tyrosine phosphatase 1B (PTPN1) gene promoter: functional characterization and association with type 2 diabetes and related metabolic traits. Clin Chem 2007; 53(9): 1585-92. [http://dx.doi.org/10.1373/clinchem.2007.088146] [PMID: 17634210]

[28]    Meshkani R, Taghikhani M, Mosapour A, *et al.* 1484insG polymorphism of the PTPN1 gene is associated with insulin resistance in an Iranian population. Arch Med Res 2007; 38(5): 556-62. [http://dx.doi.org/10.1016/j.arcmed.2007.01.010] [PMID: 17560463]

[29]    Clément S, Krause U, Desmedt F, *et al.* The lipid phosphatase SHIP2 controls insulin sensitivity. Nature 2001; 409(6816): 92-7. [http://dx.doi.org/10.1038/35051094] [PMID: 11343120]

[30]    Butler M, McKay RA, Popoff IJ, *et al.* Specific inhibition of PTEN expression reverses hyperglycemia in diabetic mice. Diabetes 2002; 51(4): 1028-34. [http://dx.doi.org/10.2337/diabetes.51.4.1028] [PMID: 11916922]

[31]    Cherrington AD. Banting Lecture 1997. Control of glucose uptake and release by the liver in vivo. Diabetes 1999; 48(5): 1198-214. [http://dx.doi.org/10.2337/diabetes.48.5.1198] [PMID: 10331429]

[32]    Taniguchi CM, Kondo T, Sajan M, *et al.* Divergent regulation of hepatic glucose and lipid metabolism by phosphoinositide 3-kinase *via* Akt and PKCλ/ζ. Cell Metab 2006; 3(5): 343-53. [http://dx.doi.org/10.1016/j.cmet.2006.04.005] [PMID: 16679292]

[33]    Puigserver P, Rhee J, Donovan J, *et al.* Insulin-regulated hepatic gluconeogenesis through FOXO1–PGC-1α interaction. Nature 2003; 423(6939): 550-5. [http://dx.doi.org/10.1038/nature01667] [PMID: 12754525]

[34]    Accili D, Arden KC. FoxOs at the crossroads of cellular metabolism, differentiation, and transformation. Cell 2004; 117(4): 421-6. [http://dx.doi.org/10.1016/S0092-8674(04)00452-0] [PMID: 15137936]

[35]    Ziolkowska S, Binienda A, Jabłkowski M, Szemraj J, Czarny P. The Interplay between Insulin Resistance, Inflammation, Oxidative Stress, Base Excision Repair and Metabolic Syndrome in Nonalcoholic Fatty Liver Disease. Int J Mol Sci 2021; 22(20): 11128. [http://dx.doi.org/10.3390/ijms222011128]

[36]    Iozzo P, Turpeinen AK, Takala T, *et al.* Defective liver disposal of free fatty acids in patients with impaired glucose tolerance. J Clin Endocrinol Metab 2004; 89(7): 3496-502. [http://dx.doi.org/10.1210/jc.2003-031142] [PMID: 15240637]

[37]    Merkel M, Eckel RH, Goldberg IJ. Lipoprotein lipase. J Lipid Res 2002; 43(12): 1997-2006. [http://dx.doi.org/10.1194/jlr.R200015-JLR200] [PMID: 12454259]

[38]    Bjorkegren J, Packard CJ, Hamsten A, *et al.* Accumulation of large very low density lipoprotein in plasma during intravenous infusion of a chylomicron-like triglyceride emulsion reflects competition for a common lipolytic pathway. J Lipid Res 1996; 37(1): 76-86.

[http://dx.doi.org/10.1016/S0022-2275(20)37637-9] [PMID: 8820104]

[39]    Chahil TJ, Ginsberg HN. Diabetic Dyslipidemia. Endocrinol Metab Clin North Am 2006; 35(3): 491-510, vii-viii.
        [http://dx.doi.org/10.1016/j.ecl.2006.06.002] [PMID: 16959582]

[40]    Horowitz BS, Goldberg IJ, Merab J, Vanni TM, Ramakrishnan R, Ginsberg HN. Increased plasma and renal clearance of an exchangeable pool of apolipoprotein A-I in subjects with low levels of high density lipoprotein cholesterol. J Clin Invest 1993; 91(4): 1743-52.
        [http://dx.doi.org/10.1172/JCI116384] [PMID: 8473514]

[41]    Vajo Z, Terry JG, Brinton EA. Increased intra-abdominal fat may lower HDL levels by increasing the fractional catabolic rate of Lp A-I in postmenopausal women. Atherosclerosis 2002; 160(2): 495-501.
        [http://dx.doi.org/10.1016/S0021-9150(01)00610-4] [PMID: 11849676]

[42]    Vega GL, Cater NB, Meguro S, Grundy SM. Influence of extended-release nicotinic acid on nonesterified fatty acid flux in the metabolic syndrome with atherogenic dyslipidemia. Am J Cardiol 2005; 95(11): 1309-13.
        [http://dx.doi.org/10.1016/j.amjcard.2005.01.073] [PMID: 15904634]

[43]    Majali KA, Cooper MB, Staels B, Luc G, Taskinen M-R, Betteridge DJ. The effect of sensitisation to insulin with pioglitazone on fasting and postprandial lipid metabolism, lipoprotein modification by lipases, and lipid transfer activities in type 2 diabetic patients. Diabetologia 2006; 49(3): 527-37.
        [http://dx.doi.org/10.1007/s00125-005-0092-4] [PMID: 16429317]

[44]    Black S, Kushner I, Samols D. C-reactive Protein. J Biol Chem 2004; 279(47): 48487-90.
        [http://dx.doi.org/10.1074/jbc.R400025200] [PMID: 15337754]

[45]    Voleti B, Agrawal A. Regulation of basal and induced expression of C-reactive protein through an overlapping element for OCT-1 and NF-kappaB on the proximal promoter. J Immunol 2005; 175(5): 3386-90.
        [http://dx.doi.org/10.4049/jimmunol.175.5.3386] [PMID: 16116232]

[46]    Young DP, Kushner I, Samols D. Binding of C/EBPbeta to the C-reactive protein (CRP) promoter in Hep3B cells is associated with transcription of CRP mRNA. J Immunol 2008; 181(4): 2420-7.
        [http://dx.doi.org/10.4049/jimmunol.181.4.2420] [PMID: 18684932]

[47]    Jialal I, Devaraj S, Venugopal SK. C-reactive protein: risk marker or mediator in atherothrombosis? Hypertension 2004; 44(1): 6-11.
        [http://dx.doi.org/10.1161/01.HYP.0000130484.20501.df] [PMID: 15148294]

[48]    Kuta AE, Baum LL. C-reactive protein is produced by a small number of normal human peripheral blood lymphocytes. J Exp Med 1986; 164(1): 321-6.
        [http://dx.doi.org/10.1084/jem.164.1.321] [PMID: 3723078]

[49]    Festa A, D'Agostino R Jr, Howard G, Mykkänen L, Tracy RP, Haffner SM. Chronic subclinical inflammation as part of the insulin resistance syndrome: the Insulin Resistance Atherosclerosis Study (IRAS). Circulation 2000; 102(1): 42-7.
        [http://dx.doi.org/10.1161/01.CIR.102.1.42] [PMID: 10880413]

[50]    Ridker PM, Buring JE, Cook NR, Rifai N. C-reactive protein, the metabolic syndrome, and risk of incident cardiovascular events: an 8-year follow-up of 14 719 initially healthy American women. Circulation 2003; 107(3): 391-7.
        [http://dx.doi.org/10.1161/01.CIR.0000055014.62083.05] [PMID: 12551861]

[51]    Pradhan AD, Manson JE, Rifai N, Buring JE, Ridker PM. C-reactive protein, interleukin 6, and risk of developing type 2 diabetes mellitus. JAMA 2001; 286(3): 327-34.
        [http://dx.doi.org/10.1001/jama.286.3.327] [PMID: 11466099]

[52]    Ridker PM, Hennekens CH, Buring JE, Rifai N. C-reactive protein and other markers of inflammation in the prediction of cardiovascular disease in women. N Engl J Med 2000; 342(12): 836-43.
        [http://dx.doi.org/10.1056/NEJM200003233421202] [PMID: 10733371]

[53] Ridker PM, Rifai N, Clearfield M, *et al*. Measurement of C-reactive protein for the targeting of statin therapy in the primary prevention of acute coronary events. N Engl J Med 2001; 344(26): 1959-65.
[http://dx.doi.org/10.1056/NEJM200106283442601] [PMID: 11430324]

[54] Ridker PM, Rifai N, Rose L, Buring JE, Cook NR. Comparison of C-reactive protein and low-density lipoprotein cholesterol levels in the prediction of first cardiovascular events. N Engl J Med 2002; 347(20): 1557-65.
[http://dx.doi.org/10.1056/NEJMoa021993] [PMID: 12432042]

[55] Yudkin JS, Stehouwer CDA, Emeis JJ, Coppack SW. C-reactive protein in healthy subjects: associations with obesity, insulin resistance, and endothelial dysfunction: a potential role for cytokines originating from adipose tissue? Arterioscler Thromb Vasc Biol 1999; 19(4): 972-8.
[http://dx.doi.org/10.1161/01.ATV.19.4.972] [PMID: 10195925]

[56] Fröhlich M, Imhof A, Berg G, *et al*. Association between C-reactive protein and features of the metabolic syndrome: a population-based study. Diabetes Care 2000; 23(12): 1835-9.
[http://dx.doi.org/10.2337/diacare.23.12.1835] [PMID: 11128362]

[57] Stehouwer CDA, Gall MA, Twisk JWR, Knudsen E, Emeis JJ, Parving HH. Increased urinary albumin excretion, endothelial dysfunction, and chronic low-grade inflammation in type 2 diabetes: progressive, interrelated, and independently associated with risk of death. Diabetes 2002; 51(4): 1157-65.
[http://dx.doi.org/10.2337/diabetes.51.4.1157] [PMID: 11916939]

[58] Van Gaal LF, Mertens IL, De Block CE. Mechanisms linking obesity with cardiovascular disease. Nature 2006; 444(7121): 875-80.
[http://dx.doi.org/10.1038/nature05487] [PMID: 17167476]

[59] Blüher M. Adipose tissue dysfunction in obesity. Exp Clin Endocrinol Diabetes 2009; 117(6): 241-50.
[http://dx.doi.org/10.1055/s-0029-1192044] [PMID: 19358089]

[60] Bays HE. Adiposopathy, diabetes mellitus, and primary prevention of atherosclerotic coronary artery disease: treating "sick fat" through improving fat function with antidiabetes therapies. Am J Cardiol 2012; 110(9) (Suppl.): 4B-12B.
[http://dx.doi.org/10.1016/j.amjcard.2012.08.029] [PMID: 23062567]

[61] Divoux A, Moutel S, Poitou C, *et al*. Mast cells in human adipose tissue: link with morbid obesity, inflammatory status, and diabetes. J Clin Endocrinol Metab 2012; 97(9): E1677-85.
[http://dx.doi.org/10.1210/jc.2012-1532] [PMID: 22745246]

[62] Spencer M, Unal R, Zhu B, *et al*. Adipose tissue extracellular matrix and vascular abnormalities in obesity and insulin resistance. J Clin Endocrinol Metab 2011; 96(12): E1990-8.
[http://dx.doi.org/10.1210/jc.2011-1567] [PMID: 21994960]

[63] Gealekman O, Guseva N, Hartigan C, *et al*. Depot-specific differences and insufficient subcutaneous adipose tissue angiogenesis in human obesity. Circulation 2011; 123(2): 186-94.
[http://dx.doi.org/10.1161/CIRCULATIONAHA.110.970145] [PMID: 21200001]

[64] Blüher M. Adipose tissue dysfunction contributes to obesity related metabolic diseases. Best Pract Res Clin Endocrinol Metab 2013; 27(2): 163-77.
[http://dx.doi.org/10.1016/j.beem.2013.02.005] [PMID: 23731879]

[65] Blüher M, Wilson-Fritch L, Leszyk J, Laustsen PG, Corvera S, Kahn CR. Role of insulin action and cell size on protein expression patterns in adipocytes. J Biol Chem 2004; 279(30): 31902-9.
[http://dx.doi.org/10.1074/jbc.M404570200] [PMID: 15131120]

[66] Skurk T, Alberti-Huber C, Herder C, Hauner H. Relationship between adipocyte size and adipokine expression and secretion. J Clin Endocrinol Metab 2007; 92(3): 1023-33.
[http://dx.doi.org/10.1210/jc.2006-1055] [PMID: 17164304]

[67] Rudich A, Kanety H, Bashan N. Adipose stress-sensing kinases: linking obesity to malfunction. Trends Endocrinol Metab 2007; 18(8): 291-9.

[http://dx.doi.org/10.1016/j.tem.2007.08.006] [PMID: 17855109]

[68]　Bashan N, Dorfman K, Tarnovscki T, *et al.* Mitogen-activated protein kinases, inhibitory-kappaB kinase, and insulin signaling in human omental versus subcutaneous adipose tissue in obesity. Endocrinology 2007; 148(6): 2955-62.
[http://dx.doi.org/10.1210/en.2006-1369] [PMID: 17317777]

[69]　Blüher M, Bashan N, Shai I, *et al.* Activated Ask1-MKK4-p38MAPK/JNK stress signaling pathway in human omental fat tissue may link macrophage infiltration to whole-body Insulin sensitivity. J Clin Endocrinol Metab 2009; 94(7): 2507-15.
[http://dx.doi.org/10.1210/jc.2009-0002] [PMID: 19351724]

[70]　Sell H, Habich C, Eckel J. Adaptive immunity in obesity and insulin resistance. Nat Rev Endocrinol 2012; 8(12): 709-16.
[http://dx.doi.org/10.1038/nrendo.2012.114] [PMID: 22847239]

[71]　Hotamisligil GS. Inflammation and metabolic disorders. Nature 2006; 444(7121): 860-7.
[http://dx.doi.org/10.1038/nature05485] [PMID: 17167474]

[72]　Weisberg SP, McCann D, Desai M, Rosenbaum M, Leibel RL, Ferrante AW Jr. Obesity is associated with macrophage accumulation in adipose tissue. J Clin Invest 2003; 112(12): 1796-808.
[http://dx.doi.org/10.1172/JCI200319246] [PMID: 14679176]

[73]　Cinti S, Mitchell G, Barbatelli G, *et al.* Adipocyte death defines macrophage localization and function in adipose tissue of obese mice and humans. J Lipid Res 2005; 46(11): 2347-55.
[http://dx.doi.org/10.1194/jlr.M500294-JLR200] [PMID: 16150820]

[74]　Harman-Boehm I, Blüher M, Redel H, *et al.* Macrophage infiltration into omental versus subcutaneous fat across different populations: effect of regional adiposity and the comorbidities of obesity. J Clin Endocrinol Metab 2007; 92(6): 2240-7.
[http://dx.doi.org/10.1210/jc.2006-1811] [PMID: 17374712]

[75]　Eizirik DL, Cardozo AK, Cnop M. The role for endoplasmic reticulum stress in diabetes mellitus. Endocr Rev 2008; 29(1): 42-61.
[http://dx.doi.org/10.1210/er.2007-0015] [PMID: 18048764]

[76]　Özcan U, Cao Q, Yilmaz E, *et al.* Endoplasmic reticulum stress links obesity, insulin action, and type 2 diabetes. Science 2004; 306(5695): 457-61.
[http://dx.doi.org/10.1126/science.1103160] [PMID: 15486293]

[77]　Zhang Y, Goldman S, Baerga R, Zhao Y, Komatsu M, Jin S. Adipose-specific deletion of *autophagy-related gene 7* ( *atg7* ) in mice reveals a role in adipogenesis. Proc Natl Acad Sci USA 2009; 106(47): 19860-5.
[http://dx.doi.org/10.1073/pnas.0906048106] [PMID: 19910529]

[78]　Kovsan J, Blüher M, Tarnovscki T, *et al.* Altered autophagy in human adipose tissues in obesity. J Clin Endocrinol Metab 2011; 96(2): E268-77.
[http://dx.doi.org/10.1210/jc.2010-1681] [PMID: 21047928]

[79]　Maixner N, Kovsan J, Harman-Boehm I, Blüher M, Bashan N, Rudich A. Autophagy in adipose tissue. Obes Facts 2012; 5(5): 710-21.
[http://dx.doi.org/10.1159/000343983] [PMID: 23108431]

[80]　Ouchi N, Kihara S, Funahashi T, Matsuzawa Y, Walsh K. Obesity, adiponectin and vascular inflammatory disease. Curr Opin Lipidol 2003; 14(6): 561-6.
[http://dx.doi.org/10.1097/00041433-200312000-00003] [PMID: 14624132]

[81]　Berg AH, Scherer PE. Adipose tissue, inflammation, and cardiovascular disease. Circ Res 2005; 96(9): 939-49.
[http://dx.doi.org/10.1161/01.RES.0000163635.62927.34] [PMID: 15890981]

[82]　Blüher M. Clinical relevance of adipokines. Diabetes Metab J 2012; 36(5): 317-27.
[http://dx.doi.org/10.4093/dmj.2012.36.5.317] [PMID: 23130315]

[83] Dahlman I, Elsen M, Tennagels N, *et al.* Functional annotation of the human fat cell secretome. Arch Physiol Biochem 2012; 118(3): 84-91.
[http://dx.doi.org/10.3109/13813455.2012.685745] [PMID: 22616691]

[84] Bays HE. Adiposopathy. J Am Coll Cardiol 2011; 57(25): 2461-73.
[http://dx.doi.org/10.1016/j.jacc.2011.02.038] [PMID: 21679848]

[85] Hegele RA, Pollex RL. Genetic and physiological insights into the metabolic syndrome. Am J Physiol Regul Integr Comp Physiol 2005; 289(3): R663-9.
[http://dx.doi.org/10.1152/ajpregu.00275.2005] [PMID: 15890790]

[86] Sutton BS, Weinert S, Langefeld CD, *et al.* Genetic analysis of adiponectin and obesity in Hispanic families: the IRAS Family Study. Hum Genet 2005; 117(2-3): 107-18.
[http://dx.doi.org/10.1007/s00439-005-1260-9] [PMID: 15843989]

[87] Jeunemaitre X, Soubrier F, Kotelevtsev YV, *et al.* Molecular basis of human hypertension: Role of angiotensinogen. Cell 1992; 71(1): 169-80.
[http://dx.doi.org/10.1016/0092-8674(92)90275-H] [PMID: 1394429]

[88] Waterworth DM, Talmud PJ, Bujac SR, Fisher RM, Miller GJ, Humphries SE. Contribution of apolipoprotein C-III gene variants to determination of triglyceride levels and interaction with smoking in middle-aged men. Arterioscler Thromb Vasc Biol 2000; 20(12): 2663-9.
[http://dx.doi.org/10.1161/01.ATV.20.12.2663] [PMID: 11116069]

[89] Pollex RL, Hegele RA. Genetic determinants of the metabolic syndrome. Nat Clin Pract Cardiovasc Med 2006; 3(9): 482-9.
[http://dx.doi.org/10.1038/ncpcardio0638] [PMID: 16932765]

[90] Rosmond R. The glucocorticoid receptor gene and its association to metabolic syndrome. Obes Res 2002; 10(10): 1078-86.
[http://dx.doi.org/10.1038/oby.2002.146] [PMID: 12376590]

[91] Kondo H, Shimomura I, Matsukawa Y, *et al.* Association of adiponectin mutation with type 2 diabetes: a candidate gene for the insulin resistance syndrome. Diabetes 2002; 51(7): 2325-8.
[http://dx.doi.org/10.2337/diabetes.51.7.2325] [PMID: 12086969]

[92] Ohashi K, Ouchi N, Kihara S, *et al.* Adiponectin I164T mutation is associated with the metabolic syndrome and coronary artery disease. J Am Coll Cardiol 2004; 43(7): 1195-200.
[http://dx.doi.org/10.1016/j.jacc.2003.10.049] [PMID: 15063429]

[93] Siffert W, Forster P, Jöckel KH, *et al.* Worldwide ethnic distribution of the G protein beta3 subunit 825T allele and its association with obesity in Caucasian, Chinese, and Black African individuals. J Am Soc Nephrol 1999; 10(9): 1921-30.
[http://dx.doi.org/10.1681/ASN.V1091921] [PMID: 10477144]

[94] Ridderstråle M, Carlsson E, Klannemark M, *et al.* FOXC2 mRNA Expression and a 5′ untranslated region polymorphism of the gene are associated with insulin resistance. Diabetes 2002; 51(12): 3554-60.
[http://dx.doi.org/10.2337/diabetes.51.12.3554] [PMID: 12453913]

[95] Kotzka J, Müller-Wieland D. Sterol regulatory element-binding protein (SREBP)-1: gene regulatory target for insulin resistance? Expert Opin Ther Targets 2004; 8(2): 141-9.
[http://dx.doi.org/10.1517/14728222.8.2.141] [PMID: 15102555]

[96] Carmelli D, Cardon LR, Fabsitz R. Clustering of hypertension, diabetes, and obesity in adult male twins: same genes or same environments? Am J Hum Genet 1994; 55(3): 566-73.
[PMID: 8079995]

[97] Edwards KL, Newman B, Mayer E, Selby JV, Krauss RM, Austin MA. Heritability of factors of the insulin resistance syndrome in women twins. Genet Epidemiol 1997; 14(3): 241-53.
[http://dx.doi.org/10.1002/(SICI)1098-2272(1997)14:3<241::AID-GEPI3>3.0.CO;2-8] [PMID: 9181354]

[98]   Austin MA, Edwards KL, McNeely MJ, *et al.* Heritability of multivariate factors of the metabolic syndrome in nondiabetic Japanese americans. Diabetes 2004; 53(4): 1166-9. [http://dx.doi.org/10.2337/diabetes.53.4.1166] [PMID: 15047637]

[99]   Lee KE, Klein BE, Klein R. Familial aggregation of components of the multiple metabolic syndrome in the Framingham Heart and Offspring Cohorts: Genetic Analysis Workshop Problem 1. BMC genetics. 2003;4 Suppl 1(Suppl 1):S94.

[100]  Pollex RL, Hegele RA. Complex trait locus linkage mapping in atherosclerosis: time to take a step back before moving forward? Arterioscler Thromb Vasc Biol 2005; 25(8): 1541-4. [http://dx.doi.org/10.1161/01.ATV.0000173307.25652.89] [PMID: 15947242]

[101]  Hegele RA. Premature atherosclerosis associated with monogenic insulin resistance. Circulation 2001; 103(18): 2225-9. [http://dx.doi.org/10.1161/01.CIR.103.18.2225] [PMID: 11342468]

[102]  Kissebah AH, Sonnenberg GE, Myklebust J, *et al.* Quantitative trait loci on chromosomes 3 and 17 influence phenotypes of the metabolic syndrome. Proc Natl Acad Sci USA 2000; 97(26): 14478-83. [http://dx.doi.org/10.1073/pnas.97.26.14478] [PMID: 11121050]

[103]  Arya R, Blangero J, Williams K, *et al.* Factors of insulin resistance syndrome--related phenotypes are linked to genetic locations on chromosomes 6 and 7 in nondiabetic mexican-americans. Diabetes 2002; 51(3): 841-7. [http://dx.doi.org/10.2337/diabetes.51.3.841] [PMID: 11872689]

[104]  Loos RJF, Katzmarzyk PT, Rao DC, *et al.* Genome-wide linkage scan for the metabolic syndrome in the HERITAGE Family Study. J Clin Endocrinol Metab 2003; 88(12): 5935-43. [http://dx.doi.org/10.1210/jc.2003-030553] [PMID: 14671193]

[105]  Langefeld CD, Wagenknecht LE, Rotter JI, *et al.* Linkage of the Metabolic Syndrome to 1q23-q31 in Hispanic Families. Diabetes 2004; 53(4): 1170-4. [http://dx.doi.org/10.2337/diabetes.53.4.1170] [PMID: 15047638]

[106]  Wu KD, Hsiao CF, Ho LT, Sheu WH, Pei D, Chuang LM, *et al.* Clustering and heritability of insulin resistance in Chinese and Japanese hypertensive families: a Stanford-Asian Pacific Program in Hypertension and Insulin Resistance sibling study. Hypertension research : official journal of the Japanese Society of Hypertension. 2002;25(4):529-36. [http://dx.doi.org/10.1291/hypres.25.529]

[107]  Guettier JM, Georgopoulos A, Tsai MY, *et al.* Polymorphisms in the fatty acid-binding protein 2 and apolipoprotein C-III genes are associated with the metabolic syndrome and dyslipidemia in a South Indian population. J Clin Endocrinol Metab 2005; 90(3): 1705-11. [http://dx.doi.org/10.1210/jc.2004-1338] [PMID: 15598690]

[108]  Pollex RL, Hanley AJG, Zinman B, Harris SB, Khan HMR, Hegele RA. Metabolic syndrome in aboriginal Canadians: Prevalence and genetic associations. Atherosclerosis 2006; 184(1): 121-9. [http://dx.doi.org/10.1016/j.atherosclerosis.2005.03.024] [PMID: 15869758]

[109]  Meirhaeghe A, Cottel D, Amouyel P, Dallongeville J. Association between peroxisome proliferator-activated receptor gamma haplotypes and the metabolic syndrome in French men and women. Diabetes 2005; 54(10): 3043-8. [http://dx.doi.org/10.2337/diabetes.54.10.3043] [PMID: 16186413]

[110]  Frederiksen L, Brødbaek K, Fenger M, *et al.* Comment: studies of the Pro12Ala polymorphism of the PPAR-gamma gene in the Danish MONICA cohort: homozygosity of the Ala allele confers a decreased risk of the insulin resistance syndrome. J Clin Endocrinol Metab 2002; 87(8): 3989-92. [PMID: 12161548]

[111]  Cao H, Hegele RA. Nuclear lamin A/C R482Q mutation in Canadian kindreds with Dunnigan-type familial partial lipodystrophy. Hum Mol Genet 2000; 9(1): 109-12. [http://dx.doi.org/10.1093/hmg/9.1.109] [PMID: 10587585]

[112] Stančáková A, Laakso M. Genetics of metabolic syndrome. Rev Endocr Metab Disord 2014; 15(4): 243-52.
[http://dx.doi.org/10.1007/s11154-014-9293-9] [PMID: 25124343]

[113] Yuan S, She D, Jiang S, Deng N, Peng J, Ma L. Endoplasmic reticulum stress and therapeutic strategies in metabolic, neurodegenerative diseases and cancer. Mol Med 2024; 30(1): 40.
[http://dx.doi.org/10.1186/s10020-024-00808-9]

[114] Kristiansson K, Perola M, Tikkanen E, *et al.* Genome-wide screen for metabolic syndrome susceptibility Loci reveals strong lipid gene contribution but no evidence for common genetic basis for clustering of metabolic syndrome traits. Circ Cardiovasc Genet 2012; 5(2): 242-9.
[http://dx.doi.org/10.1161/CIRCGENETICS.111.961482] [PMID: 22399527]

[115] Dupuis J, Langenberg C, Prokopenko I, Saxena R, Soranzo N, Jackson AU, *et al.* New genetic loci implicated in fasting glucose homeostasis and their impact on type 2 diabetes risk. Nature genetics 2010; 42(2): 105-6.

[116] Dupuis J, Langenberg C, Prokopenko I, *et al.* New genetic loci implicated in fasting glucose homeostasis and their impact on type 2 diabetes risk. Nat Genet 2010; 42(2): 105-16.
[http://dx.doi.org/10.1038/ng.520] [PMID: 20081858]

[117] Kilpeläinen TO, Zillikens MC, Stančákova A, *et al.* Genetic variation near IRS1 associates with reduced adiposity and an impaired metabolic profile. Nat Genet 2011; 43(8): 753-60.
[http://dx.doi.org/10.1038/ng.866] [PMID: 21706003]

[118] Saxena R, Hivert MF, Langenberg C, *et al.* Genetic variation in GIPR influences the glucose and insulin responses to an oral glucose challenge. Nat Genet 2010; 42(2): 142-8.
[http://dx.doi.org/10.1038/ng.521] [PMID: 20081857]

[119] Saxena R, Voight BF, Lyssenko V, *et al.* Genome-wide association analysis identifies loci for type 2 diabetes and triglyceride levels. Science 2007; 316(5829): 1331-6.
[http://dx.doi.org/10.1126/science.1142358] [PMID: 17463246]

[120] Willer CJ, Sanna S, Jackson AU, *et al.* Newly identified loci that influence lipid concentrations and risk of coronary artery disease. Nat Genet 2008; 40(2): 161-9.
[http://dx.doi.org/10.1038/ng.76] [PMID: 18193043]

[121] Stančáková A, Paananen J, Soininen P, *et al.* Effects of 34 risk loci for type 2 diabetes or hyperglycemia on lipoprotein subclasses and their composition in 6,580 nondiabetic Finnish men. Diabetes 2011; 60(5): 1608-16.
[http://dx.doi.org/10.2337/db10-1655] [PMID: 21421807]

[122] Speliotes EK, Yerges-Armstrong LM, Wu J, *et al.* Genome-wide association analysis identifies variants associated with nonalcoholic fatty liver disease that have distinct effects on metabolic traits. PLoS Genet 2011; 7(3): e1001324.
[http://dx.doi.org/10.1371/journal.pgen.1001324] [PMID: 21423719]

[123] Frayling TM, Timpson NJ, Weedon MN, *et al.* A common variant in the FTO gene is associated with body mass index and predisposes to childhood and adult obesity. Science 2007; 316(5826): 889-94.
[http://dx.doi.org/10.1126/science.1141634] [PMID: 17434869]

[124] Chambers JC, Elliott P, Zabaneh D, *et al.* Common genetic variation near MC4R is associated with waist circumference and insulin resistance. Nat Genet 2008; 40(6): 716-8.
[http://dx.doi.org/10.1038/ng.156] [PMID: 18454146]

[125] Wolffe AP, Guschin D. Review: chromatin structural features and targets that regulate transcription. J Struct Biol 2000; 129(2-3): 102-22.
[http://dx.doi.org/10.1006/jsbi.2000.4217] [PMID: 10806063]

[126] Dabelea D, Hanson RL, Lindsay RS, *et al.* Intrauterine exposure to diabetes conveys risks for type 2 diabetes and obesity: a study of discordant sibships. Diabetes 2000; 49(12): 2208-11.
[http://dx.doi.org/10.2337/diabetes.49.12.2208] [PMID: 11118027]

[127]  Nilsson E, Jansson PA, Perfilyev A, *et al.* Altered DNA methylation and differential expression of genes influencing metabolism and inflammation in adipose tissue from subjects with type 2 diabetes. Diabetes 2014; 63(9): 2962-76.
[http://dx.doi.org/10.2337/db13-1459] [PMID: 24812430]

[128]  Dayeh T, Volkov P, Salö S, *et al.* Genome-wide DNA methylation analysis of human pancreatic islets from type 2 diabetic and non-diabetic donors identifies candidate genes that influence insulin secretion. PLoS Genet 2014; 10(3): e1004160.
[http://dx.doi.org/10.1371/journal.pgen.1004160] [PMID: 24603685]

[129]  Toperoff G, Aran D, Kark JD, *et al.* Genome-wide survey reveals predisposing diabetes type 2-related DNA methylation variations in human peripheral blood. Hum Mol Genet 2012; 21(2): 371-83.
[http://dx.doi.org/10.1093/hmg/ddr472] [PMID: 21994764]

[130]  Milagro FI, Gómez-Abellán P, Campión J, Martínez JA, Ordovás JM, Garaulet M. CLOCK, PER2 and BMAL1 DNA methylation: association with obesity and metabolic syndrome characteristics and monounsaturated fat intake. Chronobiol Int 2012; 29(9): 1180-94.
[http://dx.doi.org/10.3109/07420528.2012.719967] [PMID: 23003921]

[131]  Zhang Y, Kent JW II, Lee A, *et al.* Fatty acid binding protein 3 (fabp3) is associated with insulin, lipids and cardiovascular phenotypes of the metabolic syndrome through epigenetic modifications in a northern european family population. BMC Med Genomics 2013; 6(1): 9.
[http://dx.doi.org/10.1186/1755-8794-6-9] [PMID: 23510163]

[132]  Rottiers V, Näär AM. MicroRNAs in metabolism and metabolic disorders. Nat Rev Mol Cell Biol 2012; 13(4): 239-50.
[http://dx.doi.org/10.1038/nrm3313] [PMID: 22436747]

[133]  Ge Q, Brichard S, Yi X, Li Q. microRNAs as a new mechanism regulating adipose tissue inflammation in obesity and as a novel therapeutic strategy in the metabolic syndrome. Journal of immunology research. 2014; 2014.

[134]  Prasun P. Mitochondrial dysfunction in metabolic syndrome. Biochim Biophys Acta Mol Basis Dis 2020; 1866(10): 165838.
[http://dx.doi.org/10.1016/j.bbadis.2020.165838] [PMID: 32428560]

[135]  Lee HK, Cho YM, Kwak SH, Lim S, Park KS, Shim EB. Mitochondrial dysfunction and metabolic syndrome—looking for environmental factors. Biochim Biophys Acta, Gen Subj 2010; 1800(3): 282-9.
[http://dx.doi.org/10.1016/j.bbagen.2009.11.010] [PMID: 19914351]

[136]  Furukawa S, Fujita T, Shimabukuro M, *et al.* Increased oxidative stress in obesity and its impact on metabolic syndrome. J Clin Invest 2004; 114(12): 1752-61.
[http://dx.doi.org/10.1172/JCI21625] [PMID: 15599400]

[137]  Henriksen EJ, Diamond-Stanic MK, Marchionne EM. Oxidative stress and the etiology of insulin resistance and type 2 diabetes. Free Radic Biol Med 2011; 51(5): 993-9.
[http://dx.doi.org/10.1016/j.freeradbiomed.2010.12.005] [PMID: 21163347]

[138]  Masschelin PM, Cox AR, Chernis N, Hartig SM. The Impact of Oxidative Stress on Adipose Tissue Energy Balance. Front Physiol 2020; 10: 1638.
[http://dx.doi.org/10.3389/fphys.2019.01638] [PMID: 32038305]

[139]  Lee BC, Lee J. Cellular and molecular players in adipose tissue inflammation in the development of obesity-induced insulin resistance. Biochim Biophys Acta Mol Basis Dis 2014; 1842(3): 446-62.
[http://dx.doi.org/10.1016/j.bbadis.2013.05.017] [PMID: 23707515]

[140]  Pagel-Langenickel I, Bao J, Pang L, Sack MN. The role of mitochondria in the pathophysiology of skeletal muscle insulin resistance. Endocr Rev 2010; 31(1): 25-51.
[http://dx.doi.org/10.1210/er.2009-0003] [PMID: 19861693]

[141]  Fex M, Nicholas LM, Vishnu N, *et al.* The pathogenetic role of β-cell mitochondria in type 2 diabetes.

J Endocrinol 2018; 236(3): R145-59.
[http://dx.doi.org/10.1530/JOE-17-0367] [PMID: 29431147]

[142] Rius-Pérez S, Torres-Cuevas I, Millán I, Ortega ÁL, Pérez S. PGC-1 α, Inflammation, and Oxidative Stress: An Integrative View in Metabolism. Oxid Med Cell Longev 2020; 2020: 1-20.
[http://dx.doi.org/10.1155/2020/1452696] [PMID: 32215168]

[143] Park KS, Lee KU, Song JH, *et al.* Peripheral blood mitochondrial DNA content is inversely correlated with insulin secretion during hyperglycemic clamp studies in healthy young men. Diabetes Res Clin Pract 2001; 52(2): 97-102.
[http://dx.doi.org/10.1016/S0168-8227(00)00237-0] [PMID: 11311963]

[144] Song J, Oh JY, Sung YA, Pak YK, Park KS, Lee HK. Peripheral blood mitochondrial DNA content is related to insulin sensitivity in offspring of type 2 diabetic patients. Diabetes Care 2001; 24(5): 865-9.
[http://dx.doi.org/10.2337/diacare.24.5.865] [PMID: 11347745]

[145] Lim S, Kim SK, Park KS, *et al.* Effect of exercise on the mitochondrial DNA content of peripheral blood in healthy women. Eur J Appl Physiol 2000; 82(5-6): 407-12.
[http://dx.doi.org/10.1007/s004210000238] [PMID: 10985594]

[146] Park KS, Chan JC, Chuang LM, *et al.* A mitochondrial DNA variant at position 16189 is associated with type 2 diabetes mellitus in Asians. Diabetologia 2008; 51(4): 602-8.
[http://dx.doi.org/10.1007/s00125-008-0933-z] [PMID: 18251004]

[147] Das S, Bennett AJ, Sovio U, *et al.* Detailed analysis of variation at and around mitochondrial position 16189 in a large Finnish cohort reveals no significant associations with early growth or metabolic phenotypes at age 31 years. J Clin Endocrinol Metab 2007; 92(8): 3219-23.
[http://dx.doi.org/10.1210/jc.2007-0702] [PMID: 17535991]

[148] 't Hart LM, Hansen T, Rietveld I, *et al.* Evidence that the mitochondrial leucyl tRNA synthetase (LARS2) gene represents a novel type 2 diabetes susceptibility gene. Diabetes 2005; 54(6): 1892-5.
[http://dx.doi.org/10.2337/diabetes.54.6.1892] [PMID: 15919814]

[149] Poekes L, Lanthier N, Leclercq IA. Brown adipose tissue: a potential target in the fight against obesity and the metabolic syndrome. Clin Sci (Lond) 2015; 129(11): 933-49.
[http://dx.doi.org/10.1042/CS20150339] [PMID: 26359253]

[150] Villarroya F, Cereijo R, Gavaldà-Navarro A, Villarroya J, Giralt M. Inflammation of brown/beige adipose tissues in obesity and metabolic disease. J Intern Med 2018; 284(5): 492-504.
[http://dx.doi.org/10.1111/joim.12803] [PMID: 29923291]

[151] Bhatt PS, Dhillo WS, Salem V. Human brown adipose tissue — function and therapeutic potential in metabolic disease. Curr Opin Pharmacol 2017; 37: 1-9.
[http://dx.doi.org/10.1016/j.coph.2017.07.004] [PMID: 28800407]

[152] da Rosa SE, Borba Neves E, Martinez EC, de Barros Sena MA, Mello DB, de Ribeiro dos Reis VMM. Comparison of brown adipose tissue activation detected by infrared thermography in men with vs without metabolic syndrome. J Therm Biol 2023; 112: 103459.
[http://dx.doi.org/10.1016/j.jtherbio.2022.103459] [PMID: 36796904]

[153] Blaton V. How is the Metabolic Syndrome Related to the Dyslipidemia? EJIFCC 2007; 18(1): 15-22.
[PMID: 29632463]

[154] Chan DC, Watts GF. Dyslipidemia in the metabolic syndrome. J Drug Eval 2004; 2(1): 3-34.
[http://dx.doi.org/10.3109/14791130410001728524]

[155] Grundy SM. Atherogenic dyslipidemia associated with metabolic syndrome and insulin resistance. Clin Cornerstone 2006; 8 (Suppl. 1): S21-7.
[http://dx.doi.org/10.1016/S1098-3597(06)80005-0] [PMID: 16903166]

# CHAPTER 9

# Modulation of Genotype-Phenotype Associations in Metabolic Syndrome

**Sinem Firtina**[1,*] and **Asli Kutlu**[2]

*¹ Department of Medical Genetics, Cerrahpasa Faculty of Medicine, Istanbul University-Cerrahpasa, Istanbul, Turkiye*

*² Department of Molecular Biology and Genetics, Faculty of Engineering and Natural Sciences, Istinye University, Istanbul, Turkiye*

**Abstract:** This chapter provides background information on the genotype-phenotype associations of MetS by highlighting the importance of genetic concepts in modulating MetS. To date, many reports on genetic and epigenetic screening of MetS within a community have been published in the literature. We also mention several reports to perform community-based screening of MetS by identifying genetic and epigenetic variants. Later, these attempts will be discussed in detail in order to explain more about the modulation of MetS from the perspectives of phenotype-genotype associations. The relationship between MetS modulation and the personalized medicine approach is emphasized more by referring to the treatment and management strategies applied in a patient-specific manner.

**Keywords:** Genetic predisposition, Modulation, Metabolic syndrome, Management strategies, Personalized medicine.

## INTRODUCTION

Our knowledge of classical genetics began with the discovery of the principle of inheritance pattern by Gregor Mendel [1]. Today, the inheritance pattern of more than 6000 monogenic disorders can be explained by Mendel's rules. However, monogenic disorders are mostly rare and the majority of human diseases cannot be explained by a single gene disorder. Most diseases, including common diseases in humans, show more complex inheritance patterns. These diseases are called complex, polygenic or multifactorial, and they are not raised from any specific genomic variant like monogenic disorders [2].

* **Corresponding author Sinem Firtina:** Department of Molecular Biology and Genetics, Faculty of Engineering and Natural Sciences, Istinye University, Istanbul, Turkiye; E-mail: asli.kutlu@istinye.edu.tr

**Hafize Uzun & Seyma Dumur (Eds.)**

Multifactorial diseases are caused by the combination of more than one genomic change, environmental factors, and lifestyle conditions. Many diseases fall into this group, including some congenital defects like cleft lip/palate, congenital heart defects, hydrocephalus, neural tube defects, and several common adult-onset diseases like Alzheimer's, asthma, Diabetes Mellitus, Parkinson's disease, Multiple Sclerosis, and Metabolic Syndrome [3]. Genetic variants that are associated with complex disorders have different features according to disease-related variants in monogenic disorders. Genetic variants in monogenic disorders have a strong effect on protein structure or expression, and these variants are rare variants, *e.g.* seen in 0.1% or less of the population (minor allele frequency (MAF) is <0.01%). In contrast to Mendelian disorders, in complex disorders, we identified common variants (MAF >0.1) that have a little effect on the protein. These variants are associated with an increased risk factor and cannot be the only reason for having a multifactorial disorder. Genetic conditions are only responsible for increased or decreased risk factors for a multifactorial disease phenotype. This situation explained by "genetic predisposition" means that a variant does not have the ability to develop a disease by itself, but with other factors such as age, gender, environmental factors, and lifestyle, the individual has a high risk of developing the variant-associated trait. People who have a genetic predisposition to a disease can delay or prevent the onset of the disease. Genetic factors have varying degrees of penetrance, some genes are highly penetrant and have a high-risk association with a particular complex disorder, while others have little effects and are associated with moderate or low-risk conditions [4].

Metabolic syndrome (MetS) is a multifactorial disorder that involves a cluster of metabolic diseases such as type II diabetes, cardiovascular diseases, and cancer. Age, gender, abdominal obesity, insulin resistance, high blood pressure, dyslipidaemia, diet, daily activity, and lifestyle conditions play a key role in MetS [5 - 7].

The aetiopathogenesis of MetS is complex, heterogeneous, and still lack full understanding, and it is controlled by interactions between genetic and environmental factors [8]. In addition to modifiable environmental factors (overeating and sedentary lifestyle), genetic susceptibility (heritability) plays an important role in the aetiology of MetS. Genetic risk factors have been associated with MetS by increasing the likelihood of phenotypes such as obesity, insulin resistance, high LDL levels, and hypertension, all of which are associated with MetS. To better understand the pathophysiology and pathogenesis of the disease, it is important to consider the central features of the metabolic syndrome (or describe how they relate to each other) [9] (Fig. 1).

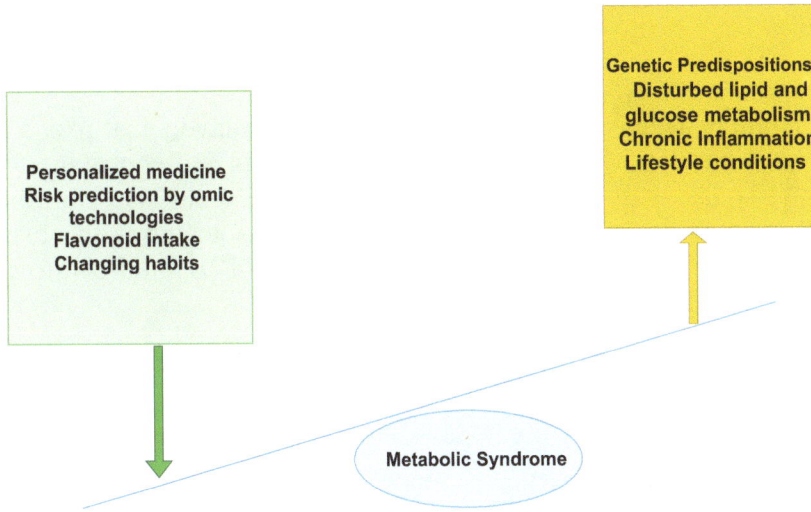

**Fig. (1).** Relationship between metabolic syndrome-related conditions and treatment or preventing strategies.

## Association between Genetic Factors and Metabolic Syndrome

Within recent decades, the focus of much research has been the investigation of genetic factors behind the phenotypic manifestations of MetS. The pathogenic mechanisms of MetS are complex by referring to the interaction between genetic and environmental factors [10]. High caloric intake and a sedentary lifestyle are among the most important triggers of chronic inflammation and insulin resistance, which are key players in the progression of MetS [11]. Insulin resistance (IR) is associated with elevations in fasting plasma glucose by enhancing the sensitivity of visceral fat cells to lipolytic hormones, thereby increasing the flux of FFA to the liver and stimulating hepatic triglyceride and apoB synthesis [12]. According to its definition, it is a fasting plasma insulin above 75% of fasting plasma IR. IR and compensatory hyperinsulinemia are linked to several abnormalities in MetS [8]. These abnormalities include dysregulated insulin signal transduction *via* the PI3K/AKT pathway, associated with serine hyperphosphorylation of the insulin receptor substrate 2 (IRS2) signalling pathway, and reduced insulin-stimulated NO production with reduced vasodilatation and prothrombotic and proatherogenic effects in atherosclerotic arteries [13, 14].

While without the presence of insulin resistance, metabolic syndrome is not diagnosed even if all other parameters are presented, more conditions must be met by patients to be diagnosed with metabolic syndrome besides IR, and these are obesity, dyslipidaemia, hypertension, and microalbuminuria. These conditions are all the key symptoms of MetS, which are mostly associated with genetic inheritance. Genetic variations in the *ADIPOQ, APOE, NR3C1, GNB3* and

*APOC3* genes have been associated with obesity, dyslipidaemia, hypertension, and IR [15, 16].

Leptin and leptin resistance (LR) are emerging as new players that play a central role in MetS. High leptin levels occur in obese patients and contribute to MetS progression [17]. LR is not only associated with obesity but also contributes to obesity and independently influences IR. Leptin is associated with obstructive sleep apnoea [18]. In addition to IR, type 2 diabetes (T2D) and cardiovascular disease (CVD) are strongly associated with MetS [19, 20].

It is estimated that 20% of patients diagnosed with MetS will develop T2DM, which is associated with the development of high-risk hypertension, accelerated atherogenesis, and subsequent CVD due to atherosclerotic stroke and coronary heart disease [13, 14]. People with CVD and T2DM have a 2-fold and 5-fold higher risk of being recognized as having MetS, respectively [21]. Till now, there has been a continuous discussion about the candidate genes regulating lipid metabolism, such as polymorphism of adiponectin, PPARγ, LPL and CETP. *GNB3, PPARG, TCF7L2, APOA5, APOC3, APOE,* and *CETP* genes have been found to be strongly associated with lipid metabolism and high risk of CVD [22]. The risk of T2D and CVD varies widely among different populations. The specific subgroups have been identified as sharing similar pathophysiology. The ongoing study on the epidemiology of MetS will also look at the high risk of type 2 diabetes (T2D) and cardiovascular disease (CVD), as well as other comorbidities (fatty liver, cholesterol gallstones, PCOS, obstructive sleep apnoea, and gout). Here, studying all these related symptoms has led to the development of treatment approaches targeting composite physiological abnormalities *via* individual criteria. To extend the definition of MetS by including certain features is the essential step to ensure the exclusion of people with individual components such as having isolated hypertension or hyperlipidaemia. There is a continuing trend to consider metabolic syndrome as a specific entity, making it possible to explore the genetic basis of susceptibility to MetS and thus to understand the underlying pathophysiology and develop treatment approaches [9].

## Modulation of Metabolic Syndrome and Risk Management

Immediately after the assessment of patients' MetS, lifestyle modifications with adopting better daily diets and more physical activity have been offered together with appropriate pharmacological management [9]. Atherosclerotic cardiovascular disease (CVD) develops in patients when certain risk conditions/factors are present. These risk factors tend to cluster and therefore respond similarly to lifestyle changes, such as reducing the risk of CVD by increasing physical activity or changing dietary patterns [9]. In many studies, risk factors for CVD have been categorised by those that cannot be changed (age, sex, family history of CVD) and those that can, including sedentary lifestyle, smoking, high cholesterol, diabetes mellitus (DM), and systolic hypertension [8].

The relationship between the components of the metabolic syndrome has been identified to better explain the pathophysiology and increased risk of CVD following the identification of patients at high risk of developing atherosclerotic CVD and type 2 diabetes. Finally, epidemiological, and pharmacological studies have been used together with the offer of lifestyle modifications and preventive treatment approaches [9, 23]. One of the most effective ways to reduce the risk of CVD is to modify the lipid profile. According to ATP III recommendations, lowering LDL is a priority because most atherogenic apoB-containing lipoproteins are found in the LDL fraction. However, many studies show that there is still a high risk of acute coronary events despite intensive therapy [24]. Lifestyle is an important determinant for MetS. A sedentary lifestyle, poor diet and smoking increase the risk of MetS by 18-30% [25]. However, changes in these habits, such as high physical activity, low carbohydrate diet, and avoidance of stress, alcohol, and smoking, significantly reduce the risk [26]. Calorie-restricted diets and supplementation control inflammation and glucose metabolism and reduce the risk of MetS by up to 50% [27].

In order to provide the necessary substrates for the methionine and folate cycles, methionine, tetrahydrofolate (THF), and vitamin B12 are supplied primarily from dietary sources. Vitamin B12 and methionine are therefore of central importance in the methionine and folate cycles. The synthesis of purine, thymidylate, and the re-methylation of homocysteine (HCY) to methionine require folate 1-carbons. It can also adenylate to S-adenosylmethionine (SAM), which is responsible for methylating the cytosine bases of DNA (important for nuclear chromatin structure), neurotransmitters, phospholipids and other protein molecules [28]. Approximately 5-7% of the general population has mild to moderate hyperhomocysteinemia (HHcy) [29]. Genetic mutations in the methyltetrahydrofolate (MTHFR) gene are known to occur in human individuals. These mutations disrupt gene function and allow the accumulation of HCY, causing HHCY. This is particularly the case when there is a deficiency of the essential B vitamins (B9, folic acid, B12 and B6). The most common variants of the MTHFR gene in humans are the primary C677T (T677T) and the secondary A1298C+C677T variants. It occurs in 10-15% of the general population [30].

## The Role of Omics-data in Personalized Medicine Approach in MetS

The genes act independently of the environmental factors involved in the aetiology of both atherogenic dyslipidaemia and the other components of the

MetS, and the variable phenotype is therefore the result of their constant interplay. Identifying the role of genetic factors in the presence of MetS-related traits, such as obesity, hypertension, and insulin resistance, is essential for understanding the multifactorial mechanisms of MetS and for patient management. The robust and high-throughput screening techniques will be used to map the genetic changes associated with MetS, identify risk factors, find new therapeutic targets, and apply early prevention strategies and gene therapy options.

Two types of studies have been used to investigate monogenic mutations that cause atherogenic dyslipidaemia and polygenic risk factors (genetic polymorphisms and environmental factors): linkage analysis (LA), candidate gene screening (CGS), whole exome or genome sequencing and association studies [31, 32]. Linkage analysis (LA) studies aim at investigating the relationship (co-segregation) between DNA polymorphisms or locations in the genome and disease. LA studies are mainly used to identify the involved gene locus and the candidate allelic variant in monogenic diseases and less so in multifactorial (polygenic) diseases with complex aetiology [31 - 33].

Candidate gene association studies (CGA) are an alternative approach to the study of polygenic diseases. Starting from the known pathogenic mechanisms of the disease in which these genes are thought to be involved, CGA analyses the association between genes and specific diseases. In MetS, genes involved in lipid metabolism, obesity, DM, lipoproteins, and hypertension have been analysed. However, this type of approach is limited by the lack of data on the highly complex pathogenic mechanisms of MetS and its components. These have provided new information on genetic inheritance in multifactorial (polygenic) diseases [31 - 33].

The need to discover new risk factors and variables will continue to increase our understanding of the MetS, along with the possibility of earlier detection for individuals and their healthcare providers to prevent the development of CVD and T2DM. Hopefully, the new findings will stimulate further research in this exciting area to reduce the risk of developing CVD and T2DM and its complications in these at-risk individuals [34].

Metabolic disorders, such as obesity, high levels of triglycerides with low high-density lipoprotein, insulin resistance, and elevated blood pressure, are considered to be a major cluster of MetS [35]. A closer look at these components has shown that they can be delayed to some extent when more details of the genetic background are available and that there is no single best therapy for the MetS [36, 37]. It is significant to remember that employing omics tools in MetS has accelerated the search for the optimal therapy for each patient rather than adapting the one-size-fits-all approach [38]. The details of personalised treatment in MetS include risk assessment with the study of MetS-related genes, especially to enable early diagnosis, molecular profiling studies to tailor the results of targeted therapy with fewer side effects or to predict the efficacy of the offered medical treatment, the use of host-microbiome interactions, and so on [39 - 41]. As noted here, the personalised medicine approach has been well-adapted to the detection, diagnosis, treatment, and management steps of MetS [42]. For the treatment and management steps of MetS, the epigenetic background of each patient must be considered as a significant factor during the assessment of the response for the applied personalised treatment since it provides control over the interactions among different cellular structures.

In the following table, the list of omics–based approaches contributing to MetS identification has been presented by short discussions of their advantages (Table **1**).

## Personalized Medicine Approach in MetS

As mentioned above, the actual causes of MetS have been attributed to both genetic and epigenetic factors. Its pathogenesis is regulated by modifiable (sedentary lifestyle, smoking, hypercholesterolaemia, diabetes mellitus (DM), and systolic hypertension) and non-modifiable (age, sex, family history of CVD) factors [8]. Mostly, the pathophysiology of MetS is described by the role of genetic factors. Together with them, the use of epidemiological and pharmacological studies, considered a collection of generalised studies, aims to determine the limits of the offered medical treatment [9, 23]. Nevertheless, it is a widely accepted idea that lifestyle modification efforts, as components of medical treatment, are key parameters to modulate MetS. They must be personalised as much as possible in order to have a lifelong and maximal impact on patient's lives. Besides the generalised offers for MetS patients, *e.g.* change of daily eating habits together with alcohol intake, effective weight control, and increase of daily physical activity, *etc.*, the identification of molecular markers, the use of data coming from clinics and omics science have highlighted the importance of adapting the personalised approach in the step of treatment and management of MetS by minimising the trial-and-error in patients' lives [43, 44].

In general, the role of personalised medicine in the MetS is defined in four steps: detection, diagnosis, treatment, and management. Among these steps, the treatment and management steps are the most promising ones for effective modulation of clinical outcomes of MetS, especially in the long term. The remaining steps, detection and diagnosis, are mainly concerned with identifying actual cases or clusters of MetS from both genetic and epigenetic perspectives.

**Table 1. Advantages of omics –based approaches in MetS.**

| Omic Technologies | Methodology | Advantages |
|---|---|---|
| Genomics | Genome-wide association study (GWAS). | Understanding the heterogeneity of MetS across different ethnicities<br>Identifying the molecular markers to clarify the aetiology and pathophysiology of MetS. |
| | Quantitative trait locus (QTL) Genetic linkage analysis. | Identification of candidate genes associated with metabolic syndrome traits, either through direct or indirect effects in MetS<br>Determination of high-priority linkage regions through mapping of multiple traits. |
| Epigenomics | CHIP or Bisulphite-method (DNA, methylation)<br>CHIP-seq (Histone modification)<br>Chromatin modifications<br>EWAS (Epigenome-wide association studies). | Enable understanding of regulatory networks and epigenetic mechanisms underlying MetS clusters<br>Tracking of the effects of environmental factors on the progression of metabolic diseases<br>Assessment of long-term disease risk, also for future generations<br>Capture daily dietary changes in RNA-mediated chromatin modifications<br>Investigation of differences in methylation profiles (understanding of the role of epigenetic variations). |
| Transcriptomics | RNA-seq. | For use in the discovery of novel biomarkers<br>Applicable for the identification of metabolic markers which may be useful as diagnostic tools in personalised medicine<br>A valid, non-invasive biological measure for the generation of information with high predictive and diagnostic content. |
| Metagenomics | Microbial sequencing. | Identify potential health problems, develop personalised treatment plans, monitor progress, and even prevent disease. |

Here, the advantages of using omics tools in MetS have accelerated the search for optimal therapy for each patient instead of adopting a one-size-fits-all concept [38]. The details of personalized treatment in MetS include the risk assessment with the study of MetS-related genes specially to enable early diagnosis, the molecular profiling studies to adjust the results of targeted treatment with fewer side effects or to predict the efficiency of the offered medical treatment, the use of host-microbiome interactions, and so on [39 - 41]. For the detection, diagnosis, treatment, and management steps of MetS, as noted here, the personalized medicine approach has been well-adapted [42]. In particular, for the treatment and management steps of MetS, the epigenetic background of the patients has to be considered as a significant parameter to evaluate the responses to the applied personalised treatment, since it is a key factor in controlling the interactions existing among different cellular structures.

So far, several treatment options for MetS have been introduced for the effective treatment of patients, but there is still a continuous search for possible MetS therapies *via* the use of natural compounds or synthetic analogues. The most important motivation for continuing to search for natural products to treat MetS is the side effects of current drugs, especially flatulence, which occurs very early in treatment and continues later [45]. Some patients have low tolerance to these side effects and it would be very challenging for them to take these common drugs for a long time. Curcumin, resveratrol, and quercetin are the best-known potential therapeutics for MetS, but they do not limit the natural treatment options for MetS [46]. Essentially, these products exert anti-diabetic effects through one or more of the following mechanisms: inhibition of glucose absorption, improvement of insulin expression to overcome its resistance, promotion of glucose utilization, regulation of carbohydrate and lipid metabolism, *etc* [47, 48]. In this context, the search for the potential targets of these natural products is based on the interactions between the molecules and the proteins, which aim to be revealed either by wet laboratory or *in silico* studies [49]. Still today, due to the lack of sufficient support based on double-blind clinical trials, the application of these natural products under the name of medical treatment is lacking.

In the following Table **2**, the list of natural products identified as potential therapeutic targets for MetS has been presented.

Table 2. The list of natural products as potential therapeutics in MetS.

| Name of Natural Products | The General Acting Mechanism in MetS | The Most Targeted Protein(s) in MetS if Exist. | Microbiome-host Interaction known |
|---|---|---|---|
| Curcumin | Anti-inflammatory, Antioxidant, Anti-diabetic. | NOS3, IL6, INS, ADIPOQ, PPAR [9]. | Yes [10] |
| Quercetin | Anti-inflammatory, Anti-diabetics, Anti-lipogenic, Anti-hyperglycaemic [11 - 13]. | SIRT1, GSK-3$\beta$, SREBP1-2 UCP-1/2/3, GLUT-4 [14]. | Yes [15] |
| Resveratrol | Anti-diabetic, Anti-obesity Anti-atherosclerosis. | SIRT1, BDNF, LXA4, AMKP, PGC-1$\alpha$, NF-$\kappa$B [16 - 19]. | Yes [20] |

*(Table 2) cont.....*

| Name of Natural Products | The General Acting Mechanism in MetS | The Most Targeted Protein(s) in MetS if Exist. | Microbiome-host Interaction known |
|---|---|---|---|
| Berberine | Anti-lipogenic, Anti-diabetic, Anti-inflammatory [21]. | PPARγ2, C/EBPα, AMPK, MAPK, GLUT-4, PPARα [22]. | Yes [23] |
| Naringenin | Antioxidant, Anti-proinflammatory. | GAL-4, PPAR γ, CPT-1, UCP-2, TNF-α, IL-6 [24 - 26]. | Yes [27, 28] |
| Capsaicin | Anti-diabetic, Anti-obesity, Antioxidant, Anti-inflammatory [29]. | PPAR-α, UCP1/2, CPT-1α, TRPV1, AMPK, GLP-1 [29]. | Yes [30, 31] |
| Emodin | Anti-inflammatory, Anti-diabetic, Antioxidant, Anti-dyslipidaemia [32 - 34]. | PPAR-γ, GLUT1, GLUT4, 11β-HSD1, ATGL, G0S2 [35, 36]. | Yes [37] |
| Gymnemic acid | Anti-diabetic [38]. | G3PDH, SGLT1, GLUT2/3/5 [39, 40]. | NA |
| Scutellarin | Anti-diabetic, Antioxidant [41]. | AMPK, SOD, GSH, Nrf2, HO-1, PI3K, AKT [41 - 44]. | NA |
| Stevioside | Antihyperglycemic Anti-obesity, anti-hyperglycaemic, anti-hypertensive, anti-hyperlipidaemic [45, 46]. | PPAR γ, SREBP-1c, C/EBP α, FAS, IRS-1, Akt, GLUT-4, AMPK [47, 48]. | Yes [49] |
| Silybin | Antioxidant, Anti-inflammatory [50]. | CYP7A1/1A2/2B6/2C8/2C9/2C19/2D6/3A4, ABCG5 and ABCG8 [51 - 53]. | NA |
| Baicalin | Anti-oxidative, Anti-dyslipidaemia, Anti-lipogenic, Anti-obesity, Anti-inflammatory, Anti-diabetic [54]. | AMPK, PPAR-α, PPAR-γ, SREBP-1, GLUT-4, DKK-1 [55]. | Yes [56] |

## CONCLUDING REMARKS

In conclusion, the main cluster of MetS is defined by the set of metabolic disorders such as obesity, high triglyceride levels with low high-density lipoprotein, insulin resistance, and increased blood pressure [25]. Molecular approaches have provided great benefits in understanding more about the genetic and epigenetic basis of these clusters. They have highlighted the importance of personalised approaches. They have also contributed to the development of therapeutic options for MetS by accelerating studies in this area [26, 27].

# REFERENCES

[1]     Stenseth NC, Andersson L, Hoekstra HE. Gregor Johann Mendel and the development of modern evolutionary biology. Proc Natl Acad Sci USA 2022; 119(30): e2201327119.
[http://dx.doi.org/10.1073/pnas.2201327119] [PMID: 35858454]

[2]     Glazier AM, Nadeau JH, Aitman TJ. Finding genes that underlie complex traits. Science 2002; 298(5602): 2345-9.
[http://dx.doi.org/10.1126/science.1076641] [PMID: 12493905]

[3]     Shi C, de Wit S, Učambarlić E, *et al.* Multifactorial Diseases of the Heart, Kidneys, Lungs, and Liver and Incident Cancer: Epidemiology and Shared Mechanisms. Cancers (Basel) 2023; 15(3): 729.
[http://dx.doi.org/10.3390/cancers15030729] [PMID: 36765688]

[4]     Forrest IS, Chaudhary K, Vy HMT, *et al.* Population-Based Penetrance of Deleterious Clinical Variants. JAMA 2022; 327(4): 350-9.
[http://dx.doi.org/10.1001/jama.2021.23686] [PMID: 35076666]

[5]     McCarthy JJ, Meyer J, Moliterno DJ, Newby LK, Rogers WJ, Topol EJ. Evidence for substantial effect modification by gender in a large-scale genetic association study of the metabolic syndrome among coronary heart disease patients. Hum Genet 2003; 114(1): 87-98.
[http://dx.doi.org/10.1007/s00439-003-1026-1] [PMID: 14557872]

[6]     Fall T, Ingelsson E. Genome-wide association studies of obesity and metabolic syndrome. Mol Cell Endocrinol 2014; 382(1): 740-57.
[http://dx.doi.org/10.1016/j.mce.2012.08.018] [PMID: 22963884]

[7]     Sookoian S, Pirola CJ. Metabolic syndrome: from the genetics to the pathophysiology. Curr Hypertens Rep 2011; 13(2): 149-57.
[http://dx.doi.org/10.1007/s11906-010-0164-9] [PMID: 20957457]

[8]     Butnariu LI, Gorduza EV, Ţarcă E, *et al.* Current Data and New Insights into the Genetic Factors of Atherogenic Dyslipidemia Associated with Metabolic Syndrome. Diagnostics (Basel) 2023; 13(14): 2348.
[http://dx.doi.org/10.3390/diagnostics13142348] [PMID: 37510094]

[9]     Nguyen HD, Kim MS. The protective effects of curcumin on metabolic syndrome and its components: *In-silico* analysis for genes, transcription factors, and microRNAs involved. Arch Biochem Biophys 2022; 727: 109326.
[http://dx.doi.org/10.1016/j.abb.2022.109326] [PMID: 35728632]

[10]   Feng W, Wang H, Zhang P, *et al.* Modulation of gut microbiota contributes to curcumin-mediated attenuation of hepatic steatosis in rats. Biochim Biophys Acta, Gen Subj 2017; 1861(7): 1801-12.
[http://dx.doi.org/10.1016/j.bbagen.2017.03.017] [PMID: 28341485]

[11]   Hosseini A, Razavi BM, Banach M, Hosseinzadeh H. Quercetin and metabolic syndrome: A review. Phytother Res 2021; 35(10): 5352-64.
[http://dx.doi.org/10.1002/ptr.7144] [PMID: 34101925]

[12]   Leiherer A, Stoemmer K, Muendlein A, *et al.* Quercetin Impacts Expression of Metabolism- and Obesity-Associated Genes in SGBS Adipocytes. Nutrients 2016; 8(5): 282.
[http://dx.doi.org/10.3390/nu8050282] [PMID: 27187453]

[13]   Rivera L, Morón R, Sánchez M, Zarzuelo A, Galisteo M. Quercetin ameliorates metabolic syndrome and improves the inflammatory status in obese Zucker rats. Obesity (Silver Spring) 2008; 16(9): 2081-7.
[http://dx.doi.org/10.1038/oby.2008.315] [PMID: 18551111]

[14] Castrejón-Tellez V, Rodríguez-Pérez J, Pérez-Torres I, *et al.* The Effect of Resveratrol and Quercetin Treatment on PPAR Mediated Uncoupling Protein (UCP-) 1, 2, and 3 Expression in Visceral White Adipose Tissue from Metabolic Syndrome Rats. Int J Mol Sci 2016; 17(7): 1069.
[http://dx.doi.org/10.3390/ijms17071069] [PMID: 27399675]

[15] Shabbir U, Rubab M, Daliri EBM, Chelliah R, Javed A, Oh DH. Curcumin, Quercetin, Catechins and Metabolic Diseases: The Role of Gut Microbiota. Nutrients 2021; 13(1): 206.
[http://dx.doi.org/10.3390/nu13010206] [PMID: 33445760]

[16] Leiro J, Arranz JA, Fraiz N, Sanmartín ML, Quezada E, Orallo F. Effect of cis-resveratrol on genes involved in nuclear factor kappa B signaling. Int Immunopharmacol 2005; 5(2): 393-406.
[http://dx.doi.org/10.1016/j.intimp.2004.10.006] [PMID: 15652768]

[17] Lagouge M, Argmann C, Gerhart-Hines Z, *et al.* Resveratrol improves mitochondrial function and protects against metabolic disease by activating SIRT1 and PGC-1alpha. Cell 2006; 127(6): 1109-22.
[http://dx.doi.org/10.1016/j.cell.2006.11.013] [PMID: 17112576]

[18] Diaz-Gerevini GT, Repossi G, Dain A, Tarres MC, Das UN, Eynard AR. Beneficial action of resveratrol: How and why? Nutrition 2016; 32(2): 174-8.
[http://dx.doi.org/10.1016/j.nut.2015.08.017] [PMID: 26706021]

[19] Elibol B, Kilic U. High Levels of SIRT1 Expression as a Protective Mechanism Against Disease-Related Conditions. Front Endocrinol (Lausanne) 2018; 9: 614.
[http://dx.doi.org/10.3389/fendo.2018.00614] [PMID: 30374331]

[20] Hu Y, Chen D, Zheng P, *et al.* The Bidirectional Interactions between Resveratrol and Gut Microbiota: An Insight into Oxidative Stress and Inflammatory Bowel Disease Therapy. BioMed Res Int 2019; 2019: 1-9.
[http://dx.doi.org/10.1155/2019/5403761] [PMID: 31179328]

[21] Och A, Och M, Nowak R, Podgórska D, Podgórski R. Berberine, a Herbal Metabolite in the Metabolic Syndrome: The Risk Factors, Course, and Consequences of the Disease. Molecules 2022; 27(4): 1351.
[http://dx.doi.org/10.3390/molecules27041351] [PMID: 35209140]

[22] Zhang Q, Xiao X, Feng K, Wang T, Li W, Yuan T, *et al.* Berberine Moderates Glucose and Lipid Metabolism through Multipathway Mechanism. Evid Based Complement Alternat Med. 2011; 2011.
[http://dx.doi.org/10.1155/2011/924851]

[23] Wang H, Zhang H, Gao Z, Zhang Q, Gu C. The mechanism of berberine alleviating metabolic disorder based on gut microbiome. Front Cell Infect Microbiol 2022; 12: 854885.
[http://dx.doi.org/10.3389/fcimb.2022.854885] [PMID: 36093200]

[24] Horiba T, Nishimura I, Nakai Y, Abe K, Sato R. Naringenin chalcone improves adipocyte functions by enhancing adiponectin production. Mol Cell Endocrinol 2010; 323(2): 208-14.
[http://dx.doi.org/10.1016/j.mce.2010.03.020] [PMID: 20363289]

[25] Cho KW, Kim YO, Andrade JE, Burgess JR, Kim YC. Dietary naringenin increases hepatic peroxisome proliferators–activated receptor α protein expression and decreases plasma triglyceride and adiposity in rats. Eur J Nutr 2011; 50(2): 81-8.
[http://dx.doi.org/10.1007/s00394-010-0117-8] [PMID: 20567977]

[26] Raja Kumar S, Mohd Ramli ES, Abdul Nasir NA, Ismail NHM, Mohd Fahami NA. Preventive Effect of Naringin on Metabolic Syndrome and Its Mechanism of Action: A Systematic Review. Evid Based Complement Alternat Med 2019; 2019: 1-11.
[http://dx.doi.org/10.1155/2019/9752826] [PMID: 30854019]

[27] Koudoufio M, Desjardins Y, Feldman F, Spahis S, Delvin E, Levy E. Insight into Polyphenol and Gut Microbiota Crosstalk: Are Their Metabolites the Key to Understand Protective Effects against Metabolic Disorders? Antioxidants 2020; 9(10): 982.
[http://dx.doi.org/10.3390/antiox9100982] [PMID: 33066106]

[28] Kasprzak-Drozd K, Oniszczuk T, Stasiak M, Oniszczuk A. Beneficial Effects of Phenolic Compounds

on Gut Microbiota and Metabolic Syndrome. Int J Mol Sci 2021; 22(7): 3715.
[http://dx.doi.org/10.3390/ijms22073715] [PMID: 33918284]

[29]   Panchal SK, Bliss E, Brown L. Capsaicin in Metabolic Syndrome. Nutrients 2018; 10(5): 630.
[http://dx.doi.org/10.3390/nu10050630] [PMID: 29772784]

[30]   Sun F, Xiong S, Zhu Z. Dietary Capsaicin Protects Cardiometabolic Organs from Dysfunction. Nutrients 2016; 8(5): 174.
[http://dx.doi.org/10.3390/nu8050174] [PMID: 27120617]

[31]   Kang C, Wang B, Kaliannan K, *et al.* Gut Microbiota Mediates the Protective Effects of Dietary Capsaicin against Chronic Low-Grade Inflammation and Associated Obesity Induced by High-Fat Diet. MBio 2017; 8(3): e00470-17.
[http://dx.doi.org/10.1128/mBio.00470-17] [PMID: 28536285]

[32]   Li L, Sheng X, Zhao S, *et al.* Nanoparticle-encapsulated emodin decreases diabetic neuropathic pain probably *via* a mechanism involving P2X3 receptor in the dorsal root ganglia. Purinergic Signal 2017; 13(4): 559-68.
[http://dx.doi.org/10.1007/s11302-017-9583-2] [PMID: 28840511]

[33]   Dong X, Fu J, Yin X, *et al.* Emodin: A Review of its Pharmacology, Toxicity and Pharmacokinetics. Phytother Res 2016; 30(8): 1207-18.
[http://dx.doi.org/10.1002/ptr.5631] [PMID: 27188216]

[34]   Wu JH, Lv CF, Guo XJ, *et al.* Low Dose of Emodin Inhibits Hypercholesterolemia in a Rat Model of High Cholesterol. Med Sci Monit 2021; 27: e929346.
[http://dx.doi.org/10.12659/MSM.929346] [PMID: 34257265]

[35]   Feng Y, Huang S, Dou W, *et al.* Emodin, a natural product, selectively inhibits 11β-hydroxysteroid dehydrogenase type 1 and ameliorates metabolic disorder in diet-induced obese mice. Br J Pharmacol 2010; 161(1): 113-26.
[http://dx.doi.org/10.1111/j.1476-5381.2010.00826.x] [PMID: 20718744]

[36]   Lu K, Xie S, Han S, *et al.* Preparation of a nano emodin transfersome and study on its anti-obesity mechanism in adipose tissue of diet-induced obese rats. J Transl Med 2014; 12(1): 72.
[http://dx.doi.org/10.1186/1479-5876-12-72] [PMID: 24641917]

[37]   Mabwi HA, Lee HJ, Hitayezu E, *et al.* Emodin modulates gut microbial community and triggers intestinal immunity. J Sci Food Agric 2023; 103(3): 1273-82.
[http://dx.doi.org/10.1002/jsfa.12221] [PMID: 36088620]

[38]   Leach MJ. Gymnema sylvestre for diabetes mellitus: a systematic review. J Altern Complement Med 2007; 13(9): 977-83.
[http://dx.doi.org/10.1089/acm.2006.6387] [PMID: 18047444]

[39]   Scow JS, Tavakkolizadeh A, Zheng Y, Sarr MG. Acute "adaptation" by the small intestinal enterocyte: A posttranscriptional mechanism involving apical translocation of nutrient transporters. Surgery 2011; 149(5): 601-5.
[http://dx.doi.org/10.1016/j.surg.2011.02.001] [PMID: 21496564]

[40]   Ishijima S, Takashima T, Ikemura T, Izutani Y. Gymnemic acid interacts with mammalian glycerol--phosphate dehydrogenase. Mol Cell Biochem 2008; 310(1-2): 203-8.
[http://dx.doi.org/10.1007/s11010-007-9681-5] [PMID: 18080092]

[41]   Gao L, Tang H, Zeng Q, Tang T, Chen M, Pu P. The anti-insulin resistance effect of scutellarin may be related to antioxidant stress and AMPKα activation in diabetic mice. Obes Res Clin Pract 2020; 14(4): 368-74.
[http://dx.doi.org/10.1016/j.orcp.2020.06.005] [PMID: 32631803]

[42]   Wang Y, Fan X, Fan B, *et al.* Scutellarin Reduce the Homocysteine Level and Alleviate Liver Injury in Type 2 Diabetes Model. Front Pharmacol 2020; 11: 538407.
[http://dx.doi.org/10.3389/fphar.2020.538407] [PMID: 33362535]

[43] Fan H, Ma X, Lin P, *et al.* Scutellarin Prevents Nonalcoholic Fatty Liver Disease (NAFLD) and Hyperlipidemia *via* PI3K/AKT-Dependent Activation of Nuclear Factor (Erythroid-Derived 2)-Like 2 (Nrf2) in Rats. Med Sci Monit 2017; 23: 5599-612.
[http://dx.doi.org/10.12659/MSM.907530] [PMID: 29172017]

[44] Yang LL, Xiao N, Liu J, *et al.* Differential regulation of baicalin and scutellarin on AMPK and Akt in promoting adipose cell glucose disposal. Biochim Biophys Acta Mol Basis Dis 2017; 1863(2): 598-606.
[http://dx.doi.org/10.1016/j.bbadis.2016.11.024] [PMID: 27903431]

[45] Carrera-Lanestosa A, Moguel-Ordóñez Y, Segura-Campos M. *Stevia rebaudiana* Bertoni: A Natural Alternative for Treating Diseases Associated with Metabolic Syndrome. J Med Food 2017; 20(10): 933-43.
[http://dx.doi.org/10.1089/jmf.2016.0171] [PMID: 28792778]

[46] Dyrskog SEU, Jeppesen PB, Colombo M, Abudula R, Hermansen K. Preventive effects of a soy-based diet supplemented with stevioside on the development of the metabolic syndrome and type 2 diabetes in Zucker diabetic fatty rats. Metabolism 2005; 54(9): 1181-8.
[http://dx.doi.org/10.1016/j.metabol.2005.03.026] [PMID: 16125530]

[47] Deenadayalan A, Subramanian V, Paramasivan V, *et al.* Stevioside Attenuates Insulin Resistance in Skeletal Muscle by Facilitating IR/IRS-1/Akt/GLUT 4 Signaling Pathways: An In Vivo and In Silico Approach. Molecules 2021; 26(24): 7689.
[http://dx.doi.org/10.3390/molecules26247689] [PMID: 34946771]

[48] Park M, Baek H, Han JY, Lee HJ. Stevioside Enhances the Anti-Adipogenic Effect and β-Oxidation by Activating AMPK in 3T3-L1 Cells and Epididymal Adipose Tissues of *db/db* Mice. Cells 2022; 11(7): 1076.
[http://dx.doi.org/10.3390/cells11071076] [PMID: 35406641]

[49] Gatea F, Sârbu I, Vamanu E. *In Vitro* Modulatory Effect of Stevioside, as a Partial Sugar Replacer in Sweeteners, on Human Child Microbiota. Microorganisms 2021; 9(3): 590.
[http://dx.doi.org/10.3390/microorganisms9030590] [PMID: 33805627]

[50] Poruba M, Matušková Z, Kazdová L, *et al.* Positive effects of different drug forms of silybin in the treatment of metabolic syndrome. Physiol Res 2015; 64 (Suppl. 4): S507-12.
[http://dx.doi.org/10.33549/physiolres.933235] [PMID: 26681080]

[51] Xie Y, Zhang D, Zhang J, Yuan J. Metabolism, Transport and Drug–Drug Interactions of Silymarin. Molecules 2019; 24(20): 3693.
[http://dx.doi.org/10.3390/molecules24203693] [PMID: 31615114]

[52] Brantley SJ, Oberlies NH, Kroll DJ, Paine MF. Two flavonolignans from milk thistle (Silybum marianum) inhibit CYP2C9-mediated warfarin metabolism at clinically achievable concentrations. J Pharmacol Exp Ther 2010; 332(3): 1081-7.
[http://dx.doi.org/10.1124/jpet.109.161927] [PMID: 19934397]

[53] Poruba M, Kazdová L, Oliyarnyk O, *et al.* Improvement bioavailability of silymarin ameliorates severe dyslipidemia associated with metabolic syndrome. Xenobiotica 2015; 45(9): 751-6.
[http://dx.doi.org/10.3109/00498254.2015.1010633] [PMID: 26068528]

[54] Fang P, Yu M, Shi M, Bo P, Gu X, Zhang Z. Baicalin and its aglycone: a novel approach for treatment of metabolic disorders. Pharmacol Rep 2020; 72(1): 13-23.
[http://dx.doi.org/10.1007/s43440-019-00024-x] [PMID: 32016847]

[55] Baradaran Rahimi V, Askari VR, Hosseinzadeh H. Promising influences of *Scutellaria baicalensis* and its two active constituents, baicalin, and baicalein, against metabolic syndrome: A review. Phytother Res 2021; 35(7): 3558-74.
[http://dx.doi.org/10.1002/ptr.7046] [PMID: 33590943]

[56]   Lin Y, Wang ZY, Wang MJ, *et al.* Baicalin attenuate diet-induced metabolic syndrome by improving abnormal metabolism and gut microbiota. Eur J Pharmacol 2022; 925: 174996.
[http://dx.doi.org/10.1016/j.ejphar.2022.174996] [PMID: 35513018]

CHAPTER 10

# The Interplay between Metabolic Syndrome and Behavior

**Shimaa Mohammad Yousof**[1,*] and **Asmaa Seddek**[2]

[1] *Department of Medical Physiology, Faculty of Medicine in Rabigh, King Abdulaziz University, Rabigh, Saudi Arabia*

[2] *Department of Medical Physiology, Faculty of Medicine, Suez Canal University, Ismailia, Egypt*

**Abstract:** Metabolic syndrome (MetS) indicates a cluster of symptoms that include abdominal obesity, dyslipidemia, hypertension, and hyperglycemia. Even though the etiology of MetS is unknown, it is thought to be multifaceted, with a complicated interaction between genetic predisposition and significant changes in lifestyle behavior, such as physical inactivity, high carbohydrate diets, and alcohol and cigarette use. The circadian system regulates many physiological and behavioral rhythms, which operate on 24-hour cycles. Circadian rhythm disturbances are also seen in various clinical disorders linked to adipose tissue functioning. In addition, night-shift employees who have their rest-activity cycles reversed are more likely to acquire MetS. Individuals with MetS experienced more seasonal variations in mood and behavior, with obesity being a substantial risk factor for metabolic syndrome. MetS has been linked to psychiatric illnesses. In those diagnosed with major depressive disorder and bipolar disorder in adulthood, disruption to biological rhythms (sleep, social activities, and eating habits) has been linked to essential components of MetS. MetS and its components were found to be connected to a higher risk of suicide. It is apparent that the relationship between behavior and MetS is bidirectional, and each component can affect the other. Awareness of MetS-related factors can aid in identifying high-risk individuals and implementing disease prevention and control strategies, as well as lifestyle adjustments. Lifestyle modification can help to improve the MetS condition and behavior.

**Keywords:** Behavior, MetS, Metabolic syndrome, Microbiota, Psychiatric illness, Stress.

## INTRODUCTION

Metabolic syndrome (MetS), also known as pattern X or insulin resistance pattern, is a cluster of disorders that include hypertension, insulin resistance, central obesity, and atherogenic dyslipidemia. MetS, a major health concern in

---

* **Corresponding author Shimaa Mohammad Yousof:** Department of Medical Physiology, Faculty of Medicine in Rabigh, King Abdulaziz University, Rabigh, Saudi Arabia; E-mail: drshimaay@gmail.com

**Hafize Uzun & Seyma Dumur (Eds.)**

Westernized ultramodern countries, was formerly a major clinical practice difficulty [1].

The International Diabetes Federation (IDF) estimates that a quarter of the world's adult population has MetS, and the observed prevalence of MetS in the National Health and Nutrition Examination Survey (NHANES) was 5% among the normal weighted subjects, 22% among the over-weighted, and 60% among the obese [2].

The diagnostic criteria for MetS include a minimum of three out of five medical problems, including abdominal obesity, hypertension, higher fasting plasma glucose, increased serum triglycerides, and reduced levels of high-density lipoprotein (HDL) cholesterol [3]. The IDF considers the abdominal circumference and two other factors, and the World Health Organization (WHO) uses the waist/hip ratio, the presence of type 2 diabetes mellitus (DM) or insulin resistance, micro-albuminuria, hypertension, and triglycerides [4].

Comorbidity and multimorbidity are clinical challenges. Combinations of several diseases are common. Cardiovascular risk factors such as high blood pressure, obesity, atherogenic dyslipidemia, diabetes, alcohol and drug misuse, smoking, and inadequate physical exercise are associated with schizophrenia and major depressive disorders. Stress, psychodrama, hypercortisolemia, and immune function abnormalities may cause MetS and other mental illnesses [5].

Extensive research has been conducted to investigate the pathophysiological processes behind MetS. Findings consistently point to two prominent factors: the intake of fast food that is high in calories and poor in fiber, and insufficient levels of physical exercise. These factors have emerged as primary contributors to the development and progression of MetS [6, 7]. The examination of genetic predispositions has also been the subject of investigation, however, it has been shown that they exert only a marginal influence [8]. The primary factor contributing to this phenomenon was a shift in dietary patterns, as individuals transitioned from consuming mostly natural and unprocessed foods to adopting a diet characterized by elevated levels of fat, sugar, and salt [9, 10].

There is a growing body of research indicating that the disparities between our "Paleolithic genome" and our present-day "modern" food and lifestyle may play a significant part in the prevailing pandemics of obesity, hypertension, diabetes, atherosclerosis, and other manifestations of MetS [11]. It was found that self-discipline measures had a significant influence on physical activity levels among individuals diagnosed with diabetes or MetS, mostly *via* the enhancement of self-efficacy [12].

MetS alters cognitive function and emotional memory by enhancing hippocampal neuroinflammation [13]. The comorbidity and relation between MetS and psychiatric diseases have been reported [14 - 19]. According to reports, the co-occurrence of MetS and mental conditions such as anxiety, depression, insomnia, and cognitive dysfunction significantly contribute to medical expenses. Consequently, it is imperative to acknowledge and address these factors [20 - 23]. The results obtained from genome association studies have mostly concentrated on investigating the potential relationship between the management of circadian rhythms, maintenance of glucose balance, and the signaling of melatonin in the pancreas. These findings provide support for the hypothesis that disturbances in the peripheral circadian clocks might potentially contribute to metabolic dysregulation in human beings. Furthermore, alterations in cortisol release in relation to the timing of eating and fasting during circadian misalignment have the potential to induce insulin resistance. During periods of alertness, leptin levels are found to be lower, whereas during sleep, they are seen to be greater, Fig. (**1**) [24].

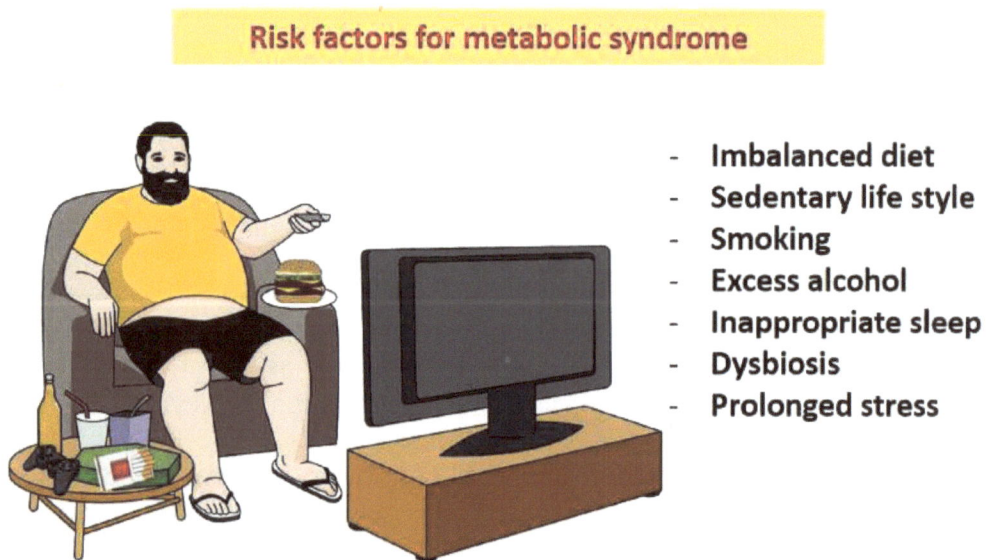

Fig. (1). Displaying the risk factors for metabolic syndrome.

A growing body of research supports the role of gut bacteria in human metabolism [25]. The gut microbiota (GM) and its effects on human health have garnered attention in recent years, particularly in the context of metabolic disorders (obesity, type 2 diabetes, dyslipidemia), which increase the risk of heart disease and deaths in industrialized nations. Diet is unquestionably one of the key elements influencing the microbiota [26 - 28].

From the aforementioned, it is evident that MetS is a syndrome with multifactorial predisposing factors, multiple effects on different body systems, and different mechanisms by which it interacts and interferes with body function. This chapter will focus on the relationship between behavior and MetS. We will discuss the behaviors that can predispose or result from MetS. Moreover, we will discuss the mechanisms underlying this relationship between behavior and MetS.

## The Relationship between MetS and Neuropsychiatric Diseases

A growing body of research suggests that persons exhibiting symptoms of depression and anxiety may have interfering effects that contribute to the development of MetS. Despite the considerable amount of research conducted on MetS, there is a shortage of information about its correlation with anxiety and depression throughout the broader community. Furthermore, the available studies on this topic have produced inconsistent and contradictory results. Previous studies have examined the correlation between MetS and anxiety [29]. However, several authors have found a weak or inconclusive link between individuals with pressure and the presence of MetS [30, 31]. Moreover, many studies have shown a favorable correlation between MetS and depression [32, 33]. Nevertheless, contrasting findings have also been reported, suggesting no significant link [29, 31].

A study by Skilton *et al.* published in 2007 reported that MetS was correlated with a higher incidence of depression, but not anxiety, in both males and females. The quantity of components associated with the MetS exhibited a positive correlation with escalating levels of depression, whereas anxiety levels did not demonstrate a similar relationship. The observed correlation between MetS and depressive symptoms remained statistically significant even after controlling for variables such as age, smoking status, socioeconomic factors, and lifestyle. The association was seen across various body mass index categories and was unaffected by anxiety [32]. In a systematic review by Tang *et al.*, published in 2017, they found 18 cross-sectional and two cohort studies. Anxiety was positively associated with MetS in cross-sectional studies (OR 1.07, 95% CI 1.01–1.12), with moderate heterogeneity ($I2 = 45.7\%$, P = 0.018). Anxiety and MetS were not significantly associated in the two cohort studies [34].

MetS and depression overlay. Predominantly, lifestyle factors, such as lack of sleep, low activity, lack of inspiration, changes in eating patterns, and sedentary lifestyle, all have an essential effect on depression [35, 36] and the MetS. Concurrently, health-related behavioral factors, such as poor diet, neurogenic hyperphagia, bulimia, and smoking, are also common risk factors for depression and MetS [37]. Similar to patients with MetS, individuals with major depressive disease display chronic, low-grade inflammation characterized by high circulating cytokine profiles. Statistical Manual of Mental Disorders (DSM) criteria for major depressive disorders have reported significant elevations in plasma levels of chemo-attractant protein (CCL2), interferon alpha, Interleukin (IL) IL-1,2,6,8,12, tumor necrosis factor and C-reactive protein [38 - 42]. A comprehensive analysis was conducted on a collection of cross-sectional and prospective cohort studies to examine the correlation between depression and MetS [43]. The findings of this analysis revealed the presence of a bidirectional link between depression and MetS [44]. Vancampfort *et al.* 2014 performed a meta-analysis to elucidate the incidence and associated factors of MetS among individuals diagnosed with major depressive disorder. Among the 5,531 persons included in the study who were diagnosed with depression, it was found that 30.5% of them satisfied the criteria for MetS.

Moreover, when comparing these people with control groups matched for age and gender, it was shown that patients diagnosed with severe depressive disorder had a greater frequency of MetS, with an odds ratio of 1.54 [43, 45]. The aforementioned results were reproduced in a subsequent meta-analysis conducted in 2015 by the same research team. In this study, it was determined that the combined prevalence of MetS among individuals with severe mental illness was 32.6% (95% CI: 30.8-34.3%; N = 198; n = 52,678) [43, 46]. Moreover, based on the analysis of the 2009-2010 National Health and Nutrition Examination Survey, Rethorst *et al.* demonstrated that a significant proportion of persons experiencing depression, namely over 29%, had heightened levels of C-reactive protein. Additionally, it was shown that 41% of these patients fulfilled the criteria for MetS. Significantly, their findings revealed a positive correlation between heightened inflammation levels and increased likelihood of obesity [47]. Meng *et al.* (2012) found that depression is associated with an elevated chance of developing high blood pressure [48]. In addition, the concurrent existence of a comorbid mental condition, such as depression, can hinder the effective treatment of diabetes by reducing medication adherence. Blood glucose testing and insulin injection are only two instances that exemplify how investigations and therapies may be impeded by conditions such as injection anxiety. Individuals with mental health disorders are also shown to be less likely to seek assistance [49].

According to many studies, individuals diagnosed with type 2 diabetes (T2D) had a higher likelihood, ranging from 1.2 to 2.3 times, of experiencing symptoms of depression compared to the general population. In contrast to individuals of average weight, obese individuals with favorable metabolic profiles exhibit a modestly elevated susceptibility to depression. However, when obesity is accompanied by metabolic disorders such as hypertension, dyslipidemia, elevated C-reactive protein levels, or insulin resistance, the likelihood of experiencing depression becomes more pronounced [47, 50, 51]. The impact of MetS on behavior is summarized is Fig. (**2**).

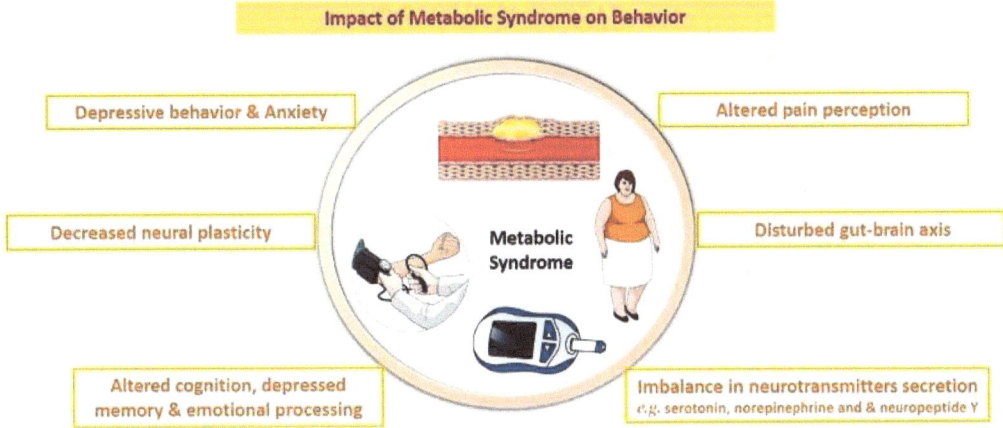

**Fig. (2).** Displaying impact of metabolic syndrome on behavior.

Hypometabolism-induced amyloid-β (Aβ) accumulation in the brain leads to neurological diseases, including Alzheimer's disease [52]. Proton magnetic resonance spectroscopy has also demonstrated that cognitive decline is associated with metabolite concentration changes in brain areas in neurometabolic illnesses such as multiple sclerosis, brain tumors, epilepsy, Alzheimer's disease, and dementia. Previous reports suggest that metabolic brain diseases may alter cognition-related brain areas. Neuronal alterations and cognitive decline occur in most metabolic illnesses [53 - 55].

## Suggested Mechanisms Beyond the Relationship between MetS and Mental Illnesses

MetS syndrome changes the equilibrium of neurotransmitters such as acetylcholine, monoamine, and GABA, resulting in anxiety, memory deficiency, and sleep disorder [35, 56]. Moreover, extensive evidence supports the notion that oxidative stress significantly contributes to the development of mental diseases and MetS [37]. The simultaneous presence of brain diseases and MetS may intensify the incidence of oxidative stress and lipid peroxidation, resulting in more pronounced brain damage and dysfunction. However, compounds with antioxidant properties have the ability to mitigate these detrimental consequences [57 - 59].

The potential association between obesity and depression has been suggested to include the neuroimmune route. The enlargement of adipocytes has the potential to induce the generation of molecules involved in inflammation, thereby impacting the central nervous system and leading to neuroinflammation in the hypothalamus and hippocampus [60]. Research findings indicate that a high-fat diet (HFD) might result in prolonged increases in cytokines and chemokines, which may induce neuroplastic changes in specific brain regions. Consequently, this can contribute to mood disturbances and weight gain. Previous research has shown that the hypothalamic-pituitary-adrenal (HPA) axis plays a significant role in the pathophysiology of depression.

Furthermore, empirical investigations have shown that individuals diagnosed with major depressive disorder (MDD) have heightened activity within the HPA axis. Existing research indicates that the HPA axis potentially impacts the body weight of persons experiencing stress *via* regulating cortisol levels [61]. Collectively, these findings shed light on the shared mechanisms between obesity, an element of MetS, and depression.

Research has shown a relationship between psychiatric problems and diabetes, wherein the presence of one condition may intensify the severity or impact of the other. Obesity and depression may be linked through neuroimmune pathways. Inflammatory mediators from adipocyte hypertrophy may produce hypothalamic and hippocampal neuroinflammation. Depression has been shown to impede the secretion of islet cells, decreasing the capacity to control glucose metabolism among individuals diagnosed with diabetes [45, 60, 62]. Consequently, this may significantly elevate the likelihood of mortality [63]. Moreover, diabetes induces a persistent state of inflammation inside the body. Similarly, depression is characterized by a chronic, low-grade inflammatory response. Patients diagnosed with depression frequently exhibit increased levels of proinflammatory cytokines. The severity of depression is correlated with the concentration of peripheral inflammatory markers. Furthermore, the administration of exogenous proinflammatory cytokines has been shown to induce depressive symptoms. It has been observed that antidepressant medications can partially mitigate inflammatory markers in individuals with depression [60].

## Metabolic Syndrome and Stress

The research suggests that stress positively correlates with the inclination of rats and humans to engage in tasks for desirable food. Furthermore, other studies indicate that stress enhances the activation of neurons in the brain's motivation and reward circuits when individuals are exposed to appetizing meals. Significantly, the consumption of tasty meals due to stress may manifest in individuals who, while reducing their overall calorie intake, experience stress [64, 65]. Chronic psychological stress has serious health consequences and is a growing public health issue. Stress may directly affect metabolic (*e.g.*, diabetes) and mental (*e.g.*, depression) disorders but also indirectly affect diet and exercise. Stress may cause binge eating and disinhibition in controlled eaters and cause dietary relapse [65]. Everyday problems have been reported to increase snacking under free-living settings, as found in experimental stress. Other stressors like student exams and workload have been linked to higher fat, energy, or unhealthy food intake. Some people are stress-eaters, whereas others decrease calorie intake due to psychological stress. The physiological cause of stress-eating and individual variance in stress-related food consumption is unclear; however, glucocorticoid and insulin signaling (*e.g.*, diabetes) may be involved [64 - 66]. A 2-year, randomized, controlled clinical trial examined the impact of significant life events on exercise adherence rates in individuals. Regardless of exercise condition, those reporting 3 or 4 considerable life events had worse maintenance phase exercise adherence than those reporting 0 or 1 [67].

Obesity, MetS, and Psychological stress are happening in a "toxic" food environment that encourages overeating, especially calorie-dense, nutrient-poor meals. Obesity, psychological stress, and eating habits are intricately linked. Because prolonged stress-induced glucocorticoid release promotes abdominal fat accumulation, stress affects abdominal obesity the most. Stress-induced eating, similarly triggered by glucocorticoids, favors sugary, fatty, and highly appealing meals. Acute and persistent stress may overlap and worsen stress eating. Chronically stressed people consume more than under acute stress, Fig. (**3**) [68 - 71].

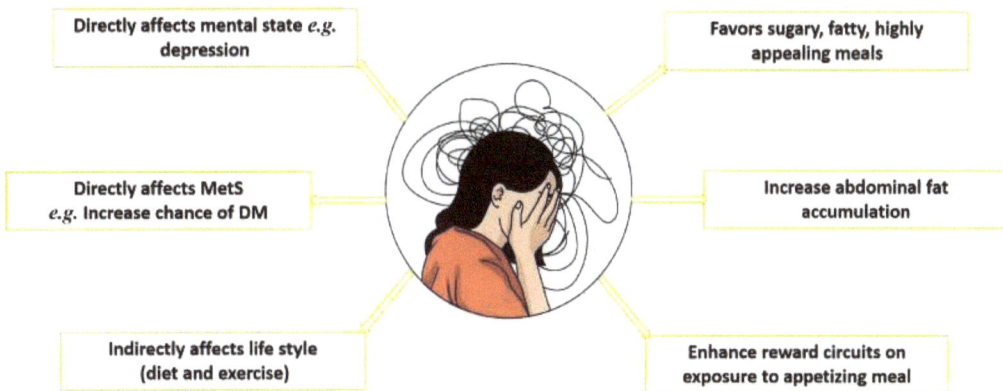

**Effects of Prolonged Stress on Metabolic Syndrome & Behavior**

Directly affects mental state *e.g.* depression

Favors sugary, fatty, highly appealing meals

Directly affects MetS *e.g.* Increase chance of DM

Increase abdominal fat accumulation

Indirectly affects life style (diet and exercise)

Enhance reward circuits on exposure to appetizing meal

**Fig. (3).** Effect of chronic prolonged stress on the metabolic syndrome and behavior.

The chance of developing diabetes mellitus is heightened by stress, particularly in persons who are overweight, since psychological stress has an impact on insulin requirements. Chronic stress has been shown to potentially contribute to atherosclerosis development, characterized by plaque accumulation in the arteries [72, 73]. This risk may be further exacerbated when chronic stress is coupled with a high-fat diet and a sedentary lifestyle. The association between stressful life events and mental disease has a greater magnitude than the association seen with medical or physical illness. The association between stress and mental disorders has the most pronounced correlation in mental diseases, followed by depression and schizophrenia [72, 74].

The sympathoadrenal system and the hypothalamic-pituitary-adrenocortical (HPA) axis are activated in response to stress. Defense responses include the release of catecholamines, withdrawal of vagal activity, secretion of cortisol, and activation of the renin-angiotensin system [75, 76]. Additionally, the defeat reaction serves as a stimulant for cortisol production. These effects offer roles that assist the person in coping with short-term stress. When individuals experience recurrent stress, they may struggle to adapt and manage effectively. This may result in a deficiency in their capacity to regulate the stress response or an insufficient reaction to stress, leading to the activation of compensating mechanisms [72, 75]. Consequently, the allostatic load, which refers to the cumulative physiological burden of stress, may become overwhelming. In turn, the adaptive processes that were initially intended to help individuals cope with stress may become maladaptive [75].

A previous meta-analysis regarding the perceived stress and the development of MetS found that the included studies provide evidence supporting a correlation between perceived stress and distress and the emergence of MetS. The analysis revealed that marital stress, particularly among women, was a significant risk factor. Evidence supports the notion that perceived stress experienced in the workplace is a risk factor for MetS. The study proposed that a strong sense of justice in the workplace serves as a protective element for males. Still, job pressure was identified as contributing to MetS among women, Fig. (**3**) [77].

*DM= diabetes mellitus.

## Metabolic Syndrome and Cognitive Function

Numerous research have provided evidence indicating that Type 2 Diabetes Mellitus (T2DM) exacerbates dysfunction in the amygdala, resulting in adverse effects on emotional, depressive, and social behaviors, as well as impairments in learning abilities [78, 79]. A decline in cognitive functioning, namely in the form of impaired episodic memory, has been also seen in association with a weakened link between the amygdala and prefrontal cortex [80, 81]. Additionally, heightened dopamine receptor activation, diminished dopamine neurotransmission, and elevated levels of anxiety have been implicated in this phenomenon [82, 83].

MetS has been shown to disrupt the metabolism of many neurotransmitters, including serotonin, norepinephrine, substance P, somatostatin, and neuropeptide Y. This disruption therefore leads to changes in cognitive function, appetite regulation, pain sensitivity, and the manifestation of depressive symptoms. The observed effects include a decrease in amygdala neuronal projections towards the medial preoptic area [84], atrophy of neuronal dendrites, and a reduction in dendritic spines inside the hippocampus and pyramidal neurons of the prefrontal cortex. These locations are known to be involved in the process of memory formation [84, 85]. Many studies have suggested that MetS induces impaired declarative memory, anxiety, and poor attention [86, 87]. Diabetes reduces neuronal connectivity in limbic brain regions related to emotional processing [88]. Several studies have reported that diabetes causes decreasing sizes of the prefrontal cortex, amygdala, and hippocampus, which is accompanied by cognitive deterioration [7, 89 - 92].

The study revealed that persons with Type 2 Diabetes Mellitus (T2DM) had decreased neutral declarative and emotional memory, which may be attributed to aberrant microvascular structure in the white matter [87]. The Mets has been shown to contribute to the development of insulin resistance, disrupted production of neurotransmitters, impaired brain synaptic plasticity, and increased accumulation of free fatty acids in the amygdala and hippocampus. These effects are believed to occur *via* many processes. The observed abnormalities in the connection between the amygdala and hippocampus are associated with cognitive decline, compromised memory consolidation, and modifications in emotional processing. These alterations have been implicated in the development of dementia and neuropsychiatric illnesses, as well as mood disturbances and anxiety. The link between the amygdala and hippocampus has an impact on the storage of both emotional and neutral memories. The presence of heightened amygdala activity in individuals with metabolic disorders has been shown to be correlated with impaired psychomotor coordination and reduced motor speed. Mets cause insulin resistance, imbalanced secretion of neurotransmitters, poor neural synaptic plasticity, and accumulation of free fatty acids through various mechanisms in the amygdala and hippocampus. These metabolic alterations in amygdala and hippocampus connectivity are linked to cognitive decline, impaired memory consolidation, and changes in emotional processing, leading to dementia and neuropsychiatric disorders, mood changes, and anxiety. Emotional memory, as well as neutral memory consolidation, are influenced by amygdala-hippocampus connectivity. Amygdala activity in MetS is associated with poor psychomotor coordination and motor speed [93]. The clinical observation revealed a correlation between hyperglycemia and a decrease in grey matter density, as well as a reduction in glucose metabolism in the frontotemporal areas of the brain [94, 95]. Furthermore, the presence of elevated inflammation and endothelial dysfunction in individuals with MetS poses a heightened risk for neurological deterioration [96]. The presence of inflammation in individuals with obesity has been implicated as a potential factor contributing to cognitive deterioration [96]. The potential consequences include progressive deterioration of the blood-brain barrier, chronic hypo perfusion, impairment of both big and small cerebral arteries, and, over time, the manifestation of cognitive decline and dementia [97, 98].

The signaling of insulin in the brain is of utmost importance in controlling several physiological processes, including food intake, body weight, reproduction, learning, and memory. Insulin injection *via* the nasal route has been shown to enhance working memory in both human and animal subjects [99]. Additionally, insulin delivery directly into the hippocampus has been shown to improve spatial working memory that relies on the hippocampus [100]. Furthermore, it has been shown that the expression of InsR mRNA and protein is elevated in the CA1 area of the hippocampus after the completion of a spatial memory task, indicating a potential enhancement of neuronal insulin sensitivity during short-term memory formation [101]. On the other hand, the impairment of insulin signaling renders neurons more susceptible to metabolic stress, hence expediting the onset of neuronal dysfunction [102]. Impaired insulin signaling has been linked to a decline in cognitive function and the onset of dementia, namely Alzheimer's disease (AD) [103]. A decrease in InsR expression and cerebrospinal fluid (CSF) insulin levels has been seen in individuals with diabetes and Alzheimer's disease (AD), which is linked to worse cognitive function [104]. Notably, the brain areas exhibiting the most concentrated presence of InsR, namely the hippocampus and temporal lobe, coincide with the primary sites of neurodegeneration seen in Alzheimer's disease (AD). Hence, the presence of altered insulin signaling resulting from insulin resistance (IR) may significantly influence cognitive deterioration and the progression of Alzheimer's disease (AD) [101].

## Metabolic Syndrome and Biological Rhythms

Circadian rhythms include a range of physiological, mental, and behavioral alterations that adhere to a 24-hour cycle. Despite the inherent ability of cells to generate independent rhythms, the suprachiasmatic nuclei (SCN) located in the hypothalamus serve as a circadian pacemaker, synchronizing rhythms across many tissues by environmental signals such as exposure to light, patterns of food, physical activity, and prevailing weather conditions [105].

Nobel laureates Jeffrey C. Hall, Michael Rosbash, and Michael W. Young have elucidated the molecular processes underlying the relationship between circadian misalignment and the development of MetS. A collection of genes exhibiting rhythmic diurnal expression was identified, including not just involvement in the regulation of metabolic pathways and hormone release, but also the regulation of several other physiological processes [106, 107]. Metabolic illnesses have been linked to internal desynchronization, characterized by the asynchronous expression of circadian genes across several organs [108, 109]. In addition to the circadian regulation of transcription factors and enzyme expression, the molecular clock also coordinates the secretion of many hormones and peptides, including melatonin, insulin, glucagon, glucagon-like-peptide-1, cortisol, leptin, adiponectin, ghrelin, and the Renin-Angiotensin-Aldosterone System (RAAS). The aforementioned hormones serve as the principal regulators of metabolism, so establishing a crucial link between the circadian rhythm and metabolic activities [110 - 115].

The primary factors that often disturb the circadian rhythm in humans are insufficient sleep, shiftwork, improper scheduling of meals, heightened nighttime activity, and the use of electronic gadgets before sleep [116, 117]. Sleep and circadian rhythms have a crucial role in the synchronization of hormones and lipids that are involved in energy metabolism. These include leptin, ghrelin, glucose, insulin, glucocorticoids, catecholamines, fatty acids, and triglycerides [56, 118 - 121]. The findings of the study indicate that there is a correlation between short-term circadian misalignment in humans and an increase in postprandial blood glucose levels. The observed outcomes may have arisen due to a reduction in pancreatic β-cell compensation or insulin sensitivity [121]. Based on the existing epidemiological research, it seems that those who are exposed to night-shift employment may face an elevated likelihood of encountering weight gain, obesity, hypertension, and an augmented vulnerability to the onset of cardiovascular disease. Although the mechanisms behind these effects are not yet fully understood, the use of animal models offers a beneficial methodology for identifying potential targets that might be targeted and utilized to mitigate the negative health consequences associated with long-term shift work [122].

**Microbiota, Metabolic Syndrome, and Behavior**

Due to its considerable metabolic activity, GM is occasionally referred to as "a new virtual metabolic organ" [123]. Previous studies have shown that GM is necessary for nutrient absorption and digestion [124], the synthesis of short-chain fatty acids (SCFAs), amines, phenols/indoles, and sulfurous compounds [125], the synthesis of vitamins B and K, the bioavailability of minerals, and the metabolism of bile acids [126]. GM works to restore damaged epithelial barriers and aids the preservation of gut health by preserving cell-cell junctions [127].

The gut-brain axis, which connects the central nervous system and gut bacteria, has garnered attention recently. Gut microbiota is increasingly linked to gastrointestinal and extragastrointestinal illnesses. Today's common mental diseases, like anxiety and depression, are connected to gut dysbiosis and inflammation [128]. Dysbiosis is defined as a raised or lowered F/B ratio, with the former identifying with obesity and the latter being associated with inflammatory bowel disease [129, 130]. Compared to healthy people, T2D patients have lower amounts of Firmicutes and Clostridia and a lower F/B ratio and phyla [131]. Changes in glucose homeostasis are connected with changes in gut microbiota and are clearly linked to type 2 diabetes mellitus (T2DM) and its consequences. Understanding the link between gut microbiota and metabolic risk provides the potential to identify vulnerable individuals and allow for early-targeted intervention. F/B ratios have a negative and substantial relationship with plasma glucose levels. Although some studies show that obese people with MetS have a greater F/B ratio than "healthy obese" individuals, this is not definitive and requires additional investigation [25, 131]. Obesity increases the likelihood of depression and anxiety, and vice versa, according to epidemiological research. These connections between illnesses with likely distinct causes reveal common pathogenic pathways. Gut microbiota mediates environmental stressors (*e.g.*, nutrition, lifestyle) and host physiology, therefore its modification may explain the cross-link between those illnesses. Westernized diets are a key cause of obesity, which promotes dysbiotic drift in the gut microbiota and obesity-related problems [132].

The interactions between a host and the microbiome are highly complex. Many elements of metabolism are influenced by intestinal bacteria, which produce metabolic precursors to hormones and neurotransmitters or directly produce active metabolites [133, 134]. Furthermore, the vagus nerve connects the enteric nervous system (ENS) to the central nervous system (CNS), providing a direct neurochemical conduit for microbial-promoted signals in the gastrointestinal tract to be transmitted to the brain [134]. The microbiota has been shown to influence the hypothalamic-pituitary-adrenal (HPA) axis, indicating a bidirectional connection between the gut and the brain that notably impacts the host's behavior [134]. According to Borre *et al.* (2014), the implications of microbiota on outcomes may be contingent upon a certain period of development and might result in persistent neurological consequences. Microbial signals can potentially influence brain function in many instances [135]. According to Clarke *et al.*

(2013), a recovery of anxiety-like behavior in adult germ-free (GF) mice to levels comparable to specific pathogen-free SPF mice is seen when they are recolonized with microbiota [136]. This finding suggests that there is a continuous communication between the microbiome and the central nervous system (CNS) that regulates anxiety behavior. The GF animals had reduced levels of brain-derived neurotrophic factor (BDNF), serotonin (5-HT; 5-hydroxytryptamine), and specific serotonin receptors, such as 5HT1A, inside the amygdala and hippocampus. The host chemicals in question are not retrieved upon the recolonization of adult mice, suggesting that the microbiota plays a role in programming certain traits during fetal development or adolescence [134, 136, 137].

Microbial endocrinology refers to the scientific study of the ability of microorganisms to produce and detect neurochemicals, which may originate from either the bacteria themselves or the host organism in which they reside. Microbial endocrinology is an interdisciplinary field that intersects the domains of microbiology and neurobiology [133]. Alterations in the gut microbiota can influence brain insulin signaling and metabolite levels, resulting in altered neurobehavior [138]. Soto *et al.*, 2018 studied the effect of diet-induced obesity on mice. They discovered that this diet causes higher levels of depression and anxiety. This was linked to reduced insulin signaling and increased amygdala and nucleus accumbens inflammation. Treatment with metronidazole or vancomycin lowered inflammation, boosted insulin signaling in the brain, and minimized anxiety and depression symptoms. These outcomes were linked to alterations in tryptophan, GABA, BDNF, amino acids, and various acylcarnitines levels [138]. According to research, it was shown that including fermentable dietary fiber in mice's diet protects against diet-induced obesity and metabolic abnormalities [139]. The study observed that the inclusion of oligofructose, which is classified as a dietary fiber, resulted in a decrease in hyperphagia, weight gain, and elevated blood triglyceride levels in rats that were subjected to a high-fat diet for 35 days. GLP-1 and GLP-2 were identified in fiber metabolites resulting from microbial fermentation, as determined by the scientists. The hormone GLP-1 has been shown to enhance glucose metabolism, whereas GLP-2 has been shown to promote the integrity of tight junctions in the intestinal epithelium [139]. Additional research has shown that laboratory-bred mice, who are genetically predisposed to obesity and hepatosteatosis, exhibited a reversal of these traits after three generations of breeding inside a controlled laboratory environment [140, 141]. Based on these findings, it can be inferred that the microbiome is significantly influenced by food and environment, suggesting that some microbial profiles may exhibit a heightened susceptibility to metabolic disease [142].

Homeostatic intestinal hormones and immune cells have diurnal fluxes [143]. Recent evidence suggests that gut microbiota alterations induced by antibiotic depletion or long-term HFD usage may disturb local circadian rhythms, promoting weight gain and abnormal glucose fluxes [143 - 145]. Leone *et al.* found that germ-free mice's brains and livers did not change their diurnal clock gene expression with a low-fat or high-fat diet. However, conventionally reared mice with intact microbiota maintained homeostatic clock gene expression on a low-fat diet [145]. High-fat, high-sugar diets disrupted these mice's circadian rhythms. Several gut bacteria species spontaneously change in abundance over the day [145]. Previous studies [146, 147] show that ad libitum eating, especially after an HFD, disrupts liver clock genes that regulate free fatty acid intake and release. Thaiss *et al.* found that intestinal mucus barrier thickness cycles with microbial richness in mice. These data suggest gut microbiota circadian rhythm disturbance may induce barrier problems [142, 148].

## Behavioral Therapy for Metabolic Syndrome & Its Comorbid Conditions

Lifestyle changes, including diet, exercise, and education, are the main ways to prevent and cure MetS. This suggests that lifestyle changes may reduce MetS risk factors. Several studies on MetS risk factors and lifestyle therapies support this approach. Lifestyle risk factors such as inadequate nutrition, excessive alcohol intake, lack of exercise, smoking, and extended sedentary behavior have been linked to metabolic syndrome [149, 150]. Recent research indicates that the length of sleep is a lifestyle component that may significantly predict an individual's health state [151, 152].

Behavioral therapy-based lifestyle change is the most effective MetS treatment [154]. Contemporary lifestyle modification therapy combines diet and exercise recommendations with behavioral and cognitive techniques [155]. Interventions might be provided in person, in groups, or individually [153]. In order to evaluate the efficacy of cognitive-behavioral therapy (CBT) in modifying lifestyle behaviors among patients diagnosed with MetS, a randomized controlled trial was undertaken. 76 MetS patients participated in this clinical trial, which included a follow-up period of 18 months. Among the participants, 45 were assigned to the experimental group and 31 to the control group. A psychologist delivered the CBT intervention in a group setting. The findings of the study revealed that the participants in the experimental group exhibited improved adherence to the Mediterranean diet, assertiveness, and reduced anger [154].

People with diabetes must follow lifestyle changes, self-management, and prescriptions to control their condition. Mental health issues make diabetes management harder for patients. Diabetes is one of the most cognitively and behaviorally demanding chronic medical illnesses, making it more likely to create mental health issues. Patients with diabetes often have problems such as schizophrenia, anxiety, and depression. An interprofessional team can diagnose and treat mental health concerns as part of diabetes care [49].

Psychotherapy and medicine have been shown to help alleviate depression among individuals with metabolic diseases. The prompt and efficient management of depression may significantly enhance the overall well-being of individuals with metabolic illnesses, reduce their psychological distress, and facilitate the successful treatment of metabolic conditions [155].

## CONCLUSION

Many ailments occur concurrently. High blood pressure, obesity, atherogenic dyslipidemia, diabetes, alcohol and drug misuse, smoking, and inactivity are associated with schizophrenia and severe depression. Stress, psychodrama, hypercortisolemia, and immunological dysfunction may cause metabolic syndrome and other mental illnesses.

Poor exercise and high-calorie/low-fiber fast food are the major causes of metabolic syndrome, according to studies. Genetic predispositions were also examined but found unimportant. Switching from a natural to a high-fat, sugar, and salt diet was the major cause for MetS. Growing data supports gut bacteria's metabolic role. Metabolic issues have highlighted the gut microbiota and its health effects. The major circadian rhythm disruptors in humans include lack of sleep, shiftwork, improper meal timing, increased nocturnal activity, and pre-bedtime electronic device use. Epidemiological study suggests that night-shift employees may be more prone to develop obesity, hypertension, and heart disease. Animal models may assist in lessening the health hazards of continuous shift work by identifying targets. MetS may cause amygdala and hippocampal insulin resistance, neurotransmitter imbalance, neural plasticity, and free fatty acid accumulation. Metabolic alterations in the amygdala-hippocampal link affect cognitive decline, memory consolidation, and emotional processing, producing dementia, neuropsychiatric illnesses, mood disorders, and anxiety. Modern lifestyle modification therapy integrates food and exercise with behavioral and cognitive methods to treat MetS properly. Individual, group, or in-person interventions are possible.

## REFERENCES

[1]    Steckhan N, Hohmann CD, Kessler C, Dobos G, Michalsen A, Cramer H. Effects of different dietary approaches on inflammatory markers in patients with metabolic syndrome: A systematic review and meta-analysis. Nutrition 2016; 32(3): 338-48.
[http://dx.doi.org/10.1016/j.nut.2015.09.010] [PMID: 26706026]

[2]     Kaur J. A comprehensive review on metabolic syndrome. Cardiol Res Pract 2014; 2014: 1-21.
        [http://dx.doi.org/10.1155/2014/943162] [PMID: 24711954]

[3]     Amihăesei IC, Chelaru L. Metabolic syndrome a widespread threatening condition; risk factors,
        diagnostic criteria, therapeutic options, prevention and controversies: an overview. Rev Med Chir Soc
        Med Nat Iasi 2014; 118(4): 896-900.
        [PMID: 25581945]

[4]     World Health O. Diet, nutrition and the prevention of chronic diseases : report of a joint WHO/FAO
        expert consultation, Geneva, 28 January - 1 February 2002. Geneva: World Health Organization;
        2003.

[5]     Lasić D, Bevanda M, Bošnjak N, Uglešić B, Glavina T, Franić T. Metabolic syndrome and
        inflammation markers in patients with schizophrenia and recurrent depressive disorder. Psychiatr
        Danub 2014; 26(3): 214-9.
        [PMID: 25191767]

[6]     Barrès R, Zierath JR. The role of diet and exercise in the transgenerational epigenetic landscape of
        T2DM. Nat Rev Endocrinol 2016; 12(8): 441-51.
        [http://dx.doi.org/10.1038/nrendo.2016.87] [PMID: 27312865]

[7]     Bird SR, Hawley JA. Update on the effects of physical activity on insulin sensitivity in humans. BMJ
        Open Sport Exerc Med 2017; 2(1): e000143.
        [http://dx.doi.org/10.1136/bmjsem-2016-000143] [PMID: 28879026]

[8]     Locke AE, Kahali B, Berndt SI, *et al.* Genetic studies of body mass index yield new insights for
        obesity biology. Nature 2015; 518(7538): 197-206.
        [http://dx.doi.org/10.1038/nature14177] [PMID: 25673413]

[9]     Lovegrove JA, Gitau R. Nutrigenetics and CVD: what does the future hold? Proc Nutr Soc 2008;
        67(2): 206-13.
        [http://dx.doi.org/10.1017/S0029665108007040] [PMID: 18412994]

[10]    Phillips C. Nutrigenetics and metabolic disease: current status and implications for personalised
        nutrition. Nutrients 2013; 5(1): 32-57.
        [http://dx.doi.org/10.3390/nu5010032] [PMID: 23306188]

[11]    Kuneš J, Zicha J. The interaction of genetic and environmental factors in the etiology of hypertension.
        Physiol Res 2009; 58 (Suppl. 2): S33-42.
        [http://dx.doi.org/10.33549/physiolres.931913] [PMID: 20131935]

[12]    Olson EA, Mullen SP, Raine LB, Kramer AF, Hillman CH, McAuley E. Integrated Social- and
        Neurocognitive Model of Physical Activity Behavior in Older Adults with Metabolic Disease. Ann
        Behav Med 2017; 51(2): 272-81.
        [http://dx.doi.org/10.1007/s12160-016-9850-4] [PMID: 27844326]

[13]    Mohamadi Y, Jameie SB, Akbari M, *et al.* Hyperglycemia decreased medial amygdala projections to
        medial preoptic area in experimental model of Diabetes Mellitus. Acta Med Iran 2015; 53(1): 1-7.
        [PMID: 25597598]

[14]    Belmaker RH, Agam G. Major depressive disorder. N Engl J Med 2008; 358(1): 55-68.
        [http://dx.doi.org/10.1056/NEJMra073096] [PMID: 18172175]

[15]    Murphy A, Chin-Dusting JP, Sviridov D, Woollard K. The anti inflammatory effects of high density
        lipoproteins. Curr Med Chem 2009; 16(6): 667-75.
        [http://dx.doi.org/10.2174/092986709787458425] [PMID: 19199930]

[16]    Valkanova V, Ebmeier KP. Vascular risk factors and depression in later life: a systematic review and
        meta-analysis. Biol Psychiatry 2013; 73(5): 406-13.
        [http://dx.doi.org/10.1016/j.biopsych.2012.10.028] [PMID: 23237315]

[17]    Taylor WD, Aizenstein HJ, Alexopoulos GS. The vascular depression hypothesis: mechanisms linking

vascular disease with depression. Mol Psychiatry 2013; 18(9): 963-74.
[http://dx.doi.org/10.1038/mp.2013.20] [PMID: 23439482]

[18]   Kivimäki M, Shipley MJ, Batty GD, *et al.* Long-term inflammation increases risk of common mental disorder: a cohort study. Mol Psychiatry 2014; 19(2): 149-50.
[http://dx.doi.org/10.1038/mp.2013.35] [PMID: 23568195]

[19]   Virtanen M, Shipley MJ, Batty GD, *et al.* Interleukin-6 as a predictor of symptom resolution in psychological distress: a cohort study. Psychol Med 2015; 45(10): 2137-44.
[http://dx.doi.org/10.1017/S0033291715000070] [PMID: 25697833]

[20]   Heiskanen TH, Niskanen LK, Hintikka JJ, *et al.* Metabolic syndrome and depression: a cross-sectional analysis. J Clin Psychiatry 2006; 67(9): 1422-7.
[http://dx.doi.org/10.4088/JCP.v67n0913] [PMID: 17017829]

[21]   Dunbar JA, Reddy P, Davis-Lameloise N, *et al.* Depression: an important comorbidity with metabolic syndrome in a general population. Diabetes Care 2008; 31(12): 2368-73.
[http://dx.doi.org/10.2337/dc08-0175] [PMID: 18835951]

[22]   Santos M, Kövari E, Hof PR, Gold G, Bouras C, Giannakopoulos P. The impact of vascular burden on late-life depression. Brain Res Brain Res Rev 2009; 62(1): 19-32.
[http://dx.doi.org/10.1016/j.brainresrev.2009.08.003] [PMID: 19744522]

[23]   Yates KF, Sweat V, Yau PL, Turchiano MM, Convit A. Impact of metabolic syndrome on cognition and brain: a selected review of the literature. Arterioscler Thromb Vasc Biol 2012; 32(9): 2060-7.
[http://dx.doi.org/10.1161/ATVBAHA.112.252759] [PMID: 22895667]

[24]   Ohnon W, Wattanathorn J, Thukham-mee W, Muchimapura S, Wannanon P, Tong-un T. The Combined Extract of Black Sticky Rice and Dill Improves Poststroke Cognitive Impairment in Metabolic Syndrome Condition. Oxid Med Cell Longev 2019; 2019: 1-19.
[http://dx.doi.org/10.1155/2019/9089035] [PMID: 30937145]

[25]   Cunningham AL, Stephens JW, Harris DA. Gut microbiota influence in type 2 diabetes mellitus (T2DM). Gut Pathog 2021; 13(1): 50.
[http://dx.doi.org/10.1186/s13099-021-00446-0] [PMID: 34362432]

[26]   Moszak M, Szulińska M, Bogdański P. You Are What You Eat—The Relationship between Diet, Microbiota, and Metabolic Disorders—A Review. Nutrients 2020; 12(4): 1096.
[http://dx.doi.org/10.3390/nu12041096] [PMID: 32326604]

[27]   Liou AP, Paziuk M, Luevano JM Jr, Machineni S, Turnbaugh PJ, Kaplan LM. Conserved shifts in the gut microbiota due to gastric bypass reduce host weight and adiposity. Sci Transl Med 2013; 5(178): 178ra41.
[http://dx.doi.org/10.1126/scitranslmed.3005687] [PMID: 23536013]

[28]   David LA, Maurice CF, Carmody RN, *et al.* Diet rapidly and reproducibly alters the human gut microbiome. Nature 2014; 505(7484): 559-63.
[http://dx.doi.org/10.1038/nature12820] [PMID: 24336217]

[29]   Akbari H, Sarrafzadegan N, Aria H, Garaei AG, Zakeri H. Anxiety but not depression is associated with metabolic syndrome: The Isfahan Healthy Heart Program. Journal of research in medical sciences : the official journal of Isfahan University of Medical Sciences. 2017; 22: 90.

[30]   Goldbacher EM, Matthews KA. Are psychological characteristics related to risk of the metabolic syndrome? A review of the literature. Annals of behavioral medicine : a publication of the Society of Behavioral Medicine. 2007; 34(3): 240-52.

[31]   Hildrum B, Mykletun A, Midthjell K, Ismail K, Dahl AA. No association of depression and anxiety with the metabolic syndrome: the Norwegian HUNT study. Acta Psychiatr Scand 2009; 120(1): 14-22.
[http://dx.doi.org/10.1111/j.1600-0447.2008.01315.x] [PMID: 19120047]

[32]   Skilton MR, Moulin P, Terra JL, Bonnet F. Associations between anxiety, depression, and the metabolic syndrome. Biol Psychiatry 2007; 62(11): 1251-7.

[http://dx.doi.org/10.1016/j.biopsych.2007.01.012] [PMID: 17553465]

[33]    Rhee SJ, Kim EY, Kim SH, *et al.* Subjective depressive symptoms and metabolic syndrome among the general population. Prog Neuropsychopharmacol Biol Psychiatry 2014; 54: 223-30.
[http://dx.doi.org/10.1016/j.pnpbp.2014.06.006] [PMID: 24975752]

[34]    Tang F, Wang G, Lian Y. Association between anxiety and metabolic syndrome: A systematic review and meta-analysis of epidemiological studies. Psychoneuroendocrinology 2017; 77: 112-21.
[http://dx.doi.org/10.1016/j.psyneuen.2016.11.025] [PMID: 28027497]

[35]    Lopresti AL, Hood SD, Drummond PD. A review of lifestyle factors that contribute to important pathways associated with major depression: Diet, sleep and exercise. J Affect Disord 2013; 148(1): 12-27.
[http://dx.doi.org/10.1016/j.jad.2013.01.014] [PMID: 23415826]

[36]    Butnoriene J, Steibliene V, Saudargiene A, Bunevicius A. Does presence of metabolic syndrome impact anxiety and depressive disorder screening results in middle aged and elderly individuals? A population based study. BMC Psychiatry 2018; 18(1): 5.
[http://dx.doi.org/10.1186/s12888-017-1576-8] [PMID: 29310620]

[37]    Marazziti D, Rutigliano G, Baroni S, Landi P, Dell'Osso L. Metabolic syndrome and major depression. CNS Spectr 2014; 19(4): 293-304.
[http://dx.doi.org/10.1017/S1092852913000667] [PMID: 24103843]

[38]    Yau PL, Javier D, Tsui W, *et al.* Emotional and neutral declarative memory impairments and associated white matter microstructural abnormalities in adults with type 2 diabetes. Psychiatry Res Neuroimaging 2009; 174(3): 223-30.
[http://dx.doi.org/10.1016/j.pscychresns.2009.04.016] [PMID: 19906514]

[39]    Sellbom KS, Gunstad J. Cognitive function and decline in obesity. J Alzheimers Dis 2012; 30(s2) (Suppl. 2): S89-95.
[http://dx.doi.org/10.3233/JAD-2011-111073] [PMID: 22258511]

[40]    Francis H, Stevenson R. The longer-term impacts of Western diet on human cognition and the brain. Appetite 2013; 63: 119-28.
[http://dx.doi.org/10.1016/j.appet.2012.12.018] [PMID: 23291218]

[41]    Wium-Andersen MK, Ørsted DD, Nielsen SF, Nordestgaard BG. Elevated C-reactive protein levels, psychological distress, and depression in 73, 131 individuals. JAMA Psychiatry 2013; 70(2): 176-84.
[http://dx.doi.org/10.1001/2013.jamapsychiatry.102] [PMID: 23266538]

[42]    Flores-Gómez AA, de Jesús Gomez-Villalobos M, Flores G. Consequences of diabetes mellitus on neuronal connectivity in limbic regions. Synapse 2019; 73(3): e22082.
[http://dx.doi.org/10.1002/syn.22082] [PMID: 30457679]

[43]    Al-Khatib Y, Akhtar MA, Kanawati MA, Mucheke R, Mahfouz M, Al-Nufoury M. Depression and Metabolic Syndrome: A Narrative Review. Cureus 2022; 14(2): e22153.
[http://dx.doi.org/10.7759/cureus.22153] [PMID: 35308733]

[44]    Pan A, Keum N, Okereke OI, *et al.* Bidirectional association between depression and metabolic syndrome: a systematic review and meta-analysis of epidemiological studies. Diabetes Care 2012; 35(5): 1171-80.
[http://dx.doi.org/10.2337/dc11-2055] [PMID: 22517938]

[45]    Vancampfort D, Correll CU, Wampers M, *et al.* Metabolic syndrome and metabolic abnormalities in patients with major depressive disorder: a meta-analysis of prevalences and moderating variables. Psychol Med 2014; 44(10): 2017-28.
[http://dx.doi.org/10.1017/S0033291713002778] [PMID: 24262678]

[46]    Vancampfort D, Stubbs B, Mitchell AJ, *et al.* Risk of metabolic syndrome and its components in people with schizophrenia and related psychotic disorders, bipolar disorder and major depressive disorder: a systematic review and meta-analysis. World Psychiatry 2015; 14(3): 339-47.

[http://dx.doi.org/10.1002/wps.20252] [PMID: 26407790]

[47]   Rethorst CD, Bernstein I, Trivedi MH. Inflammation, obesity, and metabolic syndrome in depression: analysis of the 2009-2010 National Health and Nutrition Examination Survey (NHANES). J Clin Psychiatry 2014; 75(12): e1428-32.
[http://dx.doi.org/10.4088/JCP.14m09009] [PMID: 25551239]

[48]   Meng L, Chen D, Yang Y, Zheng Y, Hui R. Depression increases the risk of hypertension incidence. J Hypertens 2012; 30(5): 842-51.
[http://dx.doi.org/10.1097/HJH.0b013e32835080b7] [PMID: 22343537]

[49]   Akhaury K, Chaware S. Relation Between Diabetes and Psychiatric Disorders. Cureus 2022; 14(10): e30733.
[PMID: 36447711]

[50]   Mezuk B, Eaton WW, Albrecht S, Golden SH. Depression and type 2 diabetes over the lifespan: a meta-analysis. Diabetes Care 2008; 31(12): 2383-90.
[http://dx.doi.org/10.2337/dc08-0985] [PMID: 19033418]

[51]   Knol MJ, Twisk JWR, Beekman ATF, Heine RJ, Snoek FJ, Pouwer F. Depression as a risk factor for the onset of type 2 diabetes mellitus. A meta-analysis. Diabetologia 2006; 49(5): 837-45.
[http://dx.doi.org/10.1007/s00125-006-0159-x] [PMID: 16520921]

[52]   Bero AW, Yan P, Roh JH, *et al.* Neuronal activity regulates the regional vulnerability to amyloid-β deposition. Nat Neurosci 2011; 14(6): 750-6.
[http://dx.doi.org/10.1038/nn.2801] [PMID: 21532579]

[53]   Kordestani-Moghadam P, Assari S, Nouriyengejeh S, Mohammadipour F, Pourabbasi A. Cognitive Impairments and Associated Structural Brain Changes in Metabolic Syndrome and Implications of Neurocognitive Intervention. J Obes Metab Syndr 2020; 29(3): 174-9.
[http://dx.doi.org/10.7570/jomes20021] [PMID: 32747611]

[54]   Kantarci K, Jicha GA. Development of $^1$H MRS biomarkers for tracking early predementia Alzheimer disease. Neurology 2019; 92(5): 209-10.
[http://dx.doi.org/10.1212/WNL.0000000000006839] [PMID: 30610092]

[55]   Carlin D, Babourina-Brooks B, Davies NP, Wilson M, Peet AC. Variation of $T_2$ relaxation times in pediatric brain tumors and their effect on metabolite quantification. J Magn Reson Imaging 2019; 49(1): 195-203.
[http://dx.doi.org/10.1002/jmri.26054] [PMID: 29697883]

[56]   Mahjoub S, Masrour-Roudsari J. Role of oxidative stress in pathogenesis of metabolic syndrome. Caspian J Intern Med 2012; 3(1): 386-96.
[PMID: 26557292]

[57]   Trottier MD, Naaz A, Li Y, Fraker PJ. Enhancement of hematopoiesis and lymphopoiesis in diet-induced obese mice. Proc Natl Acad Sci USA 2012; 109(20): 7622-9.
[http://dx.doi.org/10.1073/pnas.1205129109] [PMID: 22538809]

[58]   Ryder E, Diez-Ewald M, Mosquera J, *et al.* Association of obesity with leukocyte count in obese individuals without metabolic syndrome. Diabetes Metab Syndr 2014; 8(4): 197-204.
[http://dx.doi.org/10.1016/j.dsx.2014.09.002] [PMID: 25301008]

[59]   Yoshimura A, Ohnishi S, Orito C, *et al.* Association of peripheral total and differential leukocyte counts with obesity-related complications in young adults. Obes Facts 2015; 8(1): 1-16.
[http://dx.doi.org/10.1159/000373881] [PMID: 25765160]

[60]   Qiu W, Cai X, Zheng C, Qiu S, Ke H, Huang Y. Update on the Relationship Between Depression and Neuroendocrine Metabolism. Front Neurosci 2021; 15: 728810.
[http://dx.doi.org/10.3389/fnins.2021.728810] [PMID: 34531719]

[61]   Fu X, Wang Y, Zhao F, *et al.* Shared biological mechanisms of depression and obesity: focus on adipokines and lipokines. Aging (Albany NY) 2023; 15(12): 5917-50.

[http://dx.doi.org/10.18632/aging.204847] [PMID: 37387537]

[62]   Vancassel S, Capuron L, Castanon N. Brain Kynurenine and BH4 Pathways: Relevance to the Pathophysiology and Treatment of Inflammation-Driven Depressive Symptoms. Front Neurosci 2018; 12: 499.
[http://dx.doi.org/10.3389/fnins.2018.00499] [PMID: 30140200]

[63]   Felger JC. The Role of Dopamine in Inflammation-Associated Depression: Mechanisms and Therapeutic Implications. Curr Top Behav Neurosci 2016; 31: 199-219.
[http://dx.doi.org/10.1007/7854_2016_13] [PMID: 27225499]

[64]   Dallman MF, Pecoraro N, Akana SF, *et al.* Chronic stress and obesity: A new view of "comfort food". Proc Natl Acad Sci USA 2003; 100(20): 11696-701.
[http://dx.doi.org/10.1073/pnas.1934666100] [PMID: 12975524]

[65]   Laugero KD, Falcon LM, Tucker KL. Relationship between perceived stress and dietary and activity patterns in older adults participating in the Boston Puerto Rican Health Study. Appetite 2011; 56(1): 194-204.
[http://dx.doi.org/10.1016/j.appet.2010.11.001] [PMID: 21070827]

[66]   Dallman MF, Warne JP, Foster MT, Pecoraro NC. Glucocorticoids and insulin both modulate caloric intake through actions on the brain. J Physiol 2007; 583(2): 431-6.
[http://dx.doi.org/10.1113/jphysiol.2007.136051] [PMID: 17556388]

[67]   Oman RF, King AC. The effect of life events and exercise program format on the adoption and maintenance of exercise behavior. Health psychology : official journal of the Division of Health Psychology, American Psychological Association. 2000;19(6):605-12.
[http://dx.doi.org/10.1037/0278-6133.19.6.605]

[68]   Tomiyama AJ, Dallman MF, Epel ES. Comfort food is comforting to those most stressed: Evidence of the chronic stress response network in high stress women. Psychoneuroendocrinology 2011; 36(10): 1513-9.
[http://dx.doi.org/10.1016/j.psyneuen.2011.04.005] [PMID: 21906885]

[69]   Wadden TA, Brownell KD, Foster GD. Obesity: Responding to the global epidemic. J Consult Clin Psychol 2002; 70(3): 510-25.
[http://dx.doi.org/10.1037/0022-006X.70.3.510] [PMID: 12090366]

[70]   Dallman MF, Akana SF, Laugero KD, *et al.* A spoonful of sugar: feedback signals of energy stores and corticosterone regulate responses to chronic stress. Physiol Behav 2003; 79(1): 3-12.
[http://dx.doi.org/10.1016/S0031-9384(03)00100-8] [PMID: 12818705]

[71]   Leigh Gibson E. Emotional influences on food choice: Sensory, physiological and psychological pathways. Physiol Behav 2006; 89(1): 53-61.
[http://dx.doi.org/10.1016/j.physbeh.2006.01.024] [PMID: 16545403]

[72]   Salleh MR. Life event, stress and illness. Malays J Med Sci 2008; 15(4): 9-18.
[PMID: 22589633]

[73]   Yaribeygi H, Panahi Y, Sahraei H, Johnston TP, Sahebkar A. The impact of stress on body function: A review. EXCLI J 2017; 16: 1057-72.
[PMID: 28900385]

[74]   Bass C, Akhras F. Physical and psychological correlates of severe heart disease in men. Psychol Med 1987; 17(3): 695-703.
[http://dx.doi.org/10.1017/S0033291700025939] [PMID: 3628630]

[75]   Hjemdahl P. Stress and the metabolic syndrome: an interesting but enigmatic association. Circulation 2002; 106(21): 2634-6.
[http://dx.doi.org/10.1161/01.CIR.0000041502.43564.79] [PMID: 12438283]

[76]   Herman JP, McKlveen JM, Ghosal S, *et al.* Regulation of the Hypothalamic-Pituitary-Adrenocortical Stress Response. Compr Physiol 2016; 6(2): 603-21.

[http://dx.doi.org/10.1002/cphy.c150015] [PMID: 27065163]

[77]     Bergmann N, Gyntelberg F, Faber J. The appraisal of chronic stress and the development of the metabolic syndrome: a systematic review of prospective cohort studies. Endocr Connect 2014; 3(2): R55-80.
[http://dx.doi.org/10.1530/EC-14-0031] [PMID: 24743684]

[78]     van Bussel FCG, Backes WH, Hofman PAM, *et al.* Increased GABA concentrations in type 2 diabetes mellitus are related to lower cognitive functioning. Medicine (Baltimore) 2016; 95(36): e4803.
[http://dx.doi.org/10.1097/MD.0000000000004803] [PMID: 27603392]

[79]     Thielen JW, Gancheva S, Hong D, *et al.* Higher GABA concentration in the medial prefrontal cortex of Type 2 diabetes patients is associated with episodic memory dysfunction. Hum Brain Mapp 2019; 40(14): 4287-95.
[http://dx.doi.org/10.1002/hbm.24702] [PMID: 31264324]

[80]     Sanchez-Vega L, Juárez I, De Jesus Gomez-Villalobos M, Flores G. Cerebrolysin reverses hippocampal neural atrophy in a mice model of diabetes mellitus type 1. Synapse 2015; 69(6): 326-35.
[http://dx.doi.org/10.1002/syn.21819] [PMID: 25851531]

[81]     Xia W, Luo Y, Chen YC, *et al.* Disrupted functional connectivity of the amygdala is associated with depressive mood in type 2 diabetes patients. J Affect Disord 2018; 228: 207-15.
[http://dx.doi.org/10.1016/j.jad.2017.12.012] [PMID: 29272791]

[82]     Xiang Q, Zhang J, Li CY, *et al.* Insulin resistance-induced hyperglycemia decreased the activation of Akt/CREB in hippocampus neurons: Molecular evidence for mechanism of diabetes-induced cognitive dysfunction. Neuropeptides 2015; 54: 9-15.
[http://dx.doi.org/10.1016/j.npep.2015.08.009] [PMID: 26344332]

[83]     Choi Y, Min HY, Hwang J, Jo YH. *Magel2* knockdown in hypothalamic POMC neurons innervating the medial amygdala reduces susceptibility to diet-induced obesity. Life Sci Alliance 2022; 5(11): e202201502.
[http://dx.doi.org/10.26508/lsa.202201502] [PMID: 36007929]

[84]     Siervo M, Harrison SL, Jagger C, Robinson L, Stephan BCM. Metabolic syndrome and longitudinal changes in cognitive function: a systematic review and meta-analysis. J Alzheimers Dis 2014; 41(1): 151-61.
[http://dx.doi.org/10.3233/JAD-132279] [PMID: 24577475]

[85]     García-Casares N, Jorge RE, García-Arnés JA, *et al.* Cognitive dysfunctions in middle-aged type 2 diabetic patients and neuroimaging correlations: a cross-sectional study. J Alzheimers Dis 2014; 42(4): 1337-46.
[http://dx.doi.org/10.3233/JAD-140702] [PMID: 25024335]

[86]     Shen J, Yu H, Li K, Ding B, Xiao R, Ma W. The Association Between Plasma Fatty Acid and Cognitive Function Mediated by Inflammation in Patients with Type 2 Diabetes Mellitus. Diabetes Metab Syndr Obes 2022; 15: 1423-36.
[http://dx.doi.org/10.2147/DMSO.S353449] [PMID: 35573864]

[87]     Ferreira LSS, Fernandes CS, Vieira MNN, De Felice FG. Insulin Resistance in Alzheimer's Disease. Front Neurosci 2018; 12: 830.
[http://dx.doi.org/10.3389/fnins.2018.00830] [PMID: 30542257]

[88]     Pérez-Taboada I, Alberquilla S, Martín ED, *et al.* Diabetes Causes Dysfunctional Dopamine Neurotransmission Favoring Nigrostriatal Degeneration in Mice. Mov Disord 2020; 35(9): 1636-48.
[http://dx.doi.org/10.1002/mds.28124] [PMID: 32666590]

[89]     Bird CM, Burgess N. The hippocampus and memory: insights from spatial processing. Nat Rev Neurosci 2008; 9(3): 182-94.
[http://dx.doi.org/10.1038/nrn2335] [PMID: 18270514]

[90]     Dinel AL, André C, Aubert A, Ferreira G, Layé S, Castanon N. Cognitive and emotional alterations

are related to hippocampal inflammation in a mouse model of metabolic syndrome. PLoS One 2011; 6(9): e24325.
[http://dx.doi.org/10.1371/journal.pone.0024325] [PMID: 21949705]

[91]    Lamar M, Rubin L, Ajilore O, *et al.* What Metabolic Syndrome Contributes to Brain Outcomes in African American & Caucasian Cohorts. Curr Alzheimer Res 2015; 12(7): 640-7.
[http://dx.doi.org/10.2174/1567205012666150701102325] [PMID: 26239040]

[92]    Rebolledo-Solleiro D, Araiza LFO, Broccoli L, *et al.* Dopamine D1 receptor activity is involved in the increased anxiety levels observed in STZ-induced diabetes in rats. Behav Brain Res 2016; 313: 293-301.
[http://dx.doi.org/10.1016/j.bbr.2016.06.060] [PMID: 27374159]

[93]    Song J. Amygdala activity and amygdala-hippocampus connectivity: Metabolic diseases, dementia, and neuropsychiatric issues. Biomed Pharmacother 2023; 162: 114647.
[http://dx.doi.org/10.1016/j.biopha.2023.114647] [PMID: 37011482]

[94]    Reddy S, Reddy V, Sharma S. Physiology, Circadian Rhythm. StatPearls. Treasure Island (FL): StatPearls Publishing Copyright © 2023, StatPearls Publishing LLC.; 2023.

[95]    Froy O. Metabolism and circadian rhythms--implications for obesity. Endocr Rev 2010; 31(1): 1-24.
[http://dx.doi.org/10.1210/er.2009-0014] [PMID: 19854863]

[96]    Acosta-Rodríguez VA, Rijo-Ferreira F, Green CB, Takahashi JS. Importance of circadian timing for aging and longevity. Nat Commun 2021; 12(1): 2862.
[http://dx.doi.org/10.1038/s41467-021-22922-6] [PMID: 34001884]

[97]    Boden G, Ruiz J, Urbain JL, Chen X. Evidence for a circadian rhythm of insulin secretion. Am J Physiol 1996; 271(2 Pt 1): E246-52.
[PMID: 8770017]

[98]    Cipolla-Neto J, Amaral FG, Afeche SC, Tan DX, Reiter RJ. Melatonin, energy metabolism, and obesity: a review. J Pineal Res 2014; 56(4): 371-81.
[http://dx.doi.org/10.1111/jpi.12137] [PMID: 24654916]

[99]    van der Heide LP, Ramakers GMJ, Smidt MP. Insulin signaling in the central nervous system: Learning to survive. Prog Neurobiol 2006; 79(4): 205-21.
[http://dx.doi.org/10.1016/j.pneurobio.2006.06.003] [PMID: 16916571]

[100]   Zhao W, Chen H, Xu H, *et al.* Brain insulin receptors and spatial memory. Correlated changes in gene expression, tyrosine phosphorylation, and signaling molecules in the hippocampus of water maze trained rats. J Biol Chem 1999; 274(49): 34893-902.
[http://dx.doi.org/10.1074/jbc.274.49.34893] [PMID: 10574963]

[101]   Kim B, Feldman EL. Insulin resistance as a key link for the increased risk of cognitive impairment in the metabolic syndrome. Experimental & Molecular Medicine. 2015; 47(3): e149.
[http://dx.doi.org/10.1038/emm.2015.3]

[102]   De La Monte SM. Insulin resistance and Alzheimer's disease. BMB Rep 2009; 42(8): 475-81.
[http://dx.doi.org/10.5483/BMBRep.2009.42.8.475] [PMID: 19712582]

[103]   Duarte AI, Moreira PI, Oliveira CR. Insulin in central nervous system: more than just a peripheral hormone. J Aging Res 2012; 2012: 1-21.
[http://dx.doi.org/10.1155/2012/384017] [PMID: 22500228]

[104]   Liu Y, Liu F, Grundke-Iqbal I, Iqbal K, Gong CX. Deficient brain insulin signalling pathway in Alzheimer's disease and diabetes. J Pathol 2011; 225(1): 54-62.
[http://dx.doi.org/10.1002/path.2912] [PMID: 21598254]

[105]   Schmid SM, Jauch-Chara K, Hallschmid M, Schultes B. Mild sleep restriction acutely reduces plasma glucagon levels in healthy men. J Clin Endocrinol Metab 2009; 94(12): 5169-73.
[http://dx.doi.org/10.1210/jc.2009-0969] [PMID: 19837925]

[106] Oster H, Challet E, Ott V, *et al.* The Functional and Clinical Significance of the 24-Hour Rhythm of Circulating Glucocorticoids. Endocr Rev 2017; 38(1): 3-45.
[http://dx.doi.org/10.1210/er.2015-1080] [PMID: 27749086]

[107] Sun Q, Liu Y, Wei W, *et al.* Chronic Timed Sleep Restriction Attenuates LepRb-Mediated Signaling Pathways and Circadian Clock Gene Expression in the Rat Hypothalamus. Front Neurosci 2020; 14: 909.
[http://dx.doi.org/10.3389/fnins.2020.00909] [PMID: 33013300]

[108] Gómez-Abellán P, Gómez-Santos C, Madrid JA, *et al.* Circadian expression of adiponectin and its receptors in human adipose tissue. Endocrinology 2010; 151(1): 115-22.
[http://dx.doi.org/10.1210/en.2009-0647] [PMID: 19887569]

[109] Qian J, Morris CJ, Caputo R, Garaulet M, Scheer FAJL. Ghrelin is impacted by the endogenous circadian system and by circadian misalignment in humans. Int J Obes 2019; 43(8): 1644-9.
[http://dx.doi.org/10.1038/s41366-018-0208-9] [PMID: 30232416]

[110] Van Cauter E, Polonsky KS, Scheen AJ. Roles of circadian rhythmicity and sleep in human glucose regulation. Endocr Rev 1997; 18(5): 716-38.
[PMID: 9331550]

[111] Scheer FAJL, Hilton MF, Mantzoros CS, Shea SA. Adverse metabolic and cardiovascular consequences of circadian misalignment. Proc Natl Acad Sci USA 2009; 106(11): 4453-8.
[http://dx.doi.org/10.1073/pnas.0808180106] [PMID: 19255424]

[112] Nguyen J, Wright KP Jr. Influence of weeks of circadian misalignment on leptin levels. Nat Sci Sleep 2009; 2: 9-18.
[PMID: 23616693]

[113] Spiegel K, Tasali E, Leproult R, Scherberg N, Van Cauter E. Twenty-four-hour profiles of acylated and total ghrelin: relationship with glucose levels and impact of time of day and sleep. J Clin Endocrinol Metab 2011; 96(2): 486-93.
[http://dx.doi.org/10.1210/jc.2010-1978] [PMID: 21106712]

[114] Buxton OM, Cain SW, O'Connor SP, *et al.* Adverse metabolic consequences in humans of prolonged sleep restriction combined with circadian disruption. Sci Transl Med 2012; 4(129): 129ra43.
[http://dx.doi.org/10.1126/scitranslmed.3003200] [PMID: 22496545]

[115] Ruddick-Collins LC, Morgan PJ, Johnstone AM. Mealtime: A circadian disruptor and determinant of energy balance? J Neuroendocrinol 2020; 32(7): e12886.
[http://dx.doi.org/10.1111/jne.12886] [PMID: 32662577]

[116] Bouatia-Naji N, Bonnefond A, Cavalcanti-Proença C, *et al.* A variant near MTNR1B is associated with increased fasting plasma glucose levels and type 2 diabetes risk. Nat Genet 2009; 41(1): 89-94.
[http://dx.doi.org/10.1038/ng.277] [PMID: 19060909]

[117] Singh D, Kondepudi KK, Bishnoi M, Chopra K. Altered Monoamine Metabolism in High Fat Diet Induced Neuropsychiatric Changes in Rats. J Obes Weight Loss Ther 2014; 4: 1000234.

[118] Goldsmith JR, Kordysh E. Why dose-response relationships are often non-linear and some consequences. J Expo Anal Environ Epidemiol 1993; 3(3): 259-76.
[PMID: 8260836]

[119] Roberts CK, Sindhu KK. Oxidative stress and metabolic syndrome. Life Sci 2009; 84(21-22): 705-12.
[http://dx.doi.org/10.1016/j.lfs.2009.02.026] [PMID: 19281826]

[120] Sandoval-Salazar C, Ramírez-Emiliano J, Trejo-Bahena A, Oviedo-Solís CI, Solís-Ortiz MS. A high-fat diet decreases GABA concentration in the frontal cortex and hippocampus of rats. Biol Res 2016; 49(1): 15.
[http://dx.doi.org/10.1186/s40659-016-0075-6] [PMID: 26927389]

[121] Wattanathorn J, Ohnon W, Thukhammee W, Muchmapura S, Wannanon P, Tong-un T.

Cerebroprotective Effect against Cerebral Ischemia of the Combined Extract of *Oryza sativa* and *Anethum graveolens* in Metabolic Syndrome Rats. Oxid Med Cell Longev 2019; 2019: 1-19.
[http://dx.doi.org/10.1155/2019/9658267] [PMID: 31827714]

[122] Tamashiro KL, Sakai RR, Shively CA, Karatsoreos IN, Reagan LP. Chronic stress, metabolism, and metabolic syndrome. Stress 2011; 14(5): 468-74.
[http://dx.doi.org/10.3109/10253890.2011.606341] [PMID: 21848434]

[123] Evans JM, Morris LS, Marchesi JR. The gut microbiome: the role of a virtual organ in the endocrinology of the host. J Endocrinol 2013; 218(3): R37-47.
[http://dx.doi.org/10.1530/JOE-13-0131] [PMID: 23833275]

[124] Rinninella E, Raoul P, Cintoni M, *et al.* What is the Healthy Gut Microbiota Composition? A Changing Ecosystem across Age, Environment, Diet, and Diseases. Microorganisms 2019; 7(1): 14.
[http://dx.doi.org/10.3390/microorganisms7010014] [PMID: 30634578]

[125] Oliphant K, Allen-Vercoe E. Macronutrient metabolism by the human gut microbiome: major fermentation by-products and their impact on host health. Microbiome 2019; 7(1): 91.
[http://dx.doi.org/10.1186/s40168-019-0704-8] [PMID: 31196177]

[126] Jasirwan COM, Lesmana CRA, Hasan I, Sulaiman AS, Gani RA. The role of gut microbiota in non-alcoholic fatty liver disease: pathways of mechanisms. Biosci Microbiota Food Health 2019; 38(3): 81-8.
[http://dx.doi.org/10.12938/bmfh.18-032] [PMID: 31384519]

[127] Sommer F, Bäckhed F. The gut microbiota — masters of host development and physiology. Nat Rev Microbiol 2013; 11(4): 227-38.
[http://dx.doi.org/10.1038/nrmicro2974] [PMID: 23435359]

[128] Clapp M, Aurora N, Herrera L, Bhatia M, Wilen E, Wakefield S. Gut microbiota's effect on mental health: The gut-brain axis. Clin Pract 2017; 7(4): 987.
[http://dx.doi.org/10.4081/cp.2017.987] [PMID: 29071061]

[129] Stojanov S, Berlec A, Štrukelj B. The Influence of Probiotics on the Firmicutes/Bacteroidetes Ratio in the Treatment of Obesity and Inflammatory Bowel disease. Microorganisms 2020; 8(11): 1715.
[http://dx.doi.org/10.3390/microorganisms8111715] [PMID: 33139627]

[130] DeGruttola AK, Low D, Mizoguchi A, Mizoguchi E. Current Understanding of Dysbiosis in Disease in Human and Animal Models. Inflamm Bowel Dis 2016; 22(5): 1137-50.
[http://dx.doi.org/10.1097/MIB.0000000000000750] [PMID: 27070911]

[131] Thomas MS, Blesso CN, Calle MC, Chun OK, Puglisi M, Fernandez ML. Dietary Influences on Gut Microbiota with a Focus on Metabolic Syndrome. Metab Syndr Relat Disord 2022; 20(8): 429-39.
[http://dx.doi.org/10.1089/met.2021.0131] [PMID: 35704900]

[132] Agustí A, García-Pardo MP, López-Almela I, *et al.* Interplay Between the Gut-Brain Axis, Obesity and Cognitive Function. Front Neurosci 2018; 12: 155.
[http://dx.doi.org/10.3389/fnins.2018.00155] [PMID: 29615850]

[133] Lyte M. Microbial endocrinology and the microbiota-gut-brain axis. Adv Exp Med Biol 2014; 817: 3-24.
[http://dx.doi.org/10.1007/978-1-4939-0897-4_1] [PMID: 24997027]

[134] Sampson TR, Mazmanian SK. Control of brain development, function, and behavior by the microbiome. Cell Host Microbe 2015; 17(5): 565-76.
[http://dx.doi.org/10.1016/j.chom.2015.04.011] [PMID: 25974299]

[135] Borre YE, O'Keeffe GW, Clarke G, Stanton C, Dinan TG, Cryan JF. Microbiota and neurodevelopmental windows: implications for brain disorders. Trends Mol Med 2014; 20(9): 509-18.
[http://dx.doi.org/10.1016/j.molmed.2014.05.002] [PMID: 24956966]

[136] Clarke G, Grenham S, Scully P, *et al.* The microbiome-gut-brain axis during early life regulates the hippocampal serotonergic system in a sex-dependent manner. Mol Psychiatry 2013; 18(6): 666-73.

[http://dx.doi.org/10.1038/mp.2012.77] [PMID: 22688187]

[137]  Heijtz RD, Wang S, Anuar F, *et al.* Normal gut microbiota modulates brain development and behavior. Proc Natl Acad Sci USA 2011; 108(7): 3047-52.
[http://dx.doi.org/10.1073/pnas.1010529108] [PMID: 21282636]

[138]  Soto M, Herzog C, Pacheco JA, *et al.* Gut microbiota modulate neurobehavior through changes in brain insulin sensitivity and metabolism. Mol Psychiatry 2018; 23(12): 2287-301.
[http://dx.doi.org/10.1038/s41380-018-0086-5] [PMID: 29910467]

[139]  Cani PD, Neyrinck AM, Maton N, Delzenne NM. Oligofructose promotes satiety in rats fed a high-fat diet: involvement of glucagon-like Peptide-1. Obes Res 2005; 13(6): 1000-7.
[http://dx.doi.org/10.1038/oby.2005.117] [PMID: 15976142]

[140]  Ussar S, Griffin NW, Bezy O, *et al.* Interactions between Gut Microbiota, Host Genetics and Diet Modulate the Predisposition to Obesity and Metabolic Syndrome. Cell Metab 2015; 22(3): 516-30.
[http://dx.doi.org/10.1016/j.cmet.2015.07.007] [PMID: 26299453]

[141]  Fujisaka S, Ussar S, Clish C, *et al.* Antibiotic effects on gut microbiota and metabolism are host dependent. J Clin Invest 2016; 126(12): 4430-43.
[http://dx.doi.org/10.1172/JCI86674] [PMID: 27775551]

[142]  Dabke K, Hendrick G, Devkota S. The gut microbiome and metabolic syndrome. J Clin Invest 2019; 129(10): 4050-7.
[http://dx.doi.org/10.1172/JCI129194] [PMID: 31573550]

[143]  Mukherji A, Kobiita A, Ye T, Chambon P. Homeostasis in intestinal epithelium is orchestrated by the circadian clock and microbiota cues transduced by TLRs. Cell 2013; 153(4): 812-27.
[http://dx.doi.org/10.1016/j.cell.2013.04.020] [PMID: 23663780]

[144]  Wang Y, Kuang Z. The intestinal microbiota regulates body composition through NFIL3 and the circadian clock. 2017; 357(6354): 912-6.
[http://dx.doi.org/10.1126/science.aan0677]

[145]  Leone V, Gibbons SM, Martinez K, *et al.* Effects of diurnal variation of gut microbes and high-fat feeding on host circadian clock function and metabolism. Cell Host Microbe 2015; 17(5): 681-9.
[http://dx.doi.org/10.1016/j.chom.2015.03.006] [PMID: 25891358]

[146]  Thaiss CA, Zeevi D, Levy M, *et al.* Transkingdom control of microbiota diurnal oscillations promotes metabolic homeostasis. Cell 2014; 159(3): 514-29.
[http://dx.doi.org/10.1016/j.cell.2014.09.048] [PMID: 25417104]

[147]  Zarrinpar A, Chaix A, Yooseph S, Panda S. Diet and feeding pattern affect the diurnal dynamics of the gut microbiome. Cell Metab 2014; 20(6): 1006-17.
[http://dx.doi.org/10.1016/j.cmet.2014.11.008] [PMID: 25470548]

[148]  Thaiss CA, Levy M, Korem T, *et al.* Microbiota Diurnal Rhythmicity Programs Host Transcriptome Oscillations. Cell 2016; 167(6): 1495-1510.e12.
[http://dx.doi.org/10.1016/j.cell.2016.11.003] [PMID: 27912059]

[149]  Park YS, Kang SH, Jang SI, Park EC. Association between lifestyle factors and the risk of metabolic syndrome in the South Korea. Sci Rep 2022; 12(1): 13356.
[http://dx.doi.org/10.1038/s41598-022-17361-2] [PMID: 35922546]

[150]  Poortinga W. The prevalence and clustering of four major lifestyle risk factors in an English adult population. Prev Med 2007; 44(2): 124-8.
[http://dx.doi.org/10.1016/j.ypmed.2006.10.006] [PMID: 17157369]

[151]  Hall MH, Muldoon MF, Jennings JR, Buysse DJ, Flory JD, Manuck SB. Self-reported sleep duration is associated with the metabolic syndrome in midlife adults. Sleep 2008; 31(5): 635-43.
[http://dx.doi.org/10.1093/sleep/31.5.635] [PMID: 18517034]

[152]  Moradi Y, Albatineh AN, Mahmoodi H, Gheshlagh RG. The relationship between depression and risk

of metabolic syndrome: a meta-analysis of observational studies. Clin Diabetes Endocrinol 2021; 7(1): 4.
[http://dx.doi.org/10.1186/s40842-021-00117-8] [PMID: 33648597]

[153]  Marchesini G, Calugi S, Centis E, Marzocchi R, El Ghoch M, Marchesini G. Lifestyle modification in the management of the metabolic syndrome: achievements and challenges. Diabetes Metab Syndr Obes 2010; 3: 373-85.
[http://dx.doi.org/10.2147/DMSO.S13860] [PMID: 21437107]

[154]  Garcia-Silva J, Borrego IRS, Navarrete NN, Peralta-Ramirez MI, Águila FJ, Caballo VE. Efficacy of cognitive-behavioural therapy for lifestyle modification in metabolic syndrome: a randomised controlled trial with a 18-months follow-up. 2022:1-21.

[155]  Luo H, Jiang ZL, Ren Y. Therapy Management of Metabolic Disorder Comorbidity With Depression. Front Psychol 2021; 12: 683320.
[http://dx.doi.org/10.3389/fpsyg.2021.683320] [PMID: 34408704]

# CHAPTER 11

# Neutrogenomic Strategies in Metabolic Syndrome

**Noura Ramadan Abdel-hamid[1,*]**

[1] *Department of Histology and Cell Biology, Faculty of Medicine, Suez Canal University, Ismailia, 41522, Egypt*

**Abstract:** In the last 2 decades, the relation between nutrition and health has aroused great interest. In this chapter, the background information about the Complex gene-environment interactions that contribute to MetS will be introduced by highlighting several Neutrogenomic strategies. The role of nutrition is a significant modifiable element modulating the expression of many genes involved in metabolism. This chapter will present the current state of neutrogenomic research discussing the different gene-nutrient interactions in the context of metabolic disease, the molecular mechanisms underlying many of these gene-nutrient interactions, and the shift toward personalized nutrition. Novel modern technologies in Neutrogenomics regarding transcriptomics and metabolomics will be explained.

**Keywords:** Genomics, MetS, Metabolomics, Nutrients, Transcriptomics.

## INTRODUCTION

Many studies have been carried out on nutrients' role in health and diseases, and the genes interacting with them. Neutrogenomics is a branch of science that involves scientific and biological approaches that describe how nutrition interacts with gene expression and function with the application of transcriptomics and metabolomics technologies. Neutrogenomics shows a recent way of working with nutrition and how food interferes with the genetic code [1].

According to disease ontology, MetS is a syndrome that is characterized by abdominal obesity, insulin resistance or diabetes, blood lipid disorders, inflammation, and an increased risk of developing cardiovascular disease [2].

MalaCards (Human disease database) integrated aliases for Abdominal Obesity as Metabolic Syndrome Quantitative Trait Locus 2 and described its inheritance as an autosomal dominant trait. According to the OMIM database, it is an autosomal

---

[*] **Corresponding author Noura Ramadan Abdel-hamid:** Department of Histology and Cell Biology, Faculty of Medicine, Suez Canal University, Ismailia, 41522, Egypt; E-mail: nora.ramadan@med.suez.edu.eg

**Hafize Uzun & Seyma Dumur (Eds.)**

dominant trait with abdominal obesity, hypertension, and elevated fasting glucose levels [2]. Many genes are associated with this trait as the AOMS1 gene, in relation to important pathways, such as IL-9 Signaling Pathways and PPARA Pathway [3].

## GENES RELATED TO METS

Genome-wide association (GWA) and linkage analysis studies revealed the presence of a number of gene variants for the MetS. Some variants are located near genes involved in the lipid metabolism pathway. Other variants have pleiotropic effects on multiple MetS-related traits. Epigenetic changes play a significant role in MetS pathogenesis especially in the area of DNA methylation and histone modification, increasing the risk of acquiring the disease [4].

Candidate genes for regulating processes relevant to the MetS:

- *AOMS1* gene: Aliases for AOMS1 Gene are Abdominal Obesity-Metabolic Syndrome QTL1 and SYNX. Its locus is on the long arm of chromosome 3, region 2, band 7 (3q27), according to (GRCh38/hg38) 2019) [5]. This gene locus is related to six phenotypic traits in MetS and interestingly, it exhibited possible epistatic interaction with another QTL gene on chromosome 17 (17p12) that is strongly linked to plasma leptin levels, which have an important role in biological pathways of MetS [6].
- MTTP gene: Microsomal Triglyceride Transfer Protein, is a Protein Coding gene. Its locus is on the long arm of chromosome 4 (4q23), includes 59,917 bases starting at 99,564,081, and ends at 99,623,997bp from other according to Latest Assembly (GRCh38/hg38) 2019), (Fig. **1**).

**Fig. (1).** MTTP gene chromosomal location (**www.GeneCards.org**).

MTTP gene is involved in some pathways like lipoprotein assembly, remodeling and clearance. Also, it plays an important role in cholesterol biosynthesis. This gene annotation includes protein heterodimerization and lipid transporter activity [7 - 9].

- *MIR122* Gene: This gene is related to the microRNAs family that are short nucleotides not exceeding 24. They are non-coding RNAs that do not code for protein but are involved in post-transcriptional regulation of gene expression.

Its locus is on the long arm of chromosome 18 (18q21.31), (GRCh38/hg38) 2019) (Fig. **2**).

Fig. (**2**). *MIR-122* gene chromosomal location (**www.GeneCards.org**).

*miR-122* is a key regulator of cholesterol and fatty-acid metabolism in the adult liver and recent research revealed its role as a target in metabolic disease [10]. Therefore, it is a key target gene in MetS.

- *MIR33A* Gene: It is found on the long arm of chromosome 22, region 1, band 3 (22q13.2), according to (GRCh38/hg38) 2019) (Fig. **3**). It contributes to the regulation of cholesterol homeostasis [11].
- *MEG3* Gene: The maternally expressed 3 gene is one of the experimental evidence genes involved in metabolic syndrome. It regulates the expression of the HDAC7 gene through post-transcriptional regulation. In MetS, it up-regulates the expression level of HDAC7, protecting the endothelial cells [12].
- INS (Insulin), LEP (Leptin), HSD11B1(Hydroxysteroid 11-Beta Dehydrogenase 1), ADIPOQ Gene (Adiponectin, C1Q, and Collagen Domain Containing) and PPARG (Peroxisome Proliferator-Activated Receptor Gamma): They are protein-coding genes and involved in the MetS pathway interaction.

Fig. (**3**). *MIR-33A* gene chromosomal location (**www.GeneCards.org**)

## PATHWAYS INVOLVED IN METS

According to the GeneCards database, there are several pathways involved in MetS as metabolism pathway, IL-9 Signaling Pathways, Nuclear receptors meta-pathway, *etc*. PPARA activates gene expression, AMP-activated protein kinase signaling, Nuclear receptors, FOXA2 and FOXA3 transcription factor networks, and PPAR signaling pathway [5] (Figs. **4, 5**).

- STRING interaction network for Metabolism Pathway:

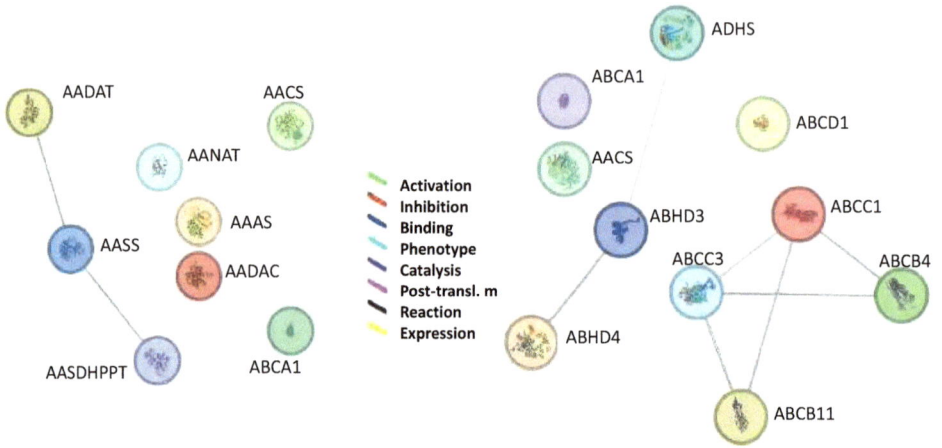

**Fig. (4).** Pathways in metabolism (Reactome database).

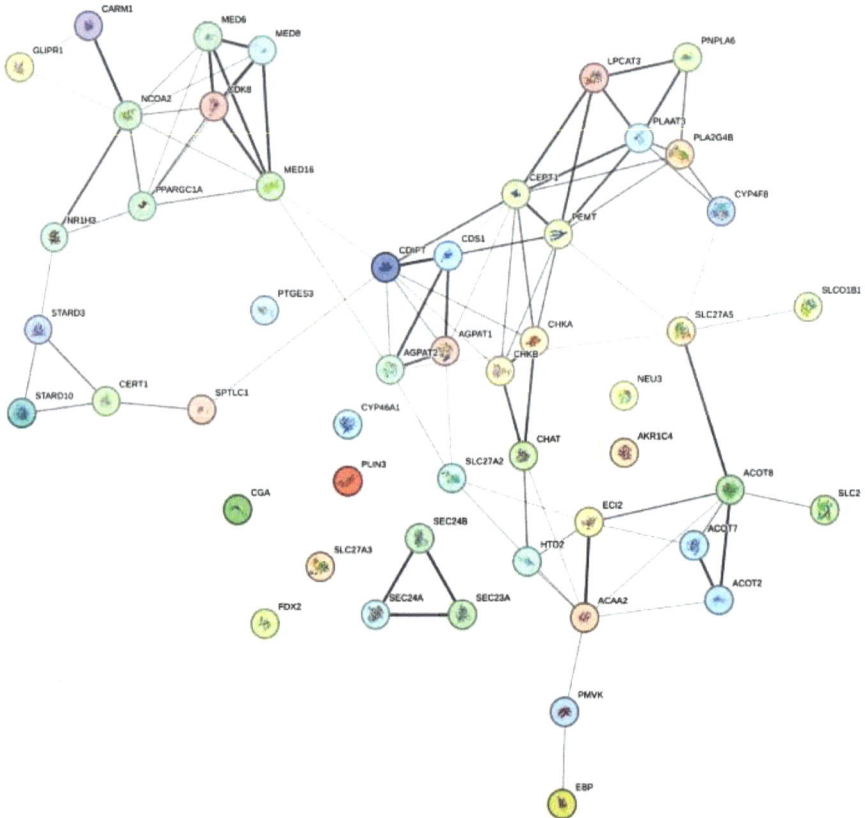

**Fig. (5).** Pathways related to Abdominal Obesity-Metabolic Syndrome 1(Reactome database) [13, 14].

## GENETIC REGULATION IN METS

Regulation of genes, insulin, and fat deposition is a cornerstone strategy for MetS. GWAS revealed many loci involved in obesity in relation to Mets phenotypic traits. One of these important loci is the rs2943634 variant that is found near *IRS1*, which is a protein-coding gene, encodes the insulin receptor 1, which acts mainly in reduced fat deposition and insulin signaling pathway, but is also associated with increasing visceral fat, insulin resistance, dyslipidemia, cardiac diseases, and decreased adiponectin levels [15]. Clinical trials on the *IRSI* gene revealed that animal models that lack it, had delayed growth and developed insulin resistance [20]. Another susceptible locus in *GCKR* was found to be involved in increasing blood glucose, triglycerides, and lipoprotein levels [15, 16].

Obesity-susceptible loci within *FTO, GRB14,* and *MC4R* genes are also linked to fat deposition, cholesterol level, insulin resistance, and diabetes. The rs8050136 variant that is found near *FTO* is associated with fat deposition and insulin regulation [18].

A few susceptible loci within ADAMTS9 and CDKAL1 are found to be linked to insulin resistance and diabetes [17, 18].

*MC4R* is protein-coding gene for leptin. Several variants are involved in dysregulating this gene pathway interacting with them [19].

Epigenetic heritable changes in gene expression do not involve alterations in the DNA sequence, but rather involve chromatin-based molecular signals like DNA methylation, histone variants, and modifications [20, 21]. They possibly mediate the effects of environmental exposures on the metabolism. Epigenetics plays a significant role in changing the regulatory pattern of many pathways involved in metabolism. Epigenetic changes in FTO and IRSI genes are linked to the risk of insulin resistance and diabetes mellitus [22].

Pleiotropic genes for metabolic syndrome are significantly present as the single gene may have multiple phenotypes with multiple body system affection. There were about 130 pleiotropic gene-associated SNPs linked to metabolic inflammatory markers like *LOC646736IRS1, COBLL1, MACF1 GRB14, TFAP2B, FTO, GCKR, MACF1, PTPN11,* and *MC4R* [23].

## NEUTROGENOMIC STRATEGIES IN METS

The emergence of neutrogenomics comes from the recent challenges in reducing the risk of food-related diseases to support health and well-being. By using the basics of bioinformatics, the field of nutrition and genetic alteration has expanded.

Moreover, in MetS, every minor diet change is related to the varying severity of the disorder.

The genetic strategies and tools in the field of 'Omics' technologies would show a comprehensive picture of transcriptomes, proteomics and metabolomics of nutrient-gene interactions [24]. (Fig. **6**)

| | |
|---|---|
| **Genomics** | • DNA<br>• Genome |
| **Transcriptomic** | • RNA<br>• Transcriptome<br>• Transcriptional regulation |
| **Proteomics** | • Protein<br>• proteome |
| **Metabolomics** | • Metabolites<br>• Metabolome |
| **Precision nutrition** | • Body composition analysis<br>• Biochemical profile of sera<br>• Physiological measures (sleep, lifestyle)<br>• Quantity of energy expenses |

**Fig. (6).** Genotype-phenotype interaction [25].

## Transcriptomics Tools

They are used to measure gene expression levels. Polymerase Chain Reaction (PCR), quantitative real-time (RT-PCR), RNA-sequencing and DNA microarray technologies can measure these changes in genetic expression. The use of microarray technologies in the neutrogenomics field allows revealing any gene and chromosome structure abnormalities related to different phenotypic traits on MetS [26, 27]. Foods rich in omega-3 polyunsaturated fatty acids, one of the nutrients under transcriptomic tools, are relating them to MetS [27].

## Proteomics Tools

To measure the proteins, their interactions, and different structures, proteomics tools are used. The use of electrophoresis techniques added a novel idea about the protein composition, the effect of dietary methionine on protein deposition, and the safe use of genetically engineered crops in animal feeding.

## Metabolomic Tools

They detect the level of metabolites, and identify biomarkers, or targets and their clinical relevance. Also, they allowed the detection of changes in the biochemical profiles of plasma and urine for the determination of metabolite profiles [28].

## Epigenetic Tools

They are used for detecting differential gene expression by analyzing methylation patterns and histone modifications by gene-specific analysis or genome-wide scans [29].

Bioinformatics science in Mets adds a novel area of science due to helping in annotating genes related to metabolism pathways. Using alignment tools of next-generation sequencing can predict changes in either genes or proteins [29, 30].

The integration of the Omics technologies with bioinformatics tools in MetS represents a novel focus on gene-nutrients especially with recent changes in macronutrients and micronutrients, involved as confounding factors in DNA synthesis and replication [27, 31].

## Lipids

Polyunsaturated fatty acids (PUFAs) are one of the components that are involved in (omics) tools. Omega 6 PUFAs especially linoleic acid and omega 3 PUFAs with their role in producing or decreasing the inflammation of several metabolic disorders [32].

Increasing omega 3 PUFAs in the daily diet is related to reducing the activity of sterol regulatory element-binding proteins (SREBP)-1 transcription factor, and upregulating the genes of fatty acid oxidation, leading to great improvement in lipid profile [32].

## Carbohydrates

Regarding carbohydrates, a diet rich in fructose becomes evident that one of the recent strategies in reducing inflammatory processes in metabolic disease due to the pleiotropic role of fructose-involved genes [33].

## Proteins

Neutrogenomics tools on proteins are recently being given attention with respect to metabolic diseases. Recent research now revealed upregulation in the expression level of genes involved in autophagy regulation, as p62, p53,

ATG7and beclin-1. Moreover, the role of sarcopenia in triggering the upregulation of PPAR-α, SREBP-1, and acetyl-CoA carboxylase was also correlated to increasing fatty acid synthesis responsible for muscle cellular fat accumulation [34].

## CONCLUDING REMARKS

On the Way of a Genetic-Based Dietary Approach, Thanks to the recent tools and technologies, it may be a genetic-based nutritional recommendation for a tailored MetS therapeutic management.

Due to the novelty of the topic and the promising, scientific evidence, it is not possible to transfer the results of the studies in the routine clinical practice as well as compare the therapeutic outcome of conventional general healthy diet recommendation to a genetic-based approach.

## REFERENCES

[1] Drayna D. Human taste genetics. Annu Rev Genomics Hum Genet 2005; 6(1): 217-35.
[http://dx.doi.org/10.1146/annurev.genom.6.080604.162340] [PMID: 16124860]

[2] Després JP, Lemieux I. Abdominal obesity and metabolic syndrome. Nature 2006; 444(7121): 881-7.
[http://dx.doi.org/10.1038/nature05488] [PMID: 17167477]

[3] OMIM® and Online Mendelian Inheritance in Man® are registered trademarks of Johns Hopkins University. Copyright® 1966-2023 Johns Hopkins University. Available from: https://omim.org/clinicalSynopsis/605572

[4] Stančáková A, Laakso M. Genetics of metabolic syndrome. Rev Endocr Metab Disord 2014; 15(4): 243-52.
[http://dx.doi.org/10.1007/s11154-014-9293-9] [PMID: 25124343]

[5] Genecards database: https://www.genecards.org/cgi-bin/carddisp.pl?gene=AOMS1#disorders-addl

[6] Kissebah AH, Sonnenberg GE, Myklebust J, *et al.* Quantitative trait loci on chromosomes 3 and 17 influence phenotypes of the metabolic syndrome. Proc Natl Acad Sci U S A 2000; 19;97(26): 14478-83.
[http://dx.doi.org/10.1073/pnas.97.26.14478]

[7] Khatun I, Walsh MT, Hussain MM. Loss of both phospholipid and triglyceride transfer activities of microsomal triglyceride transfer protein in abetalipoproteinemia. J Lipid Res 2013; 54(6): 1541-9.
[http://dx.doi.org/10.1194/jlr.M031658] [PMID: 23475612]

[8] Miller SA, Burnett JR, Leonis MA, McKnight CJ, van Bockxmeer FM, Hooper AJ. Novel missense MTTP gene mutations causing abetalipoproteinemia. Biochim Biophys Acta Mol Cell Biol Lipids 2014; 1841(10): 1548-54.
[http://dx.doi.org/10.1016/j.bbalip.2014.08.001] [PMID: 25108285]

[9] Khatun I, Walsh MT, Hussain MM. Loss of both phospholipid and triglyceride transfer activities of microsomal triglyceride transfer protein in abetalipoproteinemia. J Lipid Res 2013; 54(6): 1541-9.
[http://dx.doi.org/10.1194/jlr.M031658] [PMID: 23475612]

[10] Esau C, Davis S, Murray SF, *et al.* miR-122 regulation of lipid metabolism revealed by in vivo antisense targeting. Cell Metab 2006; 3(2): 87-98.
[http://dx.doi.org/10.1016/j.cmet.2006.01.005] [PMID: 16459310]

[11]   Rayner KJ, Suárez Y, Dávalos A, *et al.* MiR-33 contributes to the regulation of cholesterol homeostasis. Science 2010; 328(5985): 1570-3.
[http://dx.doi.org/10.1126/science.1189862] [PMID: 20466885]

[12]   Liu HZ, Wang QY, Zhang Y, *et al.* Pioglitazone up-regulates long non-coding RNA MEG3 to protect endothelial progenitor cells *via* increasing HDAC7 expression in metabolic syndrome. Biomed Pharmacother 2016; 78: 101-9.
[http://dx.doi.org/10.1016/j.biopha.2016.01.001] [PMID: 26898430]

[13]   2023. Pathcards database: https://pathcards.genecards.org/Pathway/660 Copyright © 2023, Weizmann Institute of Science. Version 5.16.984.0, Updated 2023 May 31.

[14]   Reactome database. Available from: https://reactome.org/PathwayBrowser/#/R-HSA-1430728

[15]   Kilpeläinen TO, Zillikens MC, Stančákova A, *et al.* Genetic variation near IRS1 associates with reduced adiposity and an impaired metabolic profile. Nat Genet 2011; 43(8): 753-60.
[http://dx.doi.org/10.1038/ng.866] [PMID: 21706003]

[16]   Dupuis J, Langenberg C, Prokopenko I, *et al.* New genetic loci implicated in fasting glucose homeostasis and their impact on type 2 diabetes risk. Nat Genet 2010; 42(2): 105-16.
[http://dx.doi.org/10.1038/ng.520] [PMID: 20081858]

[17]   Kawajiri T, Osaki Y, Kishimoto T. Association of gene polymorphism of the fat mass and obesity associated gene with metabolic syndrome: a retrospective cohort study in Japanese workers. Yonago Acta Med 2012; 55(2): 29-40.
[PMID: 24031137]

[18]   Tschritter O, Preissl H, Yokoyama Y, Machicao F, Häring HU, Fritsche A. Variation in the FTO gene locus is associated with cerebrocortical insulin resistance in humans. Diabetologia 2007; 50(12): 2602-3.
[http://dx.doi.org/10.1007/s00125-007-0839-1] [PMID: 17917711]

[19]   Butler AA, Cone RD. The melanocortin receptors: Lessons from knockout models. Neuropeptides 2002; 36(2-3): 77-84.
[http://dx.doi.org/10.1054/npep.2002.0890] [PMID: 12359499]

[20]   Tamemoto H, Kadowaki T, Tobe K, *et al.* Insulin resistance and growth retardation in mice lacking insulin receptor substrate-1. Nature 1994; 372(6502): 182-6.
[http://dx.doi.org/10.1038/372182a0] [PMID: 7969452]

[21]   Wolffe AP, Guschin D. Review: chromatin structural features and targets that regulate transcription. J Struct Biol 2000; 129(2-3): 102-22.
[http://dx.doi.org/10.1006/jsbi.2000.4217] [PMID: 10806063]

[22]   Nilsson E, Jansson PA, Perfilyev A, *et al.* Altered DNA methylation and differential expression of genes influencing metabolism and inflammation in adipose tissue from subjects with type 2 diabetes. Diabetes 2014; 63(9): 2962-76.
[http://dx.doi.org/10.2337/db13-1459] [PMID: 24812430]

[23]   Rajesh S, Varanavasiappan S. Nutrigenomics: Insights and Implications for Genome-Based Nutrition. In: S. V., R., Praveen, S. (eds) Conceptualizing Plant-Based Nutrition. Springer, Singapore. 2022.
[http://dx.doi.org/10.1007/978-981-19-4590-8_10]

[24]   Blasbalg TL, Hibbeln JR, Ramsden CE, Majchrzak SF, Rawlings RR. Changes in consumption of omega-3 and omega-6 fatty acids in the United States during the 20th century. Am J Clin Nutr 2011; 93(5): 950-62.
[http://dx.doi.org/10.3945/ajcn.110.006643] [PMID: 21367944]

[25]   Santos-Marcos JA, Perez-Jimenez F, Camargo A. The role of diet and intestinal microbiota in the development of metabolic syndrome. J Nutr Biochem 2019; 70: 1-27.
[http://dx.doi.org/10.1016/j.jnutbio.2019.03.017] [PMID: 31082615]

[26]     Neeha VS, Kinth P. Nutrigenomics research: a review. J Food Sci Technol 2013; 50(3): 415-28.
         [http://dx.doi.org/10.1007/s13197-012-0775-z] [PMID: 24425937]

[27]     Chirita-Emandi A, Niculescu M. Methods for global nutrigenomics and precision nutrition.Principles
         of nutrigenetics and nutrigenomics. Cambridge, MA: Academic Press 2020; pp. 49-58.
         [http://dx.doi.org/10.1016/B978-0-12-804572-5.00007-0]

[28]     Mayer B. Bioinformatics for Omics data. Humana Press in Springer Science 2011; pp. 379-547.
         [http://dx.doi.org/10.1007/978-1-61779-027-0]

[29]     Mullins VA, Bresette W, Johnstone L, Hallmark B, Chilton FH. Genomics in Personalized Nutrition:
         Can You "Eat for Your Genes"? Nutrients 2020; 12(10): 3118.
         [http://dx.doi.org/10.3390/nu12103118] [PMID: 33065985]

[30]     Wu H, Jang J, Dridi S, *et al.* Net protein balance correlates with expression of autophagy,
         mitochondrial biogenesis, and fat metabolism□related genes in skeletal muscle from older adults.
         Physiol Rep 2020; 8(19): e14575.
         [http://dx.doi.org/10.14814/phy2.14575] [PMID: 33063954]

[31]     Wang L, Zhang H, Zhou J, *et al.* Betaine attenuates hepatic steatosis by reducing methylation of the
         MTTP promoter and elevating genomic methylation in mice fed a high-fat diet. J Nutr Biochem 2014;
         25(3): 329-36.
         [http://dx.doi.org/10.1016/j.jnutbio.2013.11.007] [PMID: 24456734]

[32]     Zduńczyk Z, Pareek C. Application of nutrigenomics tools in animal feeding and nutritional research.
         J Anim Feed Sci 2009; 18(1): 3-16.
         [http://dx.doi.org/10.22358/jafs/66361/2009]

[33]     Rajesh S, Varanavasiappan S. Nutrigenomics: Insights and Implications for Genome-Based Nutrition.
         In: S. V., R., Praveen, S. (eds) Conceptualizing Plant-Based Nutrition. Springer, Singapore. 2022.
         [http://dx.doi.org/10.1007/978-981-19-4590-8_10]

[34]     Neeha VS, Kinth P. Nutrigenomics research: a review. J Food Sci Technol 2013; 50(3): 415-28.
         [http://dx.doi.org/10.1007/s13197-012-0775-z] [PMID: 24425937]

# CHAPTER 12

# Multitarget Pharmacotherapeutic Strategies for Metabolic Syndrome and Related Disorders: Perspectives on Personalized Medicine Using a Pharmacology Network Approach

**Samah M. Elaidy[1,\*], Fatma S. Samman[1] and Samar Imbaby[1]**

*[1] Department of Clinical Pharmacology, Faculty of Medicine, Suez Canal University, 41522 Ismailia, Egypt*

**Abstract:** One of the most common metabolic illnesses worldwide is the MetS. In the MetS and its related disorders, rationalized and evidence-based pharmacotherapeutic strategies are corner stones in the mitigation of polypharmacy. The pharmacology network approach and enhanced bioinformatics tools related to the epigenetic, genomic, transcriptomics, proteomic, and metabolomic levels are considered useful bench-side tools for the exploration of molecular preventive and therapeutic multitargets. Molecular multitarget therapy is regarded as a novel pharmacological strategy that forms the foundation of personalized and precision medicine. That will decrease the socioeconomic burden and will improve the health-related quality of life.

**Keywords:** Bioinformatic analysis, Gene Expression Omnibus (GEO) database, Hub genes, Insulin resistance, Metabolic syndrome, Mmolecular multi-target therapy, Next Generation Sequencing (NGS), Polypharmacy, Protein-Protein Interaction (PPI) network, Precision medicine, Personalized medicine, Pharmacology network, Receiver operating characteristic curve (ROC) analysis.

## INTRODUCTION

One of the metabolic illnesses that are occurring at an alarming rate worldwide is the MetS; insulin resistance syndrome and X syndrome are two more names for this condition. MetS is a major global health issue with a high morbidity and mortality rate due to numerous severe comorbid disorders [1, 2]. In order to deliver effective preventative and therapeutic measures to improve patient outcomes, this significant socioeconomic burden urgently requires population-

---

\* **Corresponding author Samah M. Elaidy:** Department of Clinical Pharmacology, Faculty of Medicine, Suez Canal University, 41522 Ismailia, Egypt; E-mail: samah_elaidi@med.suez.edu.eg

**Hafize Uzun & Seyma Dumur (Eds.)**

and system-based solutions, multitargeted pharmacotherapy, as well as the interdisciplinary collaboration of different health experts [1, 3].

## METABOLIC SYNDROME AND RELATED DISORDERS

Metabolic syndrome is linked to chronic inflammation interfering with many of the body's regulatory systems. It does this by raising plasma-free fatty acids, causing insulin resistance, and upregulating inflammatory cytokines, chemokines, and mediators like adiponectin, leptin, and resistin [4, 5]. Different educational and academic organizations propose a range of diagnostic criteria for MetS, with considerable differences in the sensitivity of these criteria [6]. Obesity in the abdomen, hypertension, poor glucose metabolism, and atherogenic dyslipidaemia are the four criteria recommended by guidelines for the diagnosis of MetS [2, 7].

The multifactorial MetS was accompanied by a wide range of reciprocal disorders, including liver dysfunction, kidney dysfunction, cardiovascular events, obstructive sleep apnea, polycystic ovary syndrome, sympathetic stimulation, and hyperuricemia, in addition to type 2 diabetes mellitus (T2DM) and hypertension [7, 8]. All of these multifactor start chronic inflammatory pathways leading to diverse complications in the form of nephropathy, neuropathy, and retinopathy as examples [9 - 12].

Metabolic-associated fatty liver disease (MAFLD), an inflammatory liver disease characterized by more than 5% hepatic steatosis, has the potential to proceed to non-alcoholic steatohepatitis (NASH), fibrosis and cirrhosis. Patients with MFALD are at an increased risk of developing hepatocellular carcinoma (HCC), T2DM, cardiovascular disease, and colorectal and breast cancers [7, 13, 14]. MAFLD is different from non-alcoholic fatty liver disease (NAFLD). Any patient with MetS and hepatic steatosis (as was displayed in diagnostic imaging, elastography or histopathology) will be diagnosed with MAFLD regardless of alcohol consumption [14].

Obesity-related kidney damage and dysfunction are clearly associated with MetS. Inflammatory, hemodynamic, and metabolic difficulties and fat-induced physical compression activate the sympathetic nerve and renin-angiotensin-aldosterone system and cause glomerular hyperfiltration and nephron loss [15, 16]. Due to the suppression of nitric oxide and the subsequent induction of endothelial dysfunction, as well as an increase in insulin resistance, patients with hyperuricemia, defined as a serum uric acid level greater than 7 mg/dl (420 mol/l), are more likely to develop and progress through the various components of the MetS, such as hypertension, T2DM, fatty liver disease, and chronic kidney disease [17, 18]. Polycystic ovarian syndrome is one of the most prevalent endocrine problems in MetS female patients, and it has been extensively connected to cardiovascular risks and insulin resistance, underlining the need for medical intervention [19, 20].

Heart failure with restricted ejection fraction or left ventricular dysfunction is one of the disorders associated with MetS. Obesity and insulin resistance promote inflammation and exacerbate coronary microcirculation, causing concentric left ventricular hypertrophy and stiffness [21 - 23]. Furthermore, sympathetic overstimulation and tachycardia are linked to MetS since inflammation and insulin resistance impair central modulation of sympathetic and parasympathetic activity, causing autonomic imbalance and tachycardia, a risk factor for cardiovascular disease [24, 25].

## POLYPHARMACY APPROACH FOR METS AND RELATED DISORDERS

MetS cannot be treated with a single therapeutic agent due to its complex multifactorial pathogenesis, necessitating a multi-targeted approach for intensive management of all components of MetS in conjunction with initiating a healthy lifestyle modification consisting of diet, exercise, and behavioral therapy as the first therapeutic option in MetS [3, 26, 27]. MetS must be treated and prevented by encouraging healthy nutrition, physical activity, and good sleep hygiene [7, 28].

Polypharmacy, a multidrug regimen including at least five drugs being prescribed for MetS, involves anti-dyslipidemic agents, anti-diabetic and anti-obesity therapies, anti-hypertensive and heart failure drugs. The rate of polypharmacy is increasing and could elevate higher than 60% in diabetic elderly patients. The majority of patients use at least one anti-diabetic medication, a lipid-lowering medication, and at least one anti-hypertensive medication. Therefore, polypharmacy poses a big problem in the treatment of patients with MetS due to many adverse effects of drugs that could have central and peripheral effects and drug-drug interactions, which reduce the patient compliance and prescriptions especially with elderly [29, 30]. Peroxisome proliferator-activated receptor-γ (PPAR) agonist, one of the efficient antidiabetic medicines, is associated with edema, which limits its usage in MetS patients with T2DM and heart failure [31]. Furthermore, most anti-obesity drugs work centrally on the central nervous system to decrease the appetite and peripherally by modulating glucose and lipid metabolism, leading to central and peripheral adverse effects that could vary from minimal to severe adverse effects, lowering the patient's adherence. Rimonabant is one of the anti-obesity drugs, which was withdrawn due to its associated high depression and suicide rates [32 - 34].

The best therapeutic approach for polypharmacy in patients with MetS is to develop and use drugs with multi-actions to target several components of the MetS implying adequate comprehensive and effective therapeutic approaches that could reduce each of blood glucose and lipid levels, blood pressure, and inflammation to optimize health outcomes [1, 35].

In the current work, we focused on the MetS drugs that have multi-actions at various multiple targets to launch the introduction of novel multifunctional efficacious therapeutic agents to combat the various aspects of MetS manifestations, comorbidities, and complications.

Statins like atorvastatin, simvastatin, and rosuvastatin block 3-hydroxy-3-methylglutaryl-coenzyme A (HMG-CoA) reductase, a rate-limiting enzyme in the cholesterol synthesis pathway. They can reduce plasma levels of cholesterol and apoB-containing lipoproteins in hypercholesterolemic patients through various techniques, affecting various parameters in the lipid pathway [2, 36]. They are the most effective hypolipidemic compounds with multiple pleiotropic effects that reduce lipid abnormalities in MetS patients, in addition to their direct anti-inflammatory activity by lowering C-reactive protein levels, anti-oxidant and anti-apoptotic effects, and vasodilatory effects by increasing the bioavailability of nitric oxide and ameliorating endothelial dysfunction [11, 37, 38]. Also, they have cardio-beneficial effects by increasing the HDL cholesterol plasma levels in patients with hyperlipidemia with anti-atherogenic action and subsequently reducing the risk of development and progression of atherosclerosis and coronary heart disease [38, 39]. Patients with nondiabetic MetS were randomly assigned to receive either 10 mg of rosuvastatin or 10 mg of atorvastatin for 6 weeks in a randomized trial. Rosuvastatin outperformed atorvastatin in achieving NCEP ATP III LDL-C targets in these patients [40].

Ezetimibe is an inhibitor of intestinal cholesterol absorption and can be taken with statin to attain the desired LDL cholesterol level (below 100 mg/dL) in patients with MetS [27, 36].

GLP-1 receptor agonists and dipeptidyl peptidase-4 (DPP4) inhibitors are a very important family of drugs that have recently acquired importance in T2DM and MetS therapy regimens due to their pleiotropic effects [2, 7]. Gliptins, DPP4 inhibitors, increase glucose absorption by inhibiting the DPP4 enzyme while maintaining the GLP-1 effect [41]. The two most significant incretin hormones, GLP-1 and glucose-dependent insulinotropic peptide (GIP) play critical roles in diabetes and other metabolic illnesses by stimulating insulin secretion in a dose-dependent manner after oral glucose uptake and decreasing glucagon production [42]. However, GLP-1 is rapidly destroyed in the human body by DPP4, making it difficult to be targeted [43]. Controlling hyperglycemia and decreasing weight will be associated with improvements in various MetS measures, including blood pressure, lipid profiles, and liver enzyme levels, implying a reduction in lipid infiltration into the liver and relief of MetS's many symptoms [2, 44]. GLP-1 receptor agonists are advised for patients who have most of the components of MetS (overweight and obesity, pre-diabetes, T2DM, hypertension, atherosclerosis) and the clinical implications that come with it (obstructive sleep apnea, fatty liver disease, and polycystic ovarian syndrome) [7].

GLP-1RA or sodium-glucose co-transporter 2 (SGLT2) inhibitors possess adequate cardio-protective effects on cardiovascular risk and renal beneficial activity and can be used alone as a monotherapy in diabetic patients without concomitant complications. Dual therapy with one of these medications (GLP-1RA or SGLT2 inhibitor) is recommended in diabetic individuals with overweight/obesity, atherosclerotic cardiovascular disease, or chronic renal illness [45, 46].

The biguanide metformin, another potential poly-target compound, is extensively used for T2DM and MetS [11, 36]. In addition to its main modulatory action on hepatic glucose output and insulin resistance, it displayed pleiotropic functions to combat various MetS-related disorders such as hypertension, hyperlipidemia, obesity, polycystic ovary, and many inflammatory conditions in addition to its anti-psychotic, and anti-depressive actions [1, 47, 48]. It also lowers circulation plasminogen activator inhibitor-1 levels, which may help prevent cardiovascular illnesses linked with T2DM and MetS [11, 36, 48].

Another multi-target agent for MetS is PPAR agonists. PPAR receptors, known as lipid and insulin sensors, participate in the modulation of metabolic homeostasis. They are transcription factors (TFs) that regulate the expression of many genes involved in glucose and lipids' use, storage, and inflammation. Also, they protect the vascular endothelium by elevating the nitric oxide bioavailability and lowering the endothelial oxidative stress [49, 50]. PPAR agonists could have efficacious therapeutic approaches in different components of MetS involving T2DM (as insulin-sensitizing agents), atherosclerotic complications, and inflammation [1, 36, 42, 51]. There have been some trials to develop compounds that can work on multiple PPARs involving PPAR-α, -γ, and -δ for treating metabolic diseases [36, 51]. Although these dual-acting PPARs were not licensed for treating metabolic illnesses, the PPAR activity was used to develop innovative multi-target medicines for MetS [49].

Bezafibrate is an agonist for PPAR-α, -γ, and -δ. The European Atherosclerosis Society has approved it for treating secondary hyperlipidemias when diet and lifestyle changes such as increased activity or weight loss are ineffective. This includes categories IIa, IIb, III, IV, and V of primary hyperlipidaemia. Clofibrate, fenofibrate, and gemfibrozil have high molecular agonistic affinities to PPAR-α. When diet, hyperlipidemia, and high cholesterol are insufficient in treating primary dysbetalipoproteinemia (Type III hyperlipidemia), clofibrate is a therapeutic option. Adults with primary hypercholesterolemia or mixed dyslipidemia (Fredrickson Types IIa and IIb) may benefit from fenofibrate when combined with dietary adjustments to reduce elevated levels of LDL-C, total-C, triglycerides, and apo B while increasing HDL-C. Adults with hyperlipidemia and pancreatitis risk due to high blood triglyceride levels (types IV and V hyperlipidemia) who have not responded to a low-fat diet are prescribed gemfibrozil. Pioglitazone, a PPAR-γ agonist, is an approved therapeutic modality for T2DM [52].

Because there are currently no approved drugs for treating many metabolic diseases in humans, such as NAFLD and fibrotic diseases, urgent investigations to uncover novel molecules, such as farnesoid X receptor (FXR) agonists, were done [3, 53, 54]. FXR stimulation decreases the lipid accumulation in the liver with anti-fibrotic and anti-inflammatory actions suggesting beneficial effects in those diseases [3, 54]. Although obeticholic acid, an FXR agonist, is being researched for NASH and NAFLD, it has been proven to have some detrimental effects in high total cholesterol levels and an elevated HDL-c/non-HDL-c ratio [55, 56].

## ROLES OF PRECISION MEDICINE IN METS AND RELATED DISORDERS

Disease prevention and treatment in the context of precision, also known as personalized medicine, is revolutionary because it considers individual variations in genes, surroundings, and lifestyles. Precision medicine aims to provide the most appropriate care to each patient at the most optimal moment [57 - 60]. With the use of personalized medicine informed by genomics and omics, doctors may be better able to treat patients with MetS by implementing appropriate influence on patient behavior, lifestyle, or even pharmaceutical treatment [61]. Advantages of precision medicine extend beyond patients and extend to hospitals, doctors, and insurance companies. This allows for more accurate and fast diagnosis of patients at lower cost [62].

The risk of developing MetS may be estimated with the use of precision medicine by evaluating the risk genes. This information allows for tailored medication in the form of targeted medicines with fewer side effects. Moreover, the ability to monitor therapeutic efficacy and illness progression is further facilitated by elucidating the molecular mechanisms behind MetS [63, 64].

Omics is a catchall term for any biological discipline with a -omics suffix, including genomics, transcriptomics, proteomics, and metabolomics. The purpose of omics research is to identify potential biomarkers that might be utilized as an early diagnostic tool to identify a subset of persons at high risk of developing MetS [65].

A lengthy trip is required for drug development to obtain the ideal authorised one in terms of safety and effectiveness. Through this journey, *in silico* methods like a bench-side investigation play a significant part. It may also scan different cellular and extracellular targeted proteins using the pharmacology network and numerous bioinformatic methods. After substantial pre-clinical and clinical research, these proteins have been discovered as possible preventive and therapeutic targets for key disease categories, including MetS.

## PHARMACOLOGY NETWORK APPROACH FOR POTENTIAL TARGET EXPLORATION IN METS AND RELATED DISORDERS

Genetic and metabolic disorders are frequent causes of metabolic blockages and illnesses. Understanding the reaction pathways that are directly and indirectly affected by the encoded genes and the effect of reaction step modification and metabolite depletion on overall reaction networks is essential for developing bioinformatics methods and concepts for analyzing metabolic disorders. The Human Genome Project and related clinical efforts have gathered an enormous quantity of vital biological data. Numerous public databases house massively collected knowledge in the fields of biology and medicine. These databases include the results of extensive efforts to identify, isolate, sequence, and assemble information on genes, enzymes, and metabolic pathways [66].

Combining pharmacological and sickness data is a significant advantage of network-based research, which can also be used to analyze the complexity of biological systems *in silico* and evaluate the interactions among the various actors involved. Recent network-based biology systems have looked for unexplored uses for already available medications, anticipated novel anticancer therapies, and discovered novel therapeutic targets [65, 67, 68].

### Common Workflow for Pharmacology Network Approach and Bioinformatics Analytical Tools Used in MetS and Related Disorders

Several databases and platforms are now being utilized to investigate the various omics levels in various diseases and disorders, including the predictable complications. These databases use a number of analytical methods and methodologies that aid in the finding of single or combined molecular targets and pathways for preventive and therapeutic discoveries.

Limited bioinformatic studies have been published till now. The databases and bioinformatic analyses used in different studies provide wildly different lists of key targets. In light of this, it is clear that picking the right databases and analytical tools is crucial.

What also gives attention is how the researchers choose their starting point. From the traditional theoretical point of view, the drug development process begins with preclinical research and progresses to clinical trials. However, current applications of network pharmacology assist researchers in selecting their beginning point in reverse. Some researchers choose to locate their target in clinical individuals, and then use bioinformatic analysis to investigate the interacting biomolecules and their accompanying pathways.

Many researchers start their target identification methods by searching the Gene Expression Omnibus (GEO) database (Fig. **1**), a conceptual foundation for the pharmacology network approach. GEO is a database that stores information regarding gene expression and RNA methylation. GEO archives and openly distributes microarray, next-generation sequencing, and other high-throughput functional genomic data from the scientific community. It is run by the National Center for Biotechnology Information (NCBI): https://www.ncbi.nlm.nih.gov/geo/ [69]. A query was submitted to the GEO database to obtain the data set for expression profiling by high throughput sequencing. A permanent and unique identifier for each sample record is called a GEO accession number (GSMxxx). You may include the same Sample in numerous Series, but it can only ever relate to one Platform.

Additional information is provided by means of next-generation sequencing (NGS). Differently expressed genes (DEGs) were identified between diseased subjects and healthy controls. Gene Ontology (GO) enrichment analysis, REACTOME pathway analysis, KEGG pathway analysis, and Protein-Protein interaction (PPI) network analysis are approaches extensively available for evaluating DEGs. GO is the most popular ontology for describing where genes in humans and model organisms are located, what they do, and how they fit into biological processes; http://geneontology.org/ [70, 71]. REACTOME is a free, open-source, curated, and peer-reviewed route database aimed to aid fundamental research, genomic analysis, modeling, systems biology, and education by providing simple bioinformatics tools for displaying, understanding, and analyzing pathway data. https://reactome.org/ [72]. KEGG (Kyoto Encyclopedia of Genes and Genomes) provides insight into biological systems' higher-level functions and utility by using large-scale molecular datasets obtained by genome sequencing and other high-throughput experimental technologies. They are a free and open-source software platform for analyzing and visualizing molecular interaction networks, biological pathways, annotations, gene expression patterns, and other state data types; cells, creatures, and ecosystems, for example; https://www.genome.jp/kegg/ [73].

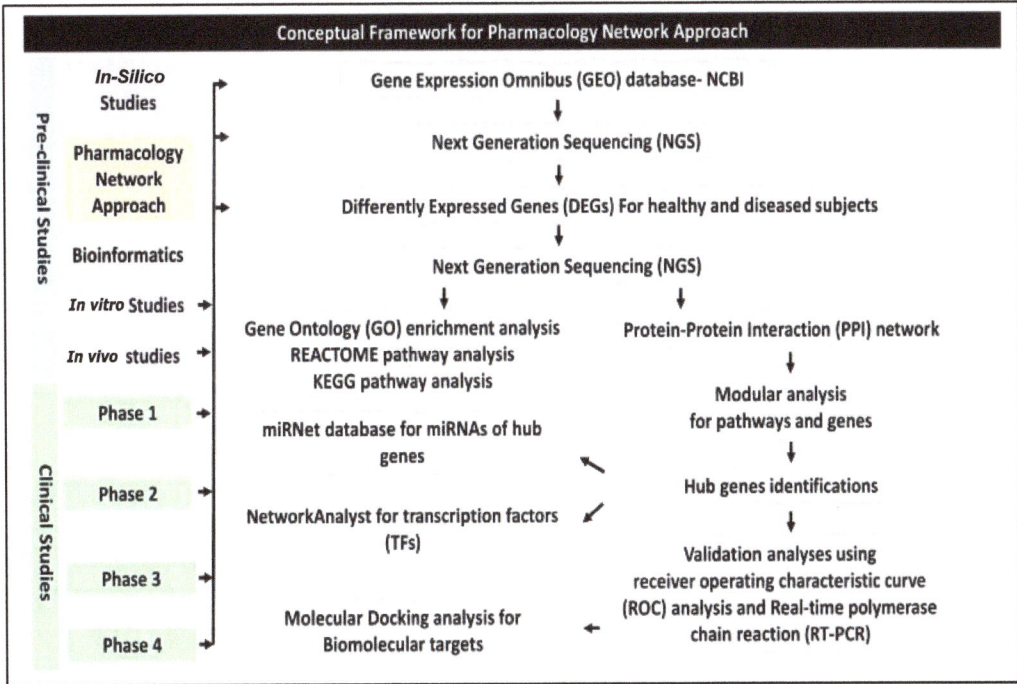

**Fig. (1).** Conceptual framework for Pharmacology Network approach and bioinformatic analysis in MetS and related disorders.

For protein-protein interaction analysis, functional protein association networks, and proteomic analysis, several software are available such as STRING; https://string-db.org/ [74] and cytoscape platform; https://cytoscape.org/ [75]. They are a software platform for analyzing and visualizing molecular interaction networks, biological pathways, and gene expression patterns that is free and open-source. This software and platform help in the selection of hub genes. Hub genes are highly connected nodes in gene networks and often serve an important function in gene regulation or other biological processes [76]. For further analysis, hub gene microRNA (miR) candidates were proposed by the miRNet database: https://www.mirnet.ca/miRNet/ [77 - 79]. TFs that control the expression of hub genes were identified using NetworkAnalyst; https://www.networkanalyst.ca/ [80]. Many researchers rely on validation analyses of the receiver operating characteristic curve (ROC) and real-time polymerase chain reaction (RT-PCR) as their final approach for identifying disease-targeted biomolecules. Molecular docking methods are employed by a small number of scientists to provide predictions about which ligands could be effective in binding to newly identified targets; these predictions are then used to inform *in vitro*, *in vivo*, and clinical studies (Fig. **1**).

## POTENTIAL MOLECULAR MULTITARGETS FOR PHARMACOTHERAPEUTICS IN METS AND RELATED DISORDERS

Patients with MetS would benefit most from a multi-target medicine that treats several pathophysiological paths for MetS and related disorders at once. This section will focus on the multi-target in common overlapping presentations associated to the MetS, drawing on information gathered from the pharmacology network and bioinformatics. In the current section, we will focus on the core genes and other targets including the epigenetic, transcriptional, and metabolic levels for the common MetS disorders. The authors will also focus on the co-occurring conditions that are indicative of MetS.

### Type 2 Diabetes Mellitus

Several studies have revealed a plethora of primary targets for T2DM. Vastrad & Vastrad, 2021 discovered ten T2DM hub genes and biomarkers, including JUN, VCAM1, RELA, U2AF2, ADRB2, FN1, CDK1, TK1, A2M, and ACTA2. The GEO database was examined for expression profiling by high throughput sequencing data set GSE154126 for their methodological outflow. The genes discovered to be differentially expressed in T2DM *versus* the control group were identified. They then performed a REACTOME pathway analysis and a GO functional enrichment research. DEGs were used to investigate the PPI network and module.

Furthermore, the miRNet database discovered potential hub gene miRNA candidates. NetworkAnalyst uncovered the TFs that regulate the expression of hub genes. RT-PCR and ROC analyses were used for additional validation. In total, 925 DEGs were discovered to be linked to T2DM. According to the functional enrichment analysis, the up-regulated DEGs were highly enriched in defensive response, neutrophil degranulation, cell adhesion, and extracellular matrix structure [81].

Data from a microarray study using laser capture microdissection (GSE201966) to separate beta cells in tissue samples from 10 healthy people and 10 people with T2DM were evaluated in another investigation. The network analysis of PPI revealed 83 potential genes involved in T2DM. An inflammatory response and lipid metabolic process were both active for 46 upregulated candidate genes in a literature search, whereas positive control of cell death and proliferation was active for 37 downregulated candidate genes. The PI3K/Akt signaling pathway, the Rap1 signaling pathway, the Ras signaling network, and the MAPK signaling pathway have all been associated with T2DM. The datasets miRNet and NetworkAnalyst were used to construct miR and TF-target gene regulatory networks. Specifically, hsa-miR-192, -124, and -335-5p were found to be involved in T2DM by potentially regulating the expression of candidate genes such as procollagen C-endopeptidase enhancer 2, connective tissue growth factor and family with sequence similarity 105, member A, protein phosphatase 1 regulatory inhibitor subunit 1 A, and C-C motif chemokine receptor 4. The TFs Smad5 and Bcl6 are regulated by ankyrin repeat domain 23 and transmembrane protein 37, respectively [82].

In one intriguing study, T2DM patients had higher plasma circulating miRNA-126 and miRNA-28-3p levels. The researcher utilized bioinformatics to determine the most relevant target genes for these microRNAs, which included VEGFA, SPRED1, PIK3R2, PARP16, SLC7A5, IGF1, IGF2R, MAP2K3, MAPK1, and RAF1 [83]. To uncover anticipated target genes for miRNA-126 and miRNA-2-3p, target bioinformatics tools such as targetScan, the GCBI online database, microRNA.org, and miRanda were employed. Basic bioinformatics activities, probable regulatory signaling pathways, and associated circular RNAs (circRNAs) and long non-coding RNAs (lncRNAs) were predicted using KEGG pathway and starBase (lncRNA). Furthermore, the researchers used CircNet to evaluate the data and create a map. MiRNAMap2 can estimate the expression levels of miRNA-126 and miRNA-28-3p in various tissues. The introns, exons, and polymorphism sites of miRNA-126 and miRNA-28-3p were predicted using the UCSC Genome Browser [83].

## Obesity & T2DM

Increases in both weight and waist size are important indicators of MetS. Identification of many hub genes for people with T2DM and obesity was shown in the published literature. Notably, the hub genes found are distinct from those in T2DM patients. These results support the hypothesis that manipulating several molecular targets and pathways has promise as a treatment strategy. Yet, in order to determine the clinical conceptualization of these therapies, extensive investigative studies are required.

Ganekal *et al.*, 2023 found MYH9, FLNA, DCTN1, CLTC, ERBB2, TCF4, VIM, LRRK2, IFI16, and CAV1 as probable hub genes in diabetic obese patients. The GEO database obtained GSE132831 NGS data. ToppGene was used to investigate DEG functional enrichment. The target gene-TF regulatory network, the PPI network, and the miRNet database were all explored. ROC analysis verified 872 DEGs, including 439 up-regulated and 433 down-regulated genes. The important activities of these DEGs were identified in functional enrichment research as axon guidance, neutrophil degranulation, plasma membrane-bounded cell projection organization, and cell activation [84].

Furthermore, the hub genes CEBPD, TP73, ESR2, Table **1**, MAP 3K5, FN1, UBD, RUNX1, PIK3R2, and TNF may be involved in T2DM caused by obesity. Prashanth *et al.*, 2021 demonstrated these findings. The researchers collected data from a high-throughput sequencing screen for T2DM-related symptoms (GSE143319). The GO and REACTOME databases were used to enrich pathways. They created and tested PPI networks, miRNA-target gene regulatory networks, and TF-target gene regulatory networks to find the hub and target genes. ROC curve analysis and RT-PCR were used to validate the hub genes. Finally, molecular docking analysis was employed among the over-expressed proteins to find small drug targets [85].

**Table 1. Potentially useful medications for treating MetS and related disorders.**

| Generic Name | Target and Pharmacodynamic Affinity |
|:---:|:---:|
| Adapalene | RARG, RXRB; Agonist. |
| Alitretinoin | RARG; Agonist. |
| Crizotinib | MET; Inhibitor. |
| Doconexent | RXRA; Activator. |
| Erlotinib | NR1I2; Agonist. |
| Ibrutinib | BTK; Inhibitor. |
| Rucaparib | PARP1; Antagonist. |
| Ruxolitinib | JAK1; Inhibitor. |
| Tofacitinib | JAK1, JAK2; Antagonist, inhibitor respectively. |

Data is retrieved from DrugBank (https://go.drugbank.com/).

Adapalene, afatinib, alitretinoin, belinostat, bosutinib, crizotinib, dequalinium, doconexent, erlotinib, ibrutinib, lapatinib, nintedanib, panobinostat, rucaparib, and ruxolitin were the subsequent bioinformatics analyses of DrugBank (https://go.drugbank.com/). Table **1** shows these medications' pharmacodynamic activity and targets [52]. Following that, a final prioritization phase was carried out to establish whether the tissue expression of the targets corresponded to illness presentations. Only ibrutinib target bruton tyrosine kinase (BTK) and the erlotinib target nuclear receptor subfamily 1 group I member 2 (NR1I2) revealed tissue-specific expression important for MetS. According to the Human Protein Atlas [86], GTEx [87], and FANTOM5 [88] databases, BTK gene expression is consistently elevated in immune-related tissues, and NR1I2 expression is enriched in the liver, although the other targets showed no tissue-specificity.

The BTK inhibitor ibrutinib is discovered as a possible therapeutic for lowering the chronic inflammatory illness associated with obesity by applying this computational paradigm to MetS. Ibrutinib's ability to diminish obesity-associated inflammation in zebrafish larvae by decreasing macrophage accumulation adds to its potential for repurposing in the context of obesity [52].

## Ischemia And Diabetes

Myocardial ischemia (MI) is a type of coronary heart disease in which the heart muscles lose their ability to pump blood accurately. Although diabetes and MI are unrelated, they share similar biological actions. A bioinformatics strategy based on a bio-molecular signature discovered that 144 genes in both illnesses overlap. According to the GO analysis, most genes were associated with the cytokine-mediated signaling pathway and cytokine activity. Based on their connectivity range, the PPI network found genes such as IL6, TNF, VEGFA, IL10, CCL2, IL1B, CXCL8, and ICAM1. The findings show genetic and biological functional connections between diabetes and MI. The study's findings will aid in developing future diabetes and MI medicines [89].

Several miRNAs were presented by Pordzik *et al.*, 2019 that were investigated in relation to T2DM and platelet reactivity. They discovered that miRNAs in T2DM all target the same gene (PRKAR1A), which is involved in glucose metabolism, blood coagulation, and insulin signaling. Furthermore, data from the electronic database GO was used to construct networks of miRNA-target gene interactions. According to their findings, miR-30a-5p, miR-30d-5p, and miR-30c-5p are the most frequently regulated miRNAs across all ontologies tested, making them excellent candidates for future clinical research on T2DM biomarkers [90].

## Diabetes and Nephropathy

Some publications have been made using proteome and peptidomic analysis of diabetic participants' urine in quest of a biomarker that predicts the development of nephropathy. The proteins and PPI in urine were studied to learn more about the molecular mechanisms at each stage of diabetic nephropathy. Proteomic and peptidomic studies demonstrated that fibrotic pathways in the kidney were engaged before the onset of microalbuminuria in simple diabetes. Changes in glomerular permselectivity and tubular reabsorption, at least in part, account for the proteins and peptides detected in urine when albumin excretion rates were aberrant in early nephropathy, according to proteomic and peptidomic investigations. Finally, proteins involved in wound healing, chronic fibrosis, and inflammation characterize overt nephropathy. The results suggest that people with diabetes experience a number of biochemical changes. Protein network analysis may be more illuminating than assessing individual indicators in determining disease stage and prognosis in diabetic kidney disease, according to a review of the available literature [91].

## CONCLUSION

The ideal impending set-up for MetS diagnosis and treatment involves a patient visiting a clinic, the doctor filling out a health questionnaire about the patient's lifestyle choices, and the laboratory then determining genetic-metabolic and proteomic biomarkers. Precision medicine, which considers the entire patient's condition, is one step ahead of individualized treatment. Precision medicine, or better therapeutic individualization, is thus conceivable. Integration and accessibility, as well as training healthcare providers to use the deluge of data, would be crucial. Understanding the pathophysiology of difficulties may also enable approaches to target certain medications that are effective while avoiding major issues. Predictable hurdles for using precision medicine in patients with MetS include the availability and cost of laboratory procedures. Furthermore, the ability to shed light on the molecular mechanism underlying the aetiology of MetS and to discover treatment alternatives for individual and combination illnesses is, in a nutshell, a major impedance. Because of this, studies into the molecular mechanism of the revealed hub genes and macromolecules, as well as their therapeutic use as biomarkers, are warranted. Finally, keep in mind that MetS develops and progresses over time, beginning with overweight and obesity and progressing to specific MetS components. The earlier the effective intervention is used, the slower the progression of MetS to its components and the occurrence of problems.

## REFERENCES

[1]     Lillich FF, Imig JD, Proschak E. Multi-Target Approaches in Metabolic Syndrome. Front Pharmacol 2021; 11: 554961.
[http://dx.doi.org/10.3389/fphar.2020.554961] [PMID: 33776749]

[2]     Binesh Marvasti T, Adeli Kh. Pharmacological management of metabolic syndrome and its lipid complications. Daru 2010; 18(3): 146-54.
[PMID: 22615610]

[3]     Oseini AM, Sanyal AJ. Therapies in non-alcoholic steatohepatitis ( NASH ). Liver Int 2017; 37(S1) (Suppl. 1): 97-103.
[http://dx.doi.org/10.1111/liv.13302] [PMID: 28052626]

[4]     Gateva A, Assyov Y, Tsakova A, Kamenov Z. Classical (adiponectin, leptin, resistin) and new (chemerin, vaspin, omentin) adipocytokines in patients with prediabetes. Horm Mol Biol Clin Investig 2018; 34(1): 20170031.
[http://dx.doi.org/10.1515/hmbci-2017-0031] [PMID: 29332012]

[5]     Di Lorenzo C, Dell'Agli M, Colombo E, Sangiovanni E, Restani P. M D, E C, E S, P R. Metabolic

syndrome and inflammation: a critical review of *in vitro* and clinical approaches for benefit assessment of plant food supplements. Evid Based Complement Alternat Med 2013; 2013: 1-10.
[http://dx.doi.org/10.1155/2013/782461]

[6]     Adibi N, Robati RM. Skin and metabolic syndrome. J Res Med Sci 2021; 26(1): 16.
[http://dx.doi.org/10.4103/jrms.JRMS_585_20] [PMID: 34084195]

[7]     Dobrowolski P, Prejbisz A, Kuryłowicz A, *et al.* Metabolic syndrome – a new definition and management guidelines. Arch Med Sci 2022; 18(5): 1133-56.
[http://dx.doi.org/10.5114/aoms/152921] [PMID: 36160355]

[8]     Villarroel-Vicente C, Gutiérrez-Palomo S, Ferri J, Cortes D, Cabedo N. Natural products and analogs as preventive agents for metabolic syndrome *via* peroxisome proliferator-activated receptors: An overview. Eur J Med Chem 2021; 221: 113535.
[http://dx.doi.org/10.1016/j.ejmech.2021.113535] [PMID: 33992930]

[9]     Esser N, Legrand-Poels S, Piette J, Scheen AJ, Paquot N. Inflammation as a link between obesity, metabolic syndrome and type 2 diabetes. Diabetes Res Clin Pract 2014; 105(2): 141-50.
[http://dx.doi.org/10.1016/j.diabres.2014.04.006] [PMID: 24798950]

[10]    Forbes JM, Cooper ME. Mechanisms of diabetic complications. Physiol Rev 2013; 93(1): 137-88.
[http://dx.doi.org/10.1152/physrev.00045.2011] [PMID: 23303908]

[11]    Dandona P, Aljada A, Chaudhuri A, Mohanty P, Garg R. Metabolic Syndrome. Circulation 2005; 111(11): 1448-54.
[http://dx.doi.org/10.1161/01.CIR.0000158483.13093.9D] [PMID: 15781756]

[12]    Bernardi S, Marcuzzi A, Piscianz E, Tommasini A, Fabris B. The Complex Interplay between Lipids, Immune System and Interleukins in Cardio-Metabolic Diseases. Int J Mol Sci 2018; 19(12): 4058.
[http://dx.doi.org/10.3390/ijms19124058] [PMID: 30558209]

[13]    Targher G, Corey KE, Byrne CD, Roden M. The complex link between NAFLD and type 2 diabetes mellitus — mechanisms and treatments. Nat Rev Gastroenterol Hepatol 2021; 18(9): 599-612.
[http://dx.doi.org/10.1038/s41575-021-00448-y] [PMID: 33972770]

[14]    Eslam M, Sanyal AJ, George J, *et al.* MAFLD: A Consensus-Driven Proposed Nomenclature for Metabolic Associated Fatty Liver Disease. Gastroenterology 2020; 158(7): 1999-2014.e1.
[http://dx.doi.org/10.1053/j.gastro.2019.11.312] [PMID: 32044314]

[15]    Hall JE, Mouton AJ, da Silva AA, *et al.* Obesity, kidney dysfunction, and inflammation: interactions in hypertension. Cardiovasc Res 2021; 117(8): 1859-76.
[http://dx.doi.org/10.1093/cvr/cvaa336] [PMID: 33258945]

[16]    Mouton AJ, Li X, Hall ME, Hall JE. Obesity, Hypertension, and Cardiac Dysfunction. Circ Res 2020; 126(6): 789-806.
[http://dx.doi.org/10.1161/CIRCRESAHA.119.312321] [PMID: 32163341]

[17]    Soltani Z, Rasheed K, Kapusta DR, Reisin E. Potential role of uric acid in metabolic syndrome, hypertension, kidney injury, and cardiovascular diseases: is it time for reappraisal? Curr Hypertens Rep 2013; 15(3): 175-81.
[http://dx.doi.org/10.1007/s11906-013-0344-5] [PMID: 23588856]

[18]    Kanbay M, Jensen T, Solak Y, *et al.* Uric acid in metabolic syndrome: From an innocent bystander to a central player. Eur J Intern Med 2016; 29: 3-8.
[http://dx.doi.org/10.1016/j.ejim.2015.11.026] [PMID: 26703429]

[19]    Chen W, Pang Y. Metabolic Syndrome and PCOS: Pathogenesis and the Role of Metabolites. Metabolites 2021; 11(12): 869.
[http://dx.doi.org/10.3390/metabo11120869] [PMID: 34940628]

[20]    Pasquali R. Metabolic Syndrome in Polycystic Ovary Syndrome. Front Horm Res 2018; 49: 114-30.
[http://dx.doi.org/10.1159/000485995] [PMID: 29894990]

[21]    Savji N, Meijers WC, Bartz TM, *et al.* The Association of Obesity and Cardiometabolic Traits With Incident HFpEF and HFrEF. JACC Heart Fail 2018; 6(8): 701-9.
[http://dx.doi.org/10.1016/j.jchf.2018.05.018] [PMID: 30007554]

[22]    Watson WD. Response to 'Prevalence and correlates of coronary microvascular dysfunction in heart failure with preserved ejection fraction: PROMIS-HFpEF'. Eur Heart J 2019; 40(41): 3434-4.
[http://dx.doi.org/10.1093/eurheartj/ehz473] [PMID: 31292627]

[23]    Packer M, Lam CSP, Lund LH, Maurer MS, Borlaug BA. Characterization of the inflammatory-metabolic phenotype of heart failure with a preserved ejection fraction: a hypothesis to explain influence of sex on the evolution and potential treatment of the disease. Eur J Heart Fail 2020; 22(9): 1551-67.
[http://dx.doi.org/10.1002/ejhf.1902] [PMID: 32441863]

[24]    Willerson JT, Ridker PM. Inflammation as a cardiovascular risk factor. Circulation 2004; 109(21_suppl_1) (Suppl. 1): II2-II10.
[http://dx.doi.org/10.1161/01.CIR.0000129535.04194.38] [PMID: 15173056]

[25]    Inoue T, Iseki K, Iseki C, Ohya Y, Kinjo K, Takishita S. Effect of heart rate on the risk of developing metabolic syndrome. Hypertens Res 2009; 32(9): 801-6.
[http://dx.doi.org/10.1038/hr.2009.109] [PMID: 19644506]

[26]    Tabatabaei-Malazy O, Larijani B, Abdollahi M. Targeting metabolic disorders by natural products. J Diabetes Metab Disord 2015; 14(1): 57.
[http://dx.doi.org/10.1186/s40200-015-0184-8] [PMID: 26157708]

[27]    Grundy SM. Drug therapy of the metabolic syndrome: minimizing the emerging crisis in polypharmacy. Nat Rev Drug Discov 2006; 5(4): 295-309.
[http://dx.doi.org/10.1038/nrd2005] [PMID: 16582875]

[28]    Visseren FLJ, Mach F, Smulders YM, *et al.* 2021 ESC Guidelines on cardiovascular disease prevention in clinical practice. Eur J Prev Cardiol 2022; 29(1): 5-115.
[http://dx.doi.org/10.1093/eurjpc/zwab154] [PMID: 34558602]

[29]    Alwhaibi M, Balkhi B, Alhawassi TM, *et al.* Polypharmacy among patients with diabetes: a cross-sectional retrospective study in a tertiary hospital in Saudi Arabia. BMJ Open 2018; 8(5): e020852.
[http://dx.doi.org/10.1136/bmjopen-2017-020852] [PMID: 29794097]

[30]    Noale M, Veronese N, Perin PC, *et al.* Reply to Letter to the Editor "Polypharmacy in elderly people with diabetes admitted to hospital". Acta Diabetol 2016; 53(5): 859-60.
[http://dx.doi.org/10.1007/s00592-015-0819-8] [PMID: 26607826]

[31]    Stafylas PC, Sarafidis PA, Lasaridis AN. The controversial effects of thiazolidinediones on cardiovascular morbidity and mortality. Int J Cardiol 2009; 131(3): 298-304.
[http://dx.doi.org/10.1016/j.ijcard.2008.06.005] [PMID: 18684530]

[32]    Després JP, Van Gaal L, Pi-Sunyer X, Scheen A. Efficacy and safety of the weight-loss drug rimonabant. Lancet 2008; 371(9612): 555.
[http://dx.doi.org/10.1016/S0140-6736(08)60261-5] [PMID: 18280320]

[33]    Christensen R, Kristensen PK, Bartels EM, Bliddal H, Astrup A. Efficacy and safety of the weight-loss drug rimonabant: a meta-analysis of randomised trials. Lancet 2007; 370(9600): 1706-13.
[http://dx.doi.org/10.1016/S0140-6736(07)61721-8] [PMID: 18022033]

[34]    Kumar M, Kaushik D, Kaur J, *et al.* A Critical Review on Obesity: Herbal Approach, Bioactive Compounds, and Their Mechanism. Appl Sci (Basel) 2022; 12(16): 8342.
[http://dx.doi.org/10.3390/app12168342]

[35]    Morphy R, Rankovic Z. Z R. Designed multiple ligands. An emerging drug discovery paradigm. J Med Chem 2005; 48(21): 6523-43.
[http://dx.doi.org/10.1021/jm058225d]

[36]    Bianchi C, Penno G, Romero F, Del Prato S, Miccoli R. Treating the metabolic syndrome. Expert Rev Cardiovasc Ther 2007; 5(3): 491-506.
[http://dx.doi.org/10.1586/14779072.5.3.491] [PMID: 17489673]

[37]    Ginsberg HN. REVIEW: Efficacy and mechanisms of action of statins in the treatment of diabetic dyslipidemia. J Clin Endocrinol Metab 2006; 91(2): 383-92.
[http://dx.doi.org/10.1210/jc.2005-2084] [PMID: 16291700]

[38]    Bland AR, Payne FM, Ashton JC, Jamialahmadi T, Sahebkar A. The cardioprotective actions of statins in targeting mitochondrial dysfunction associated with myocardial ischaemia-reperfusion injury. Pharmacol Res 2022; 175: 105986.
[http://dx.doi.org/10.1016/j.phrs.2021.105986] [PMID: 34800627]

[39]    Stone NJ, Robinson JG, Lichtenstein AH, *et al.* 2013 ACC/AHA guideline on the treatment of blood cholesterol to reduce atherosclerotic cardiovascular risk in adults: a report of the American College of Cardiology/American Heart Association Task Force on Practice Guidelines. Circulation 2014; 129(25_suppl_2) (Suppl. 2): S1-S45.
[http://dx.doi.org/10.1161/01.cir.0000437738.63853.7a] [PMID: 24222016]

[40]    Park JS, Kim YJ, Choi JY, *et al.* Comparative study of low doses of rosuvastatin and atorvastatin on lipid and glycemic control in patients with metabolic syndrome and hypercholesterolemia. Korean J Intern Med (Korean Assoc Intern Med) 2010; 25(1): 27-35.
[http://dx.doi.org/10.3904/kjim.2010.25.1.27] [PMID: 20195400]

[41]    Scheen AJ. The safety of gliptins : updated data in 2018. Expert Opin Drug Saf 2018; 17(4): 387-405.
[http://dx.doi.org/10.1080/14740338.2018.1444027] [PMID: 29468916]

[42]    Dhankhar S, Chauhan S, Mehta DK, *et al.* Novel targets for potential therapeutic use in Diabetes mellitus. Diabetol Metab Syndr 2023; 15(1): 17.
[http://dx.doi.org/10.1186/s13098-023-00983-5] [PMID: 36782201]

[43]    Tomlinson B, Hu M, Zhang Y, Chan P, Liu ZM. Investigational glucagon-like peptide-1 agonists for the treatment of obesity. Expert Opin Investig Drugs 2016; 25(10): 1167-79.
[http://dx.doi.org/10.1080/13543784.2016.1221925] [PMID: 27563838]

[44]    Klonoff DC, Buse JB, Nielsen LL, *et al.* Exenatide effects on diabetes, obesity, cardiovascular risk factors and hepatic biomarkers in patients with type 2 diabetes treated for at least 3 years. Curr Med Res Opin 2008; 24(1): 275-86.
[http://dx.doi.org/10.1185/030079908X253870] [PMID: 18053320]

[45]    Araszkiewicz A, Bandurska-Stankiewicz E, Borys S, *et al.* 2021 Guidelines on the management of patients with diabetes. A position of Diabetes Poland. Clinical Diabetology 2021; 10(1): 1-113.
[http://dx.doi.org/10.5603/DK.2021.0001]

[46]    17. Diabetes Advocacy: *Standards of Medical Care in Diabetes—2022*. Diabetes Care 2022; 45 (Suppl. 1): S254-5.
[http://dx.doi.org/10.2337/dc22-S017] [PMID: 34964878]

[47]    Atici Y, Baskol G, Bayram F. A new approach for the pleiotropic effect of metformin use in type 2 diabetes mellitus. Turk Biyokim Derg 2022; 47(6): 775-82.
[http://dx.doi.org/10.1515/tjb-2022-0013]

[48]    Forouzandeh F, Salazar G, Patrushev N, *et al.* Metformin beyond diabetes: pleiotropic benefits of metformin in attenuation of atherosclerosis. J Am Heart Assoc 2014; 3(6): e001202.
[http://dx.doi.org/10.1161/JAHA.114.001202] [PMID: 25527624]

[49]    Ammazzalorso A, Maccallini C, Amoia P, Amoroso R. Multitarget PPARγ agonists as innovative modulators of the metabolic syndrome. Eur J Med Chem 2019; 173: 261-73.
[http://dx.doi.org/10.1016/j.ejmech.2019.04.030] [PMID: 31009912]

[50]    Maccallini C, Mollica A, Amoroso R. The Positive Regulation of eNOS Signaling by PPAR Agonists in Cardiovascular Diseases. Am J Cardiovasc Drugs 2017; 17(4): 273-81.

[http://dx.doi.org/10.1007/s40256-017-0220-9] [PMID: 28315197]

[51]  Jain MR, Giri SR, Bhoi B, *et al.* Dual PPAR α/γ agonist saroglitazar improves liver histopathology and biochemistry in experimental NASH models. Liver Int 2018; 38(6): 1084-94.
[http://dx.doi.org/10.1111/liv.13634] [PMID: 29164820]

[52]  Misselbeck K, Parolo S, Lorenzini F, *et al.* A network-based approach to identify deregulated pathways and drug effects in metabolic syndrome. Nat Commun 2019; 10(1): 5215.
[http://dx.doi.org/10.1038/s41467-019-13208-z] [PMID: 31740673]

[53]  Ali AH, Carey EJ, Lindor KD. Recent advances in the development of farnesoid X receptor agonists. Ann Transl Med 2015; 3(1): 5.
[http://dx.doi.org/10.3978/j.issn.2305-5839.2014.12.06] [PMID: 25705637]

[54]  Sumida Y, Yoneda M. Current and future pharmacological therapies for NAFLD/NASH. J Gastroenterol 2018; 53(3): 362-76.
[http://dx.doi.org/10.1007/s00535-017-1415-1] [PMID: 29247356]

[55]  Han C. Update on FXR Biology: Promising Therapeutic Target? Int J Mol Sci 2018; 19(7): 2069.
[http://dx.doi.org/10.3390/ijms19072069] [PMID: 30013008]

[56]  Mudaliar S, Henry RR, Sanyal AJ, *et al.* Efficacy and safety of the farnesoid X receptor agonist obeticholic acid in patients with type 2 diabetes and nonalcoholic fatty liver disease. Gastroenterology 2013; 145(3): 574-582.e1.
[http://dx.doi.org/10.1053/j.gastro.2013.05.042] [PMID: 23727264]

[57]  Vicente AM, Ballensiefen W, Jönsson JI. How personalised medicine will transform healthcare by 2030: the ICPerMed vision. J Transl Med 2020; 18(1): 180.
[http://dx.doi.org/10.1186/s12967-020-02316-w] [PMID: 32345312]

[58]  International Consortium for Personalised Medicine - ICPerMed n.d. https://www.icpermed.eu/ (accessed August 14, 2023).

[59]  Personalized Medicine. GenomeGov n.d. https://www.genome.gov/genetics-glossary/Personalize--Medicine (accessed August 14, 2023).

[60]  Health C for D and R. Precision Medicine. FDA 2022. https://www.fda.gov/medical-devices/in-vit-o-diagnostics/precision-medicine (accessed August 14, 2023).

[61]  Gharipour M, Nezafati P, Sadeghian L, Eftekhari A, Rothenberg I, Jahanfar S. Precision medicine and metabolic syndrome. ARYA Atheroscler 2022; 18(4): 1-10.
[http://dx.doi.org/10.22122/arya.2022.26215] [PMID: 36817343]

[62]  Jakka S, Rossbach M. An economic perspective on personalized medicine. HUGO J 2013; 7(1): 1.
[http://dx.doi.org/10.1186/1877-6566-7-1]

[63]  Savoia C, Volpe M, Grassi G, Borghi C, Agabiti Rosei E, Touyz RM. Personalized medicine—a modern approach for the diagnosis and management of hypertension. Clin Sci (Lond) 2017; 131(22): 2671-85.
[http://dx.doi.org/10.1042/CS20160407] [PMID: 29109301]

[64]  Guest FL, Guest PC. Point-of-Care Testing and Personalized Medicine for Metabolic Disorders.Investigations of Early Nutrition Effects on Long-Term Health: Methods and Applications. New York, NY: Springer 2018; pp. 105-14.
[http://dx.doi.org/10.1007/978-1-4939-7614-0_6]

[65]  Quezada H, Guzmán-Ortiz AL, Díaz-Sánchez H, Valle-Rios R, Aguirre-Hernández J. Omics-based biomarkers: current status and potential use in the clinic. Bol Méd Hosp Infant México 2017; 74(3): 219-26.
[http://dx.doi.org/10.1016/j.bmhimx.2017.03.003] [PMID: 29382490]

[66]  Chen M, Hofestädt R. A medical bioinformatics approach for metabolic disorders: Biomedical data prediction, modeling, and systematic analysis. J Biomed Inform 2006; 39(2): 147-59.

[http://dx.doi.org/10.1016/j.jbi.2005.05.005] [PMID: 16023895]

[67]    Sridhar A, Saremy S, Bhattacharjee B. Elucidation of molecular targets of bioactive principles of black cumin relevant to its anti-tumour functionality - An Insilico target fishing approach. Bioinformation 2014; 10(11): 684-8.
[http://dx.doi.org/10.6026/97320630010684] [PMID: 25512684]

[68]    Ramachandra Sridhar G, Lakshmi G. Bioinformatics, Genomics and Diabetes.Computational Intelligence Techniques in Health Care. Singapore: Springer 2016; pp. 1-18.
[http://dx.doi.org/10.1007/978-981-10-0308-0_1]

[69]    Home - GEO - NCBI n.d. https://www.ncbi.nlm.nih.gov/geo/ (accessed August 15, 2023).

[70]    Tomczak A, Mortensen JM, Winnenburg R, *et al.* Interpretation of biological experiments changes with evolution of the Gene Ontology and its annotations. Sci Rep 2018; 8(1): 5115.
[http://dx.doi.org/10.1038/s41598-018-23395-2] [PMID: 29572502]

[71]    Gene Ontology Resource. Gene Ontology Resource n.d. http://geneontology.org/ (accessed August 15, 2023).

[72]    Home - Reactome Pathway Database n.d. https://reactome.org/ (accessed August 15, 2023).

[73]    KEGG: Kyoto Encyclopedia of Genes and Genomes n.d. https://www.genome.jp/kegg/ (accessed August 15, 2023).

[74]    STRING: functional protein association networks n.d. https://string-db.org/ (accessed August 15, 2023).

[75]    Otasek D, Morris JH, Bouças J, Pico AR, Demchak B. Cytoscape Automation: empowering workflow-based network analysis. Genome Biol 2019; 20(1): 185.
[http://dx.doi.org/10.1186/s13059-019-1758-4] [PMID: 31477170]

[76]    Yu D, Lim J, Wang X, Liang F, Xiao G. Enhanced construction of gene regulatory networks using hub gene information. BMC Bioinformatics 2017; 18(1): 186.
[http://dx.doi.org/10.1186/s12859-017-1576-1] [PMID: 28335719]

[77]    Chang L, Zhou G, Soufan O, Xia J. miRNet 2.0: network-based visual analytics for miRNA functional analysis and systems biology. Nucleic Acids Res 2020; 48(W1): W244-51.
[http://dx.doi.org/10.1093/nar/gkaa467] [PMID: 32484539]

[78]    Fan Y, Xia J. miRNet—Functional Analysis and Visual Exploration of miRNA–Target Interactions in a Network Context. In: Von Stechow L, Santos Delgado A, editors. Computational Cell Biology, vol. 1819, New York, NY: Springer New York; 2018, p. 215–33.
[http://dx.doi.org/10.1007/978-1-4939-8618-7_10]

[79]    Fan Y, Siklenka K, Arora SK, Ribeiro P, Kimmins S, Xia J. miRNet - dissecting miRNA-target interactions and functional associations through network-based visual analysis. Nucleic Acids Res 2016; 44(W1): W135-41.
[http://dx.doi.org/10.1093/nar/gkw288] [PMID: 27105848]

[80]    Zhou G, Soufan O, Ewald J, Hancock REW, Basu N, Xia J. NetworkAnalyst 3.0: a visual analytics platform for comprehensive gene expression profiling and meta-analysis. Nucleic Acids Res 2019; 47(W1): W234-41.
[http://dx.doi.org/10.1093/nar/gkz240] [PMID: 30931480]

[81]    Vastrad B, Vastrad C. Bioinformatics analysis of potential key genes and mechanisms in type 2 diabetes mellitus 2021; 03.28.: 437386.
[http://dx.doi.org/10.1101/2021.03.28.437386]

[82]    Lu Y, Li Y, Li G, Lu H. Identification of potential markers for type 2 diabetes mellitus *via* bioinformatics analysis. Mol Med Rep 2020; 22(3): 1868-82.
[http://dx.doi.org/10.3892/mmr.2020.11281] [PMID: 32705173]

[83]    Nie H, Zhang K, Xu J, Liao K, Zhou W, Fu Z. Combining Bioinformatics Techniques to Study

Diabetes Biomarkers and Related Molecular Mechanisms. Front Genet 2020; 11: 367.
[http://dx.doi.org/10.3389/fgene.2020.00367] [PMID: 32425976]

[84]    Ganekal P, Vastrad B, Kavatagimath S, Vastrad C, Kotrashetti S. Bioinformatics and Next-Generation
        Data Analysis for Identification of Genes and Molecular Pathways Involved in Subjects with Diabetes
        and Obesity. Medicina (Kaunas) 2023; 59(2): 309.
        [http://dx.doi.org/10.3390/medicina59020309] [PMID: 36837510]

[85]    Prashanth G, Vastrad B, Tengli A, Vastrad C, Kotturshetti I. Investigation of candidate genes and
        mechanisms underlying obesity associated type 2 diabetes mellitus using bioinformatics analysis and
        screening of small drug molecules. BMC Endocr Disord 2021; 21(1): 80.
        [http://dx.doi.org/10.1186/s12902-021-00718-5] [PMID: 33902539]

[86]    Uhlén M, Fagerberg L, Hallström BM, *et al.* Tissue-based map of the human proteome. Science 2015;
        347(6220): 1260419.
        [http://dx.doi.org/10.1126/science.1260419] [PMID: 25613900]

[87]    Battle A, Brown CD, Engelhardt BE, Montgomery SB. Genetic effects on gene expression across
        human tissues. Nature 2017; 550(7675): 204-13.
        [http://dx.doi.org/10.1038/nature24277] [PMID: 29022597]

[88]    Lizio M, Harshbarger J, Shimoji H, *et al.* Gateways to the FANTOM5 promoter level mammalian
        expression atlas. Genome Biol 2015; 16(1): 22.
        [http://dx.doi.org/10.1186/s13059-014-0560-6] [PMID: 25723102]

[89]    Hasan MT, Hassan M, Ahmed K, *et al.* Network based study to explore genetic linkage between
        diabetes mellitus and myocardial ischemia: Bioinformatics approach. Gene Rep 2020; 21: 100809.
        [http://dx.doi.org/10.1016/j.genrep.2020.100809]

[90]    Pordzik J, Jakubik D, Jarosz-Popek J, *et al.* Significance of circulating microRNAs in diabetes mellitus
        type 2 and platelet reactivity: bioinformatic analysis and review. Cardiovasc Diabetol 2019; 18(1):
        113.
        [http://dx.doi.org/10.1186/s12933-019-0918-x] [PMID: 31470851]

[91]    Van JAD, Scholey JW, Konvalinka A. Insights into Diabetic Kidney Disease Using Urinary
        Proteomics and Bioinformatics. J Am Soc Nephrol 2017; 28(4): 1050-61.
        [http://dx.doi.org/10.1681/ASN.2016091018] [PMID: 28159781]

## CHAPTER 13

# Role of Exercise in Metabolic Syndrome

**Seyma Dumur**[1,*]

[1] *Department of Medical Biochemistry, Faculty of Medicine, Istanbul Atlas University, Istanbul, Turkey*

**Abstract:** Metabolic syndrome (MetS) is a primary and increasing public health problem as a result of worldwide urbanization, excessive energy intake, and increasing sedentary lifestyles. MetS is a combination of the interrelated risk factors of cardiovascular disease, diabetes and obesity. These factors are dysglycemia, dyslipidemia, elevated blood pressure, insulin resistance or type 2 diabetes, and low HDL levels. Clinical and epidemiological studies show that these factors are strongly associated with cardiovascular risk factors. The worldwide incidence of MetS varies, depending on the region, urban or rural situation, as well as the gender, age, race, and ethnicity of the population studied. Effective preventive approaches include weight loss, dietary habits with high content of industrialized foods, the use of appropriate pharmacological agents, and exercise to reduce specific risk factors of MetS. Many physicians treat each of the components of MetS separately. But instead, a solution should be found to address all these factors together. As discussed in this chapter, exercise plays a very crucial role in controlling insulin activity, reducing the risk of cardiovascular disease, and maintaining weight control. Various studies have proven that effective exercise provides positive results in treating MetS components. The aim of this chapter is to explain the effects of physical activity on MetS in light of current information about MetS.

**Keywords:** Exercise, Insulin resistance, Metabolic syndrome, Physical activity.

## INTRODUCTION

According to the Metabolic Syndrome Working Group of the Turkish Society of Endocrinology and Metabolism, Metabolic Syndrome (MetS) is a lethal endocrinopathy accompanied by regular disorders such as abdominal obesity, glucose intolerance or diabetes, high blood pressure, and coronary artery disease, driven by insulin resistance [1]. MetS is a combination of the interrelated risk factors of cardiovascular disease and diabetes. These factors are dysglycemia, high blood pressure, low HDL levels, and obesity [2].

---

\* **Corresponding author Seyma Dumur:** Department of Medical Biochemistry, Faculty of Medicine, Istanbul Atlas University, Istanbul, Turkey; E-mail: seyma.dumur@atlas.edu.tr

The association of these factors has been known for years. Although its pathogenesis remains unclear, recent attention has focused on the possible impact of insulin resistance as an important factor, as well as on the establishment of diagnostic criteria. MetS is a condition in which physiological, biochemical, clinical and metabolic factors are linked to each other like a constellation and directly increases the risk of cardiovascular disease and type 2 diabetes and their associated mortality [1 - 4].

With the increase in obesity and sedentary lifestyle in the world, the prevalence of MetS will increase. In this respect, MetS is both a public health problem and a clinical problem. In the last ten years, different diagnostic criteria have been proposed by different organizations [5, 6]. Organizations such as the World Health Organization (WHO), the International Diabetes Federation (IDF), and the National Adult Cholesterol Education Program Adult Treatment Panel III (NCEP-ATP III) have conducted research on MetS diagnostic criteria. As a result of the researches, the most known and accepted one for the diagnosis of MetS is the diagnostic criteria table performed by NCEP-ATP III. Qualification for the diagnosis of MetS in this diagnostic criteria table is the presence of three of the five criteria [7 - 9].

Although MetS can be observed in all ages, it is more common in older ages. Also, it is estimated that the incidence of MetS is more obvious, especially in women, and that this issue is related to abdominal obesity [10, 11]. According to the 2012 data of the Turkish Adult Heart Disease and Risk Factors Screening study related to the prevalence of MetS in Turkey, the prevalence of MetS in Turkish men is 45.1%, while it is 54.5% in Turkish women [12, 13]. Additionally, to investigate whether the distribution of "at risk" clusters of MetS components differed cross-culturally, a study of 34,821 individuals from 12 cohorts from 10 European countries and 1 US participant in the MARE (Metabolic syndrome and Arteries Research) Consortium found a prevalence of MetS of 24.3% (8468 subjects) (23.9% in men *vs* 24.6% in women, $p<0.001$) and an age-related increase in prevalence in all cohorts [14].

It is now known that a fructose-rich diet increases the risk of cardiovascular disease and leads to the development of pathological conditions such as MetS, which is caused by a physically inactive lifestyle and irregular or excessive nutrition. Fructose is found naturally in honey and fruits, and as a sweetener in industrial products [15]. Since liver tissue is the main tissue where fructose is metabolized, it is the tissue where the negative effects of high fructose diet are most intense [16].

Studies in the literature have adopted a high fructose diet in rats to create an experimental example of MetS. There are studies reporting the occurrence of MetS like problems such as fatty liver and glucose intolerance in rats depending on the proportion of fructose in these diets, how it is used and its duration [17 - 20].

The aim of this chapter is to explain the effects of physical activity on MetS in the light of current information about MetS, which is a combination of various diseases that disrupts the quality of life of individuals and even puts their lives in danger. The main goal of MetS treatment is to change lifestyle and diet habits while simultaneously improving physical activity.

## METABOLIC SYNDROME AND EXERCISE

MetS is a complex disease with a high mortality risk, characterized by inflammation that starts with insulin resistance and is accompanied by abdominal obesity, glucose intolerance and/or diabetes mellitus, high blood pressure, dyslipidemia, hypertriglyceridemia and coronary artery disease [1, 2].

Pro-inflammatory cytokines associated with MetS can cause physical inactivation that becomes a cycle of chronic inflammation. Physical activity becomes psychologically and physically undesirable when inflammation is present. "Inflammation-based disease state", which is revealed by using experimental animals, is in a size to support this hypothesis [21 - 25].

Calorie restriction diet and exercise studies are studies that trigger further improvement by leading to the activation of anti-inflammatory effects, improving biological and exercise ability. Although it has been observed that there are negative effects of overproduction, the regular operation of the skeletal muscle and the free radicals produced at a low limit activates the enzyme activities that prevent oxidative destruction and help to create power against oxidative stress by creating special adaptations [26, 27].

Studies revealing the link between physical inactivity and obesity indicate that there is a statistically negative correlation depending on body mass index, waist thickness and waist-hip balance parameters. These results reveal the necessity of maintaining a physically active lifestyle and reducing intra-abdominal fat in order to prevent the progression of the MetS [28].

Reducing fat mass may support raising adiponectin levels and enhancing the cytokine profile associated with MetS. The release and control of two cytokines, tumor necrosis factor-α (TNF-α) and interleukin-6 (IL-6) aid the normal maintenance effects of physical activity. The increase in the levels of the first cytokine IL-6 released into the circulation during exercise is the result of the response to exercise. IL-6 is a cytokine that elicits both pro-inflammatory and anti-inflammatory effects [29, 30].

Regular exercise elicits regulating effects on insulin function and glucose tolerance in ordinary healthy individuals, as well as in patients with obesity, MetS, and diabetes. One of the main effects of exercise is that it increases the amount of lipid oxidation in skeletal muscles and results in an increase in lipid oxidation in the whole body [31, 32].

Systematic exercises produce a moderate antihypertensive effect [33, 34]. Aerobic exercises likewise regularly reduce blood pressure in overweight people. In this context, reductions in systolic and diastolic blood pressure were associated with weight loss in overweight individuals [35]. Weight loss and exercise studies affect functional and structural regulation of the palate system, including blood pressure. Variations in the renin-angiotensin system affect the sympathetic nervous system with decreased stimuli and increased insulin sensitivity [36]. Exercise has important effects on the morphological structures of different blood vessels. This structural differentiation is followed by functional variations that increase blood flow. Exercises like this stimulate angiogenesis and support the growth of capillaries, the regulation of capillary resistance arteries, and the growth of existing vessels [37, 38].

**Physical Exercise**

Those who do less than 150 minutes of physical activity per week are defined as physically inactive or sedentary [39]. Before starting physical exercise programs, various medical examinations should be performed in order to determine diabetes control and whether there are progressive serious complications in diabetic patients. Exercise is an important component of MetS treatment. Exercise not only improves the plasma lipid profile (increased triglyceride and decreased HDL ratios) but also has positive effects on other risk factors [39].

Physical exercise has been shown to reduce skeletal muscle lipid levels and insulin resistance, regardless of BMI [40, 41]. Regular exercise has been shown to increase insulin sensitivity, decrease plasma triglyceride levels, and reduce cardiovascular morbidity and mortality [42].

In a study conducted by Young Kim *et al.*, they observed a significant improvement in obesity indices and metabolic risk factors (weight, BMI, waist circumference, systolic blood pressure, diastolic blood pressure and triglyceride) in a 24-week regular walking exercise program [43].

There are studies showing that high-intensity aerobic interval exercise is more effective in reducing cardiovascular risk factors related to MetS than moderate-intensity continuous exercise. However, both exercise programs were found to be equally effective in reducing body weight and fat content. These results show that exercise reduces the effects of MetS, and the magnitude of this effect depends on the exercise intensity [44].

Owens and Gutin argue that vigorous physical activity has a beneficial effect on the MetS components, especially in children. They also think that high mechanical loads of intense physical activity compared with moderate or light activity probably differentiate stem cells into lean tissue types (muscle or bone) rather than fat cells [45].

## Endocrinological and Metabolic Effects of Exercise

During physical exercise, glucose uptake to the working muscles increases depending on the intensity of the work done [40]. Intense exercise increases the release of anti-insulin hormones such as glucagon and catecholamines. Therefore, blood sugar levels may increase after intense physical exercise [40]. Improvements in body composition, bone mineral density, cardiovascular risk factors, and quality of life have been reported with growth hormone therapy [42]. While there are reports of exercise-induced growth hormone increases, there is little evidence to confirm the effects of growth hormone increases on MetS factors.

Growth hormone release was found to be higher in those who did 12-week aerobic and strength exercises together compared to those who did only aerobic exercise [43]. Growth hormone release was found to be higher in those who did 12-week aerobic and strength exercises together compared to those who did only aerobic exercise.

Studies examining the endocrinological and metabolic effects of exercise have shown that physical exercise increases the use of blood sugar and free fatty acids in the muscles and lowers blood sugar levels in well-controlled diabetic patients. Long-term, light, regular jogging increases the effect of insulin on carbohydrate and lipid metabolism without affecting BMI or maximal oxygen use [31].

## Effects of Training

Continued physical exercise improves insulin IGT (Improved Glucose Tolerance) tissue sensitivity and type 2 diabetes [40]. Nagasawa *et al.*, in their study in 1990, showed that insulin sensitivity, which developed due to physical exercise, decreased within 3 days and disappeared after 7 days [46]. Dela *et al.* showed an increase in muscle GLUT4 protein and mRNA in patients with Type II diabetes who responded to physical exercise and in control subjects [47].

Yoo *et al.* conducted a study examining the effects of exercises on MetS in a study combining water exercises and muscle strengthening exercises with elastic tera bands in the elderly with MetS. It was determined that triglyceride levels and waist circumference were significantly reduced in the group in which combined exercises were applied, compared to tera band and in-water exercises. The amount of HDL cholesterol increased significantly in the combined group compared to the muscle-strengthening group. The results show that combined exercise is more effective in improving dyslipidemia and abdominal obesity [48].

In a 12-week study of obese middle-aged women combining strength exercises and aerobic exercises, significant benefits were obtained in terms of body composition and MetS factors, and visfatin levels were reduced [3].

In another study investigating the effects of yoga exercises in Korean postmenopausal women, it was observed that adiponectin levels, serum lipids and MetS risk factors improved. It was concluded that yoga exercises can be effective in preventing cardiovascular diseases in Korean obese postmenopausal women [49].

The standard exercise recommendation is a minimum of 30 minutes of moderate-intensity physical activity daily [50]. As an exercise prescription, moderate intensity light aerobic exercises such as walking and jogging are recommended for 10-30 minutes a day, 3-5 days a week. Mild strength training with the use of light dumbbells and stretching cables should be combined with aerobic exercises in older people with reduced muscle strength [51]. The amount of exercise can be easily determined with a pedometer carried by the patient, 10000 steps (at least 7500 steps) should be taken during a day [41].

## Strength Exercises

Skeletal muscle accounts for approximately 40% and 30% of humans' total body weight, and evidence suggests that it may be effective in modifying metabolic risk factors through the enhancement of muscle mass [52, 53]. Decreased muscle mass has metabolic consequences, and normal aging and decreased physical activity can lead to an increase in the incidence of metabolic disorders [54, 55].

There is evidence in the literature for the concept that strength exercises are as effective as aerobic exercise in reducing some important cardiovascular disease risk factors. Furthermore, there are findings in the literature showing that after aerobic exercise and diet, strength exercises can be a good alternative for obese patients to improve their body composition and reduce fat mass [56 - 58].

Studies in the literature have shown that it would be reasonable to determine the potential effect of strength training, which changes the general exercise volume, on individuals with metabolic syndrome and low-grade inflammation markers over a long period of time [59 - 61]. It is thought that greater training frequency will lead to greater reductions in body fat mass and more positive changes in metabolic syndrome markers and low-grade inflammation levels in a group of healthy men and women over the age of 65 [59].

In a study where Botezelli *et al.* aimed to compare the effects of aerobic, strength, and combined training on metabolic disorders caused by a fructose-rich diet, they found that strength training prevented hyperinsulinemia, insulin resistance and inflammation in fructose-fed animals, and independent of weight loss [62].

It has been shown that strength exercises mobilize subcutaneous and visceral fat tissue in the abdomen [63, 64]. Reducing fat mass, ensuring glycemic control, and improving the blood lipid profile are important in reducing microvascular and macrovascular complications in people with MetS [50, 65]. From this perspective, strength exercises will be an additional aid in treatment in reducing the biggest known risk factors for MetS.

## The Effect of Exercise on Metabolic Syndrome Components

Components such as obesity, hypertension, glucose metabolism disorder (diabetes and insulin resistance) and dyslipidemia due to insufficient physical activity, inactive lifestyle, and excessive nutrition play a major role in MetS [66].

Furthermore, exercise is a very effective practice in the treatment of obesity in obese individuals [67]. Supporting physical activity with healthy nutrition is the cornerstone of lifestyle changes, which are the primary treatment for individuals with obesity [68]. In order to get effective results from physical activity, calorie restriction is also necessary. Energy expenditure through physical activity helps maintain energy balance [69, 70]. Obese individuals who have generally adopted a sedentary life should transition to a physically active life [71, 72]. Obese individuals should schedule their exercise time for a certain period of time after eating and should be physically active throughout the day. In obese people, the maximum heart rate level should be calculated and 80% of the maximum heart rate level should be reached with exercises [73, 74]. In individuals who are very accustomed to a sedentary life and have no exercise history, the duration and intensity of physical activity should be started low and gradually increased [68 -

73]. In a study conducted by Wataru *et al.* on healthy young individuals, it was reported that low-intensity exercise performed after a meal prevented the increase in post-meal triglyceride concentration [75].

Physical activity is also very important in the control and treatment of type 2 diabetes, which is the other component of MetS. As a result of the exercises, it has been observed that insulin resistance decreases, the individual's insulin sensitivity increases and blood sugar is balanced [76, 77]. Many studies have shown that physical activity has a positive effect on MetS. Physical activity has a significant effect on treating the components of MetS and reducing their incidence [78 - 80]. It has been observed that the incidence of MetS is lower in individuals who are more physically active. The basic physical activity recommendation of 150 minutes of low or 75 minutes of moderate intensity exercise per week reduces the risk of MetS [81, 82]. Increasing the number of daily steps every 2000 steps also reduces the risk of MetS [83, 84].

## CONCLUSION

Metabolic syndrome is defined as a set of biochemical, physiological, clinical, cardiovascular disease and diabetes. Studies have shown that most of the risk factors associated with metabolic syndrome are positively affected by exercise. It also shows that regular physical activity is effective in preventing cardiovascular disease, diabetes and premature deaths. In order to maintain the effect of exercise on insulin sensitivity, a sedentary lifestyle should be abandoned and exercise should be done regularly. In addition, if there are no contraindications, strength exercises should be added to exercise programs.

## REFERENCES

[1]     Kaur J. A comprehensive review on metabolic syndrome. Cardiol Res Pract 2014; 2014: 1-21.
[http://dx.doi.org/10.1155/2014/943162] [PMID: 24711954]

[2]     Reisinger C, Nkeh-Chungag BN, Fredriksen PM, Goswami N. The prevalence of pediatric metabolic syndrome—a critical look on the discrepancies between definitions and its clinical importance. Int J Obes 2021; 45(1): 12-24.
[http://dx.doi.org/10.1038/s41366-020-00713-1] [PMID: 33208861]

[3]     Seo DI, Jun TW, Park KS, Chang H, So WY, Song W. 12 weeks of combined exercise is better than aerobic exercise for increasing growth hormone in middle-aged women. Int J Sport Nutr Exerc Metab 2010; 20(1): 21-6.
[http://dx.doi.org/10.1123/ijsnem.20.1.21] [PMID: 20190348]

[4]     Guembe MJ, Fernandez-Lazaro CI, Sayon-Orea C, Toledo E, Moreno-Iribas C. RIVANA Study Investigators. Risk for cardiovascular disease associated with metabolic syndrome and its components: a 13-year prospective study in the RIVANA cohort. Cardiovasc Diabetol. 2020; 19(1): 195.
[http://dx.doi.org/10.1186/s12933-020-01166-6]

[5]     Haverinen E, Paalanen L, Palmieri L, *et al.* Comparison of metabolic syndrome prevalence using four different definitions - a population-based study in Finland. Arch Public Health. 2021; 79(1): 231.
[http://dx.doi.org/10.1186/s13690-021-00749-3]

[6]     Jemal A, Girum T, Kedir S, *et al.* Metabolic syndrome and its predictors among adults seeking medical care: A trending public health concern. Clin Nutr ESPEN 2023; 54: 264-70.
[http://dx.doi.org/10.1016/j.clnesp.2023.01.034] [PMID: 36963872]

[7]     Saif-Ali R, Kamaruddin NA, Al-Habori M, Al-Dubai SA, Ngah WZW. Relationship of metabolic syndrome defined by IDF or revised NCEP ATP III with glycemic control among Malaysians with Type 2 Diabetes. Diabetol Metab Syndr. 2020;12:67.
[http://dx.doi.org/10.1186/s13098-020-00575-7]

[8]     Ulaganathan V, Kandiah M, Shariff ZM. A case-control study of the association between metabolic syndrome and colorectal cancer: a comparison of International Diabetes Federation, National Cholesterol Education Program Adults Treatment Panel III, and World Health Organization definitions. J Gastrointest Oncol 2018; 9(4): 650-63.
[http://dx.doi.org/10.21037/jgo.2018.04.01] [PMID: 30151261]

[9]     Kim S, So WY. Prevalence of Metabolic Syndrome among Korean Adolescents According to the National Cholesterol Education Program, Adult Treatment Panel III and International Diabetes Federation. Nutrients. 2016; 8(10): 588.
[http://dx.doi.org/10.3390/nu8100588]

[10]    Falkner B, Cossrow NDFH. Prevalence of metabolic syndrome and obesity-associated hypertension in the racial ethnic minorities of the United States. Curr Hypertens Rep 2014; 16(7): 449.
[http://dx.doi.org/10.1007/s11906-014-0449-5] [PMID: 24819559]

[11]    Azimi-Nezhad M, Aminisani N, Ghasemi A, *et al.* Sex-specific prevalence of metabolic syndrome in older adults: results from the Neyshabur longitudinal study on aging, Iran. J Diabetes Metab Disord. 2022; 21(1): 263-273.
[http://dx.doi.org/10.1007/s40200-022-00969-6]

[12]    Atik D, Atik C, Karatepe H. Metabolic syndrome in patients undergoing coronary angiography. Acta Inform Med 2014; 22(6): 360-4.
[http://dx.doi.org/10.5455/aim.2014.22.360-364] [PMID: 25684840]

[13]    Onat A, Yüksel M, Köroğlu B, *et al.* Turkish Adult Risk Factor Study survey 2012: overall and coronary mortality and trends in the prevalence of metabolic syndrome. Turk Kardiyol Dern Ars 2013; 41(5): 373-8.
[http://dx.doi.org/10.5543/tkda.2013.15853] [PMID: 23917000]

[14]    Scuteri A, Laurent S, Cucca F, *et al.* Metabolic syndrome across Europe: Different clusters of risk factors. Eur J Prev Cardiol 2015; 22(4): 486-91.
[http://dx.doi.org/10.1177/2047487314525529] [PMID: 24647805]

[15]    Hernandez-Castillo C, Shuck SC. Diet and Obesity-Induced Methylglyoxal Production and Links to Metabolic Disease. Chem Res Toxicol 2021; 34(12): 2424-40.
[http://dx.doi.org/10.1021/acs.chemrestox.1c00221] [PMID: 34851609]

[16]    Hannou SA, Haslam DE, McKeown NM, Herman MA. Fructose metabolism and metabolic disease. J Clin Invest 2018; 128(2): 545-55.
[http://dx.doi.org/10.1172/JCI96702] [PMID: 29388924]

[17]    Chan AML, Ng AMH, Mohd Yunus MH, *et al.* Recent Developments in Rodent Models of High-Fructose Diet-Induced Metabolic Syndrome: A Systematic Review. Nutrients 2021; 13(8): 2497.
[http://dx.doi.org/10.3390/nu13082497]

[18]    Bentanachs R, Blanco L, Montesinos M, *et al.* Adipose Tissue Protects against Hepatic Steatosis in Male Rats Fed a High-Fat Diet plus Liquid Fructose: Sex-Related Differences. Nutrients 2023; 15(18): 3909.
[http://dx.doi.org/10.3390/nu15183909] [PMID: 37764693]

[19]    Moreno-Fernández S, Garcés-Rimón M, Vera G, Astier J, Landrier JF, Miguel M. High Fat/High Glucose Diet Induces Metabolic Syndrome in an Experimental Rat Model. Nutrients 2018; 10(10):

1502.
[http://dx.doi.org/10.3390/nu10101502] [PMID: 30322196]

[20]    Buniam J, Chansela P, Weerachayaphorn J, Saengsirisuwan V. Dietary Supplementation with 20-Hydroxyecdysone Ameliorates Hepatic Steatosis and Reduces White Adipose Tissue Mass in Ovariectomized Rats Fed a High-Fat, High-Fructose Diet. Biomedicines 2023; 11(7): 2071.
[http://dx.doi.org/10.3390/biomedicines11072071] [PMID: 37509710]

[21]    Burini RC, Anderson E, Durstine JL, Carson JA. Inflammation, physical activity, and chronic disease: An evolutionary perspective. Sports Med Health Sci 2020; 2(1): 1-6.
[http://dx.doi.org/10.1016/j.smhs.2020.03.004]

[22]    Furman D, Campisi J, Verdin E, *et al.* Chronic inflammation in the etiology of disease across the life span. Nat Med 2019; 25(12): 1822-32.
[http://dx.doi.org/10.1038/s41591-019-0675-0] [PMID: 31806905]

[23]    Bennett JM, Reeves G, Billman GE, Sturmberg JP. Inflammation-Nature's Way to Efficiently Respond to All Types of Challenges: Implications for Understanding and Managing "the Epidemic" of Chronic Diseases. Front Med (Lausanne). 2018; 5: 316.
[http://dx.doi.org/10.3389/fmed.2018.00316]

[24]    Monteiro R, Azevedo I. Chronic inflammation in obesity and the metabolic syndrome. Mediators Inflamm 2010; 2010: 1-10.
[http://dx.doi.org/10.1155/2010/289645] [PMID: 20706689]

[25]    Milano W, Carizzone F, Foia M, *et al.* Obesity and Its Multiple Clinical Implications between Inflammatory States and Gut Microbiotic Alterations. Diseases 2022; 11(1): 7.
[http://dx.doi.org/10.3390/diseases11010007] [PMID: 36648872]

[26]    Simioni C, Zauli G, Martelli AM, *et al.* Oxidative stress: role of physical exercise and antioxidant nutraceuticals in adulthood and aging. Oncotarget. 2018; 9(24): 17181-17198.
[http://dx.doi.org/10.18632/oncotarget.24729]

[27]    Wu Q, Gao ZJ, Yu X, Wang P. Dietary regulation in health and disease. Signal Transduct Target Ther 2022; 7(1): 252.
[http://dx.doi.org/10.1038/s41392-022-01104-w]

[28]    Slentz CA, Houmard JA, Kraus WE. Exercise, abdominal obesity, skeletal muscle, and metabolic risk: evidence for a dose response. Obesity (Silver Spring) 2009; 17(S3) (Suppl. 3): S27-33.
[http://dx.doi.org/10.1038/oby.2009.385] [PMID: 19927142]

[29]    Longo M, Zatterale F, Naderi J, *et al.* Adipose Tissue Dysfunction as Determinant of Obesity-Associated Metabolic Complications. Int J Mol Sci. 2019; 20(9): 2358.
[http://dx.doi.org/10.3390/ijms20092358]

[30]    Zorena K, Jachimowicz-Duda O, Ślęzak D, Robakowska M, Mrugacz M. Adipokines and Obesity. Potential Link to Metabolic Disorders and Chronic Complications. Int J Mol Sci 2020; 21(10): 3570.
[http://dx.doi.org/10.3390/ijms21103570] [PMID: 32443588]

[31]    Bird SR, Hawley JA. Update on the effects of physical activity on insulin sensitivity in humans. BMJ Open Sport Exerc Med 2017; 2(1): e000143.
[http://dx.doi.org/10.1136/bmjsem-2016-000143]

[32]    Henderson GC. Plasma Free Fatty Acid Concentration as a Modifiable Risk Factor for Metabolic Disease. Nutrients. 2021; 13(8): 2590.
[http://dx.doi.org/10.3390/nu13082590]

[33]    Ghadieh AS, Saab B. Evidence for exercise training in the management of hypertension in adults. Can Fam Physician 2015; 61(3): 233-9.
[PMID: 25927108]

[34]    Rodrigues GD, Lima LS, da Silva NCS, *et al.* Are home-based exercises effective to reduce blood pressure in hypertensive adults? A systematic review. Clin Hypertens 2022; 28(1): 28.

[http://dx.doi.org/10.1186/s40885-022-00211-8]

[35]    Ritchie LD, Campbell NC, Murchie P. New NICE guidelines for hypertension. BMJ 2011; 343(sep07 1): d5644.
[http://dx.doi.org/10.1136/bmj.d5644] [PMID: 21900351]

[36]    Francischetti EA, Genelhu VA. Obesity-hypertension: an ongoing pandemic. Int J Clin Pract 2007; 61(2): 269-80.
[http://dx.doi.org/10.1111/j.1742-1241.2006.01262.x] [PMID: 17263714]

[37]    Nystoriak MA, Bhatnagar A. Cardiovascular Effects and Benefits of Exercise. Front Cardiovasc Med. 2018; 5: 135.
[http://dx.doi.org/10.3389/fcvm.2018.00135]

[38]    Hotta K, Behnke BJ, Arjmandi B, *et al.* Daily muscle stretching enhances blood flow, endothelial function, capillarity, vascular volume and connectivity in aged skeletal muscle. J Physiol 2018; 596(10): 1903-17.
[http://dx.doi.org/10.1113/JP275459] [PMID: 29623692]

[39]    The Diabetes Prevention Program (DPP): description of lifestyle intervention. Diabetes Care 2002; 25(12): 2165-71.
[http://dx.doi.org/10.2337/diacare.25.12.2165] [PMID: 12453955]

[40]    Sato Y. Diabetes and life-styles: role of physical exercise for primary prevention. Br J Nutr 2000; 84(6) (Suppl. 2): 187-90.
[http://dx.doi.org/10.1079/096582197388662] [PMID: 11242467]

[41]    Koplan JP, Dietz WH. Caloric imbalance and public health policy. JAMA 1999; 282(16): 1579-81.
[http://dx.doi.org/10.1001/jama.282.16.1579] [PMID: 10546699]

[42]    Molitch ME, Clemmons DR, Malozowski S, Merriam GR, Vance ML. Evaluation and treatment of adult growth hormone deficiency: an Endocrine Society clinical practice guideline. J Clin Endocrinol Metab 2011; 96(6): 1587-609.
[http://dx.doi.org/10.1210/jc.2011-0179] [PMID: 21602453]

[43]    Kim DY, Seo BD, Kim DJ. Effect of Walking Exercise on Changes in Cardiorespiratory Fitness, Metabolic Syndrome Markers, and High-molecular-weight Adiponectin in Obese Middle-aged Women. J Phys Ther Sci 2014; 26(11): 1723-7.
[http://dx.doi.org/10.1589/jpts.26.1723] [PMID: 25435686]

[44]    Haram PM, Kemi OJ, Lee SJ, *et al.* Aerobic interval training *vs.* continuous moderate exercise in the metabolic syndrome of rats artificially selected for low aerobic capacity. Cardiovasc Res 2008; 81(4): 723-32.
[http://dx.doi.org/10.1093/cvr/cvn332] [PMID: 19047339]

[45]    Gutin B, Owens S. The influence of physical activity on cardiometabolic biomarkers in youths: a review. Pediatr Exerc Sci 2011; 23(2): 169-85.
[http://dx.doi.org/10.1123/pes.23.2.169] [PMID: 21633131]

[46]    Nagasawa J, Sato Y, Ishiko T. Effect of training and detraining on *in vivo* insulin sensitivity. Int J Sports Med 1990; 11(2): 107-10.
[http://dx.doi.org/10.1055/s-2007-1024772] [PMID: 2187003]

[47]    Dela F, Handberg A, Mikines KJ, Vinten J, Galbo H. GLUT 4 and insulin receptor binding and kinase activity in trained human muscle. J Physiol 1993; 469(1): 615-24.
[http://dx.doi.org/10.1113/jphysiol.1993.sp019833] [PMID: 8271219]

[48]    Yoo YK, Kim SK, Song MS. Effects of muscular and aqua aerobic combined exercise on metabolic indices in elderly women with metabolic syndrome. J Exerc Nutrition Biochem 2013; 17(4): 133-41.
[http://dx.doi.org/10.5717/jenb.2013.17.4.133] [PMID: 25566424]

[49]    Lee JA, Kim JW, Kim DY. Effects of yoga exercise on serum adiponectin and metabolic syndrome factors in obese postmenopausal women. Menopause 2012; 19(3): 296-301.

[http://dx.doi.org/10.1097/gme.0b013e31822d59a2] [PMID: 22089179]

[50]   Colberg SR, Sigal RJ, Yardley JE, *et al.* Physical Activity/Exercise and Diabetes: A Position Statement of the American Diabetes Association. Diabetes Care 2016; 39(11): 2065-79. [http://dx.doi.org/10.2337/dc16-1728] [PMID: 27926890]

[51]   Sato Y, Nagasaki M, Kubota M, Uno T, Nakai N. Clinical aspects of physical exercise for diabetes/metabolic syndrome. Diabetes Res Clin Pract 2007; 77(3) (Suppl. 1): S87-91. [http://dx.doi.org/10.1016/j.diabres.2007.01.039] [PMID: 17498834]

[52]   Csapo R, Gumpenberger M, Wessner B. Skeletal Muscle Extracellular Matrix - What Do We Know About Its Composition, Regulation, and Physiological Roles? A Narrative Review. Front Physiol. 2020; 11: 253. [http://dx.doi.org/10.3389/fphys.2020.00253]

[53]   McPherron AC, Guo T, Bond ND, Gavrilova O. Increasing muscle mass to improve metabolism. Adipocyte 2013; 2(2): 92-8. [http://dx.doi.org/10.4161/adip.22500] [PMID: 23805405]

[54]   Grevendonk L, Connell NJ, McCrum C, *et al.* Impact of aging and exercise on skeletal muscle mitochondrial capacity, energy metabolism, and physical function. Nat Commun. 2021; 12(1): 4773. [http://dx.doi.org/10.1038/s41467-021-24956-2]

[55]   Bowden Davies KA, Pickles S, Sprung VS, *et al.* Reduced physical activity in young and older adults: metabolic and musculoskeletal implications. Ther Adv Endocrinol Metab. 2019; 10. [http://dx.doi.org/10.1177/2042018819888824]

[56]   Pinckard K, Baskin KK, Stanford KI. Effects of Exercise to Improve Cardiovascular Health. Front Cardiovasc Med. 2019; 6: 69. [http://dx.doi.org/10.3389/fcvm.2019.00069]

[57]   Lopez-Jaramillo P, Lopez-Lopez JP, Tole MC, Cohen DD. Muscular Strength in Risk Factors for Cardiovascular Disease and Mortality: A Narrative Review. Anatol J Cardiol 2022; 26(8): 598-607. [http://dx.doi.org/10.5152/AnatolJCardiol.2022.1586] [PMID: 35924286]

[58]   Williams MA, Haskell WL, Ades PA, *et al.* Resistance exercise in individuals with and without cardiovascular disease: 2007 update: a scientific statement from the American Heart Association Council on Clinical Cardiology and Council on Nutrition, Physical Activity, and Metabolism. Circulation 2007; 116(5): 572-84. [http://dx.doi.org/10.1161/CIRCULATIONAHA.107.185214] [PMID: 17638929]

[59]   Ihalainen JK, Inglis A, Mäkinen T, *et al.* Strength Training Improves Metabolic Health Markers in Older Individual Regardless of Training Frequency. Front Physiol. 2019; 10: 32. [http://dx.doi.org/10.3389/fphys.2019.00032]

[60]   Makarewicz A, Jamka M, Geltz J, *et al.* Comparison of the Effect of Endurance, Strength, and Endurance-Strength Training on Inflammatory Markers and Adipokines Levels in Overweight and Obese Adults: Systematic Review and Meta-Analysis of Randomised Trials. Healthcare (Basel). 2022; 10(6): 1098. [http://dx.doi.org/10.3390/healthcare10061098]

[61]   Sandsdal RM, Juhl CR, Jensen SBK, *et al.* Combination of exercise and GLP-1 receptor agonist treatment reduces severity of metabolic syndrome, abdominal obesity, and inflammation: a randomized controlled trial. Cardiovasc Diabetol. 2023; 22(1): 41. [http://dx.doi.org/10.1186/s12933-023-01765-z]

[62]   Botezelli JD, Coope A, Ghezzi AC, *et al.* Strength Training Prevents Hyperinsulinemia, Insulin Resistance, and Inflammation Independent of Weight Loss in Fructose-Fed Animals. Sci Rep. 2016; 6: 31106. [http://dx.doi.org/10.1038/srep31106]

[63]   Zotti T, Giacco A, Cuomo A, *et al.* Exercise Equals the Mobilization of Visceral *versus* Subcutaneous

Adipose Fatty Acid Molecules in Fasted Rats Associated with the Modulation of the AMPK/ATGL/HSL Axis. Nutrients 2023; 15(14): 3095.
[http://dx.doi.org/10.3390/nu15143095] [PMID: 37513513]

[64]  Wedell-Neergaard AS, Lang Lehrskov L, Christensen RH, *et al.* Exercise-Induced Changes in Visceral Adipose Tissue Mass Are Regulated by IL-6 Signaling: A Randomized Controlled Trial. Cell Metab 2019; 29(4): 844-855.e3.
[http://dx.doi.org/10.1016/j.cmet.2018.12.007] [PMID: 30595477]

[65]  Pedersen BK, Saltin B. Exercise as medicine – evidence for prescribing exercise as therapy in 26 different chronic diseases. Scand J Med Sci Sports 2015; 25(S3) (Suppl. 3): 1-72.
[http://dx.doi.org/10.1111/sms.12581] [PMID: 26606383]

[66]  Rochlani Y, Pothineni NV, Kovelamudi S, Mehta JL. Metabolic syndrome: pathophysiology, management, and modulation by natural compounds. Ther Adv Cardiovasc Dis 2017; 11(8): 215-25.
[http://dx.doi.org/10.1177/1753944717711379] [PMID: 28639538]

[67]  Stone T, DiPietro L, Stachenfeld NS. Exercise Treatment of Obesity. In: Feingold KR, Anawalt B, Blackman MR, *et al.*, editors. Endotext [Internet]. South Dartmouth (MA): MDText.com, Inc. 2000; 15. Available from: https://www.ncbi.nlm.nih.gov/books/NBK278961/

[68]  Wadden TA, Tronieri JS, Butryn ML. Lifestyle modification approaches for the treatment of obesity in adults. Am Psychol 2020; 75(2): 235-51.
[http://dx.doi.org/10.1037/amp0000517] [PMID: 32052997]

[69]  Westerterp KR. Control of energy expenditure in humans. Eur J Clin Nutr 2017; 71(3): 340-4.
[http://dx.doi.org/10.1038/ejcn.2016.237] [PMID: 27901037]

[70]  Pons V, Riera J, Capó X, *et al.* Calorie restriction regime enhances physical performance of trained athletes. J Int Soc Sports Nutr. 2018; 15: 12.
[http://dx.doi.org/10.1186/s12970-018-0214-2]

[71]  Park JH, Moon JH, Kim HJ, Kong MH, Oh YH. Sedentary Lifestyle: Overview of Updated Evidence of Potential Health Risks. Korean J Fam Med 2020; 41(6): 365-73.
[http://dx.doi.org/10.4082/kjfm.20.0165] [PMID: 33242381]

[72]  Franklin BA, Eijsvogels TMH, Pandey A, Quindry J, Toth PP. Physical activity, cardiorespiratory fitness, and cardiovascular health: A clinical practice statement of the American Society for Preventive Cardiology Part II: Physical activity, cardiorespiratory fitness, minimum and goal intensities for exercise training, prescriptive methods, and special patient populations. Am J Prev Cardiol. 2022; 12: 100425.
[http://dx.doi.org/10.1016/j.ajpc.2022.100425]

[73]  Izquierdo M, Merchant RA, Morley JE, *et al.* International Exercise Recommendations in Older Adults (ICFSR): Expert Consensus Guidelines. J Nutr Health Aging 2021; 25(7): 824-53.
[http://dx.doi.org/10.1007/s12603-021-1665-8] [PMID: 34409961]

[74]  Sigal RJ, Kenny GP, Wasserman DH, Castaneda-Sceppa C. Physical Activity/Exercise and Type 2 Diabetes. Diabetes Spectr 2005; 18(2): 88-101.
[http://dx.doi.org/10.2337/diaspect.18.2.88]

[75]  Aoi W, Yamauchi H, Iwasa M, *et al.* Combined light exercise after meal intake suppresses postprandial serum triglyceride. Med Sci Sports Exerc 2013; 45(2): 245-52.
[http://dx.doi.org/10.1249/MSS.0b013e31826f3107] [PMID: 22914246]

[76]  Lee SC, Hairi NN, Moy FM. Metabolic syndrome among non-obese adults in the teaching profession in Melaka, Malaysia. J Epidemiol 2017; 27(3): 130-4.
[http://dx.doi.org/10.1016/j.je.2016.10.006] [PMID: 28142038]

[77]  Kikuchi A, Monma T, Ozawa S, Tsuchida M, Tsuda M, Takeda F. Risk factors for multiple metabolic syndrome components in obese and non-obese Japanese individuals. Prev Med 2021; 153: 106855.
[http://dx.doi.org/10.1016/j.ypmed.2021.106855] [PMID: 34687728]

[78]    Jo H, Kim JY, Jung MY, Ahn YS, Chang SJ, Koh SB. Leisure Time Physical Activity to Reduce Metabolic Syndrome Risk: A 10-Year Community-Based Prospective Study in Korea. Yonsei Med J 2020; 61(3): 218-28.
[http://dx.doi.org/10.3349/ymj.2020.61.3.218] [PMID: 32102122]

[79]    Kim HL, Chung J, Kim KJ, *et al.* Lifestyle Modification in the Management of Metabolic Syndrome: Statement From Korean Society of CardioMetabolic Syndrome (KSCMS). Korean Circ J 2022; 52(2): 93-109.
[http://dx.doi.org/10.4070/kcj.2021.0328] [PMID: 35128848]

[80]    Walker TJ, Tullar JM, Diamond PM, Kohl HW III, Amick BC III. Association of Self-Reported Aerobic Physical Activity, Muscle-Strengthening Physical Activity, and Stretching Behavior With Presenteeism. J Occup Environ Med 2017; 59(5): 474-9.
[http://dx.doi.org/10.1097/JOM.0000000000000978] [PMID: 28379877]

[81]    Cleven L, Krell-Roesch J, Schmidt SCE, *et al.* Longitudinal association between physical activity and the risk of incident metabolic syndrome in middle-aged adults in Germany. Sci Rep. 2022; 12(1): 19424.
[http://dx.doi.org/10.1038/s41598-022-24052-5]

[82]    Bull FC, Al-Ansari SS, Biddle S, *et al.* World Health Organization 2020 guidelines on physical activity and sedentary behaviour. Br J Sports Med 2020; 54(24): 1451-62.
[http://dx.doi.org/10.1136/bjsports-2020-102955] [PMID: 33239350]

[83]    Kraus W, Janz KF, Powell K, *et al.* Daily Step Counts for Measuring Physical Activity Exposure and Its Relation to Health. Med Sci Sports Exerc 2019; 51(6): 1206-12.
[http://dx.doi.org/10.1249/MSS.0000000000001932] [PMID: 31095077]

[84]    Paluch AE, Gabriel KP, Fulton JE, *et al.* Steps per Day and All-Cause Mortality in Middle-aged Adults in the Coronary Artery Risk Development in Young Adults Study. JAMA Netw Open. 2021; 4(9): e2124516.
[http://dx.doi.org/10.1001/jamanetworkopen.2021.24516]

# CHAPTER 14

# Chronic Obstructive Pulmonary Disease and Metabolic Syndrome

## Pelin Uysal[1,*]

[1] *Department of Pulmonary Medicine, Faculty of Medicine, Istanbul Atlas University, Istanbul, Turkey*

**Abstract:** Chronic obstructive pulmonary disease (COPD) is a clinical condition characterized by progressive airflow limitation caused by an abnormal inflammatory response of the lungs to harmful particles or gases that is not fully reversible. Smoking is largely responsible for the development of the disease. Systemic inflammation induced by smoking contributes to the natural history and clinical manifestations of COPD by causing chronic heart failure, metabolic syndrome (MetS) and other chronic diseases. MetS is a collection of interrelated clinical and biochemical disorders. MetS includes abdominal obesity, elevated triglycerides and low high-density lipoprotein (HDL) (atherogenic dyslipidemia), elevated blood pressure, insulin resistance, prothrombotic and proinflammatory markers (elevated C-reactive protein (CRP), fibrinogen, and other coagulation factors) with or without glucose intolerance. In patients with COPD, one or more components of MetS may be present in comorbidities that develop as a result of systemic inflammation. The prevalence of metabolic syndrome in COPD patients was found to be 30% and the prevalence of type 2 diabetes (T2DM) was found to be between 10-23%. Especially oral steroids used in the treatment of COPD exacerbations increase the risk of T2DM. Treatment of MetS and T2DM in patients with COPD does not differ.

**Keywords:** Comorbidities, Chronic obstructive pulmonary disease, Metabolic syndrome, Smoking, Systemic inflammation.

## INTRODUCTION

Metabolic syndrome (MetS) is an endocrinopathy of unknown etiopathogenesis that leads to diabetes and cardiovascular disease. MetS is a health problem whose prevalence is increasing worldwide and negatively affects people's lives. Although MetS, which is based on insulin resistance, is not recognized as a disease, it is a combination of many risk factors that force the body's metabolism to work abnormally. In the formation of MetS, sedentary lifestyle, and nutrition in addition to factors such as hereditary factors are also of great importance [1].

---

* **Corresponding author Pelin Uysal:** Department of Pulmonary Medicine, Faculty of Medicine, Istanbul Atlas University, Istanbul, Turkey; E-mail: drpelinuysal@gmail.com

**Hafize Uzun & Seyma Dumur (Eds.)**

Visceral adiposity, lipid profile disorder, endothelial dysfunction, arterial hypertension, chronic stress, insulin resistance, and hypercoagulability are the parameters that constitute MetS. The prevalence of MetS is on the rise globally. In the past few decades, several international organizations have provided the definitions of MetS. MetS has been proposed as a definition rather than a diagnosis [2, 3].

Chronic obstructive pulmonary disease (COPD) is a common, preventable and treatable disease characterized by persistent airflow limitation due to impaired airway and/or alveolar structure caused by host factors including exposure to harmful particles or gases and abnormal lung development. COPD is a lung disease characterized by chronic respiratory symptoms (shortness of breath, cough, sputum production and/or exacerbations) due to abnormalities of the airways (bronchitis, bronchiolitis) and/or alveoli (emphysema) that cause permanent, often progressive airflow obstruction [4]. Smoking is largely responsible for the development of the disease. Smoking not only causes inflammation in the airways and lungs, but also systemic cellular and humoral inflammation, systemic oxidative stress, altered vasomotor and endothelial function, and increased procoagulant factors. Systemic inflammation induced by smoking contributes to the natural history and clinical manifestations of COPD by causing chronic heart failure, MetS, and other chronic diseases [5].

**Metabolic Syndrome**

*Definition*

MetS is a proinflammatory, prothrombotic condition associated with the development of cardiovascular disease and type 2 diabetes mellitus (T2DM), which is caused by a combination of risk factors such as impaired glucose and insulin metabolism, obesity, dyslipidemia, and hypertension. There are problems in the diagnosis of metabolic syndrome due to the different definitions proposed. In 2005, the International Diabetes Federation (IDF) modified the ATP III criteria, noting that abdominal obesity is correlated with insulin resistance. The IDF noted ethnic differences in the correlation between MetS risk factors and abdominal obesity and defined abdominal obesity differently. There are problems in the diagnosis of MetS due to the different definitions proposed [6]. Table **1** shows the NCEP-ATP III metabolic syndrome diagnostic criteria [7].

*Risk Factors of Metabolic Syndrome*

Met Sis a cluster of conditions that occur together, increasing the risk of heart disease, stroke, and T2DM. Several risk factors contribute to the development of MetS [7 - 11].

**Table 1. NCEP-ATP III metabolic syndrome diagnostic criteria.**

| Parameter | Criteria |
|---|---|
| Abdominal obesity. | Waist circumference (WC). ≥ 102 cm (M). ≥88 cm (FM). |
| Triglyceride (TG). | ≥150 mg/dL or taking medication for hypertriglyceridemia. |
| High-density lipoprotein (HDL). | <40 mg/dL (M). <50 mg/dL (FM) or being treated for low HDL. |
| Blood pressure (BP). | Systolic blood pressure ≥130 mmHg or Diastolic blood pressure ≥85 mmHg or taking antihypertensive medication in a patient with a history of hypertension. |
| Fasting blood glucose. | ≥100 mg/dL or taking medication for the treatment of high blood glucose. |

- **Obesity:** Excess body fat, particularly around the waistline (abdominal obesity), is a significant risk factor for metS.
- **Insulin Resistance:** Insulin resistance occurs when cells in your body do not respond effectively to insulin, a hormone that helps control blood sugar levels. This leads to high blood sugar levels, which can contribute to the development of T2DM.
- **Physical Inactivity:** Lack of physical activity is associated with obesity and insulin resistance, both of which are key components of MetS.
- **Unhealthy Diet:** Consuming a diet high in processed foods, refined sugars, saturated fats, and cholesterol can contribute to obesity, insulin resistance, high blood pressure, and abnormal lipid levels—all components of MetS.
- **Genetics:** Family history and genetics can play a role in the development of MetS.
- **Age:** The risk of MetS increases with age, partly because muscle mass tends to decrease with age, leading to a decrease in metabolic rate.
- **Ethnicity:** Certain ethnic groups, such as African Americans, Hispanics, Native Americans, and Asians, have a higher risk of developing MetS.
- **Hormonal Imbalances:** Conditions such as polycystic ovary syndrome (PCOS) and Cushing's syndrome, which affect hormone levels, can increase the risk of MetS.
- **Sleep Apnea:** Sleep apnea, a condition characterized by pauses in breathing during sleep, is associated with MetS.
- **Smoking:** Smoking cigarettes is linked to insulin resistance and abdominal obesity, both of which are risk factors for MetS.

- **Stress:** Chronic stress can lead to overeating, physical inactivity, and unhealthy coping mechanisms such as smoking or excessive alcohol consumption, all of which contribute to MetS.
- **Metaflammation:** Metaflammation is a term that combines "metabolic" and "inflammation" and refers to low-grade chronic inflammation that occurs in the context of metabolic dysfunction, such as obesity, insulin resistance, and metabolic syndrome. This type of inflammation differs from acute inflammation, which is the body's natural response to injury or infection. In conditions like obesity and type 2 diabetes, adipose tissue (fat tissue) becomes dysfunctional and releases pro-inflammatory molecules called cytokines and adipokines. These molecules can trigger inflammation throughout the body, affecting various organs and systems, including the liver, pancreas, blood vessels, and immune system.

Managing these risk factors through lifestyle changes such as maintaining a healthy diet, regular physical activity, weight management, and avoiding smoking can help reduce the risk of developing metabolic syndrome. Additionally, medication may be prescribed to manage specific components of metabolic syndrome, such as high blood pressure or high cholesterol. Regular check-ups and screenings are important for early detection and management of MetS.

### *Components of Metabolic Syndrome*

MetS is characterized by a cluster of interconnected metabolic abnormalities that increase the risk of cardiovascular disease, T2DM, and other health problems. The key components of MetS typically include [12 - 15]:

- **Abdominal Obesity:** This is often measured by waist circumference. In men, abdominal obesity is defined as a waist circumference (WC) of 102 cm or more, while in women, it is defined as a waist circumference of 88 cm or more.
- **Insulin Resistance:** This occurs when the body's cells don't respond effectively to insulin, a hormone that regulates blood sugar levels. As a result, blood sugar levels rise, leading to hyperglycemia.
- **High Blood Pressure (Hypertension):** Blood pressure is considered high if it consistently measures 130/85 mmHg or higher. Hypertension strains the heart, arteries, and other organs, increasing the risk of heart disease and stroke.
- **High Blood Sugar (Hyperglycemia):** Elevated fasting blood sugar levels, indicative of impaired glucose metabolism, are often seen in MetS. A fasting blood glucose level of 100 mg/dL or higher is considered indicative of hyperglycemia.

- **High Triglyceride Levels:** Triglycerides are a type of fat found in the blood. Levels above 150 mg/dL are considered high. High triglyceride levels are associated with an increased risk of cardiovascular disease.
- **Low HDL Cholesterol Levels:** High-density lipoprotein (HDL) cholesterol is often referred to as "good" cholesterol because it helps remove excess cholesterol from the bloodstream. HDL levels below 40 mg/dL in men and below 50 mg/dL in women are considered low and are associated with increased cardiovascular risk.

Having three or more of these components typically leads to a diagnosis of MetS. The presence of MetS significantly increases the risk of developing cardiovascular disease (CVD), T2DM, and other health problems. Lifestyle modifications such as regular exercise, a healthy diet, weight loss, and medication (if necessary) can help manage the components of MetS and reduce the associated health risks.

The constellation of MetS, except for when defined with ATP III definition, is a marker for identifying individuals at higher risk for sudden cardiac death (SCD); however, not independent of its components. Among MetS components, abdominal obesity using the population-specific cutoff point, high glucose component (JIS/IDF definitions), and high blood pressure (WHO definition) were independent predictors of SCD [16].

**Chronic obstructive pulmonary disease (COPD)**

*Definition*

The first change in the Global Initiative for Chronic Obstructive Lung Disease (GOLD) 2023 is the definition of the disease. Accordingly, GOLD 2023 defines COPD as a heterogeneous lung condition characterized by chronic respiratory symptoms (dyspnea, cough, expectoration and/or exacerbations) due to abnormalities of the airways (bronchitis, bronchiolitis) and/or alveoli (emphysema) that cause persistent, often progressive, airflow obstruction [17].

Compared to the previous definition, the new definition emphasizes heterogeneity and symptoms but does not include a statement referring to etiology or pathogenesis. From this perspective, it is clear that there is still room for improvement. On the other hand, the concept of "GETomics", which was included in the GOLD statements for the first time, is a practical approach as it is an acrostic summarizing the complex processes in the emergence of the disease. According to this concept, COPD is caused by the interaction of genes (Gene=G) and environment (Environment=E) with the normal or aging or damaged lung of the individual (omics) throughout his/her life (life Time=T) (GETomics) [18].

## Taxonomy

In addition, for the first time in this report, "COPD taxonomy" successfully emphasized etiology and proposed to classify COPD into 7 categories according to their etiology using the short title "etiotypes" (Table 1) [17, 19]. It aims to raise awareness about nonsmoking-related COPD and to stimulate research on the mechanisms and corresponding diagnostic, preventive or therapeutic approaches for these other etiotypes of COPD, which are highly prevalent around the globe [20].

## Risk factors

Several risk factors contribute to the development and progression of COPD:

- **Smoking:** Smoking is the most studied risk factor for COPD, but it is not the only risk factor for this disease. It is known that non-smokers may also have airway restrictions [21]. However, it has been found that the course of the disease is milder and the inflammatory burden is less in non-smokers compared to smokers [22].
- **Environmental Exposure to Air Pollutants:** Prolonged exposure to indoor and outdoor air pollutants, such as particulate matter, chemicals, dust, and fumes, can contribute to the development of COPD. Occupational exposures in certain industries, such as mining, construction, agriculture, and manufacturing, pose a risk for COPD due to inhalation of hazardous substances [22].

**Table 2. Classification of COPD based on etiology [19].**

| Classification | Description |
|---|---|
| Genetically defined COPD (COPD-G). | Alpha-1 Antitrypsin deficiency (AATD). Other genetic variants. |
| COPD due to abnormal lung development (COPD-D). | Early life events (including prematurity and low birth weight). |
| Environmental COPD. - Smoking-related COPD (COPD-C). - Biomass and pollution exposure COPD (COPD-P). | • Smoking (active, passive, in-utero). • Vaping or e-cigarettes. • Cannabis. • Indoor and outdoor air pollution. • Forest fires. • Occupational hazards. |
| Infection due to COPD (COPD-I). | Childhood infection, TB-related COPD, HIV-related COPD. |
| COPD and asthma (COPD-A). | Especially childhood asthma. |
| COPD of unknown cause (COPD-U). | - |

- **Genetic Factors:** Genetic predisposition can influence an individual's susceptibility to COPD. Alpha-1 antitrypsin deficiency (AATD) is a hereditary condition that predisposes individuals to early-onset COPD, particularly in nonsmokers or those with minimal smoking history. Alpha-1 antitrypsin is a protein that protects the lungs from damage caused by inflammatory enzymes. Deficiency of this protein can lead to lung tissue damage and COPD, especially when combined with environmental exposures. Although AATD is the best-known genetic factor, it has been associated with lung damage in very few individuals [23]. However, many genetic studies have been conducted on COPD and these genes or the structures they produce have not been directly linked to the development of COPD [24 - 29].
- **Aging:** Age is always an independent risk factor for COPD. Aging is associated with physiological changes in the lungs, including decreased elasticity of lung tissue and weakening of respiratory muscles. These age-related changes can impair lung function and increase susceptibility to COPD. However, it is not known whether the increase in the prevalence of COPD with increasing age is due to the effect of environmental accumulation or changes caused by aging [30].
- **Gender:** Although male gender is thought to carry a higher risk for COPD, recent studies have shown that smoking tendencies determine this [31]. Again, recent studies have shown that women are more susceptible to the damage caused by cigarette smoking and that a more severe disease picture occurs in the female gender as a result of equal smoking [32 - 34]. This contrary view has also been confirmed by animal studies and human pathologic samples [35, 36].

**Chronic Asthma:** Individuals with poorly controlled or severe asthma are at an increased risk of developing COPD. Chronic inflammation and airway remodeling associated with asthma can lead to irreversible airflow limitation and COPD-like symptoms over time. Studies have shown that 20% of patients with asthma have permanent airway restriction and the prevalence of COPD has increased 12-fold compared to the normal population [37, 38]. This suggests that asthma is a risk factor for COPD. However, the usual airway hyperresponsiveness seen in asthma has been shown to be a risk factor for COPD in non-asthmatic patients [39, 40].

**Respiratory Infections:** Recurrent respiratory infections, particularly during childhood, may increase the risk of developing COPD later in life [41]. Infections caused by viruses (such as respiratory syncytial virus and influenza) and bacteria (such as *Streptococcus pneumoniae* and *Haemophilus influenzae*) can cause lung damage and inflammation, contributing to COPD pathogenesis. Although infections are known to cause attacks in COPD patients, their effect on the development of COPD is not fully known. However, tuberculosis can be considered among COPD risk factors [42].

## COPD AND COMORBIDITIES

Comorbidities in COPD affect symptoms, quality of life, complications, disease management, economic burden and mortality [43]. COPD is a progressive lung disease characterized by airflow limitation that is not fully reversible. Common comorbidities associated with COPD include cardiovascular diseases (such as hypertension, coronary artery disease, and heart failure), osteoporosis, anxiety, depression, and metabolic disorders like diabetes and MetS [43].

Overall, recognizing and effectively managing comorbidities in COPD patients is essential for optimizing their care and improving outcomes. A comprehensive approach that addresses both COPD and its associated comorbidities can help improve symptom control, quality of life, and overall health outcomes for individuals living with this chronic condition [44 - 46].

Comorbidities can be divided into the pulmonary and the extrapulmonary [45]:

### Major Pulmonary Comorbidities

Several major pulmonary comorbidities commonly occur alongside COPD. These comorbidities can significantly impact the progression and management of COPD. Some of the major pulmonary comorbidities in COPD include [45]:

***Pulmonary Hypertension (PH):*** PH is a condition characterized by increased pressure in the pulmonary arteries. In COPD, chronic inflammation and narrowing of the pulmonary blood vessels can lead to PH. This condition can exacerbate symptoms such as dyspnea (shortness of breath) and fatigue and can significantly worsen prognosis [47].

**Bronchial asthma:** Bronchial asthma is the most common pulmonary comorbidity in COPD. The prevalence of bronchial asthma in patients with COPD has been estimated at 27% in observational studies [43].

***Chronic Bronchitis:*** Chronic bronchitis is a type of COPD characterized by persistent inflammation and narrowing of the bronchial tubes, leading to increased mucus production and cough. While chronic bronchitis is often considered a component of COPD itself, it can also exist as a separate comorbidity alongside COPD, further exacerbating respiratory symptoms [48].

***Emphysema:*** Emphysema is another form of COPD characterized by damage to the alveoli (air sacs) in the lungs, leading to air trapping and reduced lung function. Although emphysema is typically considered part of COPD, severe cases may be distinguished as a separate comorbidity, contributing to worsened lung function and respiratory symptoms [49].

***Bronchiectasis:*** Bronchiectasis is a chronic lung condition characterized by abnormal widening and scarring of the bronchi (airways), leading to recurrent infections and mucus buildup. It can often coexist with COPD, particularly in patients with a history of chronic respiratory infections or severe airflow limitation [50]. Bronchiectasis is associated with productive cough, bronchial infections, and abnormal bronchial dilatation. In patients with COPD, bronchiectasis is associated with a reduced body mass index, more advanced age, and increased sputum production and exacerbations. Bronchiectasis is associated with productive cough, bronchial infections, and abnormal bronchial dilatation. In patients with COPD, bronchiectasis is associated with a reduced body mass index, more advanced age, and increased sputum production and exacerbations [43].

***Asthma-COPD Overlap Syndrome (ACOS):*** ACOS refers to a condition where patients exhibit features of both asthma and COPD, including airflow limitation and respiratory symptoms such as wheezing, cough, and dyspnea. This overlap syndrome can complicate diagnosis and management, requiring a tailored approach to treatment [51].

***Interstitial Lung Disease (ILD):*** ILD encompasses a group of disorders characterized by inflammation and scarring of the lung tissue. While not as common as other pulmonary comorbidities in COPD, ILD can occur concurrently with COPD, leading to progressive lung function decline and respiratory symptoms [52].

These pulmonary comorbidities often contribute to worsening respiratory symptoms, decreased lung function, and increased risk of exacerbations and hospitalizations in COPD patients. Proper identification and management of these comorbidities are crucial for optimizing treatment outcomes and improving the quality of life for individuals living with COPD [45].

## Major Extrapulmonary Comorbidities

These comorbidities can significantly impact the overall health and prognosis of COPD patients. It is one of the leading comorbidities accompanying COPD [43]. The importance of comorbidities stems from their effects on the outcomes of COPD. The most common comorbidities found in COPD are cardiovascular, endocrinologic, psychological, and lung cancer. At least 50% of COPD patients have three or more comorbidities. However, there is no conclusive evidence that active treatment of these comorbidities affects the outcome of COPD. On the other hand, comorbidities such as cardiovascular disease and lung cancer have a significant impact on COPD mortality. Several studies have shown that the Charlson comorbidity index or the COPD-specific comorbidity index (COTE) is associated with COPD mortality [53].

Some of the major extrapulmonary comorbidities in COPD include:

*I- Cardiovascular disease:* It is one of the leading comorbidities accompanying COPD. It can be said to be the most important and most common comorbidity. COPD patients have an increased risk of cardiovascular conditions such as coronary artery disease, heart failure, hypertension, and arrhythmias. Shared risk factors such as smoking, inflammation, and reduced physical activity contribute to the development of cardiovascular comorbidities [54].

### *Ischemic Heart Disease*

Most of the risk factors for ischemic heart disease are also present in COPD patients, which is why the rate of ischemic heart disease is high in COPD patients [55 - 57]. Myocardial damage may be overlooked in COPD patients, so there is evidence that it is not diagnosed accurately enough [58]. There is no different recommendation for the treatment of COPD in patients with ischemic heart disease; they should be treated as they are normally treated. Use of beta-blockers following an acute coronary syndrome (ACS) admission was much lower than expected based on the findings of general audits of ACS management in New Zealand. Along with the higher proportions using aspirin and statins, and the differences in beta-blocker dispensing by COPD severity, this suggests a particular reluctance to prescribe beta-blockers to patients with COPD [59]. Similarly, there is no different recommendation for the treatment of ischemic heart disease in COPD patients. The use of cardioselective β1 blockers is said to be more safe [60].

### *Heart Failure*

Heart failure is a common comorbidity. Even in patients with stable COPD, approximately 32% have heart failure [61]. Similarly, approximately 35% of patients with heart failure have COPD [62]. In fact, COPD is often the reason for hospitalization due to acute heart failure. There is no different recommendation for the treatment of heart failure in COPD patients; heart failure treatment should continue according to the recommendations of heart failure guidelines. Although selective β 1 blocker therapy has a significant effect on survival in patients with heart failure, the presence of COPD interferes with this treatment and is an important barrier to optimal treatment in these patients [63].

## Hypertension

Hypertension is probably the most common comorbidity in COPD patients and affects prognosis [64]. There is no specific treatment recommendation for the treatment of hypertension in patients with COPD nor for the treatment of COPD in patients with hypertension. Therefore, they should be treated in accordance with existing guidelines. If β blockers are to be used in the treatment of hypertension in COPD patients, selective β 1 blockers should be preferred [65 - 68].

## II- Metabolic disorders

Metabolic disorders are common comorbidities in individuals with COPD. These disorders can have significant implications for the management and prognosis of COPD patients. Some of the key metabolic disorders associated with COPD include:

a. **Obesity:** Obesity is prevalent among COPD patients and is associated with increased systemic inflammation, reduced exercise tolerance, and worsened respiratory symptoms. Obesity can also contribute to the development of MetS and insulin resistance, further complicating COPD management. the benefits of nutritional therapies including macro- and micro-nutrient supplementation, nutritional management during acute exacerbation, and management of obesity in COPD [69]. In patients with advanced COPD, it is well known that overweight and obese patients have better survival compared to normal-weight patients. Previous studies showed that obesity was associated with an increased risk of all-cause mortality in patients with mild-to-moderate COPD compared to normal BMI patients with comparable disease severity [70].

b. **Dyslipidemia:** Dyslipidemia, characterized by abnormal levels of cholesterol and triglycerides, is more common in COPD patients. Dyslipidemia is associated with systemic inflammation and oxidative stress, which contribute to the progression of COPD and cardiovascular diseases. Statin therapy, commonly used to manage dyslipidemia, may have beneficial effects on COPD outcomes. Systemic inflammation, along with smoking and oxidative stress, plays an important role in the development of dyslipidemia in COPD [71]. Although hyperlipidemia is a risk factor for the development of cardiovascular comorbidities, interestingly, its presence does not appear to be associated with a worse outcome of COPD. To reduce the cardiovascular risk profile, treatment of concomitant hyperlipidemia should be based on the recommendations of the relevant professional associations [72].

c. **Type 2 Diabetes Mellitus (T2DM):** COPD patients have a higher prevalence of type 2 diabetes mellitus compared to the general population. Shared risk factors such as smoking, obesity, and systemic inflammation contribute to the development of diabetes in COPD patients. Diabetes can worsen COPD outcomes by increasing the risk of exacerbations, respiratory infections, and cardiovascular events [73]. The prevalence of diabetes mellitus in patients with stable COPD is around 15% to 17%, which is higher than in the general population [74, 75]. Apart from any side effects of respiratory medication, effects of systemic inflammation due to the underlying COPD are under discussion as a possible cause [43].

d. **Metabolic syndrome:** MetS is a cluster of metabolic abnormalities including obesity, insulin resistance, dyslipidemia, and hypertension. COPD patients are at increased risk of MetS due to factors such as systemic inflammation, physical inactivity, and corticosteroid use. MetS is associated with an elevated risk of CVDs and worsened COPD outcomes. The prevalence of metabolic syndrome among those with COPD is reported to be anywhere between 21% and 58% depending on disease severity, geographic location, definition utilized and the assessments made [76, 77]. There is a suggestion that metabolic syndrome is more prevalent in those with milder airflow obstruction, but this may in part reflect the weight loss observed in the severe stages of COPD. Single studies have reported a higher prevalence of metabolic syndrome than age- and gender-matched individuals without COPD [78, 79].

There is also intriguing evidence that T2DM and MetS through an inflammatory mechanism result in airflow obstruction [80, 81] rather than metabolic derangement occurring in COPD as a co-morbidity. Whether effective metabolic management may slow the progression of airflow limitation in patients with COPD is yet unknown. Obesity and MetS are common in patients with COPD who are symptomatic and referred for pulmonary rehabilitation.

Especially oral steroids used in the treatment of COPD exacerbations increase the risk of T2DM. Some studies have found that 11% of COPD patients using oral steroids developed T2DM. In addition, high-dose inhaled steroids used in the treatment of COPD are also reported to increase the risk of T2DM and make glucose control difficult. Treatment of MetS and T2DM in patients with COPD does not differ [82].

Management of metabolic disorders in COPD patients involves a comprehensive approach, including lifestyle modifications (such as weight management and physical activity), pharmacological interventions (such as glucose-lowering medications and statins), and treatment of COPD exacerbations and complications. Multidisciplinary care teams can help address metabolic disorders and optimize COPD management to improve patient outcomes and quality of life [83].

# CONCLUSION

As a result, comorbidities have an impact on the course of COPD. It is known that group B patients die due to comorbidities rather than COPD. Exacerbation symptoms may sometimes be due to comorbidities and may be confused with true exacerbation. The cause of death in exacerbations may be due to comorbidities and the treatment of COPD may be affected by comorbidities. Hospitalizations, economic burden, and death in COPD may be related to the type and number of comorbidities rather than FEV1. Therefore, in line with the GOLD 2023 report, GOLD recommends active investigation and good management of comorbidities in COPD.

# REFERENCES

[1]    Gesteiro E, Megía A, Guadalupe-Grau A, Fernandez-Veledo S, Vendrell J, González-Gross M. Early identification of metabolic syndrome risk: A review of reviews and proposal for defining pre-metabolic syndrome status. Nutr Metab Cardiovasc Dis 2021; 31(9): 2557-74.
[http://dx.doi.org/10.1016/j.numecd.2021.05.022] [PMID: 34244048]

[2]    Molina-Luque R, Molina-Recio G, de-Pedro-Jiménez D, Álvarez Fernández C, García-Rodríguez M, Romero-Saldaña M. The Impact of Metabolic Syndrome Risk Factors on Lung Function Impairment: Cross-Sectional Study. JMIR Public Health Surveill 2023; 9: e43737.
[http://dx.doi.org/10.2196/43737] [PMID: 37669095]

[3]    Alberti KGMM, Zimmet P, Shaw J. The metabolic syndrome—a new worldwide definition. Lancet 2005; 366(9491): 1059-62.
[http://dx.doi.org/10.1016/S0140-6736(05)67402-8] [PMID: 16182882]

[4]    Agustí A, Celli BR, Criner GJ, *et al.* Global Initiative for Chronic Obstructive Lung Disease 2023 Report: GOLD Executive Summary. Eur Respir J 2023; 61(4): 2300239.
[http://dx.doi.org/10.1183/13993003.00239-2023] [PMID: 36858443]

[5]    Mannino DM, Watt G, Hole D, *et al.* The natural history of chronic obstructive pulmonary disease. Eur Respir J 2006; 27(3): 627-43.
[http://dx.doi.org/10.1183/09031936.06.00024605] [PMID: 16507865]

[6]    Grundy SM, Brewer HB Jr, Cleeman JI, Smith SC Jr, Lenfant C. Definition of metabolic syndrome: Report of the National Heart, Lung, and Blood Institute/American Heart Association conference on scientific issues related to definition. Circulation 2004; 109(3): 433-8.
[http://dx.doi.org/10.1161/01.CIR.0000111245.75752.C6] [PMID: 14744958]

[7]    Grundy SM, Cleeman JI, Daniels SR, *et al.* Diagnosis and Management of the Metabolic Syndrome. Circulation 2005; 112(17): 2735-52.
[http://dx.doi.org/10.1161/CIRCULATIONAHA.105.169404] [PMID: 16157765]

[8]    Rochlani Y, Pothineni NV, Kovelamudi S, Mehta JL. Metabolic syndrome: pathophysiology, management, and modulation by natural compounds. Ther Adv Cardiovasc Dis 2017; 11(8): 215-25.
[http://dx.doi.org/10.1177/1753944717711379] [PMID: 28639538]

[9]    Spahis S, Borys JM, Levy E. Metabolic Syndrome as a Multifaceted Risk Factor for Oxidative Stress. Antioxid Redox Signal 2017; 26(9): 445-61.
[http://dx.doi.org/10.1089/ars.2016.6756] [PMID: 27302002]

[10]   Silveira Rossi JL, Barbalho SM, Reverete de Araujo R, Bechara MD, Sloan KP, Sloan LA. Metabolic syndrome and cardiovascular diseases: Going beyond traditional risk factors. Diabetes Metab Res Rev 2022; 38(3): e3502.
[http://dx.doi.org/10.1002/dmrr.3502] [PMID: 34614543]

[11] Mandecka A, Regulska-Ilow B. Dietary interventions in the treatment of metabolic syndrome as a cardiovascular disease risk-inducing factor. A review. Rocz Panstw Zakl Hig 2018; 69(3): 227-33.
[PMID: 30141315]

[12] Hess PL, Al-Khalidi HR, Friedman DJ, *et al.* The metabolic syndrome and risk of sudden cardiac death: the atherosclerosis risk in communities study. J Am Heart Assoc 2017; 6(8): e006103.
[http://dx.doi.org/10.1161/JAHA.117.006103] [PMID: 28835363]

[13] Alberti KGMM, Eckel RH, Grundy SM, *et al.* Harmonizing the Metabolic Syndrome. Circulation 2009; 120(16): 1640-5.
[http://dx.doi.org/10.1161/CIRCULATIONAHA.109.192644] [PMID: 19805654]

[14] Azizi F, Khalili D, Aghajani H, *et al.* Appropriate waist circumference cut-off points among Iranian adults: the first report of the Iranian National Committee of Obesity. Arch Iran Med 2010; 13(3): 243-4.
[PMID: 20433230]

[15] Hadaegh F, Zabetian A, Sarbakhsh P, Khalili D, James WPT, Azizi F. Appropriate cutoff values of anthropometric variables to predict cardiovascular outcomes: 7.6 years follow-up in an Iranian population. Int J Obes 2009; 33(12): 1437-45.
[http://dx.doi.org/10.1038/ijo.2009.180] [PMID: 19752876]

[16] Masrouri S, Moazzeni SS, Cheraghloo N, Azizi F, Hadaegh F. The clinical value of metabolic syndrome and its components with respect to sudden cardiac death using different definitions: Two decades of follow-up from the Tehran Lipid and Glucose Study. Cardiovasc Diabetol 2022; 21(1): 269.
[http://dx.doi.org/10.1186/s12933-022-01707-1] [PMID: 36463175]

[17] Celli B, Fabbri L, Criner G, *et al.* Definition and Nomenclature of Chronic Obstructive Pulmonary Disease: Time for Its Revision. Am J Respir Crit Care Med 2022; 206(11): 1317-25.
[http://dx.doi.org/10.1164/rccm.202204-0671PP] [PMID: 35914087]

[18] Agustí A, Melén E, DeMeo DL, Breyer-Kohansal R, Faner R. Pathogenesis of chronic obstructive pulmonary disease: understanding the contributions of gene–environment interactions across the lifespan. Lancet Respir Med 2022; 10(5): 512-24.
[http://dx.doi.org/10.1016/S2213-2600(21)00555-5] [PMID: 35427533]

[19] 2023. Global strategy for prevention, diagnosis and managment of COPD. Report. https://goldcopd.org/2023-gold-report-2/ (last accessed on 5 June 2023) 2023.

[20] Yang IA, Jenkins CR, Salvi SS. Chronic obstructive pulmonary disease in never-smokers: risk factors, pathogenesis, and implications for prevention and treatment. Lancet Respir Med 2022; 10(5): 497-511.
[http://dx.doi.org/10.1016/S2213-2600(21)00506-3] [PMID: 35427530]

[21] Lamprecht B, McBurnie MA, Vollmer WM, *et al.* COPD in never smokers: results from the population-based burden of obstructive lung disease study. Chest 2011; 139(4): 752-63.
[http://dx.doi.org/10.1378/chest.10-1253] [PMID: 20884729]

[22] Thomsen M, Nordestgaard BG, Vestbo J, Lange P. Characteristics and outcomes of chronic obstructive pulmonary disease in never smokers in Denmark: a prospective population study. Lancet Respir Med 2013; 1(7): 543-50.
[http://dx.doi.org/10.1016/S2213-2600(13)70137-1] [PMID: 24461615]

[23] Stoller JK, Aboussouan LS. α1-antitrypsin deficiency. Lancet 2005; 365(9478): 2225-36.
[http://dx.doi.org/10.1016/S0140-6736(05)66781-5] [PMID: 15978931]

[24] Cho Michael H, *et al.* Variants in FAM13A are associated with chronic obstructive pulmonary disease. Nature genetics 423 2010; 200.
[http://dx.doi.org/10.1038/ng.535]

[25] Cho MH, McDonald MLN, Zhou X, *et al.* Risk loci for chronic obstructive pulmonary disease: a genome-wide association study and meta-analysis. Lancet Respir Med 2014; 2(3): 214-25.

[http://dx.doi.org/10.1016/S2213-2600(14)70002-5] [PMID: 24621683]

[26]     Elkington Paul T, Cooke Graham S. Cooke. MMP12, lung function, and COPD in high-risk populations. N Engl J Med 2010; 362.13: 1241.

[27]     Pillai Sreekumar G, *et al.* A genome-wide association study in chronic obstructive pulmonary disease (COPD): identification of two major susceptibility loci 2009.
         [http://dx.doi.org/10.1371/journal.pgen.1000421]

[28]     Repapi Emmanouela, *et al.* Genome-wide association study identifies five loci associated with lung function. PLoS genetics 53 2010; e1000421.
         [http://dx.doi.org/10.1038/ng.501]

[29]     Soler Artigas M, Wain LV, Repapi E, *et al.* Effect of five genetic variants associated with lung function on the risk of chronic obstructive lung disease, and their joint effects on lung function. Am J Respir Crit Care Med 2011; 184(7): 786-95.
         [http://dx.doi.org/10.1164/rccm.201102-0192OC] [PMID: 21965014]

[30]     Mercado N, Ito K, Barnes PJ. Accelerated ageing of the lung in COPD: new concepts. Thorax 2015; 70(5): 482-9.
         [http://dx.doi.org/10.1136/thoraxjnl-2014-206084] [PMID: 25739910]

[31]     Landis SH, Muellerova H, Mannino DM, *et al.* Continuing to Confront COPD International Patient Survey: methods, COPD prevalence, and disease burden in 2012-2013. Int J Chron Obstruct Pulmon Dis 2014; 9: 597-611.
         [PMID: 24944511]

[32]     Foreman MG, Zhang L, Murphy J, *et al.* Early-onset chronic obstructive pulmonary disease is associated with female sex, maternal factors, and African American race in the COPDGene Study. Am J Respir Crit Care Med 2011; 184(4): 414-20.
         [http://dx.doi.org/10.1164/rccm.201011-1928OC] [PMID: 21562134]

[33]     Sılverman, Edwın K., *et al.* Gender-related differences in severe, early-onset chronic obstructive pulmonary disease. American journal of respiratory and critical care medicine 162.6 (2000): 2152-2158. 72.

[34]     Lopez Varela MV, Montes de Oca M, Halbert RJ, *et al.* Sex-related differences in COPD in five Latin American cities: the PLATINO study. Eur Respir J 2010; 36(5): 1034-41.
         [http://dx.doi.org/10.1183/09031936.00165409] [PMID: 20378599]

[35]     Martinez FJ, Curtis JL, Sciurba F, *et al.* Sex differences in severe pulmonary emphysema. Am J Respir Crit Care Med 2007; 176(3): 243-52.
         [http://dx.doi.org/10.1164/rccm.200606-828OC] [PMID: 17431226]

[36]     Tam A, Churg A, Wright JL, *et al.* Sex differences in airway remodeling in a mouse model of chronic obstructive pulmonary disease. Am J Respir Crit Care Med 2016; 193(8): 825-34.
         [http://dx.doi.org/10.1164/rccm.201503-0487OC] [PMID: 26599602]

[37]     Silva GE, Sherrill DL, Guerra S, Barbee RA. Asthma as a risk factor for COPD in a longitudinal study. Chest 2004; 126(1): 59-65.
         [http://dx.doi.org/10.1378/chest.126.1.59] [PMID: 15249443]

[38]     Vonk JM, Jongepier H, Panhuysen CI, Schouten JP, Bleecker ER, Postma DS. Risk factors associated with the presence of irreversible airflow limitation and reduced transfer coefficient in patients with asthma after 26 years of follow up. Thorax 2003; 58(4): 322-7.
         [http://dx.doi.org/10.1136/thorax.58.4.322] [PMID: 12668795]

[39]     Hospers JJ, Postma DS, Rijcken B, Weiss ST, Schouten JP. Histamine airway hyper-responsiveness and mortality from chronic obstructive pulmonary disease: a cohort study. Lancet 2000; 356(9238): 1313-7.
         [http://dx.doi.org/10.1016/S0140-6736(00)02815-4] [PMID: 11073020]

[40]     Rijcken B, *et al.* The relationship of nonspecific bronchial responsiveness to respiratory symptoms in a

random population sample. Am Rev Respir Dis 1987; 136(1): 62-8.74.
[http://dx.doi.org/10.1164/ajrccm/136.1.62]

[41]  de Marco R, Accordini S, Marcon A, *et al.* Risk factors for chronic obstructive pulmonary disease in a European cohort of young adults. Am J Respir Crit Care Med 2011; 183(7): 891-7.
[http://dx.doi.org/10.1164/rccm.201007-1125OC] [PMID: 20935112]

[42]  Byrne AL, Marais BJ, Mitnick CD, Lecca L, Marks GB. Tuberculosis and chronic respiratory disease: a systematic review. Int J Infect Dis 2015; 32: 138-46.
[http://dx.doi.org/10.1016/j.ijid.2014.12.016] [PMID: 25809770]

[43]  Kahnert K, Jörres RA, Behr J, Welte T. The diagnosis and treatment of COPD and its comorbidities. Dtsch Arztebl Int 2023; 120(25): 434-44.
[http://dx.doi.org/10.3238/arztebl.m2023.0027] [PMID: 36794439]

[44]  Shah T, Churpek MM, Coca Perraillon M, Konetzka RT. Understanding why patients with COPD get readmitted: a large national study to delineate the Medicare population for the readmissions penalty expansion. Chest 2015; 147(5): 1219-26.
[http://dx.doi.org/10.1378/chest.14-2181] [PMID: 25539483]

[45]  Trudzinski FC, Jörres RA, Alter P, *et al.* Sex-specific associations of comorbidome and pulmorbidome with mortality in chronic obstructive pulmonary disease: results from COSYCONET. Sci Rep 2022; 12(1): 8790.
[http://dx.doi.org/10.1038/s41598-022-12828-8] [PMID: 35610473]

[46]  Spece LJ, Epler EM, Donovan LM, *et al.* Role of comorbidities in treatment and outcomes after chronic obstructive pulmonary disease exacerbations. Ann Am Thorac Soc 2018; 15(9): 1033-8.
[http://dx.doi.org/10.1513/AnnalsATS.201804-255OC] [PMID: 30079748]

[47]  Humbert M, Kovacs G, Hoeper MM, *et al.* 2022 ESC/ERS Guidelines for the diagnosis and treatment of pulmonary hypertension. Eur Heart J 2022; 43(38): 3618-731.
[http://dx.doi.org/10.1093/eurheartj/ehac237] [PMID: 36017548]

[48]  Tana A, Zhang C, DiBardino D, Orton CM, Shah PL. Bronchoscopic interventions for chronic bronchitis. Curr Opin Pulm Med 2024; 30(1): 68-74.
[http://dx.doi.org/10.1097/MCP.0000000000001036] [PMID: 37942820]

[49]  Pahal P, Avula A, Sharma S. Emphysema.StatPearls. Treasure Island, FL: StatPearls Publishing 2023.

[50]  Chalmers JD, Shoemark A. Inhaled Corticosteroids in COPD and Bronchiectasis. Chest 2023; 164(4): 809-11.
[http://dx.doi.org/10.1016/j.chest.2023.07.013] [PMID: 37805235]

[51]  Jiang T, Li P, Wang Y. Effect of budesonide formoterol combined with tiotropium bromide on pulmonary function and inflammatory factors in patients with asthma–COPD overlap syndrome. Allergol Immunopathol (Madr) 2023; 51(4): 131-8.
[http://dx.doi.org/10.15586/aei.v51i4.876] [PMID: 37422789]

[52]  Janssen DJA, Bajwah S, Boon MH, *et al.* European Respiratory Society clinical practice guideline: palliative care for people with COPD or interstitial lung disease. Eur Respir J 2023; 62(2): 2202014.
[http://dx.doi.org/10.1183/13993003.02014-2022] [PMID: 37290789]

[53]  Figueira-Gonçalves JM, Golpe R, García-Bello MÁ, García-Talavera I, Castro-Añón O. Comparison of the prognostic capability of two comorbidity indices in patients with chronic obstructive pulmonary disease, in real-life clinical practice. Clin Respir J 2019; 13(6): 404-7.
[http://dx.doi.org/10.1111/crj.13025] [PMID: 30950184]

[54]  André S, Conde B, Fragoso E, Boléo-Tomé JP, Areias V, Cardoso J. COPD and Cardiovascular Disease. Pulmonology 2019; 25(3): 168-76.
[http://dx.doi.org/10.1016/j.pulmoe.2018.09.006] [PMID: 30527374]

[55]  Lange P, *et al.* Cardiovascular morbidity in COPD: a study of the general population 2011; 7(1): 5-10.
[http://dx.doi.org/10.3109/15412550903499506]

[56]     Global, regional, and national age–sex specific all-cause and cause-specific mortality for 240 causes of death, 1990–2013: a systematic analysis for the Global Burden of Disease Study 2013. Lancet 2015; 385(9963): 117-71.
[http://dx.doi.org/10.1016/S0140-6736(14)61682-2] [PMID: 25530442]

[57]     The top 10 causes of death, n.d. https://www.who.int/news-room/fact-sheets/detail/the-top-10-c-uses-of-death (Accessed 24 September 2020).

[58]     Brekke PH, *et al.* Underdiagnosis of myocardial infarction in COPD–Cardiac Infarction Injury Score (CIIS) in patients hospitalised for COPD exacerbation. 2008; 102(9): 1243-7.

[59]     Parkin L, Quon J, Sharples K, Barson D, Dummer J. Underuse of beta-blockers by patients with COPD and co-morbid acute coronary syndrome: A nationwide follow-up study in New Zealand. Respirology 2020; 25(2): 173-82.
[http://dx.doi.org/10.1111/resp.13662] [PMID: 31401813]

[60]     Salpeter SR, Ormiston TM, Salpeter EE. Cardioselective beta-blockers for chronic obstructive pulmonary disease. Cochrane Libr 2005; 2016(8): CD003566.
[http://dx.doi.org/10.1002/14651858.CD003566.pub2] [PMID: 16235327]

[61]     Pellicori P, Cleland JGF, Clark AL. Chronic Obstructive Pulmonary Disease and Heart Failure. Cardiol Clin 2022; 40(2): 171-82.
[http://dx.doi.org/10.1016/j.ccl.2021.12.005] [PMID: 35465891]

[62]     Iversen KK, Kjaergaard J, Akkan D, *et al.* Chronic obstructive pulmonary disease in patients admitted with heart failure. J Intern Med 2008; 264(4): 361-9.
[http://dx.doi.org/10.1111/j.1365-2796.2008.01975.x] [PMID: 18537871]

[63]     Coiro S, Girerd N, Rossignol P, *et al.* Association of beta-blocker treatment with mortality following myocardial infarction in patients with chronic obstructive pulmonary disease and heart failure or left ventricular dysfunction: a propensity matched-cohort analysis from the High-Risk Myocardial Infarction Database Initiative. Eur J Heart Fail 2017; 19(2): 271-9.
[http://dx.doi.org/10.1002/ejhf.647] [PMID: 27774703]

[64]     Buch P, Friberg J, Scharling H, Lange P, Prescott E. Reduced lung function and risk of atrial fibrillation in The Copenhagen City Heart Study. Eur Respir J 2003; 21(6): 1012-6.
[http://dx.doi.org/10.1183/09031936.03.00051502] [PMID: 12797497]

[65]     Gulea C, Zakeri R, Alderman V, Morgan A, Ross J, Quint JK. Beta-blocker therapy in patients with COPD: a systematic literature review and meta-analysis with multiple treatment comparison. Respir Res 2021; 22(1): 64.
[http://dx.doi.org/10.1186/s12931-021-01661-8] [PMID: 33622362]

[66]     Ponikowski P, Voors AA, Anker SD, *et al.* 2016 ESC Guidelines for the diagnosis and treatment of acute and chronic heart failure. Eur Heart J 2016; 37(27): 2129-200.
[http://dx.doi.org/10.1093/eurheartj/ehw128] [PMID: 27206819]

[67]     Task Force on the management of STseamiotESoC. Steg PG, James SK, Atar D, Badano LP, Blomstrom-Lundqvist C, *et al.* ESC Guidelines for the management of acute myocardial infarction in patients presenting with ST-segment elevation. Eur Heart J. 2012; 33(20): 2569-619.

[68]     Whelton       PK,       Carey       RM,       Aronow       WS,     *et      al.*       2017 ACC/AHA/AAPA/ABC/ACPM/AGS/APhA/ASH/ASPC/NMA/PCNA Guideline for the Prevention, Detection, Evaluation, and Management of High Blood Pressure in Adults: Executive Summary: A Report of the American College of Cardiology/American Heart Association Task Force on Clinical Practice Guidelines. Hypertension 2018; 71(6): 1269-324.
[http://dx.doi.org/10.1161/HYP.0000000000000066] [PMID: 29133354]

[69]     Beijers RJHCG, Steiner MC, Schols AMWJ. The role of diet and nutrition in the management of COPD. Eur Respir Rev 2023; 32(168): 230003.
[http://dx.doi.org/10.1183/16000617.0003-2023] [PMID: 37286221]

[70]   Lambert AA, Putcha N, Drummond MB, *et al.* Obesity is associated with increased morbidity in moderate to severe COPD. Chest 2017; 151(1): 68-77.
[http://dx.doi.org/10.1016/j.chest.2016.08.1432] [PMID: 27568229]

[71]   Markelić I, Hlapčić I, Rogić D, *et al.* Lipid profile and atherogenic indices in patients with stable chronic obstructive pulmonary disease. Nutr Metab Cardiovasc Dis 2021; 31(1): 153-61.
[http://dx.doi.org/10.1016/j.numecd.2020.07.039] [PMID: 32981798]

[72]   Mach F, Baigent C, Catapano AL, *et al.* 2019 ESC/EAS Guidelines for the management of dyslipidaemias: lipid modification to reduce cardiovascular risk. Eur Heart J 2020; 41(1): 111-88.
[http://dx.doi.org/10.1093/eurheartj/ehz455] [PMID: 31504418]

[73]   Park SS, Perez Perez JL, Perez Gandara B, *et al.* Mechanisms Linking COPD to Type 1 and 2 Diabetes Mellitus: Is There a Relationship between Diabetes and COPD? Medicina (Kaunas) 2022; 58(8): 1030.
[http://dx.doi.org/10.3390/medicina58081030] [PMID: 36013497]

[74]   Kahnert K, Lucke T, Biertz F, *et al.* Transfer factor for carbon monoxide in patients with COPD and diabetes: results from the German COSYCONET cohort. Respir Res 2017; 18(1): 14.
[http://dx.doi.org/10.1186/s12931-016-0499-0] [PMID: 28086884]

[75]   Worth H, Buhl R, Criée CP, Kardos P, Mailänder C, Vogelmeier C. The 'real-life' COPD patient in Germany: The DACCORD study. Respir Med 2016; 111: 64-71.
[http://dx.doi.org/10.1016/j.rmed.2015.12.010] [PMID: 26775251]

[76]   Cebron Lipovec N, Beijers RJHCG, van den Borst B, Doehner W, Lainscak M, Schols AMWJ. The prevalence of metabolic syndrome in chronic obstructive pulmonary disease: a systematic review. COPD 2016; 13(3): 399-406.
[http://dx.doi.org/10.3109/15412555.2016.1140732] [PMID: 26914392]

[77]   Watz H, Waschki B, Kirsten A, *et al.* The metabolic syndrome in patients with chronic bronchitis and COPD: frequency and associated consequences for systemic inflammation and physical inactivity. Chest 2009; 136(4): 1039-46.
[http://dx.doi.org/10.1378/chest.09-0393] [PMID: 19542257]

[78]   Marquis K, Maltais F, Duguay V, *et al.* The metabolic syndrome in patients with chronic obstructive pulmonary disease. J Cardiopulm Rehabil 2005; 25(4): 226-32.
[http://dx.doi.org/10.1097/00008483-200507000-00010] [PMID: 16056071]

[79]   James BD, Jones AV, Trethewey RE, Evans RA. Obesity and metabolic syndrome in COPD: Is exercise the answer? Chron Respir Dis 2018; 15(2): 173-81.
[http://dx.doi.org/10.1177/1479972317736294] [PMID: 29117797]

[80]   Walter RE, Beiser A, Givelber RJ, O'Connor GT, Gottlieb DJ. Association between glycemic state and lung function: the Framingham Heart Study. Am J Respir Crit Care Med 2003; 167(6): 911-6.
[http://dx.doi.org/10.1164/rccm.2203022] [PMID: 12623860]

[81]   van den BB, Gosker HR, Zeegers MP, *et al.* Pulmonary function in diabetes: a meta-analysis. Chest 2010; 138(2): 393-406.

[82]   Takahashi S, Betsuyaku T. The chronic obstructive pulmonary disease comorbidity spectrum in Japan differs from that in western countries. Respir Investig 2015; 53(6): 259-70.
[http://dx.doi.org/10.1016/j.resinv.2015.05.005]

[83]   Grosbois JM, Détrée A, Pierache A, *et al.* Impact of Cardiovascular and Metabolic Comorbidities on Long-term Outcomes of Home-based Pulmonary Rehabilitation in COPD. Int J Chron Obstruct Pulmon Dis 2023; 18: 155-67.
[http://dx.doi.org/10.2147/COPD.S381744] [PMID: 36860514]

# CHAPTER 15

# Current Perspectives on Metabolic Syndrome and Cancer

**Ravindri Jayasinghe**[1], **Umesh Jayarajah**[1,*] and **Sanjeewa Seneviratne**[1]

[1] *Department of Surgery, Faculty of Medicine, University of Colombo, Colombo, Sri Lanka*

**Abstract:** Metabolic syndrome (MetS) is a cluster of metabolic disturbances, including high body mass index (BMI), waist circumference, high blood pressure, rise in triglycerides, increased plasma glucose, and reduction in high-density lipoprotein (HDL) cholesterol, leading to increased cardiovascular morbidity and mortality along with an increased predisposition to other non-communicable diseases such as diabetes and certain cancers. Its incidence is on the rise in Western countries and is a risk factor for several common cancers. Although the individual components of metabolic syndrome are linked to cancer, studies showing a direct link between metabolic syndrome and cancer are limited. This review addresses the need to summarise the associated factors and mechanisms linking these two pathologies and to identify potential targets in therapy in patients with cancer and metabolic syndrome. Understanding this link would provide insight into the process of oncogenesis in patients with MetS. This chapter focuses on the biological and physiological alterations and specific factors associated with this process, including the insulin-like growth factor (IGF-1) pathway, estrogen signaling, visceral adiposity, hyperinsulinemia, hyperglycemia, aromatase activity, adipokinase production, angiogenesis, oxidative stress, DNA damage, and pro-inflammatory cytokines in these patients and their clinical implications in cancer therapy. New research is warranted in this area and should be systemically analyzed in all cancer types. A better understanding of this link will provide greater insight into the management of cancer patients by preventing metabolic syndrome and related alterations.

**Keywords:** Cancer, Metabolic syndrome.

## INTRODUCTION

The world is facing a pandemic of non-communicable diseases. Metabolic syndrome (MetS) is a collection of metabolic disturbances, including high body mass index (BMI), waist circumference, high blood pressure, rise in triglycerides, increased plasma glucose, and reduction in high-density lipoprotein cholesterol (HDL), leading to increased cardiovascular morbidity and mortality [1]. There are

* **Corresponding author Umesh Jayarajah:** Department of Surgery, Faculty of Medicine, University of Colombo, Colombo, Sri Lanka; E-mail: umeshe.jaya@gmail.com

**Hafize Uzun & Seyma Dumur (Eds.)**

several definitions in use, but the definition by the National Cholesterol Education Programme (NCEP) Adult Treatment Panel III is the one most widely practiced. It defines metabolic syndrome as the presence of any three risk factors of the following: abdominal obesity, elevated serum triglycerides (>=150mg/dl) or on treatment, serum high-density lipoprotein cholesterol (HDL) (40mg/dl in men and <50 mg/dl in women), hypertension or on treatment for hypertension, and fasting plasma glucose of >100 mg/dl or on treatment. It also takes impaired fasting glucose corresponding to the American Diabetes Association criteria into consideration for hyperglycemia [1, 2]. Although initially, MetS was considered to be mostly a condition of the developed countries in the West, it has now become a rising public health problem globally. MetS goes hand in hand with economic development and increasing sedentary lifestyles, leading to obesity and related health problems [3]. The prevalence of metabolic syndrome is higher in men (26.8%) than women (16.6%), and it increases with age [4, 5].

MetS is associated with other non-communicable diseases, including diabetes and cancer. Studies show almost a fivefold increased risk of developing type 2 diabetes, with a higher risk of cardiovascular disease [2]. In addition to complications related to atherosclerosis, the literature reveals several types of cancer to be associated with MetS, including breast cancer, especially in postmenopausal women, renal, prostate, pancreatic, gastrointestinal cancers, including carcinoma of the colon, stomach, and the esophagus, and hepatocellular carcinoma [3].

## METABOLIC SYNDROME AND CANCER

### Obesity and Cancer

Obesity was initially a problem predominantly in developed countries; however, an alarming increase has been observed in developing countries, especially over the last two decades. It is also a part of the cluster of disorders associated with metabolic syndrome. Obesity is, by definition, a body mass index (BMI) >/= 30 kg/m$^{2,}$ and severe obesity is a BMI of >/= 40 kg/m$^2$ or a BMI of >/=35 kg/m$^2$ with associated comorbidities [6, 7]. Literature reveals epidemiological evidence where excess body weight in the form of raised BMI or waist/hip ratio is associated with several cancers. Furthermore, a study by Calle  *et al.* revealed obesity to be associated with increased cancer mortality [8]. The common cancers associated with obesity are colorectal, hepatocellular, gallbladder, pancreatic, leukemia, non-Hodgkin's lymphoma, multiple myeloma, breast, ovarian, and endometrial cancers [9]. In keeping with these findings, a study by Reeves  *et al.*, which analyzed the association of BMI with different cancers in pre and post-menopausal women, revealed that pre-menopausal women have an increased risk of colorectal cancers and melanoma, whereas post-menopausal women show a rise in breast and endometrial cancers [10]. The possible mechanism for this causal relationship is likely to be insulin resistance, although the molecular mechanisms are still under investigation. A chronically elevated insulin level with high insulin-like growth factor 1 (IGF-1) levels, increasing oxidative stress with obesity, and lipid peroxidation of anti-carcinogenic protective factors are some of the suggested contributing factors [11]. Furthermore, obesity is a known negative prognostic indicator in cancers of the breast and the colon [11]. The higher levels of estrogen found in obese women and other associated complications of obesity such as gastroesophageal reflux disease (GORD) in the long term can lead to premalignant forms such as Barret's esophagus, which may later develop into esophageal cancer [12].

## Dyslipidemia and Cancer

Dyslipidemia is a component of metabolic syndrome. It is a known risk factor for multiple cancers. Dyslipidemia includes derangement of multiple parameters in the lipid profile with low high-density lipoprotein cholesterol (HDL-C), elevated low-density lipoprotein (LDL) cholesterol, and triglycerides (TG) [6]. Low levels of HDL cholesterol in serum are known to be associated with a risk of lung cancer and non-Hodgkin lymphoma. It is also a risk factor for breast cancer in both pre-menopausal and post-menopausal women. Furthermore, there is enough evidence that postmenopausal women with a higher BMI ($\geq 25kg/m^2$) and low HDL cholesterol are at an increased risk of developing breast cancer than women without these risk factors [13 - 15]. Raised levels of serum triglycerides are a known prognostic indicator for prostate cancer in subjects controlled for age, BMI, diabetes, and use of statins. It also revealed that the progression of prostate cancer to a higher Gleeson grade was associated with an elevated triglyceride level [16, 17]. Further studies are deemed essential to explore this association.

## Diabetes and Cancer

Diabetes is a disease with implications for multiple systems. It is also strongly associated with a cluster of metabolic disturbances included in metabolic syndrome. Several studies analyzing the relationship between diabetes and cancer have revealed diabetes to be an independent risk factor for most of the common cancers. A prospective study conducted in the United States with a 16-year follow-up revealed that type 2 diabetes, independent of other risk factors such as high BMI, posed a high mortality risk from common cancers such as breast, pancreatic, bladder, and hepatocellular cancers [18]. Mortality due to breast cancer has been shown to be prominent in women with obesity and diabetes, with diabetic women being more prone to breast and pancreatic cancers [6]. Type 2 diabetes is also a risk factor for prostate cancer. Recent genetic studies have revealed that this association is likely due to the HNF1B gene, also known as TCF2, which predisposes people to type 2 diabetes [18]. Studies show that patients with colorectal cancer and diabetes share common risk factors, which contributes to the increased risk of colon cancer in patients with type 2 diabetes, affecting both sexes equally [19].

## Hypertension and Cancer

There is a lack of sufficient evidence to establish hypertension as a risk factor for cancer. However, a few studies show a positive correlation with hypertension when controlling for BMI. Systolic blood pressure was found to be associated with increased mortality from cancer. Of the types of cancers associated, renal cell and endometrial cancer were the most significant. Furthermore, it was also found that there is a 23% increase in overall cancer mortality [20 - 22]. The mechanisms of this association are yet to be discovered. At present, there is not enough evidence to determine an increased risk of cancer with hypertension when taken as an independent risk factor. Therefore, further high-quality research is necessary to establish a proper association.

## PATHOPHYSIOLOGICAL BASIS OF METABOLIC SYNDROME AND CANCER

Adipose tissue is of growing scientific interest as it has been found to play a key role in the pathophysiology of metabolic syndrome. Although previously, it was considered to be merely a storage organ, it is now considered an organ with endocrine function that plays a key role in systemic metabolism. It is known to secrete bioactive mediators such as adipokines [23]. To mediate these actions, adipose tissue is known to exhibit important features that have come to light in the recent past. Visceral and subcutaneous fatty deposits secrete adipocytokines and are known to comprise different metabolic capacities [24]. The adipose tissue comprises different types of cells, inclusive of immune cells. Adipocytokines are cytokines released by adipose tissue, specifically visceral fat. The blood vessels disseminate these cytokines to distant tissues where they exert a systemic deleterious effect involved with visceral obesity. The adipocytokines responsible include tumor necrosis factor α (TNF-α), which remodels adipose tissue, contributes to insulin resistance, and reduces insulin signaling and leptin. Leptin contributes to increased angiogenesis and increased cell proliferation. Interleukin-6 (IL-6) stimulates lipolysis and release of C-reactive protein. Other adipocytokines include monocyte chemotactic protein (MCP-1), plasminogen activator inhibitor (PAI-1), angiotensinogen retinal binding protein-4 (RBP-4), visfatin, and resistin [25].

Obesity is considered a state of low-grade chronic inflammation triggered by these bioactive molecules. Obesity is a state of anabolism; however, inflammation is predominantly catabolic. There is a homeostasis between these two mechanisms. However, in these individuals, the process of homeostasis is deranged. In order to control the growing mass of adipose tissue, the organism switches to catabolism *via* inflammation and there is a resistance to anabolic signals. This, in turn, worsens the metabolic state and promotes insulin resistance [25]. Lipolysis is stimulated in the expanding adipose tissue, releasing free fatty acids into the circulation *via* the portal vein. Free fatty acids (FFA) trigger glucose, very low-density lipoproteins (VLDL), and triglyceride synthesis, giving rise to dyslipidemia with reduced high-density lipoprotein (HDL) cholesterol and increased low-density lipoprotein (LDL) cholesterol. Free fatty acids promote insulin resistance by inhibiting glucose uptake and increasing the level of glucose in the bloodstream. It also leads to a hyperinsulinemic state by increasing pancreatic insulin secretion, leading to augmented sodium resorption, sympathetic activation, and hypertension [25]. These metabolic processors lead to a pro-inflammatory state, which, in turn, contributes to insulin resistance. The pro-inflammatory cytokines such as TNF- α and IL-6 reinforce insulin resistance and increase lipolysis further. Furthermore, IL-6 and other cytokines increase hepatic gluconeogenesis, promoting insulin resistance in muscle. In addition to this process, the liver produces fibrinogen and C reactive protein along with plasminogen activator inhibitor (PAI-1) from adipocytes creating a prothrombotic state [26]. Studies indicate the contributors to cancer are the various processes of the metabolic syndrome including, but not limited to, insulin resistance, adipocytokine production, oxidative stress, chronic inflammation, and angiogenesis [25].

## MECHANISMS INCREASING CANCER RISK

### Hyperinsulinemia and Hyperglycemia

Insulin is a potent anabolic hormone produced by the β cells of islets of Langerhans in the pancreas. It plays a vital role in glucose and fat metabolism, which increases the uptake of glucose by the liver, muscles, and adipose tissue from the blood. Furthermore, it increases glycogen synthesis in the liver and muscle, inhibits gluconeogenesis, and stimulates cell growth and differentiation [27]. The glucose homeostasis maintained in healthy individuals is by achieving a balance between the production of insulin and insulin-mediated glucose uptake in target tissue. Insulin resistance is a condition where this cellular response to insulin is altered. The β cells of islets react by secreting more insulin, resulting in high insulin concentrations in blood in order to maintain glucose homeostasis, leading to hyperinsulinemia [27]. This provides a favorable environment for neoplastic tissue and cancer stem cell survival in combination with other contributory factors such as adipokines, growth factors, reactive oxygen species, adhesion factors, and pro-inflammatory cytokines. Chronic hyperinsulinemia is associated with colorectal, endometrial, pancreatic, and breast cancers as it promotes the action of insulin-like growth factor (IGF-1) by reducing the production of its inhibitor proteins such as insulin-like growth factor binding protein 1 (IGFBP1) and 2 [28].

Hyperglycemia is also a key component of metabolic syndrome. The excess glucose in the blood is converted to macromolecular precursors for the synthesis of fatty acids, non-essential amino acids, and nucleotides. The growth of neoplastic tissue needs more substrate for proliferation. Therefore, most tumor cells have increased expression of glucose transporter proteins, such as GLUT 1 and GLUT 3, and also enzymes such as hexokinase-2 (HK-2) [3]. Tumor growth is known to be supported by certain glycolytic enzymes such as hexokinase and 6-phosphofructo-2-kinase/fructose-2,6- bisphosphatase-4 (PFKFB-4) [29]. The increased glucose uptake by the tumor correlates to a higher grade of the tumor, increased potential to metastasize, and a reduced response to treatment contributing to poor survival. This is evident in pancreatic cancer, malignant melanoma, and urothelial malignancies [30]. Studies have revealed that hyperglycemia promotes K-Ras-driven tumors that show accelerated growth and a more malignant behavior, mostly in lung cancer. Furthermore, hyperglycemia is a known contributing factor for breast cancer as it reduces the generation of reactive oxygen species and increases tumor cell survival with increased proliferation [31].

## Role of Insulin and IGF 1

Metabolic syndrome is a state that causes the overstimulation of insulin receptors and the IGF-1 receptor (IGF1R). The insulin receptor comprises two parts: IR-A, which is involved in intracellular signaling for mitotic responses, and IR-B, which is involved in the metabolic response of insulin [32]. IGF 1R is homologous to insulin receptors and regulates cell proliferation and survival. Other ligands, such as insulin growth factor 1 and 2 (IGF1, IGF-1), can also bind to these receptors. IGF-1 functions as an autocrine, paracrine, and endocrine hormone, which is released by the liver. It mediates growth hormone promoting protein synthesis and cell proliferation. Its formation is increased by a state of hyperinsulinemia. IGF-2 is a fetal growth factor acting *via* IRA and IGF1R receptors, leading to mitogenic signaling and division [32]. IGF-1 and IGF2 are bound to IGF-binding proteins (IGFBP) produced by the liver, which protect them from destruction. IGFBPs are stimulated by growth hormones and inhibited by insulin. Therefore, hyperinsulinemic states in metabolic syndrome reduce the production of IGFBPs and result in chronically high levels of free IGF acting on their receptors, causing the overstimulation of the IGF receptors. These increasing levels of insulin, IGF-1, and IGF-2 causing receptor overstimulation leads to carcinogenesis in patients with metabolic syndrome. IR-A, IGF-1, and IGF1R receptor stimulation causes autophosphorylation and interaction with insulin receptor substrates (IRS) 1-4, leading to the activation of phosphoinositide-3-kinase (PI3K) and protein kinase B (PKB). These, in turn, inhibit Bcl-2 associated death promoter (BAD), leading to reduced apoptosis. PKB is phosphorylated, and it inhibits tuberous sclerosis complex (TSC1/2), which stimulates protein synthesis by promoting mammalian target of rapamycin (mTOR) [33]. The pTEN gene, a tumor suppressor, antagonizes PI3K by a mutation, which reduces apoptosis and promotes cell growth. The presence of a hyperinsulinemic state in patients with metabolic syndrome promotes this process, causing carcinogenesis [6]. The propagation of cancer cells, maintenance, and prevention of rejection are mediated by insulin through the polarization of effector T cells, increasing type II T helper cell production [25].

## Estrogen Signaling

Adipose tissue generates endogenous sex steroids and is the principal site of estrogen synthesis in postmenopausal women and men. Following menopause, estradiol secretion by the ovaries is halted, and estrogen is mainly supplied by peripheral conversion at the adipose tissues [34]. Therefore, with increasing age and increasing adiposity in the body, the total circulating estrogen levels increase. With increasing visceral adiposity, there is a decrease in hepatic synthesis of sex hormone-binding globulin (SHBG), which has a high affinity to estradiol, resulting in a rise in bioavailable estradiol [35]. The risk of breast cancer and endometrial cancer with increasing adiposity and increasing age is explained by this association, as estrogens are responsible for the regulation of cell differentiation, proliferation, and induction of apoptosis [36]. Estrogen is known to stimulate cell proliferation through ER-αagonism, angiogenesis, and vascular endothelial growth factor, and its mutagenic effects through genotoxic metabolites [37]. Literature reveals that SHBG levels play a vital role in the prediction of the risk of estrogen receptor-positive breast cancer in postmenopausal women, where low plasma levels are related to increased risk of endometrial cancer in both pre and postmenopausal women [38].

## Role of Hormones and Proinflammatory Cytokines

Metabolic syndrome involves several hormonal alterations that contribute to the process of carcinogenesis. Leptin is one such hormone playing a profound role in obesity, later known to have effects on the inflammatory response, carcinogenesis, and insulin signaling [25]. Other proteins and cytokines such as adiponectin, IL-6, acute phase proteins, and TNF-α are also known to play a vital role in this process.

## Visceral Adiposity

Adipose tissue is of two types: brown adipose tissue (BAT) and white adipose tissue (WAT). WAT is categorized into subcutaneous and visceral adipose tissue. Visceral adipose tissue protects organs from mechanical forces, and it stores energy in the form of triglycerides. Visceral adiposity is strongly related to the development of cancer, including colorectal carcinoma, breast cancer in postmenopausal women, oesophageal, gastric, endometrial cancer, and cholangiocarcinoma [8]. White adipose tissue can be considered an endocrine organ secreting hormones with local and systemic action, such as leptin, adiponectin, and cytokines including TNF-α and IL-6, which, in turn, interact with growth factors such as IGF-1, insulin-like growth factor-binding protein (IGFBP), and transforming growth factor (TGF-β) [39].

## Leptin

Leptin is a hormone that is elevated in obese individuals, which often results in leptin resistance. It is produced predominantly by white adipocytes and several other tissues such as the placenta, ovaries, brown adipose tissue, skeletal muscle, fundal glands of the stomach, pituitary gland, liver, and mammary epithelium [6]. It is known to produce the sensation of satiety and acts *via* its receptors in the hypothalamus. The dysfunction of the leptin receptor or the absence of leptin is known to lead to obesity due to uncontrolled intake. Obesity, which is a condition associated with metabolic syndrome, is known to manifest high leptin levels in plasma due to leptin resistance [40]. Leptin resistance is known to cause disturbances in several leptin-induced processors. Leptin is a hormone that is crucial in increasing the hepatic response to insulin by reducing lipogenesis, causing free fatty acid oxidation, and decreasing gluconeogenesis, which is known to improve the lipotoxic environment and insulin resistance in these individuals [41]. It also reduces liponeogenesis, thus reducing the lipid stores in the liver and muscle.

The role of leptin in carcinogenesis is limited. However, it is known to contribute to carcinogenesis through several processes and is known to be associated with the development of colorectal, oesophageal, breast, and prostate cancer and acute myeloid leukemia (AML). It reduces apoptosis by facilitating cytokines in MO7E and TF1 cell types in colon cancer and AML. Leptin is known to upregulate VEGF with the help of NF-kB and HIF-1α in breast cancer patients. It stimulates cell proliferation in the cell lines of oesophageal, breast, and prostate carcinomas

[42 - 44]. Further research is needed to determine the detailed role of leptin in carcinogenesis.

## Adiponectin

Adiponectin is one of the most predominant proteins secreted by the adipose tissue. It is known to have anti-neoplastic properties owing to its anti-inflammatory and anti-proliferative effects and its action of antagonizing insulin resistance [45]. Females are known to express adiponectin more than men. It regulates glucose and lipid metabolism and contributes to maintaining energy homeostasis. It is found to be elevated in normal metabolic states and is reduced in obese individuals. The levels are inversely associated with the percentage of body fat. Therefore, weight loss is shown to cause a rise in adiponectin levels in circulation [46, 47]. Some studies suggest a reduction in adiponectin due to a downregulation following hypoxia and by the secretion of certain cytokines such as TNF- α, which reduce the mRNA levels of adiponectin [48]. The level of adiponectin is shown to be low in diabetic patients in comparison to healthy individuals, as it is known to correlate with systemic insulin sensitivity. These insulin-sensitizing effects are mediated through receptors Adipo R1 and Adipo R2 [49]. Its action by activating the AMP-activated protein kinase (AMPK) pathway suppressing mTOR is known to inhibit colorectal cancer cell growth, along with regulating glucose utilization and fatty acid oxidation. The anticancer effects of adiponectin are largely from its anti-inflammatory effects and negative regulation of angiogenesis [50, 51]. Adiponectin is known to cause an inhibitory effect on gastric cancer proliferation, where an intraperitoneal infusion of adiponectin is shown to suppress the formation of peritoneal metastasis [52].

## Inflammatory Factors

Adipose tissue, in altered metabolic states secretes inflammatory cytokines such as IL-6 and TNF- α in combination with macrophages. Cytokines, in the context of inflammation, play a major role in the process of carcinogenesis, which include loss of tumor suppression, promotion of oncogene expression, and increased levels of cell cycling. Furthermore, the presence of reactive oxygen species(ROS) and inflammatory mediators such as TNF- α and COX-2 are also increased [11].

## IL-6

Interleukin-6 is a promoter of angiogenesis. Its secretion from adipocytes rises profoundly with the increase in body mass index (BMI). Higher levels are found in patients with insulin resistance and estrogen receptor-positive breast cancer. Hormone-resistant prostate cancer is shown to demonstrate higher IL-6 levels than its hormone dependent variety [53]. It is strongly related to obesity and is also known to play a role in the maturation of plasma cells by differentiating immature plasmoblasts into mature plasma cells [53]. This explains the fact that obesity predisposes to B cell lymphoma and multiple myeloma.

## TNF- α

Tumor necrosis factor – α is an inflammatory mediator associated with sepsis, chronic inflammation, and cancer. Obesity is known to increase the expression of TNF- α, which positively correlates with insulin resistance and waist circumference. Its effects are the inhibition of mTOR and the synthesis of proteins by the IkB kinase (IKK) and MAPK pathways, which promote apoptosis. It is also known to contribute to cell death by necrosis and phosphorylation of IRS-1 and IRS-2 interfering with the signaling of the tyrosine kinase receptor contributing to insulin resistance [53, 54]. Furthermore, it is known to contribute to the transcription of various proteins playing a role in inflammation, cell survival, proliferation, and apoptosis prevention *via* NFkB and MAPK pathways [53].

## CRP

C-reactive protein is an acute phase protein secreted by the liver, which is used as a sensitive, non-specific marker of inflammation, tissue injury, and inflammation. It is known to exert its effect by complement activation by binding to exogenous and autologous molecules with phosphocholine (PC) released from damaged cells [55]. Increased levels are found in obesity (BMI>30kg/m2), with a female predominance (60%). CRP is known to correlate with the amount of adipose tissue, which is the main source of other pro-inflammatory mediators, inclusive of IL6, TNF- α, and leptin. IL-6 is the main regulator of CRP synthesis by the liver. It is enhanced by the increased adipose tissue in obesity, causing a higher CRP concentration in blood. It is found to increase obesity two-fold compared to healthy controls [56]. CRP is also a predictor of the development of type II diabetes in obese subjects and acts as the link between obesity and diabetes. Furthermore, it is known to contribute towards carcinogenesis, associated with several cancers such as colorectal, ovarian, and cervical carcinomas. However, further research is needed to strengthen the evidence for this association [57, 58].

## Transcription Factors

### NF-kB

The nuclear factor 'kappa-light-chain- enhancer' of activated B-cells (NF-kB) is a transcription factor present in the cytoplasm of most cells when inactive. It is involved in the response to harmful cellular stimuli, and therefore, it is activated by several cytokines, bacterial or viral antigens such as bacterial lipopolysaccharides (LPS), reactive oxygen species (ROS), and ionizing radiation. The activation of NF-kB enhances cell survival by promoting cell proliferation and inhibiting apoptosis. Therefore, several tumor types have deregulated NF-kB function [59].

## HIF-1α

Hypoxia-inducible factor 1 alpha (HIF-1α) is a hypoxia-induced transcriptional factor controling gene expression. It leads to an increase in the vascularization of tumors by hydroxylation of prolyl residues. The level of HIF-1α in blood is regulated by ubiquitination and degradation of proteasome, leading to a very short half-life of less than five minutes. Decreased ubiquitination induced by EGF, insulin, and IGFs *via* PI3K-AKT and MAPK pathways will result in high HIF-1α levels in the blood [48]. HIF-1α can be activated in normoxic conditions by bacterial lipopolysaccharide, which initiates inflammatory response. It links hypoxia to inflammation by interacting with the NF-kB pathway. Higher levels of HIF-1α are found in solid tumors as oncogenes, and the loss of action of tumor suppressor genes stabilizes HIF-1α, causing increased metastasis and invasiveness of the tumor. The inhibition of HIF-1α is known to improve the tumour's sensitivity to radiation [60].

## PPARs

Peroxisome proliferator-activated receptors (PPARs) are a part of the nuclear hormone receptor superfamily and are transcription factors activated by ligands. There are three subtypes of PPARs, namely PPARα, commonly found in the liver and activates fatty acid catabolism; PPAR β, causing oxidation and differentiation of keratinocytes; and PPARγ, which plays a role in glucose metabolism and improves insulin resistance. It is also known to play a role in the differentiation of adipose tissue. PPARγ is identified as a pro-differentiation factor and an anti-tumorigenic factor. However, PPAR β is known to act as a tumorigenic factor [11].

## Other Factors

## COX 2

Cyclooxygenase-2 (COX-2) is an inducible enzyme produced by many cell types, commonly overexpressed in several types of cancer. It is known to increase the production of prostaglandins, conversion of procarcinogens to carcinogens, promotion of angiogenesis, inhibition of apoptosis, modulation of inflammation with immune function, and increasein tumor cell invasiveness [11].

## *MIF*

Macrophage migration inhibition factor (MIF), which is secreted by macrophages, lymphocytes, and macrophages, is activated by hypoxia along with HIF-1α. It acts by reducing the departure of macrophages from hypoxic tissues. The level of MIF is known to negatively correlate with insulin sensitivity, and it is increased with rising BMI. Further research is essential to understand the detailed role of MIF; however, it is known to be associated with the inflammation of adipocytes and insulin resistance, contributing to the process of carcinogenesis [48].

## TYPES OF CANCERS LINKED

### Colon Cancer

Patients with metabolic syndrome are at an increased risk of colonic adenoma and progression to colon carcinoma. Almost all the components of metabolic syndrome, including abdominal obesity, are associated with an increased risk of colonic carcinoma [61]. Other risk factors identified were an increase in weight or high BMI>/27 kg/m², waist circumference (men ≥103.0 cm, women ≥89.0 cm), and diabetes. Only a slight risk was reported with high blood pressure and hypercholesterolemia [11]. The waist circumference in women is found to be of more significance than the BMI, related to the incidence of colon cancer in women. Higher estrogen levels in obese women with hormone replacement therapy could be a contributory factor. However, evidence is still inconclusive with regard to hyperinsulinemia in enhancing IGF-1 concentrations contributing to an increased cancer risk. Therefore, more studies are needed to understand the true associations [11, 62].

### Breast Cancer

Breast cancer is proven to be associated with metabolic syndrome, especially with increasing obesity. It is also established that there is a modest risk between type 2 diabetes and the incidence of breast cancer. Women with diabetes have a 60% higher risk of having breast cancer compared to non-diabetic controls. This risk is more pronounced in post-menopausal women with diabetes [63]. Other risk factors associated with breast cancer in post-menopausal women include abdominal obesity, lipid profile, and fasting insulin levels with increased extra-glandular estrogen production and elevation of free plasma estradiol. A healthy lifestyle, maintaining a healthy body weight with regular physical activity and a healthy diet, is shown to control the growing epidemic of obesity, thus reducing type 2 diabetes, metabolic syndrome, and breast cancer [11].

**Prostate Cancer**

Metabolic syndrome is an emerging risk factor in the etiology of prostate cancer. Certain metabolic risk factors are known to have an effect on serum prostate-specific antigen (PSA). PSA level is known to be reduced with obesity [64]. Obesity is associated with a lower level of testosterone, and increasing BMI is known to contribute to reducing free testosterone concentrations. Therefore, the degree of hypogonadism is known to positively correlate with the degree of obesity in obese men [64]. The BMI and the risk of prostate cancer vary with the stage and the grade at diagnosis, where BMI is inversely associated with the risk of non-metastatic low-grade prostate cancer. However, it is positively associated with the risk of non-metastatic, high-grade prostate cancer and high-grade metastatic prostate cancer [65]. The risk of prostate cancer in type two diabetes is more complex, and further studies are needed to determine their association [11].

## CLINICAL IMPLICATIONS

Understanding the complex mechanisms by which metabolic syndrome leads to cancer will help find newer therapeutic options for treatment. For example, metformin, an anti-diabetic oral hypoglycemic agent, is known to have a protective role due to its mechanism in reducing insulin levels and insulin resistance [66]. It is known to inhibit mTOR with AMPK activation, causing reduced cell growth and decreased protein synthesis [66]. Research is directed towards adipocytokines, such as ADP355, which have been shown to reduce the proliferation of breast cancer [67]. IGF1 receptors havealso been a target of interest where monoclonal antibodies against IGF-1R have been studied in relation to solid organ malignancies and hematological cancers. Tyrosine kinase inhibitors such as imatinib mesylate, lapatinib, and vatalanib have emerged as targeted therapies for colorectal carcinomas [68]. The inhibitors for NF-kB are also studied with increasing interest and are showing promising results in their use for the treatment of multiple myeloma. mTOR inhibitors are studied with regard to renal cell carcinoma, where they have shown promising results; thus, they are now studied in relation to endometrial carcinoma, lymphoma, and sarcoma [25].

## CONCLUSION

Metabolic syndrome and its individual components are causing an epidemic of non-communicable diseases across the globe. The effects of metabolic syndrome and its progression towards carcinogenesis are discussed in this review. The complete process of these mechanisms and their associations are not fully understood at present. However, the altered metabolic status created in the body due to metabolic syndrome, including obesity, insulin resistance, hyperglycemia, and hyperinsulinemic states, is known to be involved. Understanding these mechanisms has already led to the development of targeted therapies. Therefore, further research is deemed essential and should be systemically analyzed in common cancer types. A better understanding of this link will provide greater insights into the management of cancer patients by preventing metabolic syndrome and related alterations.

## REFERENCES

[1]  Meigs JB, Nathan DM, Wolfsdorf JI, Mulder JE. The metabolic syndrome (insulin resistance syndrome or syndrome X). Available in www. UpToDate. com Accessed. 2015 Mar 16.

[2]  Alberti KGMM, Eckel RH, Grundy SM, *et al.* Harmonizing the metabolic syndrome: a joint interim statement of the international diabetes federation task force on epidemiology and prevention; national heart, lung, and blood institute; American heart association; world heart federation; international atherosclerosis society; and international association for the study of obesity. Circulation 2009; 120(16): 1640-5.
[http://dx.doi.org/10.1161/CIRCULATIONAHA.109.192644] [PMID: 19805654]

[3]  Micucci C, Valli D, Matacchione G, Catalano A. Current perspectives between metabolic syndrome and cancer. Oncotarget 2016; 7(25): 38959-72.
[http://dx.doi.org/10.18632/oncotarget.8341] [PMID: 27029038]

[4]  Hirode G, Wong RJ. Trends in the prevalence of metabolic syndrome in the United States, 2011-2016. JAMA 2020; 323(24): 2526-8.
[http://dx.doi.org/10.1001/jama.2020.4501] [PMID: 32573660]

[5]  Wilson PWF, D'Agostino RB, Parise H, Sullivan L, Meigs JB. Metabolic syndrome as a precursor of cardiovascular disease and type 2 diabetes mellitus. Circulation 2005; 112(20): 3066-72.
[http://dx.doi.org/10.1161/CIRCULATIONAHA.105.539528] [PMID: 16275870]

[6]  Braun S, Bitton-Worms K, LeRoith D. The link between the metabolic syndrome and cancer. Int J Biol Sci 2011; 7(7): 1003-15.
[http://dx.doi.org/10.7150/ijbs.7.1003] [PMID: 21912508]

[7]  Perreault L, Apovian C, Seres D. Obesity in adults: Overview of management. UpToDate, Kunins L(Accessed on April 28, 2020) 2019.

[8]  Calle EE, Rodriguez C, Walker-Thurmond K, Thun MJ. Overweight, obesity, and mortality from cancer in a prospectively studied cohort of U.S. adults. N Engl J Med 2003; 348(17): 1625-38.
[http://dx.doi.org/10.1056/NEJMoa021423] [PMID: 12711737]

[9]  Cowey S, Hardy RW. The metabolic syndrome: A high-risk state for cancer? Am J Pathol 2006; 169(5): 1505-22.
[http://dx.doi.org/10.2353/ajpath.2006.051090] [PMID: 17071576]

[10]  Reeves GK, Pirie K, Beral V, Green J, Spencer E, Bull D. Cancer incidence and mortality in relation to body mass index in the Million Women Study: cohort study. BMJ 2007; 335(7630): 1134.
[http://dx.doi.org/10.1136/bmj.39367.495995.AE] [PMID: 17986716]

[11]  Pothiwala P, Jain SK, Yaturu S. Metabolic syndrome and cancer. Metab Syndr Relat Disord 2009; 7(4): 279-88.
[http://dx.doi.org/10.1089/met.2008.0065] [PMID: 19284314]

[12]  Hampel H, Abraham NS, El-Serag HB. Meta-analysis: obesity and the risk for gastroesophageal reflux disease and its complications. Ann Intern Med 2005; 143(3): 199-211.
[http://dx.doi.org/10.7326/0003-4819-143-3-200508020-00006] [PMID: 16061918]

[13]  Michalaki V, Koutroulis G, Koutroulis G, Syrigos K, Piperi C, Kalofoutis A. Evaluation of serum lipids and high-density lipoprotein subfractions (HDL2, HDL3) in postmenopausal patients with breast cancer. Mol Cell Biochem 2005; 268(1-2): 19-24.

[http://dx.doi.org/10.1007/s11010-005-2993-4] [PMID: 15724433]

[14] Kucharska-Newton AM, Rosamond WD, Mink PJ, Alberg AJ, Shahar E, Folsom AR. HDL-cholesterol and incidence of breast cancer in the ARIC cohort study. Ann Epidemiol 2008; 18(9): 671-7.
[http://dx.doi.org/10.1016/j.annepidem.2008.06.006] [PMID: 18794007]

[15] Lim U, Gayles T, Katki HA, *et al.* Serum high-density lipoprotein cholesterol and risk of non-hodgkin lymphoma. Cancer Res 2007; 67(11): 5569-74.
[http://dx.doi.org/10.1158/0008-5472.CAN-07-0212] [PMID: 17522388]

[16] Wuermli L, Joerger M, Henz S, *et al.* Hypertriglyceridemia as a possible risk factor for prostate cancer. Prostate Cancer Prostatic Dis 2005; 8(4): 316-20.
[http://dx.doi.org/10.1038/sj.pcan.4500834] [PMID: 16158078]

[17] Hammarsten J, Högstedt B. Clinical, haemodynamic, anthropometric, metabolic and insulin profile of men with high□stage and high□grade clinical prostate cancer. Blood Press 2004; 13(1): 47-55.
[http://dx.doi.org/10.1080/08037050310025735] [PMID: 15083641]

[18] Coughlin SS, Calle EE, Teras LR, Petrelli J, Thun MJ. Diabetes mellitus as a predictor of cancer mortality in a large cohort of US adults. Am J Epidemiol 2004; 159(12): 1160-7.
[http://dx.doi.org/10.1093/aje/kwh161] [PMID: 15191933]

[19] Berster JM, Göke B. Type 2 diabetes mellitus as risk factor for colorectal cancer. Arch Physiol Biochem 2008; 114(1): 84-98.
[http://dx.doi.org/10.1080/13813450802008455] [PMID: 18465362]

[20] Furberg AS, Thune I. Metabolic abnormalities (hypertension, hyperglycemia and overweight), lifestyle (high energy intake and physical inactivity) and endometrial cancer risk in a Norwegian cohort. Int J Cancer 2003; 104(6): 669-76.
[http://dx.doi.org/10.1002/ijc.10974] [PMID: 12640672]

[21] Sung KC, Ryu SH. Insulin resistance, body mass index, waist circumference are independent risk factor for high blood pressure. Clin Exp Hypertens 2004; 26(6): 547-56.
[http://dx.doi.org/10.1081/CEH-200031833] [PMID: 15554457]

[22] Halperin RO, Sesso HD, Ma J, Buring JE, Stampfer MJ, Michael Gaziano J. Dyslipidemia and the risk of incident hypertension in men. Hypertension 2006; 47(1): 45-50.
[http://dx.doi.org/10.1161/01.HYP.0000196306.42418.0e] [PMID: 16344375]

[23] Ouchi N, Parker JL, Lugus JJ, Walsh K. Adipokines in inflammation and metabolic disease. Nat Rev Immunol 2011; 11(2): 85-97.
[http://dx.doi.org/10.1038/nri2921] [PMID: 21252989]

[24] Fain JN, Madan AK, Hiler ML, Cheema P, Bahouth SW. Comparison of the release of adipokines by adipose tissue, adipose tissue matrix, and adipocytes from visceral and subcutaneous abdominal adipose tissues of obese humans. Endocrinology 2004; 145(5): 2273-82.
[http://dx.doi.org/10.1210/en.2003-1336] [PMID: 14726444]

[25] Mendonça FM, de Sousa FR, Barbosa AL, *et al.* Metabolic syndrome and risk of cancer: Which link? Metabolism 2015; 64(2): 182-9.
[http://dx.doi.org/10.1016/j.metabol.2014.10.008] [PMID: 25456095]

[26] Maury E, Brichard SM. Adipokine dysregulation, adipose tissue inflammation and metabolic syndrome. Mol Cell Endocrinol 2010; 314(1): 1-16.
[http://dx.doi.org/10.1016/j.mce.2009.07.031] [PMID: 19682539]

[27] Bergamini E, Cavallini G, Donati A, Gori Z. The role of autophagy in aging: its essential part in the anti-aging mechanism of caloric restriction. Ann N Y Acad Sci 2007; 1114(1): 69-78.
[http://dx.doi.org/10.1196/annals.1396.020] [PMID: 17934054]

[28] Calle EE, Kaaks R. Overweight, obesity and cancer: epidemiological evidence and proposed mechanisms. Nat Rev Cancer 2004; 4(8): 579-91.

[http://dx.doi.org/10.1038/nrc1408] [PMID: 15286738]

[29] Minchenko OH, Ochiai A, Opentanova IL, *et al.* Overexpression of 6-phosphofructo-2-kinase/fructose-2,6-bisphosphatase-4 in the human breast and colon malignant tumors. Biochimie 2005; 87(11): 1005-10.
[http://dx.doi.org/10.1016/j.biochi.2005.04.007] [PMID: 15925437]

[30] Stattin P, Björ O, Ferrari P, *et al.* Prospective study of hyperglycemia and cancer risk. Diabetes Care 2007; 30(3): 561-7.
[http://dx.doi.org/10.2337/dc06-0922] [PMID: 17327321]

[31] Masur K, Vetter C, Hinz A, *et al.* Diabetogenic glucose and insulin concentrations modulate transcriptom and protein levels involved in tumour cell migration, adhesion and proliferation. Br J Cancer 2011; 104(2): 345-52.
[http://dx.doi.org/10.1038/sj.bjc.6606050] [PMID: 21179032]

[32] Arcidiacono B, Iiritano S, Nocera A, *et al.* Insulin resistance and cancer risk: an overview of the pathogenic mechanisms. Exp Diabetes Res 2012; 2012: 1-12.
[http://dx.doi.org/10.1155/2012/789174]

[33] Cohen DH, LeRoith D. Obesity, type 2 diabetes, and cancer: the insulin and IGF connection. Endocr Relat Cancer 2012; 19(5): F27-45.
[http://dx.doi.org/10.1530/ERC-11-0374] [PMID: 22593429]

[34] Key TJ, Appleby PN, Reeves GK, *et al.* Body mass index, serum sex hormones, and breast cancer risk in postmenopausal women. J Natl Cancer Inst 2003; 95(16): 1218-26.
[http://dx.doi.org/10.1093/jnci/djg022] [PMID: 12928347]

[35] Pugeat M, Crave JC, Elmidani M, *et al.* Pathophysiology of sex hormone binding globulin (SHBG): Relation to insulin. J Steroid Biochem Mol Biol 1991; 40(4-6): 841-9.
[http://dx.doi.org/10.1016/0960-0760(91)90310-2] [PMID: 1958579]

[36] Dickson RB, Stancel GM. Chapter 8: Estrogen receptor-mediated processes in normal and cancer cells. JNCI Monographs 2000, 2000(27): 135-145.

[37] Yager JD, Davidson NE. Estrogen carcinogenesis in breast cancer. N Engl J Med 2006; 354(3): 270-82.
[http://dx.doi.org/10.1056/NEJMra050776] [PMID: 16421368]

[38] Lukanova A, Lundin E, Micheli A, *et al.* Circulating levels of sex steroid hormones and risk of endometrial cancer in postmenopausal women. Int J Cancer 2004; 108(3): 425-32.
[http://dx.doi.org/10.1002/ijc.11529] [PMID: 14648710]

[39] Wellen KE, Hotamisligil GS. Obesity-induced inflammatory changes in adipose tissue. J Clin Invest 2003; 112(12): 1785-8.
[http://dx.doi.org/10.1172/JCI20514] [PMID: 14679172]

[40] Maffei M, Fei H, Lee GH, *et al.* Increased expression in adipocytes of ob RNA in mice with lesions of the hypothalamus and with mutations at the db locus. Proc Natl Acad Sci USA 1995; 92(15): 6957-60.
[http://dx.doi.org/10.1073/pnas.92.15.6957] [PMID: 7624352]

[41] Aballay LR, Eynard AR, Díaz MP, Navarro A, Muñoz SE. Overweight and obesity: a review of their relationship to metabolic syndrome, cardiovascular disease, and cancer in South America. Nutr Rev 2013; 71(3): 168-79.
[http://dx.doi.org/10.1111/j.1753-4887.2012.00533.x] [PMID: 23452284]

[42] Toyoshima Y, Gavrilova O, Yakar S, *et al.* Leptin improves insulin resistance and hyperglycemia in a mouse model of type 2 diabetes. Endocrinology 2005; 146(9): 4024-35.
[http://dx.doi.org/10.1210/en.2005-0087] [PMID: 15947005]

[43] Konopleva M, Mikhail A, Estrov Z, *et al.* Expression and function of leptin receptor isoforms in myeloid leukemia and myelodysplastic syndromes: proliferative and anti-apoptotic activities. Blood 1999; 93(5): 1668-76.

[http://dx.doi.org/10.1182/blood.V93.5.1668.405a15_1668_1676] [PMID: 10029596]

[44]    Endo H, Hosono K, Uchiyama T, *et al.* Leptin acts as a growth factor for colorectal tumours at stages subsequent to tumour initiation in murine colon carcinogenesis. Gut 2011; 60(10): 1363-71.
[http://dx.doi.org/10.1136/gut.2010.235754] [PMID: 21406387]

[45]    Dalamaga M, Diakopoulos KN, Mantzoros CS. The role of adiponectin in cancer: a review of current evidence. Endocr Rev 2012; 33(4): 547-94.
[http://dx.doi.org/10.1210/er.2011-1015] [PMID: 22547160]

[46]    Ukkola O, Santaniemi M. Adiponectin: a link between excess adiposity and associated comorbidities? J Mol Med (Berl) 2002; 80(11): 696-702.
[http://dx.doi.org/10.1007/s00109-002-0378-7] [PMID: 12436346]

[47]    Coppola A, Marfella R, Coppola L, *et al.* Effect of weight loss on coronary circulation and adiponectin levels in obese women. Int J Cardiol 2009; 134(3): 414-6.
[http://dx.doi.org/10.1016/j.ijcard.2007.12.087] [PMID: 18378021]

[48]    Ye J. Emerging role of adipose tissue hypoxia in obesity and insulin resistance. Int J Obes 2009; 33(1): 54-66.
[http://dx.doi.org/10.1038/ijo.2008.229] [PMID: 19050672]

[49]    Tsatsanis C, Zacharioudaki V, Androulidaki A, *et al.* Peripheral factors in the metabolic syndrome: the pivotal role of adiponectin. Ann N Y Acad Sci 2006; 1083(1): 185-95.
[http://dx.doi.org/10.1196/annals.1367.013] [PMID: 17148740]

[50]    Díez JJ, Iglesias P. The role of the novel adipocyte-derived protein adiponectin in human disease: an update. Mini Rev Med Chem 2010; 10(9): 856-69.
[http://dx.doi.org/10.2174/138955710791608325] [PMID: 20482500]

[51]    Bråkenhielm E, Veitonmäki N, Cao R, *et al.* Adiponectin-induced antiangiogenesis and antitumor activity involve caspase-mediated endothelial cell apoptosis. Proc Natl Acad Sci USA 2004; 101(8): 2476-81.
[http://dx.doi.org/10.1073/pnas.0308671100] [PMID: 14983034]

[52]    Ishikawa M, Kitayama J, Yamauchi T, *et al.* Adiponectin inhibits the growth and peritoneal metastasis of gastric cancer through its specific membrane receptors AdipoR1 and AdipoR2. Cancer Sci 2007; 98(7): 1120-7.
[http://dx.doi.org/10.1111/j.1349-7006.2007.00486.x] [PMID: 17459059]

[53]    Gallagher EJ, Novosyadlyy R, Yakar S, LeRoith D. The increased risk of cancer in obesity and type 2 diabetes: potential mechanisms. In: Principles of Diabetes Mellitus. edn.: Springer; 2010: 579-599.
[http://dx.doi.org/10.1007/978-0-387-09841-8_36]

[54]    Uysal KT, Wiesbrock SM, Marino MW, Hotamisligil GS. Protection from obesity-induced insulin resistance in mice lacking TNF-α function. Nature 1997; 389(6651): 610-4.
[http://dx.doi.org/10.1038/39335] [PMID: 9335502]

[55]    Thompson D, Pepys MB, Wood SP. The physiological structure of human C-reactive protein and its complex with phosphocholine. Structure 1999; 7(2): 169-77.
[http://dx.doi.org/10.1016/S0969-2126(99)80023-9] [PMID: 10368284]

[56]    Lau DCW, Dhillon B, Yan H, Szmitko PE, Verma S. Adipokines: molecular links between obesity and atheroslcerosis. Am J Physiol Heart Circ Physiol 2005; 288(5): H2031-41.
[http://dx.doi.org/10.1152/ajpheart.01058.2004] [PMID: 15653761]

[57]    Festa A, D'Agostino R Jr, Tracy RP, Haffner SM. Elevated levels of acute-phase proteins and plasminogen activator inhibitor-1 predict the development of type 2 diabetes: the insulin resistance atherosclerosis study. Diabetes 2002; 51(4): 1131-7.
[http://dx.doi.org/10.2337/diabetes.51.4.1131] [PMID: 11916936]

[58]    Erlinger TP, Platz EA, Rifai N, Helzlsouer KJ. C-reactive protein and the risk of incident colorectal cancer. JAMA 2004; 291(5): 585-90.

[http://dx.doi.org/10.1001/jama.291.5.585] [PMID: 14762037]

[59] Puszynski K, Lipniacki T, Bertolusso R. Crosstalk between p53 and nuclear factor-κB systems: pro- and anti-apoptotic functions of NF-κB. IET Syst Biol 2009; 3(5): 356-67.
[http://dx.doi.org/10.1049/iet-syb.2008.0172] [PMID: 21028926]

[60] Eltzschig HK, Carmeliet P. Hypoxia and Inflammation. N Engl J Med 2011; 364(7): 656-65.
[http://dx.doi.org/10.1056/NEJMra0910283] [PMID: 21323543]

[61] Kim JH, Lim YJ, Kim YH, *et al.* Is metabolic syndrome a risk factor for colorectal adenoma? Cancer Epidemiol Biomarkers Prev 2007; 16(8): 1543-6.
[http://dx.doi.org/10.1158/1055-9965.EPI-07-0199] [PMID: 17684126]

[62] Giovannucci E. Metabolic syndrome, hyperinsulinemia, and colon cancer: a review. Am J Clin Nutr 2007; 86(3): 836S-42S.
[http://dx.doi.org/10.1093/ajcn/86.3.836S] [PMID: 18265477]

[63] Xue F, Michels KB. Diabetes, metabolic syndrome, and breast cancer: a review of the current evidence. Am J Clin Nutr 2007; 86(3): 823S-35S.
[http://dx.doi.org/10.1093/ajcn/86.3.823S] [PMID: 18265476]

[64] McGrowder DA, Jackson LA, Crawford TV. Prostate cancer and metabolic syndrome: is there a link? Asian Pac J Cancer Prev 2012; 13(1): 1-13.
[http://dx.doi.org/10.7314/APJCP.2012.13.1.001] [PMID: 22502649]

[65] Rodriguez C, Freedland SJ, Deka A, *et al.* Body mass index, weight change, and risk of prostate cancer in the Cancer Prevention Study II Nutrition Cohort. Cancer Epidemiol Biomarkers Prev 2007; 16(1): 63-9.
[http://dx.doi.org/10.1158/1055-9965.EPI-06-0754] [PMID: 17179486]

[66] Meric-Bernstam F, Gonzalez-Angulo AM. Targeting the mTOR signaling network for cancer therapy. J Clin Oncol 2009; 27(13): 2278-87.
[http://dx.doi.org/10.1200/JCO.2008.20.0766] [PMID: 19332717]

[67] Higgins LS, Mantzoros CS. The development of INT131 as a selective PPARγ modulator: approach to a safer insulin sensitizer. PPAR research 2008.
[http://dx.doi.org/10.1155/2008/936906]

[68] Arora A, Scholar EM. Role of tyrosine kinase inhibitors in cancer therapy. J Pharmacol Exp Ther 2005; 315(3): 971-9.
[http://dx.doi.org/10.1124/jpet.105.084145] [PMID: 16002463]

# CHAPTER 16

# Otorhinolaryngology and Metabolic Syndrome

**Mohamed Salah Rashwan**[1,2,*]

[1] *Department of Otolaryngology, Faculty of Medicine, Suez Canal University, Ismailia, Egypt*

[2] *Department of Otolaryngology, Queen's Hospital, Barking, Havering and Redbridge University Hospitals NHS Trust, Romford, UK*

**Abstract:** Metabolic syndrome (MS) is a diverse condition linked to an elevated risk of cardiovascular issues. Emerging evidence from various types of research, including experimental, translational, and clinical studies, has indicated that obstructive sleep apnoea (OSA) is connected to both existing and newly developing aspects of MS. The plausible biological explanation centers primarily around one of OSA's main features, intermittent hypoxia. This leads to heightened sympathetic activity with cardiovascular consequences, increased liver glucose production, insulin resistance due to inflammation in adipose tissue, dysfunction in pancreatic β-cells, elevated lipid levels through deteriorating fasting lipid profiles, and decreased removal of triglyceride-rich lipoproteins.

While several interconnected pathways exist, the clinical evidence primarily relies on observational data, making it difficult to establish causality. The co-occurrence of visceral obesity and potential confounding factors like medications complicates the assessment of OSA's independent impact on MS. In this chapter, we re-evaluate the evidence regarding how OSA and intermittent hypoxia may contribute to adverse effects on MS parameters independently of body fat. We place particular emphasis on recent findings from intervention studies. This chapter outlines the research gaps, the challenges faced in the field, potential directions for future exploration, and the necessity for more high-quality data from intervention studies that address the influence of both established and promising therapies for OSA and obesity.

**Keywords:** Cardiovascular issues, Metabolic syndrome, Obesity, Obstructive sleep apnoea, Sleep apnoea.

## INTRODUCTION

In recent years, healthcare professionals and researchers have turned their attention to two significant health concerns: metabolic syndrome and sleep apnoea. These conditions, each complex, often coexist in individuals, creating a

* **Corresponding author Mohamed Salah Rashwan:** Department of Otolaryngology, Faculty of Medicine, Suez Canal University, Ismailia, Egypt and Department of Otolaryngology, Queen's Hospital, Barking, Havering and Redbridge University Hospitals NHS Trust, Romford, UK; E-mail: m_salaheldin@med.suez.edu.eg

web of health-related challenges. This chapter delves into the intricate relationship between metabolic syndrome and sleep apnoea, shedding light on how they interact and exacerbate each other.

## UNDERSTANDING METABOLIC SYNDROME

Metabolic syndrome is not a singular ailment; rather, it is a constellation of interconnected risk factors. It encompasses a range of health markers, including obesity, high blood pressure, elevated blood sugar levels, abnormal lipid profiles (such as high triglycerides and low HDL cholesterol), and insulin resistance. Individuals with metabolic syndrome face an elevated risk of developing serious health issues like cardiovascular diseases and type 2 diabetes [1].

Metabolic syndrome comprises five key elements, each of which contributes to its complexity:

1. **Abdominal Obesity**: Central to metabolic syndrome is the accumulation of excess fat in the abdominal region, commonly referred to as visceral fat. This type of fat isn't just a cosmetic concern; it's closely linked to insulin resistance and chronic inflammation.

2. **High Blood Pressure (Hypertension)**: Elevated blood pressure is a frequent component of metabolic syndrome and is associated with a higher risk of heart disease, stroke, and kidney disease.

3. **Elevated Blood Sugar (Hyperglycaemia)**: High fasting blood sugar levels indicate insulin resistance, a hallmark of metabolic syndrome. If not managed, this condition can progress to full-blown type 2 diabetes.

4. **Abnormal Lipid Profile:** Individuals with metabolic syndrome often exhibit high levels of triglycerides (a type of fat in the blood) and low levels of high-density lipoprotein (HDL) cholesterol, the so-called "good" cholesterol.

5. **Insulin Resistance**: This occurs when the body's cells do not effectively respond to insulin, resulting in higher blood sugar levels.

## SLEEP APNOEA: A DISRUPTIVE SLEEP DISORDER

Sleep apnoea is a sleep disorder characterized by repetitive interrupted breathing during sleep. The most common form is obstructive sleep apnea (OSA), where the airway becomes partially or completely blocked, leading to brief awakenings throughout the night. This disruptive pattern not only robs individuals of restful sleep but also often goes undiagnosed [2].

Sleep apnoea is typically categorized into three severity levels based on the number of breathing interruptions per hour of sleep:

1. **Mild**: Involves between 5 to 15 episodes of breathing interruptions per hour of sleep.

2. **Moderate**: Involves 15 to 30 episodes per hour.

3. **Severe:** Marked by over 30 episodes per hour.

## THE BIDIRECTIONAL RELATIONSHIP

The relationship between metabolic syndrome and OSA is not only one-way; it is a complex, bidirectional interaction where each condition influences and exacerbates the other.

### OSA Contributes to Metabolic Syndrome

• Significant metabolic disruptions can happen due to OSA. The frequent awakenings and drops in oxygen saturation seen in individuals with OSA trigger a cascade of stress responses. This includes heightened activity of the sympathetic nervous system, which is responsible for the body's "fight or flight" responses, and increased inflammation. These physiological changes can disrupt metabolic processes, contributing to insulin resistance, obesity, and high blood pressure [3].

• A study published in the *Journal of the American College of Cardiology* emphasized the strong association between sleep apnoea and cardiovascular diseases, including metabolic syndrome. OSA is linked to increased sympathetic activity, oxidative stress (a type of cellular damage), and systemic inflammation, all of which contribute to the development of metabolic syndrome [4].

• Furthermore, chronic sleep deprivation and frequent sleep interruptions, which are common in individuals with sleep apnoea, can lead to disruptions in hormonal regulation. This includes increased levels of cortisol, a stress hormone, and decreased levels of leptin, a hormone responsible for regulating appetite. These hormonal shifts can promote weight gain and worsen insulin resistance [5].

### Metabolic Syndrome Worsens Sleep Apnoea

• Obesity, a central element of metabolic syndrome, is a significant risk factor for the onset and progression of sleep apnoea. As individuals accumulate excess body fat, particularly in the abdominal region, fat deposits can build up in the upper airway, further obstructing normal breathing during sleep [6].

- One of the studies published in the *New England Journal of Medicine* highlighted the undeniable link between sleep-disordered breathing and hypertension, one of the components of metabolic syndrome. It showed that individuals with sleep apnoea had a significantly higher risk of developing hypertension [7].
- Particularly, central obesity, characterized by fat deposition in the neck and throat areas, heightens the risk of airway obstruction during sleep [8].

## COMMON GROUND: OBESITY

Obesity emerges as a shared factor in both metabolic syndrome and OSA, playing a substantial role in the development and progression of both conditions. Understanding the role of obesity is pivotal in effectively managing these intertwined health challenges [9].

### The Role of Obesity

**Metabolic Syndrome**: Obesity is at the heart of metabolic syndrome. Excessive body fat, particularly visceral fat, sets off a chain reaction of inflammation and insulin resistance, which are two critical drivers of metabolic syndrome. Inflammation in adipose tissue, the body's fat stores, releases pro-inflammatory molecules known as cytokines, which interfere with insulin signaling and promote insulin resistance [10].

**Sleep Apnea**: Obesity stands out as the primary risk factor for OSA. As individuals gain weight, the accumulation of excess fat in the upper airway can lead to airway constriction or complete blockage. Notably, the likelihood of developing sleep apnoea significantly increases with weight gain [11].

## DIAGNOSTIC CHALLENGES

Diagnosing metabolic syndrome and sleep apnoea can be far from straightforward, as symptoms often overlap and can be subtle. Furthermore, individuals with one condition might not always recognize their risk for the other, creating diagnostic challenges for healthcare providers. It is crucial for healthcare professionals to remain vigilant in assessing patients for both conditions, especially when one is already present [12].

In summary, the intricate relationship between metabolic syndrome and OSA is a multifaceted interplay of physiological and pathological factors. Both conditions are closely related to obesity and share a bidirectional influence, with each worsening the other's impact on an individual's health. Recognizing this intricate connection is vital for healthcare providers and individuals alike, as it underscores the importance of a comprehensive approach to diagnosis and treatment that addresses both metabolic syndrome and sleep apnea as part of a unified whole.

## DIAGNOSTIC TESTS

**Metabolic Syndrome**: Diagnosing metabolic syndrome involves a thorough assessment using a combination of clinical criteria. These criteria encompass measurements of various health parameters, including waist circumference, blood pressure, fasting blood sugar levels, triglycerides, and high-density lipoprotein (HDL) cholesterol levels. To receive a diagnosis of metabolic syndrome, an individual typically needs to meet three or more of these criteria [13]. This comprehensive evaluation allows healthcare providers to gain insights into a person's overall metabolic health and risk factors.

**Sleep Apnoea**: Diagnosing sleep apnoea requires a specialized sleep study known as polysomnography. During this detailed assessment, numerous physiological parameters are monitored while an individual sleeps. These include airflow, blood oxygen levels, brain activity, and more. The key diagnostic metric used in determining the severity of sleep apnoea is the number of apnoea and hypopnea events per hour, known as the apnoea-hypopnea index (AHI) [14]. Polysomnography provides a comprehensive view of an individual's sleep patterns and helps identify the presence and severity of sleep aponia.

## TREATMENT APPROACHES

### Lifestyle Modifications

- Lifestyle changes are the cornerstone of managing both metabolic syndrome and sleep apnoea. These changes include weight loss, regular physical activity, and adopting a balanced, healthy diet. Weight loss plays a pivotal role in improving symptoms of sleep apnoea and may also lead to the resolution of components of metabolic syndrome [15]. Achieving and maintaining a healthy body weight is often the first line of defense in addressing these conditions.
- A study published in *Obesity* conducted a randomized controlled trial that highlighted the positive impact of lifestyle modifications. The trial demonstrated that weight loss achieved through dietary adjustments and increased physical activity can enhance insulin sensitivity and reduce blood pressure levels in individuals with metabolic syndrome [16].
- In the context of sleep apnoea, lifestyle modifications that promote weight loss are often the initial treatment strategy. Even modest weight reduction can result in significant improvements in sleep apnoea symptoms, as excess body fat can contribute to airway obstruction during sleep [17].

## 2. Continuous Positive Airway Pressure (CPAP)

- For individuals with moderate to severe sleep apnoea, Continuous Positive Airway Pressure (CPAP) therapy is a common and highly effective treatment option. CPAP involves wearing a mask that delivers a continuous stream of air, which helps keep the airway open during sleep. This prevents the repetitive interruptions in breathing characteristic of sleep apnoea and leads to enhanced sleep quality. [18]
- A comprehensive review published in *Sleep Medicine Reviews* examined the effectiveness of CPAP therapy in individuals with both sleep apnoea and metabolic syndrome. The review found that CPAP not only improved sleep-related outcomes but also modestly enhanced metabolic parameters, such as blood pressure and insulin sensitivity [19]. This suggests that CPAP therapy can positively impact both conditions simultaneously.

## 3. Pharmacotherapy

- Medications may be prescribed to manage specific components of metabolic syndrome, such as antihypertensive drugs for blood pressure control, statins to regulate lipid levels, and medications to address blood sugar irregularities. However, it is essential to emphasize that lifestyle modifications remain the primary focus of treatment, with medications considered as supplementary therapy in specific cases [20].
- A comprehensive meta-analysis published in the *Journal of the American College of Cardiology* evaluated the impact of various medications on the components of metabolic syndrome. The analysis concluded that lifestyle interventions continue to be the cornerstone of treatment. Medications are considered an adjunct when lifestyle changes alone are insufficient [21].

## SURGICAL INTERVENTIONS

In certain cases where individuals have severe obesity and have not responded adequately to other treatments, surgical interventions may be considered. Bariatric surgeries, such as gastric bypass or sleeve gastrectomy, are effective options for substantial weight loss. These surgical procedures have been shown to lead to significant improvements in both sleep apnoea and metabolic syndrome [22]. While surgery is a more invasive option, it can be a life-changing solution for those facing severe obesity-related health challenges.

## CONCLUSION

The intricate relationship between metabolic syndrome and OSA underscores the importance of taking a holistic approach to healthcare. Recognizing the bidirectional relationship of these conditions can lead to more effective management and better overall health outcomes. Healthcare providers should acknowledge the relationship between metabolic syndrome and OSA and collaborate to address both conditions comprehensively.

In summary, metabolic syndrome and OSA are deeply interconnected in a complex web of causation and exacerbation. Obesity stands as a common factor in this relationship, contributing to the emergence and progression of both conditions. Understanding the bidirectional impact of metabolic syndrome and OSA emphasizes the need for a multifaceted treatment approach, which includes lifestyle modifications, CPAP therapy, and when deemed appropriate, pharmacological interventions. The goal is to mitigate the health risks associated with these conditions and enhance the overall quality of life for affected individuals. By addressing these conditions holistically, individuals can work toward achieving better health and well-being.

## REFERENCES

[1]     Grundy SM. Metabolic syndrome pandemic. Arterioscler Thromb Vasc Biol 2008; 28(4): 629-36.
        [http://dx.doi.org/10.1161/ATVBAHA.107.151092] [PMID: 18174459]

[2]     Young T, Peppard PE, Gottlieb DJ. Epidemiology of obstructive sleep apnea: a population health perspective. Am J Respir Crit Care Med 2002; 165(9): 1217-39.
        [http://dx.doi.org/10.1164/rccm.2109080] [PMID: 11991871]

[3]     Somers VK, White DP, Amin R, *et al.* Sleep Apnea and Cardiovascular Disease. J Am Coll Cardiol 2008; 52(8): 686-717.
        [http://dx.doi.org/10.1016/j.jacc.2008.05.002] [PMID: 18702977]

[4]     Tasali E, Ip MSM. Obstructive sleep apnea and metabolic syndrome: alterations in glucose metabolism and inflammation. Proc Am Thorac Soc 2008; 5(2): 207-17.
        [http://dx.doi.org/10.1513/pats.200708-139MG] [PMID: 18250214]

[5]     Peppard PE, Young T, Palta M, Skatrud J. Prospective study of the association between sleep-disordered breathing and hypertension. N Engl J Med 2000; 342(19): 1378-84.
        [http://dx.doi.org/10.1056/NEJM200005113421901] [PMID: 10805822]

[6]     Després JP, Lemieux I. Abdominal obesity and metabolic syndrome. Nature 2006; 444(7121): 881-7.
        [http://dx.doi.org/10.1038/nature05488] [PMID: 17167477]

[7]     Grundy SM. Obesity, metabolic syndrome, and cardiovascular disease. J Clin Endocrinol Metab 2004; 89(6): 2595-600.
        [http://dx.doi.org/10.1210/jc.2004-0372] [PMID: 15181029]

[8]     Tuomilehto HPI, Seppä JM, Partinen MM, *et al.* Lifestyle intervention with weight reduction: first-line treatment in mild obstructive sleep apnea. Am J Respir Crit Care Med 2009; 179(4): 320-7.
        [http://dx.doi.org/10.1164/rccm.200805-669OC] [PMID: 19011153]

[9]     Heffernan A, Duplancic D, Kumric M, Ticinovic Kurir T, Bozic J. Metabolic Crossroads: Unveiling the Complex Interactions between Obstructive Sleep Apnoea and Metabolic Syndrome. Int J Mol Sci 2024; 25(6): 3243.
        [http://dx.doi.org/10.3390/ijms25063243]

[10]    Grundy SM, Brewer HB Jr, Cleeman JI, Smith SC Jr, Lenfant C. Definition of metabolic syndrome: Report of the National Heart, Lung, and Blood Institute/American Heart Association conference on

scientific issues related to definition. Circulation 2004; 109(3): 433-8.
[http://dx.doi.org/10.1161/01.CIR.0000111245.75752.C6] [PMID: 14744958]

[11] Jehan S, Zizi F, Pandi-Perumal SR, *et al*. Obstructive Sleep Apnea and Obesity: Implications for Public Health. Sleep Med Disord 2017; 1(4): 00019.

[12] American Academy of Sleep Medicine. The AASM Manual for the Scoring of Sleep and Associated Events: Rules, Terminology and Technical Specifications (Version 20). Darien, IL: American Academy of Sleep Medicine 2014.

[13] Fahed G, Aoun L, Bou Zerdan M, *et al*. Metabolic Syndrome: Updates on Pathophysiology and Management in 2021. Int J Mol Sci 2022; 23(2): 786.
[http://dx.doi.org/10.3390/ijms23020786]

[14] Serrano Alarcón Á, Martínez Madrid N, Seepold R. A Minimum Set of Physiological Parameters to Diagnose Obstructive Sleep Apnea Syndrome Using Non-Invasive Portable Monitors. A Systematic Review Life (Basel) 2021; 11(11): 1249.
[http://dx.doi.org/10.3390/life11111249]

[15] Epstein LJ, Kristo D, Strollo PJ Jr, *et al*. Clinical guideline for the evaluation, management and long-term care of obstructive sleep apnea in adults. J Clin Sleep Med 2009; 5(3): 263-76.
[http://dx.doi.org/10.5664/jcsm.27497] [PMID: 19960649]

[16] Weaver TE, Grunstein RR. Adherence to continuous positive airway pressure therapy: the challenge to effective treatment. Proc Am Thorac Soc 2008; 5(2): 173-8.
[http://dx.doi.org/10.1513/pats.200708-119MG] [PMID: 18250209]

[17] Drager LF, Bortolotto LA, Krieger EM. Recent advances in the pathophysiology of sleep apnea-hypopnea syndrome. *. Chest 2007; 132(4): 1322-36.
[PMID: 17934118]

[18] Pi-Sunyer FX, Aronne LJ, Heshmati HM, Devin J, Rosenstock J, RIO-North America Study Group . Effect of rimonabant, a cannabinoid-1 receptor blocker, on weight and cardiometabolic risk factors in overweight or obese patients: RIO-North America: a randomized controlled trial. JAMA 2006; 295(7): 761-75.
[http://dx.doi.org/10.1001/jama.295.7.761] [PMID: 16478899]

[19] Mottillo S, Filion KB, Genest J, *et al*. The metabolic syndrome and cardiovascular risk a systematic review and meta-analysis. J Am Coll Cardiol 2010; 56(14): 1113-32.
[http://dx.doi.org/10.1016/j.jacc.2010.05.034] [PMID: 20863953]

[20] Naha S, Gardner MJ, Khangura D, *et al*. Hypertension in Diabetes. [Updated 2021 Aug 7]. In: Feingold KR, Anawalt B, Blackman MR, *et al*., editors. Endotext [Internet]. South Dartmouth (MA): MDText.com, Inc.; 2000-. Available from: https://www.ncbi.nlm.nih.gov/books/NBK279027/

[21] Wing RR, Lang W, Wadden TA, *et al*. Benefits of modest weight loss in improving cardiovascular risk factors in overweight and obese individuals with type 2 diabetes. Diabetes Care 2011; 34(7): 1481-6.
[http://dx.doi.org/10.2337/dc10-2415] [PMID: 21593294]

[22] Crossan K, Sheer AJ. Surgical Options in the Treatment of Severe Obesity. [Updated 2023 Feb 9]. In: StatPearls [Internet]. Treasure Island (FL): StatPearls. Available from: https://www.ncbi.nlm.nih.gov/books/NBK576372/

# CHAPTER 17

# Microbiota and Metabolic Syndrome

**Fatma Köksal Çakırlar**[1,*]

[1] *Istanbul University-Cerrahpasa, Cerrahpasa medicine Faculty, Istanbul, Turkey*

**Abstract:** Composed of trillions of microorganisms, the human GutM plays a key role in maintaining general health and metabolic homeostasis. MetS is a complex and common health condition characterized by a number of metabolic abnormalities, including obesity, insulin resistance, hypertension, and dyslipidemia. Evidence emerging in recent years indicates that human GutM plays a crucial role in the pathophysiology of MetS. In this chapter, we will discuss the composition and functionality of GutM, as well as the dynamic and complex relationship between GutM's influence on metS development and progression. By reviewing relevant studies and literature, we will try to shed light on potential therapeutic strategies and innovative approaches targeting GutM, mitigating the negative effects of MetS.

**Keywords:** Microbiota, Metabolic syndrome.

## INTRODUCTION

Microbiota refers to the trillions of microorganisms, including bacteria, viruses, fungi, and other microbes, that live in and on the human body. The "microbiome" comprises all of the genetic material within a microbiota. These two terms are used interchangeably. Microbiota or microbiome is the internal ecosystem of our body. Every part of our body (mouth, nose, throat, intestines, urogenital system, skin, mucous membranes around organs, and surfaces associated with the external environment) has different microbiota.

Within the scope of "the Human Microbiome Project", which started in 2007 and was completed in 2016 by the US National Institutes of Health (NIH) and the US National Institute for Genetic Research (NHGRI), extensive research has been conducted to understand the structure and functions of microorganisms (such as bacteria, viruses, fungi, *etc.*). The results of this project have been an important resource for the understanding of health and disease in the human microbiome.

---

* **Corresponding author Fatma Köksal Çakırlar:** Istanbul University-Cerrahpasa, Cerrahpasa medicine Faculty, Istanbul, Turkey; E-mail: fatma.koksal@iuc.edu.tr

**Hafize Uzun & Seyma Dumur (Eds.)**

The major population of microorganisms in the human body is found in the gastrointestinal tract (GIS). In recent years, the role of the gut microbiota in human health has received great attention from the scientific community. Emerging evidence suggests that it plays a crucial role in a variety of physiological processes, including metabolic homeostasis. The gut microbiota (GutM) influences human physiology and pathology by modulating host nutrition and energy harvesting. Many recent studies of the human microbiota have revealed the complexity and diversity of these microbial communities and their profound impact on human health. As research into the human microbiota continues to expand, new technologies and methodologies are emerging that promise to shed even more light on these complex microbial communities. Advances in metagenomics, microbiome engineering, and other microbiota research areas may open new avenues for understanding and manipulating these bacterial communities. The future of microbiota research is an exciting and rapidly evolving field that has the potential to transform our understanding of human health and disease. Although the microbiota is essential for human health, imbalances in these microbial communities can have detrimental effects on the body. Recent research has linked GutM changes to insulin resistance, inflammation, and metabolic syndrome (MetS).

MetS is defined as a combination of interconnected physiological, biochemical, and metabolic factors that increase the risk of developing cardiovascular diseases and type 2 diabetes (T2D). Risk factors that cause both T2D and cardiovascular diseases are called cardiometabolic risk factors. Many of the cardiometabolic risk factors are preventable risk factors. This syndrome is a group of disease states defined by the hallmark of clinical signs, including obesity, high blood pressure, high blood sugar, and high cholesterol or triglycerides and dyslipidemia (high serum triglycerides and low-high-density lipoprotein cholesterol). The worldwide prevalence of MetS is <10% to 84%, which may vary depending on the geographic region and the definition criteria applied [1].

Understanding the role of the microbiota in disease is important in identifying new treatments and preventive strategies. Understanding the complex interactions between GutM and MetS is a growing area of research, and scientists are exploring potential treatments that target the microbiota to improve metabolic health.

This chapter will provide an overview of the microbiota and its extraordinary relationship with the MetS.

# GUT MICROBIOTA

## GutM Composition and Diversity

The human GutM is a complex ecosystem, which includes bacteria, viruses, fungi, and other microorganisms that perform many important tasks and have an impact on human health. The composition of each individual's microbiota may vary depending on personal characteristics such as age, gender, lifestyle, dietary habits, geographic location, and genetic factors. In a healthy individual, the gut microbiota is highly diverse, with hundreds of different bacterial species coexisting in a balanced ecosystem. The intestinal microbiota is the area with the most bacterial diversity and the most studied and clinical experience. There is a community of microorganisms living with us in our microbiota, constituting approximately 2-3% of our body weight. It contains 10 times more genes than our own cells and 150-200 times more genes than the entire human genome.

Firmicutes, Bacteroidetes, Proteobacteria, Fusobacteria, Verrucomicrobia, Cyanobacteria, and Actinobacteria are the most abundant bacterial phyla in the gut. Additionally, they are found in minority populations such as archaea, eukaryotes, and viruses. The two most abundant bacterial phyla are Firmicutes (Gram-positive 60% -80%) and Bacteroidetes (Gram-negative 20% - 40%) [2]. These microorganisms are in a symbiotic relationship with their hosts. They play important roles in various physiological processes, such as the production of vitamins and amino acids, fermentation of indigestible substrates such as dietary fiber, the production of short-chain fatty acids (SCFA), conversion of cholesterol and bile acids, the maturation of the immune system, and protection against pathogens. They also play a vital role in maintaining human health by suppressing the growth of pathogenic microorganisms.

GutM is considered an organ in its own right with impressive metabolic ability and functional flexibility. For this reason, it has been considered a "metabolic organ". These bacteria, which have an enormous metabolic capacity and diversity, are also defined as "human-bacterial superorganisms" together with their host. This evolutionary reciprocal partnership between host and microbiota provides better digestive protection. Recent research shows that GutM has a major impact on health and disease. Microbiota imbalance has been linked to a variety of health problems, including intestinal inflammation, obesity, diabetes, allergies, and immune system diseases. Understanding the complexity of GutM and protecting this complex ecosystem is crucial for human health.

## Functions of GutM in Host Metabolism

The function of GutM is very diverse and has important effects on human health [3 - 9].

### Digestion and Fermentation

GuM plays an important role in digestion, especially contributing to the extraction of energy from dietary components by secreting enzymes that can digest complex carbohydrates and some fibers that are not otherwise digestible by human enzymes. Thus, it meets the energy needs of intestinal cells. It modulates the storage and use of energy. It affects energy balance and regulates energy homeostasis by influencing host fat deposition and regulating appetite. It metabolizes nutrients through fermentation, turning them into useful products.

### Nutrient Absorption

GutM influences the absorption of nutrients and minerals by interacting with the intestinal epithelium, affecting nutrient uptake and metabolism.

### Immune System Regulation

It plays a critical role in training and modulating the host's immune system. When kept in the right balance, GutM can interact with immune cells to maintain immune homeostasis and have a protective effect against infections and inflammation.

### Vitamin and Nutrient Synthesis

Intestinal microbes produce vitamins (for example, B and K) and other bioactive compounds that contribute to the nutritional status and general health of the host.

### Metabolism of Bile Acids

GutM can metabolize bile acids required for lipid digestion and absorption, and these metabolites can also affect host lipid metabolism.

### Intestinal Barrier Function

The microbiota maintains intestinal integrity by contributing to the formation of the mucus layer, which strengthens the connections between intestinal epithelial cells and supports the intestinal barrier.

## Neurological Effects

There is a communication pathway called the gut-brain axis between the gutM and the brain. In this pathway, the microbiota can influence emotional state and behavior by producing certain compounds that act on the nervous system.

## Metabolic Health

The balance of GutM has an impact on metabolic health. Research shows that a healthy microbiota can play an important role in the development of certain diseases such as obesity, diabetes, and MetS.

The exact functioning of GutM is not yet fully understood. This area is still an active research topic for scientists. However, due to the complexity of the microbiota, research on the subject continues.

## Factors Affecting GutM Composition

Microbiota is highly dynamic depending on the region, and changes in microbiota composition can affect the physiology and health of the organism.

In the first culture-based microbiota studies, it was suggested that intestinal bacterial species constitute the "core microbiota" in healthy individuals, and it was thought that the same/similar microorganisms in the intestines of different adults constitute a "core microbiome". In studies determining the core cluster of phylotypes (which have 97% sequence similarity by 16S rRNA sequencing) in the microbiota at the species level, the main components, including *Faecalibacterium prausnitzii*, *Roseburia intestinalis*, and Bacteroides uniformis, were shown. Despite the consistency of the main components, differences in the relative species and proportions in adults have also been reported. After culture-based microbiota studies, next-generation sequencing studies, on the other hand, enabled the detection of large microbial diversity contrary to the concept of nuclei. Studies covering a wide age range from newborns to elderly individuals in different countries have partially weakened the core/common microorganism cluster view in terms of species in the gut microbiota. Even if it is predicted that each individual's microbiota is unique to the individual (such as "fingerprint") at the genus and species level, it has been reported that different microbiota may show some similarity [10, 11].

The changes that occur throughout a person's life (endogenous and exogenous factors such as diet, genetic structure and type of birth, age, geographical region, personal hygiene, presence of toxins, surgical interventions, depression and lifestyle, smoking, past diseases, antibiotic, and other drug use) are important in shaping the microbiota.

## Diet

Diet plays an important role in shaping GutM composition and function. It affects metabolic health. The type and quality of food consumed significantly affect GutM and are important factors in the formation of microbial abundance and diversity. Food choices can affect the level of inflammation in the gut. Chronic inflammation can upset the balance of the microbiota and affect the immune system response. It also affects body weight and metabolic health. Research shows that some types of microbiota can affect weight management. A Western-style diet high in refined sugars, saturated fats, and processed foods has been associated with gut dysbiosis (unbalanced microbiota) and an increased risk of MetS. A diet rich in fiber, whole grains, fruits, and vegetables promotes a more diverse and beneficial GutM, potentially reducing the risk of MetS. Compounds that support gut health, such as probiotics and prebiotics, are important for the nutrition of microorganisms. Probiotics are live bacteria species and are found in fermented foods (such as yogurt, kefir, and pickles). These probiotic bacteria perform beneficial functions in the gut and support the microbiota balance. Prebiotics, on the other hand, are non-digestible types of fiber and support the growth and activity of GutM. Foods such as onions, garlic, and bananas are rich in prebiotics. A varied diet that includes different types of nutrients can increase microbiota diversity. Fat and protein types can also have an impact on the microbiota. For example, excessive consumption of saturated fat or over-processed meat products can increase certain types of harmful bacteria. Excessive consumption of sugary or processed foods can also increase certain types of harmful bacteria. This can negatively affect gut health [12, 13].

## Genetic Factors

Individual genetic makeup can affect the composition and stability of GutM. Genetic factors can influence how the host responds to different dietary components and how the gut environment interacts with microbes [14, 15].

## Birth and Breastfeeding

The process of birth and breastfeeding affects the formation of GutM in the baby. GutM develops throughout life with different compositions at different stages of development. For example, Firmicutes bacteria increase from infancy to old age, while Bacteriodetes decrease. Factors such as mode of delivery (vaginal birth / cesarean section) and breastfeeding affect early microbiota colonization [16].

## Age

There may be differences in GutM between infants, adults, and older individuals. The development of the microbiota usually begins at birth. Microorganisms colonize the outer surfaces of the baby after birth. The genus Bifidobacterium gradually becomes dominant in the infant microbiota. In the early period of life, two main phyla, "Actinobacteria and Proteobacteria", dominate. Illness, antibiotic therapy, and dietary modification increase the diversity in GutM. Up to three years of age, the composition, diversity, and functional abilities of the infant microbiota are similar to the adult microbiota. The diversity of microorganisms increases with age. The microbiota of older individuals is slightly more diverse than that of younger individuals. Individuals over 65 years of age have an increase in Bacteroidetes and Clostridium in GutM. Microbiota-derived SCFA production was found to be decreased in the elderly [17, 18].

## Antibiotics and Drugs

The use of antibiotics and some drugs, especially those that affect intestinal motility, can disrupt GutM and lead to dysbiosis [19, 20].

## Gender

Many studies show that gender may play a role in GutM composition [21 - 24].

## Geography and Environmental Factors

GutM may vary depending on geographic location and environmental factors. For example, polluted air, water, and food can adversely affect GutM composition [25, 26].

## Depression and Lifestyle

Factors such as exercise, sleep patterns, psychological stress, and lifestyle can affect GutM. Disrupted sleep patterns and insufficient sleep have been associated with MetS, including intestinal dysbiosis and insulin resistance. Chronic stress may affect GutM and its function, potentially promoting gut dysbiosis and contributing to the development of MetS [27, 28].

Studies show that human GutM is governed by gram-positive Firmicutes (Lactobacillus, Clostridium, Eubacterium, Ruminococcus, Butyrivibrio, Roseburia, Anaerostipes and Faecalibacterium) and gram-negative Bacteroidetes and to a lesser extent gram positive Actinobacteria (Bifidobacterium genera) and gram-negative Proteobacteria [12]. Among the members of Firmicutes,

Fecalibacterium, Eubacterium, and Roseburia are butyrate producers. Bacteroides, Prevotella, and Xylanibacter genera are effective decomposers of dietary fiber.

The Bacteroides enterotype is thought to be associated with diets rich in protein and lipids, whereas the Prevotella enterotype is associated with diets rich in carbohydrates and sugar. Bifidobacterium and Actinobacteria have probiotic effects when consumed with food or supplements.

Proteobacteria include Escherichia, Desulfovibrio (sulfate-reducing bacteria), and Akkermansia muciniphila, a mucin-degrading member of the phylum Verrucomicrobia. The abundance of this bacterium in the human intestinal tract is inversely proportional to several disease states. A. muciniphila is located in the mucus layer of the large intestine, where it plays a role in maintaining intestinal integrity. An inverse correlation between the abundance of A. muciniphila and the presence of T2D or obesity has been reported in mouse and human studies. The administration of A. muciniphila has been shown to improve body weight and biomarkers of liver dysfunction in obese and overweight individuals [29 - 31].

The Firmicutes/Bacteroidetes (F/B) ratio is associated with normal intestinal homeostasis and is dependent on endogenous and exogenous factors that change throughout a person's life [1].

Numerous studies have demonstrated that the composition and diversity of GutM differs significantly between healthy individuals and those with metabolic syndrome [32, 33].

An increase or decrease in the F/B ratio is considered dysbiosis. An elevated F/B ratio has been associated with obesity and a decreased F/B ratio with inflammatory bowel disease. Compared to normal individuals, the F/B ratio is decreased in T2D patients, and the phylum differs.

It has been shown that F/B ratios have been shown to be significantly related to plasma glucose concentration. Although some studies have shown that obese patients with MetS have a higher F/B ratio compared to "healthy obese" individuals, this is not conclusive and requires further research [1, 34].

## MICROBIOTA AND METABOLIC SYNDROME

Microbiota and MetS are among the important issues related to human health. About 200 years ago, Redi, Virchow, Pasteur, Lister, Koch, and many other researchers changed the theory and practice of medicine with their experiments showing the role of microbes in disease. Theodor Escherich discovered Escherichia coli isolated from the colons of healthy children in 1885. Previously, there was no evidence of gut-resident bacteria. Escherichia showed that some strains of *E. coli* are harmless, while others are responsible for infant gastroenteritis. This study introduced not only the concept of the natural gut microbiota but also the concept of strain variation of a bacterium in different situations and individuals [31, 35, 36].

In their 1977 article, arguably one of the most influential and groundbreaking microbiology publications to date, Carl Woese and George Fox showed that the ribosomal RNA (rRNA) of all living things is divided into three categories: archaea, bacteria, and eukaryotes.

The work by Norman Pace *et al.* showed that molecular tools can be used to reliably identify bacteria in mixed populations of organisms based on 16S rRNA [37, 38].

Since the first use of the term "Microbiome/Microbiome (the ecological community of commensal, symbiotic, and pathogenic microorganisms that fully share our body space)" by Lederberg J in the early 2000s, many scientific papers describing the microbiota have been published [39].

Despite the introduction of tools to characterize previously uncultured microbial life in environments such as the human gut with the development of high-throughput sequencing technologies, precise mechanisms in human cohorts are difficult to pinpoint in detail due to the susceptibility of the microbiota to environmental disturbances and the difficulty of accessing certain body regions.

GutM's role in both the protection of health and the development of disease began to gain importance. GutM dysbiosis, for example, can lead to excessive SCFA production, which can lead to insulin resistance and metabolic dysregulation. Therefore, today, instead of a single disease, MetS, which is a cluster of risk factors, is tried to be approached by decomposing the risk factors in the microbiota, for example, by investigating whether there are microbial connections with cardiovascular disease, obesity, or dyslipidemia.

Previously, the gut was completely ignored in the definition of MetS, but as the microbiome area has come to the fore, data from the last decade have shown that the mechanisms leading to MetS risk factors may be associated with GutM. The term "Metabolic Syndrome" was first coined in the 1970s by Herman Haller, who was doing research on atherosclerosis. In the early 1920s, the association of dysmetabolism with cardiovascular risk factors was documented. Gerald Reaven proposed a new name for the MetS, "syndrome X," in 1988. The term now highlights insulin resistance among the set of risk factors [31].

One study on mice found that the development of insulin resistance was associated with changes in GutM [40].

Over the past decade, substantial evidence from both animal and human studies shows a clear link between GutM in chronic diseases, including inflammatory autoimmune disorders, intestinal inflammation-related disorders, and cardiometabolic diseases [41, 42].

## Relationship between GutM and MetS

The relationship between GutM and MetS is quite complex. Although a causal relationship can be established between gut microbial profiles and MetS in animal experiments, the relationship between them is still controversial in humans.

Studies have shown that individuals with MetS tend to have less diverse GutM compared to healthy individuals. These individuals have an abundance of harmful bacteria, such as Firmicutes and Proteobacteria, and a shortage of beneficial bacteria, such as Bacteroidetes and *Faecalibacterium prausnitzii*. It has been emphasized that this may potentially contribute to weight gain and obesity-related problems.

The first evidence of a gut-centered MetS theory emerged in 2007, when Cani *et al.*, in a series of studies in rodents and humans, found that chronic consumption of a high-fat diet leads to intestinal barrier defects that facilitate intestinal lumen permeability. This condition has been termed metabolic endotoxemia due to the low-grade inflammation caused by bacteria or bacterial by-products, especially bacterial lipopolysaccharide (LPS) entering the systemic circulation, and its inhibitory effect on normal glycemic function.

This study is also the first report to show that bacterial LPS activation of Toll-like receptors (TLRs) elicits an immune response that impairs insulin sensitivity. The study on factors affecting intestinal permeability is one of the most promising areas of microbiota research [31, 43].

Given the close relationship between GutM and MetS, scientists are exploring various therapeutic strategies targeting the microbiota for potential disease management. Probiotics, prebiotics, and dietary interventions are among the approaches aimed at restoring the intestinal microbiota balance and improving metabolic health.

Research offers promising results suggesting that manipulating GutM can serve as a complementary approach in the management of MetS [44, 45].

## GutM Dysbiosis and MetS

Various factors caused by the dysbiosis of GutM lead to extensive physiological changes and increase the risk of MetS. Intestinal dysbiosis refers to an imbalance in the composition and function of GutM, characterized by a reduction in beneficial microbes and an overgrowth of potentially harmful ones. Emerging evidence suggests that gut dysbiosis is closely related to the development and progression of MetS.

Various mechanisms, including inflammation, energy metabolism, and intestinal barrier function, come to the fore to explain how GutM affects MetS.

### *Inflammation*

GutM plays a crucial role in modulating the immune system. GutM can affect the body's inflammatory response in many ways. Some gut bacteria can produce metabolites such as LPS or endotoxins that trigger immune responses and low-grade inflammation. Increased levels of these substances in the bloodstream have been associated with insulin resistance, obesity, and other components of the MetS. In addition, some gut bacteria may affect systemic inflammation and contribute to metabolic dysfunction by affecting the balance of pro-inflammatory and anti-inflammatory molecules [4].

### *Regulation of Energy Homeostasis*

GutM may affect the efficiency of energy generation from the diet. Some microbes break down complex carbohydrates and dietary fibers that human enzymes cannot digest and produce SCFA as byproducts that can affect the body's energy metabolism. These SCFAs serve as a source of energy to intestinal cells and can also increase feelings of fullness by sending signals to the brain. In this way, a microbiota that produces the right amounts of SCFA can regulate energy intake, reducing the tendency to overeat. Therefore, SCFAs have been associated with improved insulin sensitivity and regulation of appetite. A healthy microbiota can help insulin enter cells more effectively and regulate blood sugar, thereby reducing the risk of insulin resistance and T2D. Dysbiosis can disrupt the gut-brain axis, affecting appetite regulation and energy balance, leading to weight gain and obesity, a key component of MetS. Furthermore, imbalances in GutM, such as reduced microbial diversity or overgrowth of certain bacteria, can lead to greater energy extraction from the diet, potentially contributing to weight gain and obesity. The balance of GutM can affect the effects of the hormone insulin in the body. An imbalance in GutM can affect fat storage regulations in the body. In particular, an unbalanced microbiota profile may affect fat storage mechanisms, leading to obesity. At the same time, an unhealthy microbiota can increase systemic inflammation and contribute to other components of MetS.

## Barrier Dysfunction

The intestinal barrier is a protective layer in the digestive system that prevents harmful microbial components from entering the systemic circulation from outside and acts as a very important defense mechanism. The intestinal barrier consists of elements such as the tight junctions between intestinal cells and the mucus layer. It plays a crucial role in maintaining the balance between the GutM and the host. GutM can promote the growth of some microorganisms that can support mucosal integrity. The dysbiosis of GutM compromises the integrity of the gut barrier, resulting in the formation of an impaired gut barrier, also known as a "leaky gut". As a result of the complex interactions of these mechanisms, LPS and other microbial products from the cell walls of bacteria that contribute to MetS pathogenesis may enter the bloodstream, triggering an immune response and further promoting inflammation. Chronic low-grade inflammation plays a crucial role in insulin resistance and the development of MetS [3, 46, 47].

The relationships between GutM and MetS are not fully understood, and research on the subject continues.

## Hormonal Regulation

The gutM may also interact with hormones involved in metabolism and appetite regulation. For example, some gut bacteria can affect the production of hormones such as ghrelin and glucagon-like peptide-1 (GLP-1), which play a role in appetite control and insulin secretion. Changes in gut composition may, therefore, affect hormonal signals related to metabolism.

## Microbial Metabolites

GutM produces a wide variety of metabolites as part of its metabolic activities. These metabolites can have far-reaching effects on host physiology. It has been shown that microbiota metabolites interfere with mitochondrial oxidative/nitrosative stress and autophagosome formation, thereby regulating the activation of inflammatory cytokines and the production of inflammatory cytokines involved in chronic metabolic disorders [48].

For example, bile acids, SCFAs, and metabolites such as trimethylamine N-oxide (TMAO) and indole derivatives are known to affect metabolism, inflammation, and cardiovascular health. The types and levels of these metabolites are affected by the composition and activity of GutM.

- *Secondary Bile Acids*: Bile acids are synthesized in the liver and are also metabolized into secondary bile acids by intestinal bacteria. These secondary bile acids can affect host lipid and glucose metabolism through interactions with bile acid receptors such as the farnesoid X receptor (FXR) and G-protei--coupled bile acid receptor 1 (also known as TGR5). They also affect gut barrier integrity and inflammation. Activation of TGR5 leads to higher secretion of GLP1, thereby increasing insulin sensitivity and obesity. In addition to binding to TGR5 and FXR, bile acids can interact with mitochondria and regulate metabolic processes associated with MetS [49].
- *Short Chain Fatty Acids* (**SCFAs**): SCFAs such as acetate, propionate, and butyrate are produced by gut bacteria through the fermentation of dietary fibers. They play an important role in the regulation of host energy metabolism, glucose homeostasis, and lipid metabolism. SCFAs act as signaling molecules by interacting with G-protein-coupled receptors and regulating the secretion of gut hormones such as GLP-1 and peptide YY (PYY), which affect appetite and insulin sensitivity [34, 50].
- *Trimethylamine N-Oxide (TMAO)*: TMAO is produced in the gut by specific gut bacteria from dietary choline and carnitine. High TMAO levels are associated with cardiovascular disease risk. TMAO supports atherosclerosis by affecting cholesterol metabolism and increasing foam cell formation in the arterial wall [51].
- *Indole Derivatives*: Indole derivatives are microbial metabolites released as a result of the breakdown of dietary tryptophan by intestinal bacteria. These metabolites have been shown to affect host metabolism and immune function. For example, indole-3-acetic acid has been found to improve glucose tolerance and insulin sensitivity.

## SOME MECHANISMS THAT ASSOCIATE GUTM WITH METS

### The Relationship between GutM and Obesity

Recent studies show that GutM is associated with obesity and may affect obesity. This relationship works in a complex way and is not fully understood; GutM can ferment indigestible nutrients and release energy during this process. This can result in extra calorie intake and increase the risk of obesity. Some research shows that abnormal GutM is associated with low-grade inflammation. Chronic inflammation can trigger obesity and obesity-related health problems. GutM can affect the way the body absorbs and stores the energy it receives. Some microorganisms cause greater energy absorption, while others may contribute to less energy absorption. Some components of GutM can affect appetite and satiety hormones. This can affect a person's eating behavior and eating habits. In obese individuals, a decrease in diversity in GutM and an increase in certain bacterial strains have been observed. These changes can have an impact on metabolism and weight management. Excessive and unnecessary use of antibiotics can adversely affect GutM. This can increase the risk of obesity by disrupting the metabolic balance. Nutritional habits can also affect GutM. Consuming high-fiber foods, probiotics, and fermented foods can help support a healthy microbiota balance. Karlsson *et al.* study showed that women with normal glucose control had different GutM compositions compared to diabetics [52].

Qin *et al.* study determined that certain types of GutM were increased or decreased in T2D individuals [7].

Another study shows changes in GutM with the progression of glucose intolerance [53].

All these points show that the relationship between GutM and obesity is quite complex.

The following various factors may affect this relationship;

### *Role of the Microbiota in the Regulation of Energy Harvest from the Diet*

GutM plays an important role in regulating energy harvesting from the diet, and its dysregulation plays a role in the development of obesity and MetS.GuM helps break down complex dietary components that are not otherwise digestible by the human body. Some microbes have the ability to ferment dietary fibers and other carbohydrates, producing SCFAs as a byproduct. SCFAs such as acetate, propionate, and butyrate are absorbed by intestinal cells and contribute to the host's energy supply. They can also affect food intake by affecting appetite regulation and satiety. In addition, intestinal microbes are involved in the metabolism of bile acids, which are necessary for fat digestion and absorption. Changes in gutM composition can affect bile acid metabolism, leading to changes in fat absorption and, ultimately, energy balance.

### *Gut-Brain Axis in Obesity and MetS*

The gut-brain axis and GutM play an important role in the regulation of metabolism and the development of MetS. The gut-brain axis is a bidirectional communication system between the GIS and the central nervous system that includes hormonal, neural, and immune pathways. GutM plays a crucial role in modulating this axis and can affect a variety of brain functions, including those related to appetite, mood, and behavior. Research has shown that certain gut microbes can produce neurotransmitters and metabolites that affect the brain's reward system and appetite regulation. For example, some gut bacteria produce molecules that affect the release of hormones such as leptin and ghrelin, which are crucial in signals of hunger and fullness. These hormones can activate neurons in the hypothalamus, leading to increased food intake, decreased energy expenditure, and weight gain. Furthermore, inflammation triggered by dysbiosis in GutM has been associated with insulin resistance, a hallmark of MetS. This chronic low-grade inflammation may contribute to the development of obesity and related metabolic disorders. Understanding the complex interplay between these systems can provide new insights into the prevention and treatment of MetS and related conditions [3, 54 - 57].

As obesity increases the risk of diabetes, changes similar to obesity are detected in diabetic patients with GutM. In metagenomic studies in T2D patients, a decrease in butyrate-producing Clostridiales bacteria (*Roseburia intestinalis* and *Faecalibacterium praustnitzii*) and an increase in Proteobacteria, *Lactobacillus gasseri*, and *Streptococcus mutans* were found [58].

## GutM's Insulin Resistance and Glucose Metabolism

It has been shown by various mechanisms that GutM can affect insulin resistance and glucose homeostasis.

### *Microbiota-mediated iNsulin Resistance Mechanisms*

Intestinal bacteria ferment dietary fibers to produce SCFAs such as acetate, propionate, and butyrate. SCFAs have been shown to increase insulin sensitivity by stimulating the release of gut hormones (GLP-1 and PYY), which increase insulin secretion and improve glucose uptake in peripheral tissues [59].

Disruptions in the intestinal barrier can cause bacterial products to pass into the bloodstream, triggering inflammation and insulin resistance [60].

Some gut bacteria metabolize dietary choline and L-carnitine to trimethylamine (TMA), which is converted to TMAO in the liver. High TMAO levels have been associated with insulin resistance and cardiovascular disease [61].

GutM can affect the production of proinflammatory cytokines, which can impair insulin signaling and contribute to insulin resistance [3].

Intestinal bacteria can affect signaling functions by altering the bile acid composition. Bile acids regulate glucose metabolism by interacting with nuclear receptors such as FXR and TGR5 [49].

GutM can affect energy balance, glucose metabolism, and insulin sensitivity by affecting the endocannabinoid system [62].

The effect of GutM on glucose metabolism and insulin resistance is a complex and dynamic area of research.

## Intestinal-Kidney Axis of GutM in Hypertension and Metabolic Syndrome

Research has uncovered important links between GutM and hypertension and MetS. Hypertension, or high blood pressure, is a common cardiovascular condition that increases the risk of heart disease, stroke, and other serious health problems. Certain bacteria in the gut can produce bioactive compounds that affect blood pressure levels. For example, overgrowth of certain bacteria can lead to the production of vasoactive compounds that affect blood vessel function and blood pressure. An important aspect of this relationship is the gut-kidney axis between GutM and the kidneys, which can affect blood pressure regulation and metabolic function. Studies have shown that the intestinal-kidney axis can affect hypertension and MetS through various mechanisms.

The gut-kidney axis refers to the bidirectional communication between the gut and the kidneys and enables the exchange of signaling molecules, metabolites, and inflammatory mediators that can affect kidney function and blood pressure regulation. GutM and its metabolites have a significant effect on kidney function. Therefore, disruptions in this axis caused by imbalances in GutM can lead to hypertension and other related conditions.

Some other mechanisms also contribute to the development of hypertension;

### *Inflammation and Immune Activation*

GutM plays an important role in inflammation and immune system regulation in the gut. Dysbiosis in the gut can lead to the production of proinflammatory molecules that can enter the bloodstream and contribute to systemic inflammation. It can impair blood vessel function, insulin sensitivity, and kidney function, which are linked to inflammation, hypertension, and MetS. Increased low-level inflammation in MetS may be associated with changes in GutM [43].

*SCFAs:* Produced by some intestinal bacteria through the fermentation of dietary fibers, SCFAs are reported to increase insulin sensitivity by influencing the production of hormones that regulate blood pressure, thus having various health benefits. Studies have shown that SCFAs produced from dietary fiber in GutM and SCFAs such as butyrate, propionate, and acetate produced from fermentation of resistant starch can affect lipid metabolism by modulating hepatic cholesterol synthesis and fatty acid metabolism. It has been stated that SCFAs can also interact with specific receptors by acting as G-protein-coupled receptors (GPCRs), affecting lipid metabolism in peripheral tissues [50, 63, 64].

## Hormonal and Metabolic Signaling

GutM can affect blood pressure regulation and the release of hormones and metabolites that affect metabolism. For example, gut bacteria can affect the renin-angiotensin-aldosterone system (RAAS), which plays a central role in regulating blood pressure. Disruption of this system can cause hypertension.

## Endotoxemia

Increased intestinal permeability can cause bacterial components to enter the bloodstream. Known as endotoxemia, this condition triggers an immune response and inflammation that can affect blood vessel function and contribute to metabolic abnormalities [65 - 75].

## GutM and Dyslipidemia

Dyslipidemia is a condition of abnormal levels of fat in the blood and can lead to serious health problems such as heart disease. Various studies show that GutM can affect lipid metabolism and thus contribute to the development of dyslipidemia. Mechanisms underlying this association include the interaction of bile acids, cortisol, endotoxins, and other biological signals. In their study on mice, Jiao *et al.* showed that certain intestinal bacteria species can change the lipid profile, and these changes may contribute to the development of dyslipidemia [76].

There is also evidence that regulation of GutM is a potential avenue for the treatment of dyslipidemia. In a study by Li *et al.*, it was determined that probiotic supplementation positively affected lipid profiles and reduced cardiovascular risk factors in dyslipidemia patients [77].

## Microbial modulation of Lipid Metabolism

The effects of GutM on the digestion, absorption, storage, and energy balance of lipids are a complex process. Some bacteria in GutM may alter cholesterol levels by affecting lipid metabolism [78].

SCFAs, which GutM produces by breaking down indigestible fibers, pectin, and some carbohydrates, are used as an energy source by colon cells and may also affect lipid metabolism. For example, propionic acid can reduce cholesterol synthesis in the liver and promote the breakdown of triglycerides. GutM's influence on lipid metabolism may play an important role in the development of metabolic diseases such as obesity, diabetes, and cardiovascular diseases. Research shows that GutM affects lipid metabolism in several ways. In particular, it has been observed that GutM affects triglyceride and cholesterol levels by regulating lipid absorption [49, 56, 79 - 82].

GutM can directly affect cholesterol levels by metabolizing dietary cholesterol and bile acids. It may affect cholesterol absorption in the intestine through various mechanisms, such as the expression of transporters responsible for cholesterol uptake. Increased cholesterol absorption efficiency, leading to high cholesterol levels in the blood, has been associated with specific gut bacteria [83].

Many studies show the complex relationship between GutM and dyslipidemia, especially in terms of cholesterol metabolism. Manipulating GutM with diet or other interventions holds promise for the development of new therapeutic strategies to manage dyslipidemia and reduce cardiovascular disease risk. In addition, In addition, bile acids synthesized in the liver and required for fat absorption are converted into secondary bile acids by GutM.This process can affect cholesterol homeostasis, leading to changes in blood cholesterol levels [84].

Another study describes how GutM can affect cardiovascular disease through phosphatidylcholine metabolism [6].

An altered GutM composition may lead to increased inflammation, impaired lipid metabolism, and alterations in bile acid metabolism, which may contribute to dyslipidemia [85].

The potential benefits and risks of microbial modulation of lipid metabolism will be better understood with more data and clinical trials.

**Effect of Immune System and Inflammation on MetS**

The immune system and inflammation play an important role in the development and progression of MetS. Inflammation is a natural response of the immune system to injury, infection, or other harmful stimuli. Chronic low-grade inflammation can contribute to insulin resistance, high blood pressure, and abnormal cholesterol levels, which are key components of the MetS. Insulin resistance occurs when body cells become less sensitive to insulin, a hormone that helps regulate blood sugar levels, and the body produces more insulin to compensate, leading to high blood sugar levels and an increased risk of T2D. It may also contribute to the development of other components of the MetS, such as chronic low-grade inflammation, high blood pressure, and abnormal cholesterol levels. Inflammatory cytokines, which are molecules produced by the immune system, can lead to plaque buildup in the arteries, increasing the risk of heart disease and stroke. A healthy diet and regular physical activity can help reduce inflammation and improve metabolic health.

## Effect of Antibiotic Use on GutM and MetS

Antibiotics are used to treat bacterial infections. However, they can also cause undesirable consequences on the body's microbiota, which includes trillions of microorganisms living in the intestine. Antibiotic use can lead to changes in the intestinal environment and affect the balance of microbial populations, leading to dysbiosis. This may lead to reduced microbial diversity and overgrowth of harmful bacteria, contributing to the development of MetS. The effect of antibiotics on GutM is not always negative. In some cases, antibiotics may be necessary to treat bacterial infections that can cause serious harm if left untreated. The use of antibiotics may have beneficial effects on GutM in certain situations, such as cases of Clostridium difficile infection, where antibiotics may help restore microbial balance.

Short-term use of antibiotics has been associated with changes in glucose metabolism and insulin sensitivity, potentially increasing the risk of MetS. Long-term or frequent use of antibiotics has been associated with an increased risk of obesity, T2D, and MetSr. In addition, antibiotic-induced changes in GutM may potentially contribute to the development of MetS by affecting the production of microbial metabolites and host metabolism. Many studies have highlighted the relationship between antibiotic exposure and metabolic disorders [86 - 90].

While antibiotics are an important tool in the treatment of bacterial infections, their use must be carefully considered to minimize the risk of upsetting the delicate balance of GutM and potentially contributing to the development of MetS.

## THERAPEUTIC STRATEGIES TARGETING MICROBIOTA IN METABOLIC SYNDROME

Developing techniques or algorithms that provide accurate prediction of drug, host, and microbiome interactions is critical to modern microbiome research and precision medicine. Understanding the complex interactions between the microbiota and MetS is a growing area of research.

The study by Wu *et al.* shows how metformin alters the GutM of individuals with T2D who have not started treatment and how these changes contribute to the therapeutic effects of the drug [91].

Potential therapeutic strategies targeting GutM to improve metabolic health have received considerable attention from scientists in the management of MetS. There are some basic therapeutic approaches and many studies supporting their effectiveness [92].

Sáez-Lara *et al.* examined the effects of probiotics and synbiotics (a combination of probiotics and prebiotics) on components of metabolic syndrome, including obesity, insulin resistance, T2D, and nonalcoholic fatty liver disease (NALFD), and as co-adjuvants for the prevention and treatment of these disorders. They reported that oral intake of probiotics and synbiotics gave partially good results [93].

In another study, probiotics were shown to alleviate metabolic syndrome by affecting GutM in mice fed a high-fat diet [94].

Another study examining the role of probiotics in managing MetS discussed the potential of probiotics in managing metabolic syndrome, focusing on their ability to inhibit angiotensin-converting enzyme (ACE), which is involved in blood pressure regulation and metabolic processes [95].

One review highlighted the impact of GutM on T2D and MetS and the potential of probiotics and prebiotics to modulate GutM to improve metabolic health [44].

There are hundreds of human clinical studies that demonstrate the safety and sometimes effectiveness of probiotic bacteria. There are new strains and bioengineered probiotic organisms available in commerce that provide a range of activities from neurotransmitter production to metabolizing alcohol. However, many countries have strict regulations limiting certain health claims and limited guidance on the types and doses of probiotic products to consume for the intended benefits. Although research on the use of probiotics and prebiotics to manage MetS shows promising results, it is not yet conclusive. Probiotics have not been widely adopted for clinical use by the mainstream medical community except in limited circumstances [96 - 98].

More research is needed to fully understand the specific strains, dosages, and long-term effects of probiotics and prebiotics on MetS management [99].

Only a small number of microbiota-based biotherapeutics have received U.S. Food and Drug Administration (FDA) approval following more than two decades of research. The FDA granted its initial approval to Rebiotix's standardized capsules for fecal microbiota transplantation (FMT) in November 2022. Despite evidence of its effectiveness, FMT is still regarded in many parts of the world as a "for research purposes" method of treating recurring *C. difficile* infections. This limits patients' access to the FMT procedure. A recent study in Europe reported that this treatment is only applicable to approximately 10% of all patients for whom it is indicated [100, 101].

Developing techniques or algorithms that provide accurate prediction of host-microbiome and drug-microbiome interactions is critical to modern microbiome research and precision medicine. Metagenomic studies have facilitated GutM-targeted drug discovery and efforts to improve human health management. With the development of various *in vitro* GutM culturing models such as HuMiX, SHIME, and RapidAIM, the effects of drugs against individual GutM can be rapidly screened. GutM metabolites can be measured directly using analytical techniques such as metabolomics, nuclear magnetic resonance (NMR) spectroscopy, or mass spectrometry (MS). These technologies provide an in-depth look at the proteome-level insights of the microbiome [102].

Another challenge is to encourage the scientific community, including publishers, to adopt the standards. For this, it is important to improve repeatability and consistency in reporting with the development of a tool called "Strengthening the Organization and Reporting of Microbiome Studies or STORMS". Widespread adoption of STORMS can increase the real-world impact of microbiota researchers [103, 104].

NALFD has been frequently associated with metabolic disorders in obese and diabetic patients. It is a leading cause of chronic liver disease. Cirrhosis is an important risk factor for hepatocellular carcinoma and liver-related deaths. NAFLD has numerous clinical challenges related to both diagnosis and treatment. A growing body of evidence suggests a complex link between GutM and the pathogenesis of NAFLD [105].

Current knowledge of the gut-liver axis in NAFLD provides evidence that it can be used as a non-invasive biomarker for diagnosis and staging. Developing personalized approaches based on GutM will become an integral component of personalized medicine in the coming years, especially in multifactorial chronic metabolic disorders such as GutM and NAFLD. Drugs for the treatment of T2D, such as metformin, GLP-1 agonists, and sodium-glucose cotransporter (SGLT) inhibitors, are effective in regulating glucose homeostasis and reducing liver fat content and inflammation. Thus, GutM composition was associated with progression towards a healthy phenotype.

Bariatric surgery can significantly alter GutM with a parallel improvement in the histological features of NAFLD due to modification of the gastrointestinal anatomy.

A growing body of evidence suggests a complex link between GutM and the pathogenesis of NAFLD. With many options showing promising effects in reprogramming the gut-liver axis, such as FMT and next-generation probiotics, a broader understanding of GutM in the future may lead to personalized drug selection [106].

Gan *et al.* have demonstrated that high alcohol-producing Klebsiella pneumoniae (HAPKpn) may be one of the causes of NAFLD in GutM. In this study, it was found that HAPKpn-specific phage therapy could reduce HAPKpn-induced steatohepatitis in male mice, including hepatic dysfunction, expression of cytokines, and lipogenic gene expression [107].

## Fecal Microbiota Transplant (FMT) as a Potential Treatment

FMT targeting whole GutM involves the transfer of fecal matter from a healthy donor to the recipient for a balanced and healthy GutM. In this system, stool from the donor is transferred to the recipient in the form of a nasogastric tube, colonoscope, enema, capsule, or a combination of these. While FMT is still in its infancy for the treatment of MetS, it has shown success in the treatment of some gastrointestinal disorders. It was first used in 1958 in the treatment of patients with pseudomembranous enterocolitis [108].

Therapeutically, this method has shown remarkable success in curing colitis due to recurrent *C. difficile* infection. This success has raised the question of whether FMT can be used for other indications, and evidence demonstrates its potential in modulating GutM in managing MetS and related disorders [31, 109].

In recent years, it has been used in the treatment of gastrointestinal system-related diseases such as irritable bowel syndrome, chronic constipation, diarrhea, and inflammatory bowel disease. It has become the current subject of studies even in metabolic diseases such as diabetes and obesity. Animal studies show that the transplanted microbiota acts at a level that alters the metabolic phenotype. In the study of Ridaura *et al.*, when fecal microbiota from obese and lean phenotype twin rats was transferred to sterile mice and monitored, it was shown that adipose tissue increased significantly and bacterial diversity decreased in microbiota areas from obese rats [79].

In a study investigating the effect of fecal transplantation in obese patients diagnosed with T2D from healthy lean individuals, it was observed that insulin sensitivity and butyrate-producing intestinal flora were significantly increased, and the SCFA ratio decreased in allogeneic fecal transplant recipients compared to autologous fecal transplant recipients [109].

Although fecal transplantation seems to be a very promising treatment modality, randomized controlled studies on metabolic diseases in humans are insufficient. In addition, more research is needed on metabolic diseases due to the difficulty of the method of administration, the subjectivity of the healthy microbiota, and the unknown long-term effects. In the near future, with a better understanding of the effect of microbiota on metabolic diseases, FMT can be used more safely on metabolic diseases.

## Dietary Interventions for Gut Microbiota Modulation

Diet plays a crucial role in shaping GutM composition and function. Certain dietary patterns and certain food components can promote the growth of beneficial bacteria and inhibit harmful ones, potentially improving metabolic parameters in individuals with MetS [110].

While these therapeutic strategies are promising, more research is needed to fully understand the mechanisms involved and to determine their efficacy and safety in managing MetS.

## Future perspectives and Impacts on GutM Research

Much remains to be learned about which bacterial strains in the microbiota are most associated with metS and associated complications. The mechanisms behind the relationship between the microbiota and MetS are not yet fully understood. Because the unique nature of GutM is different in each individual, future research may focus on identifying the key bacterial species responsible for the development of MetS, which could help develop more targeted therapies. As we learn more about specific bacterial species and mechanisms, it may be possible to develop personalized treatment approaches based on an individual's unique microbiota profile.

Microbiota-modifying treatments such as probiotics, prebiotics, and postbiotics may become more useful in the treatment and prevention of diseases in the future. Such treatments can help prevent or cure diseases by restoring the healthy balance of GutM. Research into microbiota engineering will likely expand. Scientists may discover ways to modify GutM using more effective probiotics, prebiotics, or FMT to improve metabolic health and prevent MetS.

Despite significant advances, the majority of gut microbial species remain uncharacterized. The identification and study of these unknown species and their role in metabolic health can offer important insights and new therapeutic opportunities. GutM is known to have significant effects on brain functions and mental health. In the future, further research can be conducted to better understand GutM's communication with the brain and the effects of these interactions on mental health, thus leading to the development of new approaches to the treatment and prevention of depression, anxiety, and other mental disorders.

There is increasing evidence that the microbiota can interact with the epigenome, influence gene expression, and potentially contribute to the development of MetS. Future research may focus on better understanding these interactions and their potential impact on metabolic health.

The concept of functional microbiota or microbiota modulation is a new concept and is described as "developing a prototype for use in health by focusing on the missing or excess bacteria or bacterial community, their metabolites, after associating microbiota differences and changes with disease and health". Therefore, there is a need for more powerful and useful bioinformatics tools. Integrative and functional meta-omics assessments are one of the most important approaches to studying microbial metabolic pathways in GutM. Conducting long-term, large-scale longitudinal studies will further assist in establishing causal relationships between GutM and MetS.

Overall, there is much to learn about the complex interaction between the microbiota and MetS, and future research will provide important insights and new therapeutic approaches [5, 111 - 116].

## Challenges and Opportunities in GutM Research

### *Challenges in GutM Research*

GutM research has attracted great interest in recent years, and important scientific studies have been carried out in this area. It is important to understand both the chemical composition and functions of microbiota components. There are technical challenges to the complexity of GutM, the diversity and quantification of microbiota components, and their quantification and characterization. Especially, low-density microorganisms are not easy to detect and analyze. In addition, each individual's GutM is unique, and environmental factors, dietary habits, and genetic differences affect microbiota diversity. This makes it difficult to decipher the precise roles and interactions of each species in GutM research and to ensure standardization and reproducibility. Therefore, it makes it necessary to work with large-scale and representative groups of individuals. Robust protocols and greater collaborative efforts are required. Since viruses, archaea, and fungi also live in GutM, it should be considered in future research. To overcome all this complexity and difficulties, advanced computational tools and multiple "omics" approaches come to the fore. Omics studies have made it possible to identify live but non-culturable microorganisms in the gut. In addition, multi-omic techniques have begun to be used in research [117].

As GutM studies progress it is important to carefully consider ethical considerations regarding privacy, informed consent, and equitable access to potential therapeutic interventions. Microbiota research can generate a significant amount of data, and bioinformatics and statistical analysis skills need to be developed in this area in order to analyze and interpret these data correctly [118].

## *Opportunities in GutM research*

GutM's role can affect many areas, including digestive health, immune system, metabolism, and brain health. Microbiota research offers important opportunities for understanding and treating many diseases. It can help develop personalized approaches for diagnosing and treating diseases. It presents personalized medicine and nutritional approaches based on individuals' GutM. It helps in the development and understanding of the effectiveness of probiotic and prebiotic products [119 - 123].

Modulation of GutM offers a promising way to improve health and prevent various diseases. As research in this area progresses, we will be able to see personalized approaches to gut health based on an individual's unique microbiota composition and health status.

## CONCLUSION

As a result, GutM plays a crucial role in the development and progression of MetS. Changes in GutM composition and function as a result of decreased diversity and abundance of beneficial bacteria and increased harmful bacteria have been associated with the development of MetS. GutM research in the context of the MetS is a rapidly developing field with important implications for human health. GutM plays a crucial role in modulating various metabolic processes and has the potential to be used for preventive and therapeutic applications. Future sequencing and culture-based GutM studies, metagenomic and metabolomic investigations, and high-throughput human multi-omic co-analysis will exponentially increase our knowledge of interactions within the gut microbial community. While there are still challenges to overcome in understanding the complexity of GutM and ensuring reproducibility in research, personalized interventions in the prevention or treatment of MetS, new therapies such as FMT, bacteriophages, and dietary approaches that can improve metabolic health and combat MetS look promising. The effects of drugs on GutM biomass and functions are important to health. However, there is limited understanding of the effects of pharmaceuticals on the absolute abundance and function of the GutM. Little is still known about host and microbe interactions. Much remains to be done regarding the role of GutM in MetS and other cardiometabolic conditions. More research and interdisciplinary collaboration are needed to better understand the complex relationship between GutM and MetS and to develop targeted, effective microbiome-based methods.

# REFERENCES

[1]     Thomas MS, Blesso CN, Calle MC, Chun OK, Puglisi M, Fernandez ML. Dietary influences on gut microbiota with a focus on metabolic syndrome. Metab Syndr Relat Disord 2022; 20(8): 429-39.
[http://dx.doi.org/10.1089/met.2021.0131] [PMID: 35704900]

[2]     Stephens RW, Arhire L, Covasa M. Gut microbiota: from microorganisms to metabolic organ influencing obesity. Obesity (Silver Spring) 2018; 26(5): 801-9.
[http://dx.doi.org/10.1002/oby.22179] [PMID: 29687647]

[3]     Tilg H, Moschen AR. Microbiota and diabetes: an evolving relationship. Gut 2014; 63(9): 1513-21.
[http://dx.doi.org/10.1136/gutjnl-2014-306928] [PMID: 24833634]

[4]     Tremaroli V, Bäckhed F. Functional interactions between the gut microbiota and host metabolism. Nature 2012; 489(7415): 242-9.
[http://dx.doi.org/10.1038/nature11552] [PMID: 22972297]

[5]     Lynch SV, Pedersen O. The human intestinal microbiome in health and disease. N Engl J Med 2016; 375(24): 2369-79.
[http://dx.doi.org/10.1056/NEJMra1600266] [PMID: 27974040]

[6]     Wang Z, Klipfell E, Bennett BJ, *et al.* Gut flora metabolism of phosphatidylcholine promotes cardiovascular disease. Nature 2011; 472(7341): 57-63.
[http://dx.doi.org/10.1038/nature09922] [PMID: 21475195]

[7]     Qin J, Li Y, Cai Z, *et al.* A metagenome-wide association study of gut microbiota in type 2 diabetes. Nature 2012; 490(7418): 55-60.
[http://dx.doi.org/10.1038/nature11450] [PMID: 23023125]

[8]     Cani PD, Neyrinck AM, Fava F, *et al.* Selective increases of bifidobacteria in gut microflora improve high-fat-diet-induced diabetes in mice through a mechanism associated with endotoxaemia. Diabetologia 2007; 50(11): 2374-83.
[http://dx.doi.org/10.1007/s00125-007-0791-0] [PMID: 17823788]

[9]     Serino M, Fernandez-Real JM. The gut microbiota drives the impact of bile acids and fat in metabolism. Gut 2018; 67(4): 763-72.

[10]    Wang PX, Deng XR, Zhang CH, Yuan HJ. Gut microbiota and metabolic syndrome. Chin Med J (Engl) 2020; 133(7): 808-16.
[http://dx.doi.org/10.1097/CM9.0000000000000696] [PMID: 32106124]

[11]    Astudillo-García C, Bell JJ, Webster NS, *et al.* Evaluating the core microbiota in complex communities: A systematic investigation. Environ Microbiol 2017; 19(4): 1450-62.
[http://dx.doi.org/10.1111/1462-2920.13647] [PMID: 28078754]

[12]    David LA, Maurice CF, Carmody RN, *et al.* Diet rapidly and reproducibly alters the human gut microbiome. Nature 2014; 505(7484): 559-63.
[http://dx.doi.org/10.1038/nature12820] [PMID: 24336217]

[13]    Wu GD, Chen J, Hoffmann C, *et al.* Linking long-term dietary patterns with gut microbial enterotypes. Science 2011; 334(6052): 105-8.
[http://dx.doi.org/10.1126/science.1208344] [PMID: 21885731]

[14]    Goodrich JK, Waters JL, Poole AC, *et al.* Human genetics shape the gut microbiome. Cell 2014; 159(4): 789-99.
[http://dx.doi.org/10.1016/j.cell.2014.09.053] [PMID: 25417156]

[15]    Turpin W, Espin-Garcia O, Xu W, *et al.* Association of host genome with intestinal microbial composition in a large healthy cohort. Nat Genet 2016; 48(11): 1413-7.
[http://dx.doi.org/10.1038/ng.3693] [PMID: 27694960]

[16]    Ottman N, Smidt H, de Vos WM, Belzer C. The function of our microbiota: who is out there and what do they do? Front Cell Infect Microbiol 2012; 2: 104.

[http://dx.doi.org/10.3389/fcimb.2012.00104] [PMID: 22919693]

[17]    Yatsunenko T, Rey FE, Manary MJ, *et al.* Human gut microbiome viewed across age and geography. Nature 2012; 486(7402): 222-7.
[http://dx.doi.org/10.1038/nature11053] [PMID: 22699611]

[18]    Odamaki T, Kato K, Sugahara H, *et al.* Age-related changes in gut microbiota composition from newborn to centenarian: a cross-sectional study. BMC Microbiol 2016; 16(1): 90.
[http://dx.doi.org/10.1186/s12866-016-0708-5] [PMID: 27220822]

[19]    Francino MP. Antibiotics and the human gut microbiome: dysbioses and accumulation of resistances. Front Microbiol 2016; 6: 1543.
[http://dx.doi.org/10.3389/fmicb.2015.01543] [PMID: 26793178]

[20]    Le Bastard Q, Al-Ghalith GA, Grégoire M, *et al.* Systematic review: human gut dysbiosis induced by non□antibiotic prescription medications. Aliment Pharmacol Ther 2018; 47(3): 332-45.
[http://dx.doi.org/10.1111/apt.14451] [PMID: 29205415]

[21]    Yurkovetskiy L, Burrows M, Khan AA, *et al.* Gender bias in autoimmunity is influenced by microbiota. Immunity 2013; 39(2): 400-12.
[http://dx.doi.org/10.1016/j.immuni.2013.08.013] [PMID: 23973225]

[22]    Org E, Mehrabian M, Parks BW, *et al.* Sex differences and hormonal effects on gut microbiota composition in mice. Gut Microbes 2016; 7(4): 313-22.
[http://dx.doi.org/10.1080/19490976.2016.1203502] [PMID: 27355107]

[23]    Haro C, Rangel-Zúñiga OA, Alcalá-Díaz JF, *et al.* Intestinal microbiota is influenced by gender and body mass index. PLoS One 2016; 11(5): e0154090.
[http://dx.doi.org/10.1371/journal.pone.0154090] [PMID: 27228093]

[24]    Bolnick DI, Snowberg LK, Hirsch PE, *et al.* Individual diet has sex-dependent effects on vertebrate gut microbiota. Nat Commun 2014; 5(1): 4500.
[http://dx.doi.org/10.1038/ncomms5500] [PMID: 25072318]

[25]    De Filippo C, Cavalieri D, Di Paola M, *et al.* Impact of diet in shaping gut microbiota revealed by a comparative study in children from Europe and rural Africa. Proc Natl Acad Sci USA 2010; 107(33): 14691-6.
[http://dx.doi.org/10.1073/pnas.1005963107] [PMID: 20679230]

[26]    Obregon-Tito AJ, Tito RY, Metcalf J, *et al.* Subsistence strategies in traditional societies distinguish gut microbiomes. Nat Commun 2015; 6(1): 6505.
[http://dx.doi.org/10.1038/ncomms7505] [PMID: 25807110]

[27]    Bailey MT, Dowd SE, Galley JD, Hufnagle AR, Allen RG, Lyte M. Exposure to a social stressor alters the structure of the intestinal microbiota: Implications for stressor-induced immunomodulation. Brain Behav Immun 2011; 25(3): 397-407.
[http://dx.doi.org/10.1016/j.bbi.2010.10.023] [PMID: 21040780]

[28]    Allen JM, Mailing LJ, Niemiro GM, *et al.* Exercise alters gut microbiota composition and function in lean and obese humans. Med Sci Sports Exerc 2018; 50(4): 747-57.
[http://dx.doi.org/10.1249/MSS.0000000000001495] [PMID: 29166320]

[29]    Geerlings SY, Kostopoulos I, De Vos WM, Belzer C. Akkermansia muciniphila in the human gastrointestinal tract: When, where, and how? Microorganisms 2018; 6(3): 75.
[http://dx.doi.org/10.3390/microorganisms6030075] [PMID: 30041463]

[30]    Weir TL. Grand challenges: Actualizing the potential of the gut microbiome to address global nutrition challenges. Front Microbiomes 2023; 2: 1146827.
[http://dx.doi.org/10.3389/frmbi.2023.1146827]

[31]    Dabke K, Hendrick G, Devkota S. The gut microbiome and metabolic syndrome. J Clin Invest 2019; 129(10): 4050-7.
[http://dx.doi.org/10.1172/JCI129194] [PMID: 31573550]

[32]    Ley RE, Turnbaugh PJ, Klein S, Gordon JI. Human gut microbes associated with obesity. Nature 2006; 444(7122): 1022-3.
[http://dx.doi.org/10.1038/4441022a] [PMID: 17183309]

[33]    Cani P, Delzenne N. The role of the gut microbiota in energy metabolism and metabolic disease. Curr Pharm Des 2009; 15(13): 1546-58.
[http://dx.doi.org/10.2174/138161209788168164] [PMID: 19442172]

[34]    Zhao Q, Wu J, Ding Y, *et al.* Gut microbiota, immunity, and bile acid metabolism: decoding metabolic disease interactions. Life Metabolism 2023.
[http://dx.doi.org/10.1093/lifemeta/load032]

[35]    Vatanen T, Plichta DR, Somani J, *et al.* Genomic variation and strain-specific functional adaptation in the human gut microbiome during early life. Nat Microbiol 2018; 4(3): 470-9.
[http://dx.doi.org/10.1038/s41564-018-0321-5] [PMID: 30559407]

[36]    Lloyd-Price J, Mahurkar A, Rahnavard G, *et al.* Strains, functions and dynamics in the expanded Human Microbiome Project. Nature 2017; 550(7674): 61-6.
[http://dx.doi.org/10.1038/nature23889] [PMID: 28953883]

[37]    Woese CR, Fox GE. Phylogenetic structure of the prokaryotic domain: The primary kingdoms. Proc Natl Acad Sci USA 1977; 74(11): 5088-90.
[http://dx.doi.org/10.1073/pnas.74.11.5088] [PMID: 270744]

[38]    Lane DJ, Pace B, Olsen GJ, Stahl DA, Sogin ML, Pace NR. Rapid determination of 16S ribosomal RNA sequences for phylogenetic analyses. Proc Natl Acad Sci USA 1985; 82(20): 6955-9.
[http://dx.doi.org/10.1073/pnas.82.20.6955] [PMID: 2413450]

[39]    Lederberg J, McCray AT. 'Ome sweet 'omics a genealogical treasury of words. Scientist 2001; 15(7): 8.

[40]    Vijay-Kumar M, Aitken JD, Carvalho FA, *et al.* Metabolic syndrome and altered gut microbiota in mice lacking Toll-like receptor 5. Science 2010; 328(5975): 228-31.
[http://dx.doi.org/10.1126/science.1179721] [PMID: 20203013]

[41]    Mutalub YB, Abdulwahab M, Mohammed A, *et al.* Gut microbiota modulation as a novel therapeutic strategy in cardiometabolic diseases. Foods 2022; 11(17): 2575.
[http://dx.doi.org/10.3390/foods11172575] [PMID: 36076760]

[42]    Gabriel CL, Ferguson JF. Gut microbiota and microbial metabolism in early risk of cardiometabolic disease. Circ Res 2023; 132(12): 1674-91.
[http://dx.doi.org/10.1161/CIRCRESAHA.123.322055] [PMID: 37289901]

[43]    Cani PD, Amar J, Iglesias MA, *et al.* Metabolic endotoxemia initiates obesity and insulin resistance. Diabetes 2007; 56(7): 1761-72.
[http://dx.doi.org/10.2337/db06-1491] [PMID: 17456850]

[44]    Delzenne NM, Cani PD, Everard A, Neyrinck AM, Bindels LB. Gut microorganisms as promising targets for the management of type 2 diabetes. Diabetologia 2015; 58(10): 2206-17.
[http://dx.doi.org/10.1007/s00125-015-3712-7] [PMID: 26224102]

[45]    Saad MJA, Santos A, Prada PO. Linking gut microbiota and inflammation to obesity and insulin resistance. Physiology (Bethesda) 2016; 31(4): 283-93.
[http://dx.doi.org/10.1152/physiol.00041.2015] [PMID: 27252163]

[46]    Fasano A. Zonulin, regulation of tight junctions, and autoimmune diseases. Ann N Y Acad Sci 2012; 1258(1): 25-33.
[http://dx.doi.org/10.1111/j.1749-6632.2012.06538.x] [PMID: 22731712]

[47]    Cani PD, Knauf C. How gut microbes talk to organs: The role of endocrine and nervous routes. Mol Metab 2016; 5(9): 743-52.
[http://dx.doi.org/10.1016/j.molmet.2016.05.011] [PMID: 27617197]

[48]　Vezza T, Abad-Jiménez Z, Marti-Cabrera M, Rocha M, Víctor VM. Microbiota-Mitochondria inter-talk: A potential therapeutic strategy in obesity and type 2 diabetes. Antioxidants 2020; 9(9): 848.
[http://dx.doi.org/10.3390/antiox9090848] [PMID: 32927712]

[49]　Sayin SI, Wahlström A, Felin J, *et al.* Gut microbiota regulates bile acid metabolism by reducing the levels of tauro-beta-muricholic acid, a naturally occurring FXR antagonist. Cell Metab 2013; 17(2): 225-35.
[http://dx.doi.org/10.1016/j.cmet.2013.01.003] [PMID: 23395169]

[50]　den Besten G, van Eunen K, Groen AK, Venema K, Reijngoud DJ, Bakker BM. The role of short-chain fatty acids in the interplay between diet, gut microbiota, and host energy metabolism. J Lipid Res 2013; 54(9): 2325-40.
[http://dx.doi.org/10.1194/jlr.R036012] [PMID: 23821742]

[51]　Wang Z, Roberts AB, Buffa JA, *et al.* Non-lethal inhibition of gut microbial trimethylamine production for the treatment of atherosclerosis. Cell 2015; 163(7): 1585-95.
[http://dx.doi.org/10.1016/j.cell.2015.11.055] [PMID: 26687352]

[52]　Karlsson FH, Tremaroli V, Nookaew I, *et al.* Gut metagenome in European women with normal, impaired and diabetic glucose control. Nature 2013; 498(7452): 99-103.
[http://dx.doi.org/10.1038/nature12198] [PMID: 23719380]

[53]　Zhang X, Shen D, Fang Z, *et al.* Human gut microbiota changes reveal the progression of glucose intolerance. PLoS One 2013; 8(8): e71108.
[http://dx.doi.org/10.1371/journal.pone.0071108] [PMID: 24013136]

[54]　Turnbaugh PJ, Ley RE, Mahowald MA, Magrini V, Mardis ER, Gordon JI. An obesity-associated gut microbiome with increased capacity for energy harvest. Nature 2006; 444(7122): 1027-31.
[http://dx.doi.org/10.1038/nature05414] [PMID: 17183312]

[55]　Cani PD, Delzenne NM. The gut microbiome as therapeutic target. Pharmacol Ther 2011; 130(2): 202-12.
[http://dx.doi.org/10.1016/j.pharmthera.2011.01.012] [PMID: 21295072]

[56]　Bäckhed F, Manchester JK, Semenkovich CF, Gordon JI. Mechanisms underlying the resistance to diet-induced obesity in germ-free mice. Proc Natl Acad Sci USA 2007; 104(3): 979-84.
[http://dx.doi.org/10.1073/pnas.0605374104] [PMID: 17210919]

[57]　Cryan JF, Dinan TG. Mind-altering microorganisms: the impact of the gut microbiota on brain and behaviour. Nat Rev Neurosci 2012; 13(10): 701-12.
[http://dx.doi.org/10.1038/nrn3346] [PMID: 22968153]

[58]　Nadal I, Santacruz A, Marcos A, *et al.* Shifts in clostridia, bacteroides and immunoglobulin-coating fecal bacteria associated with weight loss in obese adolescents. Int J Obes 2009; 33(7): 758-67.
[http://dx.doi.org/10.1038/ijo.2008.260] [PMID: 19050675]

[59]　Canfora EE, Blaak EE. The role of polyunsaturated fatty acids (n-3 PUFAs) on body weight and insulin sensitivity. Curr Diab Rep 2017; 17(11): 1-9.

[60]　de Kort S, Keszthelyi D, Masclee AAM. Leaky gut and diabetes mellitus: what is the link? Obes Rev 2011; 12(6): 449-58.
[http://dx.doi.org/10.1111/j.1467-789X.2010.00845.x] [PMID: 21382153]

[61]　Tang WHW, Hazen SL. The contributory role of gut microbiota in cardiovascular disease. J Clin Invest 2014; 124(10): 4204-11.
[http://dx.doi.org/10.1172/JCI72331] [PMID: 25271725]

[62]　Muccioli GG, Naslain D, Bäckhed F, *et al.* The endocannabinoid system links gut microbiota to adipogenesis. Mol Syst Biol 2010; 6(1): 392.
[http://dx.doi.org/10.1038/msb.2010.46] [PMID: 20664638]

[63]　Portincasa P, Bonfrate L, Vacca M, *et al.* Gut microbiota and short chain fatty acids: Implications in

glucose homeostasis. Int J Mol Sci 2022; 23(3): 1105.
[http://dx.doi.org/10.3390/ijms23031105] [PMID: 35163038]

[64] Mazhar M, Zhu Y, Qin L. The interplay of dietary fibers and intestinal microbiota affects type 2 diabetes by generating short-chain fatty acids. Foods 2023; 12(5): 1023.
[http://dx.doi.org/10.3390/foods12051023] [PMID: 36900540]

[65] Yang T, Santisteban MM, Rodriguez V, *et al.* Gut dysbiosis is linked to hypertension. Hypertension 2015; 65(6): 1331-40.
[http://dx.doi.org/10.1161/HYPERTENSIONAHA.115.05315] [PMID: 25870193]

[66] Tang WHW, Kitai T, Hazen SL. Gut microbiota in cardiovascular health and disease. Circ Res 2017; 120(7): 1183-96.
[http://dx.doi.org/10.1161/CIRCRESAHA.117.309715] [PMID: 28360349]

[67] Adnan S, Nelson JW, Ajami NJ, *et al.* Alterations in the gut microbiota can elicit hypertension in rats. Physiol Genomics 2017; 49(2): 96-104.
[http://dx.doi.org/10.1152/physiolgenomics.00081.2016] [PMID: 28011881]

[68] Yang Y, Cai Q. The role of the gut microbiota in the pathogenesis of metabolic disorders. J Clin Invest 2019; 129(10): 4050-7.
[PMID: 31573550]

[69] Doulberis M, Papaefthymiou A, Katsinelos P. Gut microbiota profile and metabolic syndrome in patients with hypertension: A cross-sectional study. High Blood Press Cardiovasc Prev 2020; 27(3): 261-70.

[70] Li J, Zhao F, Wang Y, *et al.* Gut microbiota dysbiosis contributes to the development of hypertension. Microbiome 2017; 5(1): 14.
[http://dx.doi.org/10.1186/s40168-016-0222-x] [PMID: 28143587]

[71] Wilck N, Matus MG, Kearney SM, *et al.* Salt-responsive gut commensal modulates $T_H17$ axis and disease. Nature 2017; 551(7682): 585-9.
[http://dx.doi.org/10.1038/nature24628] [PMID: 29143823]

[72] Durgan DJ, Ganesh BP, Cope JL, *et al.* Role of the gut microbiome in obstructive sleep apnea-induced hypertension. Hypertension 2020; 75(1): 139-47.
[PMID: 31735084]

[73] Santisteban MM, Qi Y, Zubcevic J, *et al.* Hypertension-linked pathophysiological alterations in the gut. Circ Res 2017; 120(2): 312-23.
[http://dx.doi.org/10.1161/CIRCRESAHA.116.309006] [PMID: 27799253]

[74] Mell B, Jala VR, Mathew AV, *et al.* Evidence for a link between gut microbiota and hypertension in the Dahl rat. Physiol Genomics 2015; 47(6): 187-97.
[http://dx.doi.org/10.1152/physiolgenomics.00136.2014] [PMID: 25829393]

[75] Karbach SH, Croxford AL, Oelze M, *et al.* Interleukin 17 drives vascular inflammation, endothelial dysfunction, and arterial hypertension in psoriasis-like skin disease. Eur Heart J 2016; 38(11): 816-27.

[76] Jiao N, Baker SS, Chapa-Rodriguez A, *et al.* Suppressed hepatic bile acid signalling despite elevated production of primary and secondary bile acids in NAFLD. Gut 2018; 67(10): 1881-91.
[http://dx.doi.org/10.1136/gutjnl-2017-314307] [PMID: 28774887]

[77] Li J, Lin S, Vanhoutte PM, Woo CW, Xu A. Akkermansia muciniphila protects against atherosclerosis by preventing metabolic endotoxemia-induced inflammation in Apoe-/- mice. Circulation 2016; 133(24): 2434-46.
[http://dx.doi.org/10.1161/CIRCULATIONAHA.115.019645] [PMID: 27143680]

[78] Velagapudi VR, Hezaveh R, Reigstad CS, *et al.* The gut microbiota modulates host energy and lipid metabolism in mice. J Lipid Res 2010; 51(5): 1101-12.
[http://dx.doi.org/10.1194/jlr.M002774] [PMID: 20040631]

[79]     Ridaura VK, Faith JJ, Rey FE, *et al.* Gut microbiota from twins discordant for obesity modulate metabolism in mice. Science 2013; 341(6150): 1241214.
[http://dx.doi.org/10.1126/science.1241214] [PMID: 24009397]

[80]     Caesar R, Tremaroli V, Kovatcheva-Datchary P, Cani PD, Bäckhed F. Crosstalk between gut microbiota and dietary lipids aggravates WAT inflammation through TLR signaling. Cell Metab 2015; 22(4): 658-68.
[http://dx.doi.org/10.1016/j.cmet.2015.07.026] [PMID: 26321659]

[81]     Zhang Y, Zhou L, Bao YL, *et al.* The regulatory effect of butyrate on lipid metabolism and lipid formation in grass carp ctenopharyngodon idellus. Int J Mol Sci 2018; 19(5): 1482.
[PMID: 29772699]

[82]     Hassan NE, El-Masry SA, Nageeb A, *et al.* Linking gut microbiota, metabolic syndrome and metabolic health among a sample of obese egyptian females. Macedonian Journal of Medical Sciences 2021; 9(A): 1123-31.
[http://dx.doi.org/10.3889/oamjms.2021.7625]

[83]     Zhong X, Zhang Z, Wang S, *et al.* Gut microbiota-mediated anti-obesity effect of the polysaccharides from Mori Fructus in high-fat diet mice. Int J Biol Macromol 2020; 154: 511-20.

[84]     Marklund M, Wu JHY, Imamura F, *et al.* Biomarkers of dietary omega-6 fatty acids and incident cardiovascular disease and mortality: An individual-level pooled analysis of 30 cohort studies. Circulation 2015; 132(10): 927-39.
[PMID: 25679302]

[85]     Carmody RN, Gerber GK, Luevano JM Jr, *et al.* Diet dominates host genotype in shaping the murine gut microbiota. Cell Host Microbe 2015; 17(1): 72-84.
[http://dx.doi.org/10.1016/j.chom.2014.11.010] [PMID: 25532804]

[86]     Cani PD, Van Hul M. Gut microbiota and obesity: benefits of probiotics and prebiotics. Endocr Rev 2015; 36(4): 309-25.

[87]     Menni C, Jackson MA, Pallister T, Steves CJ, Spector TD, Valdes AM. Gut microbiome diversity and high-fibre intake are related to lower long-term weight gain. Int J Obes 2017; 41(7): 1099-105.
[http://dx.doi.org/10.1038/ijo.2017.66] [PMID: 28286339]

[88]     Cox LM, Blaser MJ. Antibiotics in early life and obesity. Nat Rev Endocrinol 2015; 11(3): 182-90.
[http://dx.doi.org/10.1038/nrendo.2014.210] [PMID: 25488483]

[89]     Le Roy CI. The role of the gut microbiota in mediating metabolic health effects of the impact of low-dose antibiotics. Nat Commun 2019; 10(1): 1-12.
[PMID: 30602773]

[90]     Pedersen HK, Gudmundsdottir V, Nielsen HB, *et al.* Human gut microbes impact host serum metabolome and insulin sensitivity. Nature 2016; 535(7612): 376-81.
[http://dx.doi.org/10.1038/nature18646] [PMID: 27409811]

[91]     Wu H, Esteve E, Tremaroli V, *et al.* Metformin alters the gut microbiome of individuals with treatment-naive type 2 diabetes, contributing to the therapeutic effects of the drug. Nat Med 2017; 23(7): 850-8.
[http://dx.doi.org/10.1038/nm.4345] [PMID: 28530702]

[92]     Sanchez M, Darimont C, Drapeau V, *et al.* Effect of *Lactobacillus rhamnosus* CGMCC1.3724 supplementation on weight loss and maintenance in obese men and women. Br J Nutr 2014; 111(8): 1507-19.
[http://dx.doi.org/10.1017/S0007114513003875] [PMID: 24299712]

[93]     Sáez-Lara M, Robles-Sanchez C, Ruiz-Ojeda F, Plaza-Diaz J, Gil A. Effects of probiotics and synbiotics on obesity, insulin resistance syndrome, type 2 diabetes and non-alcoholic fatty liver disease: A review of human clinical trials. Int J Mol Sci 2016; 17(6): 928.
[http://dx.doi.org/10.3390/ijms17060928] [PMID: 27304953]

[94] Wang J, Tang H, Zhang C, *et al.* Modulation of gut microbiota during probiotic-mediated attenuation of metabolic syndrome in high fat diet-fed mice. ISME J 2015; 9(1): 1-15.
[http://dx.doi.org/10.1038/ismej.2014.99] [PMID: 24936764]

[95] Javadi L, Ghavami A, Khoshbaten M, *et al.* The role of probiotics in managing metabolic syndrome: a review on their angiotensin converting enzyme inhibiting properties. Adv Pharm Bull 2019; 9(4): 484-96.

[96] Dinan TG, Stanton C, Cryan JF. Psychobiotics: a novel class of psychotropic. Biol Psychiatry 2013; 74(10): 720-6.
[http://dx.doi.org/10.1016/j.biopsych.2013.05.001] [PMID: 23759244]

[97] Lu J, Zhu X, Zhang C, Lu F, Lu Z, Lu Y. Co-expression of alcohol dehydrogenase and aldehyde dehydrogenase in Bacillus subtilis for alcohol detoxification. Food Chem Toxicol 2020; 135: 110890.
[http://dx.doi.org/10.1016/j.fct.2019.110890] [PMID: 31628963]

[98] Cunningham M, Azcarate-Peril MA, Barnard A, *et al.* Shaping the future of probiotics and prebiotics. Trends Microbiol 2021; 29(8): 667-85.
[http://dx.doi.org/10.1016/j.tim.2021.01.003] [PMID: 33551269]

[99] Su GL, Ko CW, Bercik P, *et al.* AGA clinical practice guidelines on the role of probiotics in the management of gastrointestinal disorders. Gastroenterology 2020; 159(2): 697-705.
[http://dx.doi.org/10.1053/j.gastro.2020.05.059] [PMID: 32531291]

[100] Scheeler A. Where stool is a drug: International approaches to regulating the use of fecal microbiota for transplantation. J Law Med Ethics 2019; 47(4): 524-40.
[http://dx.doi.org/10.1177/1073110519897729] [PMID: 31957572]

[101] Berry SE, Valdes AM, Drew DA, *et al.* Human postprandial responses to food and potential for precision nutrition. Nat Med 2020; 26(6): 964-73.
[http://dx.doi.org/10.1038/s41591-020-0934-0] [PMID: 32528151]

[102] Li L, Ning Z, Zhang X, *et al.* RapidAIM: a culture- and metaproteomics-based Rapid Assay of Individual Microbiome responses to drugs. Microbiome 2020; 8(1): 33.
[http://dx.doi.org/10.1186/s40168-020-00806-z] [PMID: 32160905]

[103] Mirzayi C, Renson A, Furlanello C, *et al.* Reporting guidelines for human microbiome research: the STORMS checklist. Nat Med 2021; 27(11): 1885-92.
[http://dx.doi.org/10.1038/s41591-021-01552-x] [PMID: 34789871]

[104] Sharpton SR, Schnabl B, Knight R, Loomba R. Current concepts, opportunities, and challenges of gut microbiome-based personalized medicine in nonalcoholic fatty liver disease. Cell Metab 2021; 33(1): 21-32.
[http://dx.doi.org/10.1016/j.cmet.2020.11.010] [PMID: 33296678]

[105] Cao C, Shi M, Wang X, Yao Y, Zeng R. Effects of probiotics on non-alcoholic fatty liver disease: a review of human clinical trials. Front Nutr 2023; 10: 1155306.
[http://dx.doi.org/10.3389/fnut.2023.1155306] [PMID: 37457967]

[106] Maestri M, Santopaolo F, Pompili M, Gasbarrini A, Ponziani FR. Gut microbiota modulation in patients with non-alcoholic fatty liver disease: Effects of current treatments and future strategies. Front Nutr 2023; 10: 1110536.
[http://dx.doi.org/10.3389/fnut.2023.1110536] [PMID: 36875849]

[107] Gan L, Feng Y, Du B, *et al.* Bacteriophage targeting microbiota alleviates non-alcoholic fatty liver disease induced by high alcohol-producing Klebsiella pneumoniae. Nat Commun 2023; 14(1): 3215.
[http://dx.doi.org/10.1038/s41467-023-39028-w] [PMID: 37270557]

[108] Cao Y, Zhang B, Wu Y, Wang Q, Wang J, Shen F. The Value of Fecal Microbiota Transplantation in the Treatment of Ulcerative Colitis Patients: A Systematic Review and Meta-Analysis. Gastroenterol Res Pract 2018; 2018: 1-12.
[http://dx.doi.org/10.1155/2018/5480961] [PMID: 29849592]

[109] Vrieze A, Van Nood E, Holleman F, *et al*. Transfer of intestinal microbiota from lean donors increases insulin sensitivity in individuals with metabolic syndrome. Gastroenterology 2012; 143(4): 913-916.e7.
[http://dx.doi.org/10.1053/j.gastro.2012.06.031] [PMID: 22728514]

[110] Haro C, García-Carpintero S, Rangel-Zúñiga OA, *et al*. Consumption of two healthy dietary patterns restored microbiota dysbiosis in obese patients with metabolic dysfunction. Mol Nutr Food Res 2017; 61(12): 1700300.
[http://dx.doi.org/10.1002/mnfr.201700300] [PMID: 28940737]

[111] Clemente JC, Ursell LK, Parfrey LW, Knight R. The impact of the gut microbiota on human health: an integrative view. Cell 2012; 148(6): 1258-70.
[http://dx.doi.org/10.1016/j.cell.2012.01.035] [PMID: 22424233]

[112] Belkaid Y, Hand TW. Role of the microbiota in immunity and inflammation. Cell 2014; 157(1): 121-41.
[http://dx.doi.org/10.1016/j.cell.2014.03.011] [PMID: 24679531]

[113] O'Mahony SM, Clarke G, Borre YE, Dinan TG, Cryan JF. Serotonin, tryptophan metabolism and the brain-gut-microbiome axis. Behav Brain Res 2015; 277: 32-48.
[http://dx.doi.org/10.1016/j.bbr.2014.07.027] [PMID: 25078296]

[114] Sonnenburg JL, Bäckhed F. Diet–microbiota interactions as moderators of human metabolism. Nature 2016; 535(7610): 56-64.
[http://dx.doi.org/10.1038/nature18846] [PMID: 27383980]

[115] Wu HJ, Wu E. The role of gut microbiota in immune homeostasis and autoimmunity. Gut Microbes 2012; 3(1): 4-14.
[http://dx.doi.org/10.4161/gmic.19320] [PMID: 22356853]

[116] Fan Y, Pedersen O. Gut microbiota in human metabolic health and disease. Nat Rev Microbiol 2021; 19(1): 55-71.
[http://dx.doi.org/10.1038/s41579-020-0433-9] [PMID: 32887946]

[117] Carrizales-Sánchez AK, García-Cayuela T, Hernández-Brenes C, Senés-Guerrero C. Gut microbiota associations with metabolic syndrome and relevance of its study in pediatric subjects. Gut Microbes 2021; 13(1): 1960135.
[http://dx.doi.org/10.1080/19490976.2021.1960135] [PMID: 34491882]

[118] Olofsson LE, Bäckhed F. The metabolic role and therapeutic potential of the microbiome. Endocr Rev 2022; 43(5): 907-26.
[http://dx.doi.org/10.1210/endrev/bnac004] [PMID: 35094076]

[119] Wolfe W, Xiang Z, Yu X, *et al*. The challenge of applications of probiotics in gastrointestinal diseases. Hindawi Advanced Gut 2023; Article ID 1984200. 2023.
[http://dx.doi.org/10.1155/2023/1984200]

[120] Lloyd-Price J, Abu-Ali G, Huttenhower C. The healthy human microbiome. Genome Med 2016; 8(1): 51.
[http://dx.doi.org/10.1186/s13073-016-0307-y] [PMID: 27122046]

[121] Guinane CM, Cotter PD. Role of the gut microbiota in health and chronic gastrointestinal disease: understanding a hidden metabolic organ. Therap Adv Gastroenterol 2013; 6(4): 295-308.
[http://dx.doi.org/10.1177/1756283X13482996] [PMID: 23814609]

[122] Daliri EBM, Ofosu FK, Chelliah R, Lee BH, Oh DH. Challenges and perspective in integrated multi-omics in gut microbiota studies. Biomolecules 2021; 11(2): 300.
[http://dx.doi.org/10.3390/biom11020300] [PMID: 33671370]

[123] Alveirinho M, Freitas P, Faleiro ML. Role of gut microbiota in metabolic syndrome: a review of recent evidence. Porto Biomed J 2020; 5(6): e105.
[http://dx.doi.org/10.1097/j.pbj.0000000000000105] [PMID: 33299954]

# CHAPTER 18

# The Role of Bariatric and Metabolic Surgery in the Management of Metabolic Syndrome

**Halit Eren Taşkın**[1,*] and **Hafize Uzun**[2]

[1] *Department of General Surgery, Istanbul University-Cerrahpasa Cerrahpasa Medical Faculty, 34098, Istanbul, Fatih, Turkey*

[2] *Department of Medical Biochemistry, Faculty of Medicine, Istanbul Atlas University, Istanbul, Turkey*

**Abstract:** Metabolic syndrome (MetS) is characterized by central obesity, glucose intolerance, dyslipidemia, and hypertension. This is attributed to an increased inflammatory state resulting from increased cytokine synthesis from adipose tissue. Almost all of the medical problems associated with metabolic syndrome can be more successfully remised in the long term by bariatric-metabolic surgery (BMS) compared to conservative methods. In past years, the benefits of BMS have been attributed to weight loss; however, currently, it has been well described that anti-inflammatory response and remission of T2DM and other comorbidities begin in the first weeks after procedures. Moreover, there is also sufficient evidence that BMS helps in the remission of integral components of MetS, such as hyperlipidemia, hypertension, and cardiovascular diseases, in the long term where many patients do not even require medical treatment. The International Diabetes Federation (IDF) and recent guidelines recommend that metabolic surgery may be considered if glycemic control is not achieved despite optimal treatment if the patient's body mass index (BMI) is 30kg/m2 and above.

**Keywords:** Body mass index, Bariatric surgery, Comorbidities, Metabolic syndrome, Type 2 diabetes mellitus, Weight loss.

## INTRODUCTION

### Metabolic Syndrome

Metabolic syndrome (MetS) is an endocrinopathy of unknown etiopathogenesis that leads to type 2 diabetes (T2DM) and cardiovascular disease. Visceral adiposity, lipid profile disorder, endothelial dysfunction, arterial hypertension,

---

\* **Corresponding author Halit Eren Taşkın:** Department of General Surgery, Istanbul University-Cerrahpasa Cerrahpasa Medical Faculty, 34098, Istanbul, Fatih, Turkey; E-mail: eren_taskin@hotmail.com

**Hafize Uzun & Seyma Dumur (Eds.)**

chronic stress, insulin resistance (IR), and hypercoagulability are the parameters of MetS [1].

## Definition

Reaven [2] first described MetS in his 1988 Banting lecture as "Syndrome X". Reaven suggested that insulin resistance clustered together with glucose intolerance, dyslipidemia, and hypertension to increase the risk of CVD. In 1998, the World Health Organization (WHO) was the first organization to coin the term MetS, focusing primarily on insulin resistance and hyperglycemia [3]. In 2001, the National Cholesterol Education Program Adult Treatment Panel III (NCEP ATP III) expanded the definition of the syndrome to include abdominal adiposity, particularly increased waist circumference [4]. This was followed by several published definitions from different societies, often differing in the clinical assessment of abdominal adiposity. The term MetS still includes the previous terms "syndrome X", "insulin resistance syndrome", and "cardiometabolic syndrome", which encompass the same concept. In 2015, a group of experts representing more than 20 organizations articulated three key definitions supporting the concept. Accordingly, MetS is a chronic and progressive pathophysiological state. MetS represents a cluster of risk factors and refers to a complex syndrome defined by a unifying pathophysiology. Today, the term "metabolic syndrome" is widely accepted and considered to be the most useful term.

## Prevalence of Metabolic Syndrome

The prevalence of MetS is increasing with the aging of the population, physical inactivity, and an increase in the prevalence of central obesity. The prevalence of metabolic syndrome in the United States of America (USA) was 34.5% (33.7% in men and 35.4% in women), according to the NCEP ATPIII criteria. According to the International Diabetes Federation (IDF) MetS criteria, the prevalence of MetS in the USA was found to be 39% (39.9% in men and 38.1% in women) [5]. The prevalence was 34%, 33%, and 34.7% in 1999–2006 [6], 2003–12 [7], and 2011–16 [8], respectively. This may seem surprising against the background of an obesity and diabetes epidemic, which would be expected to increase the prevalence of MetS as they are components of the syndrome [9].

## Etiopathogenesis of Metabolic Syndrome

No single genetic, infectious, or environmental factor has yet been identified to explain the etiopathogenesis of all components of the MetS. However, the etiology of metabolic syndrome can be divided into three categories: obesity/adipose tissue disorders, insulin resistance, and independent factors (such as molecules of vascular, hepatic, and immunologic origin). Although polygenic predisposition is involved, a sedentary lifestyle and high-calorie diet brought about by modern urban life exacerbate the course of the syndrome. The prevalence of MetS is increasing worldwide. The rate of increase, although significant, varies between countries [10].

The pathophysiology of the MetS encompasses several complex mechanisms that are yet to be fully elucidated. It is still debated whether the different elements of MetS form distinct pathologies by themselves or fall under a common, broader pathogenic process [11].

**Diagnosis of Metabolic Syndrome**

Over time, different diagnostic criteria have been used for metabolic syndrome. While these diagnostic criteria initially included criteria that could measure insulin resistance, later on, simpler criteria were used. The most widely accepted of these diagnostic criteria are:

- (1998-99) World Health Organization (WHO).
- (2001) National Cholesterol Education Program - Adult Treatment Panel III (National Cholesterol Education Program - Adult Treatment Panel III) (NCEP ATPIII).
- (2004) Revision, modification of NCEP ATP -III definition.
- (2004-05) International Diabetes Federation (IDF) Consensus Statement.

In addition, medical associations and institutions in many countries have their own definitions.

WHO Diagnostic Criteria for Metabolic Syndrome [3].

At least one of the following:

- Insulin resistance.
- Impaired glucose tolerance.
- Obvious diabetes mellitus.

and

At least two of the following:

- Hypertension (blood pressure > 140/90 mmHg or taking antihypertensives).
- Dyslipidemia (triglyceride level > 150 mg/dl or HDL level < 35 mg/dl in men and < 39 mg/dl in women).

- Abdominal obesity (BMI > 30 kg/m2 or waist/hip ratio > 0.90 in men and > 0.85 in women).
- Microalbuminuria (urinary albumin excretion > 20 µg/min or albumin/creatinine ratio > 30 mg/g).

After the WHO's definition, "NCEP ATP-III criteria" were defined, which do not require complex measurements such as insulin and microalbuminuria measurements and can diagnose MetS with simpler tests and measurements.

National Cholesterol Education Program (NCEP) Adult Treatment Panel III (ATP III)-2001, Diagnostic Criteria for Metabolic Syndrome [12].

At least three of the following:

- Abdominal obesity (waist circumference: > 102 cm in men, > 88 cm in women).
- Hypertriglyceridemia (≥150 mg/dl).
- Low HDL (< 40 mg/dl in men, < 50 mg/dl in women).
- Hypertension (blood pressure ≥ 130/85 mmHg).
- Hyperglycemia (fasting blood glucose ≥ 110 mg/dl).

Efforts to reconcile the different clinical definitions gave rise to the harmonized criteria with contributions from the IDF, AHA/NHLBI, World Heart Federation, International Atherosclerosis Society, and the International Association for the Study of Obesity in 2009 [13].

Any three or more of the features below:

- Elevated waist circumference (WC) WC ≥ 90 cm in men, WC ≥ 80 cm in women.
- Elevated serum triglycerides (TG) ≥150 mg/dL (1.7 mmol/L) or on serum TG treatment.
- Reduced high-density lipoprotein cholesterol (HDL-C) Men: <40 mg/dL (1.0 mmol/L), Women: <50 mg/dL (1.3 mmol/L).
- Elevated blood pressure ≥130/85 mm Hg.
- Elevated fasting glucose ≥100 mg/dL (5.6 mmol/L).

## Components of Metabolic Syndrome

### *Insulin Resistance*

IR and obesity are mostly blamed for the emergence of MetS. IR is the absence or low biological response to endogenous or exogenous insulin. Genetic factors, fetal malnutrition, physical inactivity, obesity, and advancing age cause IR. Insulin mechanisms of action can be divided into 3 phases. These are insulin binding to the receptor, intracellular signal transduction, and hormone effector systems. Defects in any of these phases may lead to IR. IR is seen in 25% of the healthy population, 60% in those with impaired glucose tolerance, and 60-75% in those with T2DM. This resistance is tried to be met with hyperinsulinemia to maintain euglycemia [14, 15].

IR is usually associated with hyperinsulinemia but not always with hyperglycemia. Hyperglycemia is the advanced stage of IR. When IR develops, the pancreas tries to compensate by increasing insulin secretion so that blood glucose levels remain normal. However, in later stages, insulin secretion of the pancreas cannot meet the needs caused by IR, and diabetes may occur as a result. Vascular and metabolic changes resulting from IR increase the risk of coronary artery disease (CAD) [16].

*Diabetes Mellitus* T2DM is an endocrinopathy characterized by a decrease in the effectiveness of insulin, a defect in insulin secretion, or both. It is reported to be observed in 5-10% in most developed countries [17]. Although not all type 2 diabetics have IR, the presence of overt T2DM or impaired glucose tolerance fulfills the first step of the diagnostic criteria for MetS, and IR is not required [18, 19].

People with impaired fasting glucose and impaired glucose tolerance are at increased risk of developing overt DM and are described as "pre-diabetic". Postprandial hyperglycemia is recognized as an independent cardiovascular risk factor [15, 20, 21].

## Hypertension

IR often underlies essential hypertension. Hypertension is present in almost 80% of patients with MetS. Hypertension and IR are often found together in people with MetS. Insulin is actually a vasodilator. The hypertensive effect expected to stimulate renal water and salt retention with increased sympathetic activity seen in IR is balanced by the hypotensive effect due to peripheral vasodilation under normal physiologic conditions. In the presence of IR, it is thought to cause hypertension with an unbalanced vasopressor effect because resistance develops to its peripheral vasodilator effect. Controversy still exists regarding the optimal antihypertensive treatment for hypertension in MetS. Due to the high prevalence of hypertension in this population, more data from clinical trials are needed in the future [22, 23].

## Dyslipidemia

Dyslipidemia in MetS is characterized by high triglyceride values and is a common component in various diagnostic criteria made by international organizations (1). In addition, low levels of HDL cholesterol are another criterion associated with MetS. Low-density lipoprotein (LDL) levels, which have a potential atherogenic effect, are usually elevated. Similar to LDL cholesterol, Apolipoprotein B also has an atherogenic effect and increases the risk of cardiovascular disease. Apolipoprotein B measurement and monitoring are not yet widely used. Dyslipidemia and obesity present common diseases that must be managed to decrease the cardiovascular risk and the risk of obesity-related complications [24].

As a result of defects in lipoproteins, the amount of free fatty acids in circulation increases. IR is caused by abdominal obesity, and this increase in free fatty acids increases triglyceride synthesis in the liver. This dyslipidemia picture that emerges in MetS leads to cardiovascular disease predisposition and endothelial damage [25, 26].

## Obesity

Abdominal obesity is the most important indicator of IR. However, obesity may not be present in some cases of MetS with IR. Adipose tissue is an active endocrine organ secreting many hormones such as leptin, resistin, adiponectin, and cytokines (TNF-a, IL-6, IL-8). Every obese patient should be screened for MetS, and waist circumference should be used as an indicator of visceral adiposity instead of body mass index (BMI). Waist circumference should be measured at the midpoint of the distance between the arcus costarium and spina iliaca anterior superior [27, 28].

## Other Components

Microalbuminuria and acanthosis nigricans, which are included in the diagnostic criteria in individuals with MetS, are reflected in the clinic as a complication of diabetes [29, 30]. However, the inclusion of microalbuminuria as an essential component of the MetS remains controversial [30]. The prothrombotic status that jeopardizes cardiovascular health in individuals with MetS is another problem that should not be overlooked. Increased platelet reactivity, cytokine, and C-reactive protein triggered by IR decrease the antiplatelet response in patients. This leads to a prothrombotic and proinflammatory state. Therefore, it is inevitable that patients with MetS are in the high-risk group in terms of venous thrombosis [31].

## Treatment of Metabolic Syndrome

It is known that the most effective approach in the treatment of MetS is lifestyle modification. Targeted weight loss as a result of lifestyle modification alleviates obesity-related metabolic disorders. MetS treatment goals include controlling the risk factors that trigger insulin resistance and receiving support from surgical treatments when necessary in addition to drug treatment in order to achieve clinical goals [32 - 34].

Although no specific pharmacologic agent has been defined for MetS, there are some applications that address symptoms and support weight loss [35]. In the treatment of obesity, endocrinologists may frequently use Sibutramine, which has appetite-suppressant properties, and Orlistat, which inhibits fat absorption from the intestines. Lifestyle modification and the combined use of these agents have been reported to be effective in achieving 5-10% weight loss. Rimonabant, known as an inhibitor of the endocannabinoid system receptor, which has an important role in appetite and eating control, also has a beneficial effect on weight loss [36, 37]. However, it was never approved in the United States because of concerns over suicidal ideation and behaviors associated with its use [38].

In MetS, symptomatic pharmacologic agents targeting components of dyslipidemia and hypertension are also commonly used. In patients with atherogenic dyslipidemia, statins, and even statin-fibrate combinations have been confirmed to be beneficial for therapeutic purposes to lower triglycerides, LDL cholesterol, and Apolipoprotein B and to raise HDL cholesterol [39]. For the treatment of hypertension, it has been reported that high doses of diuretics and β-blockers specific to MetS may worsen insulin resistance and dyslipidemia, but their use at low doses would be cardioprotective. Most clinical studies report that the favorable effect of the use of antihypertensive agents on MetS is not dependent on a specific type of drug but is a result of blood pressure reduction alone [39, 40].

Metformin group drugs are the leading drugs that reduce IR, delay the onset or provide remission of T2DM, and reduce the risk of diabetes-related cardiovascular disease (CVD). Thiazolidines have also been reported to be effective in patients with impaired glucose and IR and in the treatment of T2DM. The effect of thiazolidine group agents on diabetes-related CVDs is not yet known. The presence of MetS in patients with T2DM increases the risk of developing CVD. When both are present, the best possible glycemic control should be achieved, in addition to appropriate treatment for dyslipidemia and hypertension. The choice of drug therapy to achieve the recommended MetS goals depends on clinical judgment, but lifestyle modification is necessary for all cases [41, 42].

Another potent method in the treatment of obesity is surgical interventions. Surgical interventions to restrict oral intake and reduce nutrient absorption have been clinically proven to be effective in achieving weight loss and maintaining the current weight in the progressive process [43].

**Bariatric and Metabolic Surgery in the Management of Metabolic Syndrome**

These interventions, which are called bariatric-metabolic surgery, allow the alleviation of MetS symptoms [2]. It has been reported that weight loss after bariatric surgery benefits the remission of T2DM and hypertension in patients with co-morbidities [36, 44 - 46]. Another surgical approach, liposuction, has only been tested in animal studies and is unlikely to be accepted in humans. Since subcutaneous adipose tissue also serves an endocrine function, it is predicted that the removal of adipose tissue will not improve metabolic parameters [47].

Today, the most effective treatment for obesity and T2DM is undisputedly bariatric/metabolic surgical interventions. Surgical methods used in the treatment of MetS provide not only weight control but are also effective in the remission of T2DM in the longterm because of the release of important incretins such as Ghrelin, GLP-1, GIP, and NPYY, and the alteration of the microbiota of surgically modified gastrointestinal tract. However, it should be known that there are many methods used in surgical treatment, and all these methods have their own advantages, disadvantages, and limitations [48].

Sleeve gastrectomy (SG) as a standalone procedure provides sufficient weight loss and comorbidity remission in many patients; however, in the long term, more patients regain weight, and some patients cannot achieve favorable results compared to Roux-n-y or one anastomosis gastric bypass (OAGB) surgery [49, 50]. On the other hand, gastric bypass techniques lead to more short- and long-term complications compared to SG. Recently, it has been reported that duodenal switch (DS) and single anastomosis duodeno-ileal bypass (SADI-S) surgeries provide better remission of metabolic syndrome components in the long term compared to SG and endoscopic treatment options [51].

Surgical operations that involve the exclusion of duodenum and rapid transit of semi-digested food to the terminal ileum provide optimal results in the resolution of comorbidities. Although the effect of bariatric and metabolic surgery (BMS) is immense on the resolution of metabolic syndrome and T2DM, the success of operations depends on age, BMI, the duration of the disease, pancreatic insulin reserves of the patients, and the usage of anti-diabetic medications. Patients who have c-peptide levels of more than 1.5 ng/dL and a short duration of disease, roughly less than 10 years, have better outcomes after BMS [52].

## CONCLUSION

MetS is one of the most important and frequent causes of metabolic, cardiovascular, and renal complications with insulin resistance, visceral obesity, hyperglycemia, atherogenic hyperlipidemia, and elevated blood pressure, as well as other features such as vascular inflammation, microalbuminuria, hyperuricemia, and tendency for atherothrombosis. Lifestyle modification is the most important and effective approach in the prevention and treatment of MetS. Surgical methods can also be used in the treatment of obesity in cases where lifestyle changes and conventional medical treatment fail. BMS provides optimal outcomes, especially in patients with class-3 obesity or class-2 obesity with related comorbidities. Currently, BMS also shows promising results in patients with class-1 obesity and multiple comorbidities compared to conservative treatment methods. Surgical interventions also cause the release of incretins and modification of GI cell lines and flora, which is the main reason for the alleviation of comorbidities of obesity, even in the short term. It is evident that surgical treatment is the most potent and durable treatment option in patients with obesity and MetS, but multidisciplinary patient preparation and follow-up are necessary to prevent lethal compilations and provide optimal results in the long term.

## REFERENCES

[1]     Lam DW, LeRoith D. Metabolic Syndrome.Endotext South Dartmouth (MA): MDTextcom, Inc. Feingold, KR 2019.

[2]     Reaven GM. Banting lecture 1988. Role of insulin resistance in human disease. Diabetes 1988; 37(12): 1595-607.
[http://dx.doi.org/10.2337/diab.37.12.1595] [PMID: 3056758]

[3]     Alberti KGMM, Zimmet PZ. Definition, diagnosis and classification of diabetes mellitus and its complications. Part 1: diagnosis and classification of diabetes mellitus. Provisional report of a WHO Consultation. Diabet Med 1998; 15(7): 539-53.
[http://dx.doi.org/10.1002/(SICI)1096-9136(199807)15:7<539::AID-DIA668>3.0.CO;2-S]    [PMID: 9686693]

[4]     Expert Panel on the Detection, Evaluation, and Treatment of High Blood Cholesterol in Adults. Executive summary of the third report of the National Cholesterol Education Program (NCEP) Expert Panel on Detection, Evaluation, and Treatment of High Blood Cholesterol in Adults. JAMA 2001; 285: 2486-97.
[http://dx.doi.org/10.1001/jama.285.19.2486] [PMID: 11368702]

[5]     Ford ES. Prevalence of the metabolic syndrome defined by the International Diabetes Federation among adults in the U.S. Diabetes Care 2005; 28(11): 2745-9.
[http://dx.doi.org/10.2337/diacare.28.11.2745] [PMID: 16249550]

[6]     Mozumdar A, Liguori G. Persistent increase of prevalence of metabolic syndrome among U.S. adults: NHANES III to NHANES 1999-2006. Diabetes Care 2011; 34(1): 216-9.
[http://dx.doi.org/10.2337/dc10-0879] [PMID: 20889854]

[7]    Aguilar M, Bhuket T, Torres S, Liu B, Wong RJ. Prevalence of the metabolic syndrome in the United States, 2003-2012. JAMA 2015; 313(19): 1973-4.
[http://dx.doi.org/10.1001/jama.2015.4260] [PMID: 25988468]

[8]    Hirode G, Wong RJ. Trends in the prevalence of metabolic syndrome in the United States, 2011-2016. JAMA 2020; 323(24): 2526-8.
[http://dx.doi.org/10.1001/jama.2020.4501] [PMID: 32573660]

[9]    Grundy SM. Pre-diabetes, metabolic syndrome, and cardiovascular risk. J Am Coll Cardiol 2012; 59(7): 635-43.
[http://dx.doi.org/10.1016/j.jacc.2011.08.080] [PMID: 22322078]

[10]   Dobrowolski P, Prejbisz A, Kuryłowicz A, *et al.* Metabolic syndrome – a new definition and management guidelines A joint position paper by the Polish Society of Hypertension, Polish Society for the Treatment of Obesity, Polish Lipid Association, Polish Association for Study of Liver, Polish Society of Family Medicine, Polish Society of Lifestyle Medicine, Division of Prevention and Epidemiology Polish Cardiac Society, "Club 30" Polish Cardiac Society, and Division of Metabolic and Bariatric Surgery Society of Polish Surgeons. Arch Med Sci 2022; 18(5): 1133-56.
[http://dx.doi.org/10.5114/aoms/152921] [PMID: 36160355]

[11]   Fahed G, Aoun L, Bou Zerdan M, *et al.* Metabolic Syndrome: Updates on Pathophysiology and Management in 2021. Int J Mol Sci 2022; 23(2): 786.
[http://dx.doi.org/10.3390/ijms23020786] [PMID: 35054972]

[12]   National Institutes of Health. Executive summary. In third report of the national cholesterol education Program expert Panel on detection, evaluation, and treatment of high blood cholesterol in adults (adult treatment Panel III). Washington, DC: U.S. Govt. Printing Office; 2001. NIH publ no 01-3670).

[13]   Alberti KG, Eckel RH, Grundy SM, Zimmet PZ, Cleeman JI, Donato KA, *et al.* Harmonizing the metabolic syndrome: a joint interim statement of the international diabetes federation task force on epidemiology and prevention; national Heart, Lung, and blood Institute; American Heart association; World Heart federation; international Atherosclerosis society; and international association for the study of obesity. Circular 2009;120:1640e5.

[14]   Hayden MR. Overview and New Insights into the Metabolic Syndrome: Risk Factors and Emerging Variables in the Development of Type 2 Diabetes and Cerebrocardiovascular Disease. Medicina (Kaunas) 2023; 59(3): 561.
[http://dx.doi.org/10.3390/medicina59030561] [PMID: 36984562]

[15]   Zhao X, An X, Yang C, Sun W, Ji H, Lian F. The crucial role and mechanism of insulin resistance in metabolic disease. Front Endocrinol (Lausanne) 2023; 14: 1149239.
[http://dx.doi.org/10.3389/fendo.2023.1149239] [PMID: 37056675]

[16]   Sun H, Saeedi P, Karuranga S, *et al.* IDF Diabetes Atlas: Global, regional and country-level diabetes prevalence estimates for 2021 and projections for 2045. Diabetes Res Clin Pract 2022; 183: 109119.
[http://dx.doi.org/10.1016/j.diabres.2021.109119] [PMID: 34879977]

[17]   Kahn SE. The relative contributions of insulin resistance and beta-cell dysfunction to the pathophysiology of Type 2 diabetes. Diabetologia 2003; 46(1): 3-19.
[http://dx.doi.org/10.1007/s00125-002-1009-0] [PMID: 12637977]

[18]   Kahn SE, Hull RL, Utzschneider KM. Mechanisms linking obesity to insulin resistance and type 2 diabetes. Nature 2006; 444(7121): 840-6.
[http://dx.doi.org/10.1038/nature05482] [PMID: 17167471]

[19]   Rattarasarn C. Dysregulated lipid storage and its relationship with insulin resistance and cardiovascular risk factors in non-obese Asian patients with type 2 diabetes. Adipocyte 2018; 7(2): 1-10.
[http://dx.doi.org/10.1080/21623945.2018.1429784] [PMID: 29411678]

[20]   Ling C, Rönn T. Epigenetics in human obesity and type 2 diabetes. Cell Metab 2019; 29(5): 1028-44.

[http://dx.doi.org/10.1016/j.cmet.2019.03.009] [PMID: 30982733]

[21]    Nanavaty D, Green R, Sanghvi A, *et al.* Prediabetes is an incremental risk factor for adverse cardiac events: A nationwide analysis. Atherosclerosis Plus 2023; 54: 22-6.
[http://dx.doi.org/10.1016/j.athplu.2023.08.002] [PMID: 37789875]

[22]    Litwin M, Kułaga Z. Obesity, metabolic syndrome, and primary hypertension. Pediatr Nephrol 2021; 36(4): 825-37.
[http://dx.doi.org/10.1007/s00467-020-04579-3] [PMID: 32388582]

[23]    Katsimardou A, Imprialos K, Stavropoulos K, Sachinidis A, Doumas M, Athyros V. Hypertension in Metabolic Syndrome: Novel Insights. Curr Hypertens Rev 2020; 16(1): 12-8.
[http://dx.doi.org/10.2174/18756506OTgw7ODElTcVY] [PMID: 30987573]

[24]    Nussbaumerova B, Rosolova H. Obesity and Dyslipidemia. Curr Atheroscler Rep 2023; 25(12): 947-55.
[http://dx.doi.org/10.1007/s11883-023-01167-2] [PMID: 37979064]

[25]    Therond P. Catabolism of lipoproteins and metabolic syndrome. Curr Opin Clin Nutr Metab Care 2009; 12(4): 366-71.
[http://dx.doi.org/10.1097/MCO.0b013e32832c5a12] [PMID: 19474714]

[26]    Butnariu LI, Gorduza EV, Ţarcă E, *et al.* Current Data and New Insights into the Genetic Factors of Atherogenic Dyslipidemia Associated with Metabolic Syndrome. Diagnostics (Basel) 2023; 13(14): 2348.
[http://dx.doi.org/10.3390/diagnostics13142348] [PMID: 37510094]

[27]    Shalitin S, Giannini C. Obesity, Metabolic Syndrome, and Nutrition. World Rev Nutr Diet 2023; 126: 47-69.
[http://dx.doi.org/10.1159/000527938] [PMID: 36948174]

[28]    Masenga SK, Kabwe LS, Chakulya M, Kirabo A. Mechanisms of Oxidative Stress in Metabolic Syndrome. Int J Mol Sci 2023; 24(9): 7898.
[http://dx.doi.org/10.3390/ijms24097898] [PMID: 37175603]

[29]    Philip NE, Girisha BS, Shetty S, Pinto AM, Noronha TM. Estimation of Metabolic Syndrome in Acanthosis Nigricans - A Hospital Based Cross-Sectional Study. Indian J Dermatol 2022; 67(1): 92.
[http://dx.doi.org/10.4103/ijd.ijd_442_21] [PMID: 35656279]

[30]    Saadi MM, Roy MN, Haque R, Tania FA, Mahmood S, Ali N. Association of microalbuminuria with metabolic syndrome: a cross-sectional study in Bangladesh. BMC Endocr Disord 2020; 20(1): 153.
[http://dx.doi.org/10.1186/s12902-020-00634-0] [PMID: 33028296]

[31]    Stewart LK, Kline JA. Metabolic syndrome increases risk of venous thromboembolism recurrence after acute deep vein thrombosis. Blood Adv 2020; 4(1): 127-35.
[http://dx.doi.org/10.1182/bloodadvances.2019000561] [PMID: 31917844]

[32]    Brauer P, Gorber SC, Shaw E, *et al.* Recommendations for prevention of weight gain and use of behavioural and pharmacologic interventions to manage overweight and obesity in adults in primary care. CMAJ 2015; 187(3): 184-95.
[http://dx.doi.org/10.1503/cmaj.140887] [PMID: 25623643]

[33]    Seo MH, Kim YH, Han K, Lee WY, Yoo SJ. Prevalence of Obesity and Incidence of Obesity-Related Comorbidities in Koreans Based on National Health Insurance Service Health Checkup Data 2006-2015 (J Obes Metab Syndr 2018;27:46-52). J Obes Metab Syndr 2018; 27(3): 198-9.
[http://dx.doi.org/10.7570/jomes.2018.27.3.198] [PMID: 31089563]

[34]    Ambroselli D, Masciulli F, Romano E, *et al.* New Advances in Metabolic Syndrome, from Prevention to Treatment: The Role of Diet and Food. Nutrients 2023; 15(3): 640.
[http://dx.doi.org/10.3390/nu15030640] [PMID: 36771347]

[35]    Alberti KGMM, Zimmet P, Shaw J. Metabolic syndrome—a new world-wide definition. A Consensus Statement from the International Diabetes Federation. Diabet Med 2006; 23(5): 469-80.

[http://dx.doi.org/10.1111/j.1464-5491.2006.01858.x] [PMID: 16681555]

[36] Aronne LJ. Therapeutic options for modifying cardiometa- bolic risk factors. Am J Med 2007, 120S26–S34.

[37] Castro-Barquero S, Ruiz-León AM, Sierra-Pérez M, Estruch R, Casas R. Dietary Strategies for Metabolic Syndrome: A Comprehensive Review. Nutrients 2020; 12(10): 2983.
[http://dx.doi.org/10.3390/nu12102983] [PMID: 33003472]

[38] Weight Loss Agents. In: LiverTox: Clinical and Research Information on Drug-Induced Liver Injury. Bethesda, MD: National Institute of Diabetes and Digestive and Kidney Diseases 2020.

[39] Alberti KGMM, Zimmet P, Shaw J. The metabolic syndrome—a new worldwide definition. Lancet 2005; 366(9491): 1059-62.
[http://dx.doi.org/10.1016/S0140-6736(05)67402-8] [PMID: 16182882]

[40] Elam M, Lovato L, Ginsberg H. The ACCORD-Lipid study: implications for treatment of dyslipidemia in Type 2 diabetes mellitus. Clin Lipidol 2011; 6(1): 9-20.
[http://dx.doi.org/10.2217/clp.10.84] [PMID: 26207146]

[41] Scott R, O'Brien R, Fulcher G, *et al.* Effects of fenofibrate treatment on cardiovascular disease risk in 9,795 individuals with type 2 diabetes and various components of the metabolic syndrome: the Fenofibrate Intervention and Event Lowering in Diabetes (FIELD) study. Diabetes Care 2009; 32(3): 493-8.
[http://dx.doi.org/10.2337/dc08-1543] [PMID: 18984774]

[42] Standards of medical care in diabetes--2014. Diabetes Care 2014; 37 (Suppl. 1): S14-80.
[http://dx.doi.org/10.2337/dc14-S014] [PMID: 24357209]

[43] Grundy SM. Metabolic syndrome update Trends in Cardiovascular Medicine. Elsevier Inc. 2016; Vol. 26: pp. 364-73.

[44] Horká V, Bužga M, Macháčková J, Holéczy P, Švagera Z. The effect of bariatric-metabolic surgery on selected components of metabolic syndrome and visceral adipose tissue - the pilot study. Physiol Res 2023; 72(S5) (Suppl. 5): S523-34.
[http://dx.doi.org/10.33549/physiolres.935227] [PMID: 38165756]

[45] Ikramuddin S, Buchwald H. How bariatric and metabolic operations control metabolic syndrome. Br J Surg 2011; 98(10): 1339-41.
[http://dx.doi.org/10.1002/bjs.7652] [PMID: 21751182]

[46] Flores L, Vidal J, Canivell S, Delgado S, Lacy A, Esmatjes E. Hypertension remission 1 year after bariatric surgery: predictive factors. Surg Obes Relat Dis 2014; 10(4): 661-5.
[http://dx.doi.org/10.1016/j.soard.2013.11.010] [PMID: 24582415]

[47] Ricci C, Gaeta M, Rausa E, Macchitella YBL. Early impact of bariatric surgery on type II diabetes, hyper- tension, and hyperlipidemia: a systematic review, meta- analysis and meta-regression on 6,587 patients. Obes Surg 2014; 24(4): 522-8.

[48] Bhandari V, Kosta S, Bhandari M, Bhandari M, Mathur W, Fobi M. Bariatric metabolic surgery. J Minim Access Surg 2022; 18(3): 396-400.
[http://dx.doi.org/10.4103/jmas.JMAS_325_20] [PMID: 34259204]

[49] Wölnerhanssen BK, Peterli R, Hurme S, *et al.* Laparoscopic Roux-en-Y gastric bypass *versus* laparoscopic sleeve gastrectomy: 5-year outcomes of merged data from two randomized clinical trials (SLEEVEPASS and SM-BOSS). Br J Surg 2021; 108(1): 49-57.
[http://dx.doi.org/10.1093/bjs/znaa011] [PMID: 33640917]

[50] Balasubaramaniam V, Pouwels S. Remission of Type 2 Diabetes Mellitus (T2DM) after Sleeve Gastrectomy (SG), One-Anastomosis Gastric Bypass (OAGB), and Roux-en-Y Gastric Bypass (RYGB): A Systematic Review. Medicina (Kaunas). 2023; 59(5): 985. Published 2023 May 19.

[51] Becerril S, Cienfuegos JA, Rodríguez A, *et al.* Single anastomosis duodeno-ileal bypass with sleeve

gastrectomy generates sustained improvement of glycemic control compared with sleeve gastrectomy in the diet-induced obese rat model. J Physiol Biochem 2024; 80(1): 149-60.
[http://dx.doi.org/10.1007/s13105-023-00993-x] [PMID: 37935948]

[52]    Al M, Taskin HE. Weight Loss, Type 2 Diabetes, and Nutrition in 355 Patients with Obesity Undergoing Sleeve Gastrectomy with Transit Bipartition: Two-Year Outcomes. Obes Facts 2022; 15(5): 717-29.
[http://dx.doi.org/10.1159/000526718] [PMID: 36070685]

**CHAPTER 19**

# Pathophysiological Mechanisms in Obstructive Sleep Apnea Syndrome

**Demet Aygun[1,*]**

*[1] Department of Neurology, Medicine Faculty, Istanbul Atlas University, Istanbul, Turkey*

**Abstract:** Metabolic syndrome is a condition characterized by a cluster of risk factors associated with cardiovascular disease. These metabolic factors include abdominal obesity, high blood pressure, impaired fasting glucose, high triglyceride levels, and low HDL cholesterol levels. Obstructive sleep apnea syndrome (OSAS) is a sleep disorder in which the air passages constrict during sleep, leading to repeated breathing interruptions. The prevalence of OSAS has increased over the years, particularly among aging individuals. Although the underlying reasons for airway obstruction involve various factors, such as overweight, anatomical abnormalities, shifts in airway dynamics, pharyngeal neuropathy, and fluid redistribution, these causes remain incompletely understood.

The primary characteristics of OSAS include repetitive interruptions in breathing, resulting in heightened susceptibility to a range of chronic ailments. These interruptions lead to intermittent episodes of low oxygen levels (hypoxia) and elevated carbon dioxide levels (hypercapnia), often accompanied by sleep disruptions due to arousal.

In this yet-to-be-published exploration, I navigate the intricate dynamics of human connection in the digital age, examining how technology both bridges and divides us. Through a blend of personal reflections and sociological analysis, I aim to shed light on the complexities of virtual relationships and their impact on our sense of belonging.

**Keywords:** Intermittent hypoxia, Metabolic disorders, Pathophysiological mechanisms, Respiratory diseases.

## INTRODUCTION

Metabolic syndrome is a condition characterized by a cluster of risk factors associated with cardiovascular disease. These metabolic factors include abdominal obesity, high blood pressure, impaired fasting glucose, high triglyceride levels, and low HDL cholesterol levels.

---
*[*] **Corresponding author Demet Aygun:** Department of Neurology, Medicine Faculty, Istanbul Atlas University, Istanbul, Turkey; E-mail: demetaygun@yahoo.com

**Hafize Uzun & Seyma Dumur (Eds.)**

In this unpublished essay, I explore the intricate dance between memory and identity, delving into how our recollections shape who we are. Through personal anecdotes and philosophical musings, I aim to unravel the profound interplay between memory, perception, and the construction of the self.

Obstructive sleep apnea syndrome (OSAS) is a respiratory disorder characterized by episodes of reduced breathing (hypopnea) and pauses in breathing (apnea). This condition leads to low blood oxygen levels (hypoxemia), elevated carbon dioxide levels (hypercapnia), fragmented sleep, and frequent awakenings, which result in increased respiratory effort and heightened activity of the sympathetic nervous system [1, 2]. Epidemiological data show that OSAS is most commonly observed in individuals aged 30 to 60 years, with research indicating that 24% of affected individuals are men and 9% are women [3, 4]. One resource estimates approximately 1,000,000 OSAS cases worldwide [5].

Risk factors for obstructive sleep apnea syndrome (OSAS) include obesity, age, gender, genetics, poor diet, and a sedentary lifestyle [6, 7]. Body mass index (BMI) is a critical factor in the development of the disease; an increase in BMI causes the upper airway to narrow due to an accumulation of adipose tissue, thereby heightening the risk of OSAS [8]. OSAS can manifest at any age, but its incidence tends to increase with age [9]. Male gender is a significant standalone risk factor for OSAS, with a prevalence that is 1.5 times higher in men, although the cause of this gender difference remains unclear [10]. The prevalence of OSAS also rises in postmenopausal women, likely due to the redistribution of body fat to the upper body [11].

Clinically, OSAS can vary significantly among individuals. Polysomnography (PSG) monitoring, following the 2017 scoring guidelines, is the method used for diagnosing OSAS [12]. These guidelines define episodes of respiratory arrest as reductions in respiration lasting more than 10 seconds. Respiratory depression is characterized by at least a 50% reduction in airflow and oxygen desaturation lasting longer than 10 seconds. The severity of OSAS is assessed by the rate of apnea-hypopnea events occurring per hour during sleep, known as the apnea-hypopnea index (AHI). An AHI of less than 5 indicates no sleep apnea, an AHI of 5-15 signifies mild OSAS, an AHI of 15-30 indicates moderate OSAS, and an AHI greater than 30 denotes severe OSAS. If a patient exhibits no issues and the recorded PSG AHI is less than 15, it is considered normal [12, 13].

Recent studies have reported a connection between sleep respiratory problems and an increased risk of metabolic, cardiovascular, and neurological diseases [14, 15]. Additionally, obstructive sleep apnea syndrome (OSAS) has been linked to a range of other conditions, including nonalcoholic fatty liver disease, insulin resistance, glucose metabolism issues, kidney disease, hypertension, cancer, and gastroesophageal reflux [16 - 23].

The pathophysiology of OSAS is complex and not easily understood, affecting various systems in the body. This section will investigate the mechanisms of sleep respiratory problems, examining the connections among changes in these conditions, their pathological and physiological effects, and their systemic reflections, based on current literature. With the increase in research on OSAS, it is widely accepted that both anatomical and functional factors contribute to the mechanism of upper airway collapse.

Anatomical abnormalities in the upper respiratory tract play a significant role in sleep respiratory disorders. Nearly all patients exhibit varying degrees of upper airway anatomical irregularities, including abnormal maxillofacial bone structures. These factors significantly contribute to upper airway collapse and stenosis, which can be exacerbated by conditions leading to soft tissue hyperplasia [24]. Additionally, edema in the legs, caused by various factors, can lead to fluid shifting to the neck area while lying down at night, resulting in upper airway narrowing [25].

As individuals age, decreased mandibular size due to conditions like osteoporosis and the downward positioning of bones and soft tissues in the jaw area contribute to crowding in the oronasal space [26]. Anatomical abnormalities related to skeletal conditions, such as midface hypoplasia in Pierre Robin syndrome, craniofacial synostosis in Pfeiffer syndrome, and features observed in Crouzon and Apert syndromes, are diseases that facilitate OSAS [27].

A major factor in the narrowing of the pharyngeal area is the swelling of the soft tissues in and around the airways, which is critical for OSAS. Contributing factors include excessive or elongated sagging of the soft palate, a retruded chin, an enlarged tongue, large tonsils, increased neck fat, and excessive secretions in the mouth [28]. An enlarged soft palate and tongue, along with a thickened pharyngeal wall, affect the lateral plane, which is a crucial area of airway narrowing in most OSAS patients [29].

Obesity contributes to airway compression in the pharyngeal region, and accumulation around the chest cavity may also promote the development of OSAS [30]. Inactivity during the day can cause peripheral edema in the legs. When lying down, a shift of this fluid to the top of the body can increase e upper airway constriction, thereby increasing susceptibility to OSAS [31]. Changes in leg diameter occur due to circulation correlated with strain in the neck area and changes in neck structures [30]. Breathing problems during sleep conclude microstimulation in the brain for safety [1]. Frequent awakenings during sleep, often seen in patients with respiratory issues, are referred to as "easy microstimulation thresholds" [32]. The degree of microstimulation can vary among patients but is commonly associated with respiratory problems during sleep. To understand the mechanism behind these respiratory issues, it is essential to recognize the role of microstimulation. Microstimulation plays a crucial safety role by restoring the neck structures, allowing normal respiratory functions to continue [33]. In OSAS, microstimulation during sleep can be life-saving, as it helps prevent hypoxia. However, when microstimulation occurs too frequently in OSAS patients, it leads to repetitive awakenings, disrupting sleep continuity and diminishing the quality of deep, stable sleep [34]. The increase in pressure within the rib cage is a significant factor in triggering microstimulation. A lower response to this pressure can cause a loss of muscle function, leading to airway collapse [34].In ventilation control, loop gain measures respiratory imbalance and can contribute to an indecisive chemical reflex balance in respiration, which is an important pathophysiological feature associated with OSAS [35]. Approximately one-third of cases exhibit elevated cycle gain [36]. Cycle gain is the composite measure of control gain and cycle time. High gain indicates a strong chemoreceptor response to minor changes in $PaCO_2$, meaning that even a slight respiratory response can significantly alter $PaCO_2$ levels [37]. For instance, overstimulation of the respiratory muscles by brain respiratory centers can result in frequent breathing, leading to $CO_2$ loss. This can decrease the function of muscles essential for smooth breathing [38]. Consequently, an elevated cycle gain can cause unstable ventilation through chemical reflex imbalance.

The imbalance in chemical reflex control triggers hypotonia of the upper airways due to hypocapnia, a condition produced by hyperventilation following obstructive apnea. OSAS often leads to frequent ventilation, resulting in low carbon dioxide levels and further respiratory issues. These factors contribute to the imbalance in ventilatory chemical reflex control, elevated cycle gain, and increased levels of carbon dioxide [30].

Given the critical role of oxygen in cellular survival, mechanisms that sense fluctuations in oxygen levels and initiate adaptive responses have evolved. It is understood that an organism's ability to adapt to hypoxia depends on the activation of specific genes sensitive to oxygen levels [39]. During hypoxia, oxygen availability for HIF-1α replication decreases, reducing the activity of hydroxylation enzymes. This leads to the upregulation of multiple target genes that aid in hypoxic adaptation, with approximately one hundred HIF-1α-regulated genes identified to date [40- 43]. These genes are involved in diverse biological functions, including oxygen-independent glucose metabolism, immune response, blood cell production, metabolism, angiogenesis, cell health and apoptosis, and cancer metastasis [43 - 51]. The genes mentioned are called immediate early genes (IEGs) [52]. Within the IEG family, there are jun, myc, and fos groups. Studies have shown that the fos and jun groups are activated by chronic oxygen deficiency. Activator protein-1 (AP-1) is a transcription factor composed primarily of these gene group proteins [53]. The AP-1 binding motif is frequently found in transcriptional regulatory regions and initiates the stimulation of specific genes under hypoxic conditions. Certain enzymes are involved in this process, such as tyrosine hydroxylase (TH), which plays a crucial role in catecholamine synthesis [53]. Intermittent hypoxia-induced TH activation may partly result from increased catecholamine levels, which over time can lead to heightened sympathetic system activity [54, 55]. Moreover, elevated levels of AP-1 are associated with the production of adhesion molecules and inflammatory cytokines, suggesting that AP-1 plays a role in OSAS-induced systemic chronic inflammation [56, 57].

Individuals with periodic hypoxia due to repeated apnea, as well as rodents subjected to periodic hypoxia, exhibit autonomic irregularities that can affect the autonomic nervous system. These abnormalities include heightened hypoxic respiratory responses and increased plasma catecholamine levels. In addition, sustained activation of the sympathetic nervous system and the development of systemic hypertension are observed [58]. The immediate response to hypoxia occurs within a short time and relies entirely on the oxygen-sensing function of peripheral arterial chemoreceptors, particularly the carotid body sensors [59].

Research indicates that carotid body sensors act as the first line of defense in detecting changes in oxygen levels in arterial blood during apnea. These sensors are more sensitive and respond more rapidly than other respiratory detectors, including central ones. Due to their location and functional characteristics, intermittent hypoxia, as seen in conditions like OSAS, activates the carotid body, leading to autonomic nervous system dysfunction. When the body experiences an oxygen deficit, it rapidly increases respiration, resulting in frequent respiratory activity due to the low oxygen levels, a process known as the hypoxic ventilatory response (HVR) [60, 61]. In OSAS patients, intermittent hypoxia causes ischemia-reperfusion injury to the digestive lining and leads to an inadequate oxygen supply to the intestinal mucosa. This results in alterations to the gut microbiota, disrupting the integrity of the digestive barrier [62]. The abundance of Firmicutes, a bacterial family, significantly increases with exposure to intermittent hypoxia (IH) and exhibits mucin-degrading properties [63]. The sulfate released during Prevotella's breakdown of mucin is utilized by Desulfovibrio, further promoting mucin degradation and increasing intestinal permeability [64]. Damage to the digestive wall membrane integrity leads to the release of a small protein known as plasma intestinal fatty acid-binding protein (I-FABP), an important marker of intestinal ischemia [65]. Notably, elevated levels of this protein have been observed in such cases [65].

Additionally, plasma D-lactic acid levels in patients are closely associated with digestive mucosal opacity and the severity of mucosal damage. These levels are also positively correlated with the apnea-hypopnea index (AHI) [66]. Digestive flora alterations reduce butyrate and acetate production, leading to nutritional deficiencies in the intestinal mucosa, which may cause epithelial dysfunction [67]. Repeated cycles of hypoxia and reoxygenation further damage the epithelial layer [68]. Over time, the tight junctions between digestive epithelial cells break down, leading to increased intestinal permeability.

Endotoxins, such as lipopolysaccharides produced by Prevotella, stimulate the immune response, worsening systemic inflammation through the recruitment of monocytes and cytokines [63, 69]. Additionally, Prevotella converts trimethylamine (TMA)-containing nutrients, triggering an immune response that contributes to vascular occlusion, increased LDL levels, high blood pressure, and other vascular problems [70, 71].

Multiple analyses of intestinal microbiota have shown a reduction in bacteria associated with the production of short-chain fatty acids (SCFAs) in both animal models of OSAS and OSAS patients [72]. SCFAs are the primary nutrients and energy providers for the colon membrane and play a crucial role in modulating the immune system. They are essential for maintaining intestinal integrity and influence hormones and enzymes. The immune system is affected directly or indirectly through various receptors [73].

Recent evidence highlights that respiratory problems lead to the production of reactive oxygen species (ROS) and a reduced antioxidant capacity [74]. Oxidative stress is defined as an imbalance between oxidant-producing systems and antioxidant defense mechanisms, with OSAS-associated oxidative stress occurring when ROS production exceeds antioxidant supply [74]. Recurrent respiratory arrest, a hallmark of apnea, involves severe low oxygen events and intermittent reoxygenation, resembling recurrent ischemia-reperfusion events. This process increases ROS production, affecting cellular components and functions. Excessive ROS influx during the reperfusion period can alter metabolism and damage cellular structures and genes. Apnea attacks lead to mitochondrial damage, and activated inflammatory cells are the main contributors to ROS production [75].

Hypoxia and reoxygenation can damage metabolic processes and genes [56]. This damage affects antioxidants, which are compounds that help mitigate the harmful effects of oxidative stress in cells and tissues throughout the body. Decreased antioxidant levels have been observed in individuals with chronic sleep-disordered breathing. Oxidative stress initiates a vicious cycle that creates a systemic inflammatory state, leading to increased production of inflammatory cytokines [1]. This process contributes to sympathetic activation and stimulates the renin-angiotensin-aldosterone system (RAAS), resulting in elevated blood levels of angiotensin II and aldosterone.

Furthermore, increased sympathetic tone is a key mediator of impaired glycemic control and insulin homeostasis, which may contribute to the development of metabolic risk factors in OSAS [76]. Heightened sympathetic activity is crucial in disrupting the balance of glycemic levels and insulin, potentially leading to the emergence of metabolic risk factors in individuals with OSAS.

The main outcomes of OSAS include dysfunction in endothelial cells and an increased propensity for blood clot formation. These factors are recognized as fundamental contributors to various clinical and empirical contexts, impacting a diverse array of health conditions and diseases. However, the outcomes may vary depending on the specific organ or cellular function most affected in each disease [77]. It is estimated that more than one hundred diseases are linked to reactive oxygen species (ROS) and respiratory problems, including chronic conditions such as cerebrovascular, metabolic, and cardiovascular diseases, as well as carcinogenesis, hypertension, and vascular disorders [2].

In summary, the fundamental components of OSAS include oxygen deprivation and oxidative stress, both of which are powerful inducers of various inflammatory pathways. Intermittent oxygen deficiency is speculated to trigger the NF-κB signaling pathway, resulting in the overproduction of adhesion molecules, such as vascular cell adhesion molecule (VCAM), P-selectin, and intracellular adhesion molecule (ICAM). Additionally, this process leads to excessive production of adipokines and pro-inflammatory cytokines, such as TNF-α, IL-1, IL-6, IL-8, and CRP [78].

The initiation of these inflammatory pathways stimulates endothelial cells, leukocytes, monocytes, T lymphocytes, and platelets [78]. These activated cells can further enhance oxidative stress by increasing the presence of adhesion molecules [79]. Cytokines serve as mediators that regulate both the innate and adaptive immune systems, existing both intracellularly and extracellularly. They oversee immune cell functions and control inflammatory reactions through interactions with various transcription factors within a complex network [80].

TNF-α, produced by macrophages, functions as a key cytokine in pro-inflammatory immune responses and contributes to the development of certain infections, participating in multiple signaling pathways that lead to cell death [81].

In individuals with OSAS, levels of TNF-α are elevated in monocytes and T lymphocytes [82]. Moreover, TNF-α triggers NF-κB activation by stimulating VCAM, promoting the attachment of monocytes to the endothelial lining and initiating inflammatory reactions in endothelial cells, which can lead to atherosclerosis [83]. The induction of inflammatory mechanisms *via* increased expression of NF-κB in monocytes has also been noted [84].

The transcription of NF-κB is not modulated by CRP, but rather, CRP enhances the production of adhesion molecules involved in monocyte attachment to endothelial cells [85]. Thus, CRP plays a regulatory role in inflammation through oxidative stress [10]. In certain diseases, such as metabolic disorders, cancer, cardiovascular disease, and sleep-disordered breathing, levels of plasminogen activator inhibitor-1 (PAI-1) are elevated [86, 87]. Studies indicate that sleep-disordered breathing is linked to metabolic dysfunction. Notably, the independent association between OSAS and insulin resistance suggests that sleep-disordered breathing may be a significant risk factor for obesity, insulin resistance, hypertension, and dyslipidemia, all of which are components of type 2 diabetes.

Obesity was initially a problem predominantly observed in developed countries; however, there has been an alarming increase in its prevalence in developing countries, particularly over the last two decades. Obesity is part of a cluster of disorders associated with metabolic syndrome. By definition, obesity is characterized by a body mass index (BMI) of $\geq 30$ kg/m$^2$, while severe obesity is defined as a BMI of $\geq 40$ kg/m$^2$ or $\geq 35$ kg/m$^2$ in conjunction with lipid abnormalities, including elevated levels of blood lipids, which are proportional to oxygen deficiency [81]. Several studies have shown that OSAS is independently associated with increased levels of total cholesterol, triglycerides, and LDL. Additionally, treating OSAS with continuous positive airway pressure (CPAP) may have beneficial effects on lipid profiles [84].

Diabetes is a disease that affects multiple systems and is strongly associated with a cluster of metabolic disturbances included in metabolic syndrome. Studies have confirmed that individuals with OSAS exhibit significantly higher levels of fasting blood sugar and insulin resistance compared to those without the condition. Furthermore, the severity of sleep-disordered breathing is linked to an increase in glucose intolerance [84]. This association between OSAS and insulin resistance extends even to non-obese individuals. For each unit increase in the apnea-hypopnea index (AHI), there is a corresponding 0.5% rise in insulin resistance levels [87].The relationship between OSAS and high blood pressure (BP) is distinct, although factors such as age and gender may influence it. Understanding the interplay between OSAS and arterial hypertension—both in terms of pathophysiology and clinical manifestations—is crucial for refining treatment approaches for individuals affected by both conditions. It is essential to meticulously examine potential mechanisms, such as alterations in cardiovascular autonomic regulation, modifications in ventilation dynamics, inflammatory responses, endothelial dysfunction, and the renin-angiotensin-aldosterone system. Exploring the intricate relationship between OSAS and cardiovascular diseases is vital for understanding their complex interactions and developing effective treatment strategies.

## CONCLUSION

In summary, awareness and research on OSAS and its impact on patient's quality of life have significantly increased over the last two decades. OSAS is linked to metabolic dysfunction, although the precise relationship between OSAS and various metabolic conditions remains a topic of ongoing debate. Increasing awareness of the strong correlation and timely identification of comorbidities is imperative. As discussed earlier, research findings highlight the impact of intermittent hypoxia resulting from OSAS on activating diverse signaling pathways and its close association with oxidative damage across various tissues and organs. Future studies should prioritize in vitro and animal investigations to uncover novel mechanisms underlying the pathophysiology of OSAS.

## REFERENCES

[1]     Lévy P, Kohler M, McNicholas WT, *et al.* Obstructive sleep apnoea syndrome. Nat Rev Dis Primers 2015; 1(1): 15015.
[http://dx.doi.org/10.1038/nrdp.2015.15] [PMID: 27188535]

[2]     Lavie L. Oxidative stress in obstructive sleep apnea and intermittent hypoxia – Revisited – The bad ugly and good: Implications to the heart and brain. Sleep Med Rev 2015; 20: 27-45.
[http://dx.doi.org/10.1016/j.smrv.2014.07.003] [PMID: 25155182]

[3]     Salzano G, Maglitto F, Bisogno A, *et al.* Obstructive sleep apnoea/hypopnoea syndrome: relationship with obesity and management in obese patients. Acta Otorhinolaryngol Ital 2021; 41(2): 120-30.
[http://dx.doi.org/10.14639/0392-100X-N1100] [PMID: 34028456]

[4]     Senaratna CV, Perret JL, Lodge CJ, *et al.* Prevalence of obstructive sleep apnea in the general population: A systematic review. Sleep Med Rev 2017; 34: 70-81.
[http://dx.doi.org/10.1016/j.smrv.2016.07.002] [PMID: 27568340]

[5]     Benjafield AV, Ayas NT, Eastwood PR, *et al.* Estimation of the global prevalence and burden of obstructive sleep apnoea: a literature-based analysis. Lancet Respir Med 2019; 7(8): 687-98.
[http://dx.doi.org/10.1016/S2213-2600(19)30198-5] [PMID: 31300334]

[6]     Yaggi HK, Strohl KP. Adult obstructive sleep apnea/hypopnea syndrome: definitions, risk factors, and pathogenesis. Clin Chest Med 2010; 31(2): 179-86.
[http://dx.doi.org/10.1016/j.ccm.2010.02.011] [PMID: 20488280]

[7]     Chen X, Wang R, Zee P, *et al.* Racial/ethnic differences in sleep disturbances: the multi-ethnic study of atherosclerosis (MESA). Sleep 2015; 38(6): 877-88.
[http://dx.doi.org/10.5665/sleep.4732] [PMID: 25409106]

[8]     Young T, Skatrud J, Peppard PE. Risk factors for obstructive sleep apnea in adults. JAMA 2004; 291(16): 2013-6.

[http://dx.doi.org/10.1001/jama.291.16.2013] [PMID: 15113821]

[9]     Young T, Palta M, Dempsey J, Skatrud J, Weber S, Badr S. The occurrence of sleep-disordered breathing among middle-aged adults. N Engl J Med 1993; 328(17): 1230-5.
[http://dx.doi.org/10.1056/NEJM199304293281704] [PMID: 8464434]

[10]    Lv R, Liu X, Zhang Y, *et al.* Pathophysiological mechanisms and therapeutic approaches in obstructive sleep apnea syndrome. Signal Transduct Target Ther 2023; 8(1): 218.
[http://dx.doi.org/10.1038/s41392-023-01496-3] [PMID: 37230968]

[11]    Millman RP, Carlisle CC, McGarvey ST, Eveloff SE, Levinson PD. Body fat distribution and sleep apnea severity in women. Chest 1995; 107(2): 362-6.
[http://dx.doi.org/10.1378/chest.107.2.362] [PMID: 7842762]

[12]    Kapur VK, Auckley DH, Chowdhuri S, *et al.* Clinical practice guideline for diagnostic testing for adult obstructive sleep apnea: an American Academy of Sleep Medicine Clinical Practice Guideline. J Clin Sleep Med 2017; 13(3): 479-504.
[http://dx.doi.org/10.5664/jcsm.6506] [PMID: 28162150]

[13]    Sateia MJ. International classification of sleep disorders-third edition: highlights and modifications. Chest 2014; 146(5): 1387-94.
[http://dx.doi.org/10.1378/chest.14-0970] [PMID: 25367475]

[14]    Guo WB, Liu YP, Xu HH, *et al.* [Obstructive sleep apnea and metabolic syndrome: an association study based on a large sample clinical database]. Zhonghua Er Bi Yan Hou Tou Jing Wai Ke Za Zhi 2021; 56(12): 1263-9.
[PMID: 34963213]

[15]    Kim DH, Kim B, Han K, Kim SW. The relationship between metabolic syndrome and obstructive sleep apnea syndrome: a nationwide population-based study. Sci Rep 2021; 11(1): 8751.
[http://dx.doi.org/10.1038/s41598-021-88233-4] [PMID: 33888816]

[16]    Wang X, Yu Q, Yue H, Zhang J, Zeng S, Cui F. Circulating endocannabinoids and insulin resistance in patients with obstructive sleep apnea. BioMed Res Int 2016; 2016: 1-8.
[http://dx.doi.org/10.1155/2016/9782031] [PMID: 26904688]

[17]    Sun S, Zhai H, Zhu M, Wen P, He X, Wang H. Insulin resistance is associated with Sfrp5 in obstructive sleep apnea. Rev Bras Otorrinolaringol (Engl Ed) 2019; 85(6): 739-45.
[PMID: 30120048]

[18]    Wang X, Yu Q, Yue H, Zeng S, Cui F. Effect of intermittent hypoxia and rimonabant on glucose metabolism in rats: involvement of expression of GLUT4 in skeletal muscle. Med Sci Monit 2015; 21: 3252-60.
[http://dx.doi.org/10.12659/MSM.896039] [PMID: 26503060]

[19]    Wu J, Chu Y, Jiang Z, Yu Q. Losartan protects against intermittent hypoxia-induced peritubular capillary loss by modulating the renal renin–angiotensin system and angiogenesis factors. Acta Biochim Biophys Sin (Shanghai) 2019; 52(1): 38-48.
[http://dx.doi.org/10.1093/abbs/gmz136] [PMID: 31836883]

[20]    Liu W, Yue H, Zhang J, Pu J, Yu Q. Effects of plasma ghrelin, obestatin, and ghrelin/obestatin ratio on blood pressure circadian rhythms in patients with obstructive sleep apnea syndrome. Chin Med J (Engl) 2014; 127(5): 850-5.
[http://dx.doi.org/10.3760/cma.j.issn.0366-6999.20131425] [PMID: 24571875]

[21]    Yuan F, Zhang S, Liu X, Liu Y. Correlation between obstructive sleep apnea hypopnea syndrome and hypertension: a systematic review and meta-analysis. Ann Palliat Med 2021; 10(12): 12251-61.
[http://dx.doi.org/10.21037/apm-21-3302] [PMID: 35016417]

[22]    Kendzerska T, Povitz M, Leung RS, *et al.* Obstructive sleep apnea and incident cancer: a large retrospective multicenter clinical cohort study. Cancer Epidemiol Biomarkers Prev 2021; 30(2): 295-304.

[http://dx.doi.org/10.1158/1055-9965.EPI-20-0975] [PMID: 33268490]

[23]   Polasky C, Steffen A, Loyal K, Lange C, Bruchhage KL, Pries R. Redistribution of monocyte subsets in obstructive sleep apnea syndrome patients leads to an imbalanced PD-1/PD-L1 cross-talk with CD4/CD8 T Cells. J Immunol 2021; 206(1): 51-8.
[http://dx.doi.org/10.4049/jimmunol.2001047] [PMID: 33268482]

[24]   Mayer P, Pépin JL, Bettega G, *et al.* Relationship between body mass index, age and upper airway measurements in snorers and sleep apnoea patients. Eur Respir J 1996; 9(9): 1801-9.
[http://dx.doi.org/10.1183/09031936.96.09091801] [PMID: 8880094]

[25]   White LH, Bradley TD. Role of nocturnal rostral fluid shift in the pathogenesis of obstructive and central sleep apnoea. J Physiol 2013; 591(5): 1179-93.
[http://dx.doi.org/10.1113/jphysiol.2012.245159] [PMID: 23230237]

[26]   Neelapu BC, Kharbanda OP, Sardana HK, *et al.* Craniofacial and upper airway morphology in adult obstructive sleep apnea patients: A systematic review and meta-analysis of cephalometric studies. Sleep Med Rev 2017; 31: 79-90.
[http://dx.doi.org/10.1016/j.smrv.2016.01.007] [PMID: 27039222]

[27]   Tan HL, Kheirandish-Gozal L, Abel F, Gozal D. Craniofacial syndromes and sleep-related breathing disorders. Sleep Med Rev 2016; 27: 74-88.
[http://dx.doi.org/10.1016/j.smrv.2015.05.010] [PMID: 26454241]

[28]   Azagra-Calero E, Espinar-Escalona E, Barrera-Mora JM, Llamas-Carreras JM, Solano-Reina E. Obstructive sleep apnea syndrome (OSAS). Review of the literature. Med Oral Patol Oral Cir Bucal 2012; 17(6): e925-9.
[http://dx.doi.org/10.4317/medoral.17706] [PMID: 22549673]

[29]   Ciscar MA, Juan G, Martínez V, *et al.* Magnetic resonance imaging of the pharynx in OSA patients and healthy subjects. Eur Respir J 2001; 17(1): 79-86.
[http://dx.doi.org/10.1183/09031936.01.17100790] [PMID: 11307760]

[30]   Schütz SG, Dunn A, Braley TJ, Pitt B, Shelgikar AV. New frontiers in pharmacologic obstructive sleep apnea treatment: A narrative review. Sleep Med Rev 2021; 57: 101473.
[http://dx.doi.org/10.1016/j.smrv.2021.101473] [PMID: 33853035]

[31]   White LH, Bradley TD, Logan AG. Pathogenesis of obstructive sleep apnoea in hypertensive patients: role of fluid retention and nocturnal rostral fluid shift. J Hum Hypertens 2015; 29(6): 342-50.
[http://dx.doi.org/10.1038/jhh.2014.94]

[32]   Lee RWW, Sutherland K, Sands SA, *et al.* Differences in respiratory arousal threshold in Caucasian and Chinese patients with obstructive sleep apnoea. Respirology 2017; 22(5): 1015-21.
[http://dx.doi.org/10.1111/resp.13022] [PMID: 28303676]

[33]   Altree TJ, Chung F, Chan MTV, Eckert DJ. Vulnerability to postoperative complications in obstructive sleep apnea: importance of phenotypes. Anesth. Anesth Analg 2021; 132(5): 1328-37.
[http://dx.doi.org/10.1213/ANE.0000000000005390] [PMID: 33857975]

[34]   Eckert DJ, Younes MK. Arousal from sleep: implications for obstructive sleep apnea pathogenesis and treatment. J Appl Physiol 2014; 116(3): 302-13.
[http://dx.doi.org/10.1152/japplphysiol.00649.2013] [PMID: 23990246]

[35]   Panza GS, Alex RM, Yokhana SS, Lee Pioszak DS, Badr MS, Mateika JH. Increased oxidative stress, loop gain and the arousal threshold are clinical predictors of increased apnea severity following exposure to intermittent hypoxia. Nat Sci Sleep 2019; 11: 265-79.
[http://dx.doi.org/10.2147/NSS.S228100] [PMID: 31695534]

[36]   Eckert DJ, White DP, Jordan AS, Malhotra A, Wellman A. Defining phenotypic causes of obstructive sleep apnea. Identification of novel therapeutic targets. Am J Respir Crit Care Med 2013; 188(8): 996-1004.
[http://dx.doi.org/10.1164/rccm.201303-0448OC] [PMID: 23721582]

[37] Naughton MT. Loop gain in apnea: gaining control or controlling the gain? Am J Respir Crit Care Med 2010; 181(2): 103-5.
[http://dx.doi.org/10.1164/rccm.200909-1449ED] [PMID: 20053968]

[38] Eckert DJ, Malhotra A, Jordan AS. Mechanisms of Apnea. Prog Cardiovasc Dis 2009; 51(4): 313-23.
[http://dx.doi.org/10.1016/j.pcad.2008.02.003] [PMID: 19110133]

[39] Choudhry H, Harris AL. Advances in hypoxia-inducible factor biology. Cell Metab 2018; 27(2): 281-98.
[http://dx.doi.org/10.1016/j.cmet.2017.10.005] [PMID: 29129785]

[40] Luo Z, Tian M, Yang G, *et al.* Hypoxia signaling in human health and diseases: implications and prospects for therapeutics. Signal Transduct Target Ther 2022; 7(1): 218.
[http://dx.doi.org/10.1038/s41392-022-01080-1] [PMID: 35798726]

[41] Corrado C, Fontana S. Hypoxia and HIF signaling: one axis with divergent effects. Int J Mol Sci 2020; 21(16): 5611.
[http://dx.doi.org/10.3390/ijms21165611] [PMID: 32764403]

[42] Palazon A, Goldrath AW, Nizet V, Johnson RS. HIF transcription factors, inflammation, and immunity. Immunity 2014; 41(4): 518-28.
[http://dx.doi.org/10.1016/j.immuni.2014.09.008] [PMID: 25367569]

[43] Taylor CT, Doherty G, Fallon PG, Cummins EP. Hypoxia-dependent regulation of inflammatory pathways in immune cells. J Clin Invest 2016; 126(10): 3716-24.
[http://dx.doi.org/10.1172/JCI84433] [PMID: 27454299]

[44] Kierans SJ, Taylor CT. Regulation of glycolysis by the hypoxia-inducible factor (HIF): implications for cellular physiology. J Physiol 2021; 599(1): 23-37.
[http://dx.doi.org/10.1113/JP280572] [PMID: 33006160]

[45] McGettrick AF, O'Neill LAJ. The role of HIF in immunity and inflammation. Cell Metab 2020; 32(4): 524-36.
[http://dx.doi.org/10.1016/j.cmet.2020.08.002] [PMID: 32853548]

[46] Tomc J, Debeljak N. Molecular insights into the oxygen-sensing pathway and erythropoietin expression regulation in erythropoiesis. Int J Mol Sci 2021; 22(13): 7074.
[http://dx.doi.org/10.3390/ijms22137074] [PMID: 34209205]

[47] Infantino V, Santarsiero A, Convertini P, Todisco S, Iacobazzi V. Cancer cell metabolism in hypoxia: role of HIF-1 as key regulator and therapeutic target. Int J Mol Sci 2021; 22(11): 5703.
[http://dx.doi.org/10.3390/ijms22115703] [PMID: 34071836]

[48] Sun J, Shen H, Shao L, *et al.* HIF-1α overexpression in mesenchymal stem cell-derived exosomes mediates cardioprotection in myocardial infarction by enhanced angiogenesis. Stem Cell Res Ther 2020; 11(1): 373.
[http://dx.doi.org/10.1186/s13287-020-01881-7] [PMID: 32859268]

[49] Wang J, Wu H, Zhou Y, *et al.* HIF-1α inhibits mitochondria-mediated apoptosis and improves the survival of human adipose-derived stem cells in ischemic microenvironments. J Plast Reconstr Aesthet Surg 2021; 74(8): 1908-18.
[http://dx.doi.org/10.1016/j.bjps.2020.11.041] [PMID: 33358677]

[50] Karagiota A, Kourti M, Simos G, Mylonis I. HIF-1α-derived cell-penetrating peptides inhibit ERK-dependent activation of HIF-1 and trigger apoptosis of cancer cells under hypoxia. Cell Mol Life Sci 2019; 76(4): 809-25.
[http://dx.doi.org/10.1007/s00018-018-2985-7] [PMID: 30535970]

[51] Chen X, Li Z, Yong H, *et al.* Trim21-mediated HIF-1α degradation attenuates aerobic glycolysis to inhibit renal cancer tumorigenesis and metastasis. Cancer Lett 2021; 508: 115-26.
[http://dx.doi.org/10.1016/j.canlet.2021.03.023] [PMID: 33794309]

[52]    Roussel MF. Regulation of cell cycle entry and G1 progression by CSF-1. Mol Reprod Dev 1997; 46(1): 11-8.
[http://dx.doi.org/10.1002/(SICI)1098-2795(199701)46:1<11::AID-MRD3>3.0.CO;2-U]    [PMID: 8981358]

[53]    Premkumar DR, Adhikary G, Overholt JL, Simonson MS, Cherniack NS, Prabhakar NR. Intracellular pathways linking hypoxia to activation of c-fos and AP-1. Adv Exp Med Biol 2002; 475: 101-9.
[http://dx.doi.org/10.1007/0-306-46825-5_10] [PMID: 10849652]

[54]    Kumar GK, Rai V, Sharma SD, *et al.* Chronic intermittent hypoxia induces hypoxia-evoked catecholamine efflux in adult rat adrenal medulla *via* oxidative stress. J Physiol 2006; 575(1): 229-39.
[http://dx.doi.org/10.1113/jphysiol.2006.112524] [PMID: 16777938]

[55]    Knight WD, Little JT, Carreno FR, Toney GM, Mifflin SW, Cunningham JT. Chronic intermittent hypoxia increases blood pressure and expression of FosB/ΔFosB in central autonomic regions. Am J Physiol Regul Integr Comp Physiol 2011; 301(1): R131-9.
[http://dx.doi.org/10.1152/ajpregu.00830.2010] [PMID: 21543638]

[56]    Lavie L. Obstructive sleep apnoea syndrome – an oxidative stress disorder. Sleep Med Rev 2003; 7(1): 35-51.
[http://dx.doi.org/10.1053/smrv.2002.0261] [PMID: 12586529]

[57]    Lavie L. Sleep-disordered breathing and cerebrovascular disease: a mechanistic approach. Neurol Clin 2005; 23(4): 1059-75.
[http://dx.doi.org/10.1016/j.ncl.2005.05.005] [PMID: 16243616]

[58]    Prabhakar NR, Dick TE, Nanduri J, Kumar GK. Systemic, cellular and molecular analysis of chemoreflex-mediated sympathoexcitation by chronic intermittent hypoxia. Exp Physiol 2007; 92(1): 39-44.
[http://dx.doi.org/10.1113/expphysiol.2006.036434] [PMID: 17124274]

[59]    Prabhakar NR. Oxygen sensing by the carotid body chemoreceptors. J Appl Physiol 2000; 88(6): 2287-95.
[http://dx.doi.org/10.1152/jappl.2000.88.6.2287] [PMID: 10846047]

[60]    Pamenter ME, Powell FL. Time domains of the hypoxic ventilatory response and their molecular basis. Compr Physiol 2016; 6(3): 1345-85.
[http://dx.doi.org/10.1002/cphy.c150026] [PMID: 27347896]

[61]    Peng YJ, Yuan G, Ramakrishnan D, *et al.* Heterozygous HIF-1α deficiency impairs carotid body-mediated systemic responses and reactive oxygen species generation in mice exposed to intermittent hypoxia. J Physiol 2006; 577(2): 705-16.
[http://dx.doi.org/10.1113/jphysiol.2006.114033] [PMID: 16973705]

[62]    Valentini F, Evangelisti M, Arpinelli M, *et al.* Gut microbiota composition in children with obstructive sleep apnoea syndrome: a pilot study. Sleep Med 2020; 76: 140-7.
[http://dx.doi.org/10.1016/j.sleep.2020.10.017] [PMID: 33181474]

[63]    Poroyko VA, Carreras A, Khalyfa A, *et al.* Chronic sleep disruption alters gut microbiota, induces systemic and adipose tissue inflammation and insulin resistance in mice. Sci Rep 2016; 6(1): 35405.
[http://dx.doi.org/10.1038/srep35405] [PMID: 27739530]

[64]    Payne AN, Chassard C, Lacroix C. Gut microbial adaptation to dietary consumption of fructose, artificial sweeteners and sugar alcohols: implications for host–microbe interactions contributing to obesity. Obes Rev 2012; 13(9): 799-809.
[http://dx.doi.org/10.1111/j.1467-789X.2012.01009.x] [PMID: 22686435]

[65]    Li Q, Xu T, Zhong H, *et al.* Impaired intestinal barrier in patients with obstructive sleep apnea. Sleep Breath 2021; 25(2): 749-56.
[http://dx.doi.org/10.1007/s11325-020-02178-y] [PMID: 32845474]

[66]    Heizati M, Li N, Shao L, *et al.* Does increased serum d-lactate mean subclinical hyperpermeability of

intestinal barrier in middle-aged nonobese males with OSA? Medicine (Baltimore) 2017; 96(49): e9144.
[http://dx.doi.org/10.1097/MD.0000000000009144] [PMID: 29245360]

[67] Liu P, Wang Y, Yang G, *et al.* The role of short-chain fatty acids in intestinal barrier function, inflammation, oxidative stress, and colonic carcinogenesis. Pharmacol Res 2021; 165: 105420.
[http://dx.doi.org/10.1016/j.phrs.2021.105420] [PMID: 33434620]

[68] Singhal R, Shah YM. Oxygen battle in the gut: Hypoxia and hypoxia-inducible factors in metabolic and inflammatory responses in the intestine. J Biol Chem 2020; 295(30): 10493-505.
[http://dx.doi.org/10.1074/jbc.REV120.011188] [PMID: 32503843]

[69] Scher JU, Sczesnak A, Longman RS, *et al.* Expansion of intestinal Prevotella copri correlates with enhanced susceptibility to arthritis. eLife 2013; 2: e01202.
[http://dx.doi.org/10.7554/eLife.01202] [PMID: 24192039]

[70] Ufnal M, Zadlo A, Ostaszewski R. TMAO: A small molecule of great expectations. Nutrition 2015; 31(11-12): 1317-23.
[http://dx.doi.org/10.1016/j.nut.2015.05.006] [PMID: 26283574]

[71] Xue J, Zhou D, Poulsen O, *et al.* Intermittent hypoxia and hypercapnia accelerate atherosclerosis, partially *via* trimethylamine-oxide. Am J Respir Cell Mol Biol 2017; 57(5): 581-8.
[http://dx.doi.org/10.1165/rcmb.2017-0086OC] [PMID: 28678519]

[72] Ko CY, Liu QQ, Su HZ, *et al.* Gut microbiota in obstructive sleep apnea–hypopnea syndrome: disease-related dysbiosis and metabolic comorbidities. Clin Sci (Lond) 2019; 133(7): 905-17.
[http://dx.doi.org/10.1042/CS20180891] [PMID: 30957778]

[73] Luu M, Visekruna A. Short-chain fatty acids: Bacterial messengers modulating the immunometabolism of T cells. Eur J Immunol 2019; 49(6): 842-8.
[http://dx.doi.org/10.1002/eji.201848009] [PMID: 31054154]

[74] Maniaci A, Iannella G, Cocuzza S, *et al.* Oxidative stress and inflammation biomarker expression in obstructive sleep apnea patients. J Clin Med 2021; 10(2): 277.
[http://dx.doi.org/10.3390/jcm10020277] [PMID: 33451164]

[75] Hopps E, Canino B, Calandrino V, Montana M, Lo Presti R, Caimi G. Lipid peroxidation and protein oxidation are related to the severity of OSAS. Eur Rev Med Pharmacol Sci 2014; 18(24): 3773-8.
[PMID: 25555866]

[76] Olea E, Agapito MT, Gallego-Martin T, *et al.* Intermittent hypoxia and diet-induced obesity: effects on oxidative status, sympathetic tone, plasma glucose and insulin levels, and arterial pressure. J Appl Physiol 2014; 117(7): 706-19.
[http://dx.doi.org/10.1152/japplphysiol.00454.2014] [PMID: 25103975]

[77] Lavie L. Oxidative stress inflammation and endothelial dysfunction in obstructive sleep apnea. Front Biosci (Elite Ed) 2012; E4(4): 1391-403.
[http://dx.doi.org/10.2741/e469] [PMID: 22201964]

[78] Lavie L, Lavie P. Molecular mechanisms of cardiovascular disease in OSAHS: the oxidative stress link. Eur Respir J 2009; 33(6): 1467-84.
[http://dx.doi.org/10.1183/09031936.00086608] [PMID: 19483049]

[79] Wang J, Xu H, Guo C, *et al.* Association between severity of obstructive sleep apnea and high-sensitivity C-reactive protein in patients with hypertrophic obstructive cardiomyopathy. Clin Cardiol 2020; 43(7): 803-11.
[http://dx.doi.org/10.1002/clc.23385] [PMID: 32458487]

[80] Oberholzer A, Oberholzer C, Moldawer LL. Cytokine signaling-regulation of the immune response in normal and critically ill states. Crit Care Med 2000; 28(4) (Suppl.): N3-N12.
[http://dx.doi.org/10.1097/00003246-200004001-00002] [PMID: 10807312]

[81] McNicholas WT. Obstructive sleep apnea and inflammation. Prog Cardiovasc Dis 2009; 51(5): 392-9.

[http://dx.doi.org/10.1016/j.pcad.2008.10.005] [PMID: 19249445]

[82]   Ryan S, Taylor CT, McNicholas WT. Predictors of elevated nuclear factor-kappaB-dependent genes in obstructive sleep apnea syndrome. Am J Respir Crit Care Med 2006; 174(7): 824-30.
[http://dx.doi.org/10.1164/rccm.200601-066OC] [PMID: 16840748]

[83]   Feng YM, Thijs L, Zhang ZY, *et al.* Glomerular function in relation to circulating adhesion molecules and inflammation markers in a general population. Nephrol Dial Transplant 2018; 33(3): 426-35.
[http://dx.doi.org/10.1093/ndt/gfx256] [PMID: 28992257]

[84]   Htoo AK, Greenberg H, Tongia S, *et al.* Activation of nuclear factor κB in obstructive sleep apnea: a pathway leading to systemic inflammation. Sleep Breath 2006; 10(1): 43-50.
[http://dx.doi.org/10.1007/s11325-005-0046-6] [PMID: 16491391]

[85]   Devaraj S, Davis B, Simon SI, Jialal I. CRP promotes monocyte-endothelial cell adhesion *via* Fcγ receptors in human aortic endothelial cells under static and shear flow conditions. Am J Physiol Heart Circ Physiol 2006; 291(3): H1170-6.
[http://dx.doi.org/10.1152/ajpheart.00150.2006] [PMID: 16603696]

[86]   Zakrzewski M, Zakrzewska E, Kiciński P, *et al.* Evaluation of fibrinolytic inhibitors: alpha--antiplasmin and plasminogen activator inhibitor 1 in patients with obstructive sleep apnoea. PLoS One 2016; 11(11): e0166725.
[http://dx.doi.org/10.1371/journal.pone.0166725] [PMID: 27861608]

[87]   Altalhi R, Pechlivani N, Ajjan RA. PAI-1 in diabetes: pathophysiology and role as a therapeutic target. Int J Mol Sci 2021; 22(6): 3170.
[http://dx.doi.org/10.3390/ijms22063170] [PMID: 33804680]

# CHAPTER 20

# Evaluation of Metabolic Parameters in Cushing's Syndrome

**Naile Misirlioglu[1],*** and **Hafize Uzun[2]**

[1] *Department of Biochemistry, Gaziosmanpaşa Training and Research Hospital, University of Health Sciences, Istanbul, Turkey*

[2] *Department of Medical Biochemistry, Faculty of Medicine, Istanbul Atlas University, Istanbul, Turkey*

**Abstract:** The prevalence of metabolic syndrome (MetS) is estimated to be about one-fourth of the worldwide adult population, while Cushing's syndrome (CS) is significantly rarer (estimated incidence of 2 per million). However, linking the two has not only therapeutic but also potential public health implications. The worldwide increase of obesity and MetS poses the problem of correctly identifying patients potentially hiding CS without indiscriminately screening all patients presenting one or more symptoms consistent with cortisol excess, which showed to be not cost-effective. CS is associated with hyperglycemia, protein catabolism, immunosuppression, hypertension, weight gain, neurocognitive changes, and mood disorders. Obesity, insulin resistance, hypertension, functional hypercortisolism (Endogenous/Exogenous), and MetS are common features. Early diagnosis and treatment are important because untreated CS may result in mortality due to associated metabolic risks.

**Keywords:** Cushing's syndrome, Hypertension, Hypercortisolism, Insulin resistance, Metabolic syndrome, Obesity.

## INTRODUCTION

Metabolic syndrome (MetS) is a cluster of metabolic abnormalities that include hypertension (HT), central obesity, insulin resistance (IR), and atherogenic dyslipidemia, which increase the risk of type 2 diabetes mellitus (DM), coronary heart disease (CHD) and coronary vascular disease (CVD), morbidity and mortality. MetS is also called 'dysmetabolic syndrome', 'insulin resistance syndrome', 'syndrome X', 'hypertriglyceridemic waist', and 'the deadly quartet'. MetS is a health problem that has an increasing prevalence in the world and negatively affects people's lives [1, 2].

* **Corresponding author Naile Misirlioglu:** Department of Biochemistry, Gaziosmanpaşa Training and Research Hospital, University of Health Sciences, Istanbul, Turkey; E-mail: nailemisirlioglu@gmail.com

**Hafize Uzun & Seyma Dumur (Eds.)**

Cushing's disease (CD) is a disease caused by the secretion of adrenocorticotropic hormone (ACTH) from the pituitary gland above its normal level. CD is the most common cause of spontaneous Cushing's syndrome (CS), occurring in 60–70% of Cushing's patients. Iatrogenic CS is the name given to the condition that occurs independently of ACTH secretion in the body with the administration of glucocorticoid agents in pharmacological doses. The presence of moon face, hirsutism, buffalo hump, central obesity, hypertension, hyperglycemia, mood disorders, psychosis, immunosuppression, osteoporosis, muscle weakness, or peptic ulcer should suggest CS. No single symptom or finding is pathognomonic for CS, but the simultaneous presence of multiple signs or symptoms should be a warning sign [3].

## METABOLIC SYNDROME (METS)

It is known that environmental factors such as a sedentary lifestyle and changes in dietary habits contribute to the increase in the number of patients with metabolic syndrome, which is progressing towards a pandemic, as well as genetic predisposition. Although the causes of metabolic syndrome include obesity, hypertension, and hyperlipidemia, especially fat stored in the abdominal region and IR caused by physical inactivity, the main role is thought to belong to insulin resistance. In metabolic syndrome, there is IR in liver and muscle tissue as well as in adipose tissue. Hyperinsulinemia occurs in response to this resistance. Cardiovascular mortality and morbidity are increased in patients with metabolic syndrome [4].

There are various diagnostic criteria proposed for MetS, such as the National Cholesterol Education Program (NCEP) Adult Treatment Panel (ATP) III (NCEP-ATP III) criteria, International Diabetes Federation (IDF) criteria, World Health Organization (WHO) criteria [5 - 7]. The most commonly used criterion is the NCEP-ATP III, followed by IDF and then the WHO criteria. According to the NCEP ATP III guideline, the criteria and components of MetS are presented in Table1 [8].

**Table 1. According to the NCEP ATP III guideline, the criteria and components of MetS.**

| Component | Criteria |
|---|---|
| Abdominal obesity: Increased waist circumference. | Men: ≥ 102cm<br>Women: ≥ 88cm |
| Elevated triglycerides. | ≥ 150mg/dL |
| Reduced HDL. | Men: < 40mg/dL<br>Women: < 50mg/dL |
| Elevated blood pressure. | ≥ 130/85mmHg |

*(Table 1) cont.....*

| Component | Criteria |
|---|---|
| Elevated fasting glucose. | ≥ 100mg/dL |

## CUSHING'S SYNDROME

Cushing's syndrome (CS) is a complex of symptoms that occur with prolonged increases in plasma cortisol levels that are not due to a physiological etiology. Cortisol is a hormone that affects the body's response to stress and change. Although the most frequent cause of CS is exogenous steroid use, the estimated incidence of CS due to endogenous overproduction of cortisol ranges from 2 to 8 per million people annually [9].

### Etiology

The metabolic picture is due to the overproduction of adrenal steroids, among others [10]:

- Negative nitrogen, potassium, and phosphorus balance;
- Sodium retention, which may result in HT, edema, or both;
- Impaired glucose tolerance or overt DM;
- Increased plasma fatty acids;
- There is an increase in the number of polymorphonuclear leucocytes while the number of circulating eosinophils and lymphocytes decreases.

In patients with CS, muscle atrophy and fat accumulation in the body in an unusually new distribution, *i.e.*, trunk obesity, can be found. Loss of ACTH as a result of a tumor, infection, or pituitary infarction causes the opposite set of findings [9 - 12].

If the event is due to a pituitary adenoma, it is more commonly referred to as Cushing's disease, while those of adrenal origin or those that occur with high doses and prolonged administration of exogenous ACTH or glucocorticoids (iatrogenic Cushing's syndrome) are called CS. Although glucocorticoid excess is responsible for the clinical picture, an increase in other hormones of the adrenal cortex, mineralocorticoids, and sex steroids, which vary according to the etiological causes, may also be detected. The condition, which usually occurs between the ages of 20-60 and more frequently in women, usually results in death within 5 years if left untreated. In 90% of CS of pituitary origin, adenoma is present in 90% and hyperplasia in 10% [12]. The main tumors causing CS by secreting ectopic ACTH are small cell lung cancers (SCLCs), bronchial carcinomas, thymus carcinoids, pancreatic tumors, pheochromocytoma, and medullary thyroid cancer. Local symptoms may be seen in ACTH-dependent (pituitary origin) CS. These occur mostly in macroadenoma cases due to the effects of the mass. These include headache, visual field disturbance (due to the pressure of the adenoma on the optic chiasm), hypopituitarism, and hyperpigmentation. There are some features and differences in the clinical picture of ectopic Cushing's syndrome. Some of these are more common in men, and the most prominent symptom is weight loss. Hyperpigmentation, hypertension, peripheral edema, and diffuse muscle weakness are common [12].

CS is divided into two large groups: ACTH-dependent and ACTH-independent in terms of etiology (Table **2**) [13, 14].

Table 2. Etiology in Cushing's syndrome.

| ACTH-dependent | ACTH-independent |
|---|---|
| Pituitary ACTH over-secretion. Cushing's disease 60–70%. CRH-secreting tumors (rare). | Unilateral adrenocortical tumor. Adrenocortical adenoma 10–15%. Adrenocortical carcinoma 10–15%. |
| Non-pituitary ACTH over-secretion. Ectopic ACTH syndrome 5–10%. | Bilateral adrenocortical involvement. Primary pigmented nodular. Adrenocortical dysplasia (rare)ACTH-independent bilateral macronodular adrenocortical hyperplasia (rare). |

**CRH,** Corticotropin-Releasing Hormone; **ACTH,** Adrenocorticotropic hormone.

## Clinical features of Cushing's syndrome

The clinical findings associated with hypercortisolemia may be related to the severity and degree of hypercortisolemia, the age of the patient, and the duration of the disease. Proximal muscle weakness, opportunistic infections, osteopenia/osteoporosis, cataracts, hypertension, change in fat distribution in men and women, and increase in adipose tissue in visceral compartments subcutaneous tissue in the face, neck and intraabdominal region lead to truncal obesity. The clinical reflection of truncal obesity causes a 'buffalo hump' appearance due to fat accumulation in the face and dorsocervical region [14 - 20].

Gonadal dysfunction, menstrual problems, psychological and cognitive changes, depression, neuropsychiatric problems (mânia, anxiety, cognitive dysfunction, insomnia, *etc.*), and psychoses can be seen. Main complaints and physical examination findings in patients with Cushing's syndrome are presented in Table3 [15].

**Table 3. Main complaints and physical examination findings in patients with Cushing's syndrome.**

| | |
|---|---|
| Moon face. | Buffalo hump, lethargy. |
| Depression. | Low back pain. |
| Psychosis. | Headache. |
| Weight gain. | Fatigue. |
| Hyperpigmentation. | Thinning of the skin and easy bleeding. |
| Purple stria. | Acne. |
| Edema. | Recurrent infections. |
| Supraclavicular fat accumulation. | Hair loss. |
| Centripetal obesity. | Proximal muscle weakness. |
| Hypertension. | Irregularity in menstruation. |
| Loss of libido. | Hirsutism. |

## DIAGNOSTIC PROCEDURES

CS is one of the most diagnostically challenging diseases in clinical endocrinology.

Tests used in the differential diagnosis of Cushing's Syndrome are presented in Table **4**.

**Table 4. Tests used in the differential diagnosis of Cushing's Syndrome.**

| |
|---|
| • Imaging methods. |
| • Plasma ACTH level. |
| • Dexamethasone Suppression Test. |
| • Salivary cortisol. |
| • Metyrapone test. |
| • CRH test. |
| • Inferior Petrosal Sinus Sampling (IPSS). |

## Imaging Methods

Imaging Methods Gadalinium diethylene pentacetic acid sella magnetic resonance (MR) has a sensitivity of 50-60% for pituitary CS. The main problem in imaging is whether the lesion can be held responsible for the clinic in detected microadenomas. Because of the frequency of incidental tumors, lesions detected by imaging methods, especially those below 4 mm, usually require further investigations. For microadenomas below 6 mm, only 52% of patients are correlated with surgery, and some diagnostic procedures, such as bilateral inferior petrosal or cavernous sinus sampling, are needed. However, if a tumor over 6 mm is detected by MRI, surgical confirmation is 75% to 98%. MRI remains the imaging modality of choice for the localization of ACTH-secreting pituitary adenomas and, when conducted in a specialist unit with access to the full complement of sequences, will identify the causative lesion in many cases. However, when uncertainty persists, molecular PET imaging may allow the causative lesion to be located [21 - 23]. In CS of adrenal origin, a CT examination of the adrenal glands may be sufficient. Since most ectopic ACTH-secreting tumors originate from the lung, high-resolution CT scanning is reliable [21]. However, some tumors cannot be visualized and localized despite all imaging and diagnostic methods. Some carcinoid tumors, small cell lung tumors, and ectopic ACTH-secreting neoplasms, such as medullary thyroid cancer, express high-affinity somatostatin receptors. With radioactively labeled octreotide, it is possible to determine both the activity and location of the lesion or to exclude a lesion that cannot be detected by imaging methods [23, 24]. Fluorine-18-fluorodeoxyglucose positron emission tomography (FDG PET/CT) has recently been increasingly used in the diagnosis of carcinoid tumors. It is useful in evaluating the malignancy potential and metastatic status of carcinoid tumors rather than early-stage diagnosis [25].

## Determination of Salivary Cortisol

Cortisol-binding globulin (CBG) is absent in saliva, and salivary cortisol measurement is a sensitive alternative method that does not require hospitalization. The diagnostic accuracy of a single midnight salivary cortisol level has been demonstrated in several studies. Salivary cortisol concentration shows diurnal variability. It has been found to be approximately 5.6 ng/ml (15.4 nmol/L) at 8-9 pm and approximately 1 ng/ml (2.8 nmol/L) at 23 pm. Salivary cortisol and cortisone in late-night samples and after the dexamethasone suppression test showed high accuracy for diagnosing CS, with salivary cortisone being slightly but significantly better [26 - 28]. The threshold values of the test vary depending on the method used. In one study, a salivary cortisol value higher than 2.0 ng/ml (5.5 nmol/L) was reported to have 100% sensitivity and 96% specificity for the diagnosis of CS [26, 29, 30]. The important point is that midnight salivary cortisol tends to increase in cardiovascular comorbid conditions such as age, diabetes, and hypertension; therefore, its discriminatory power decreases in the elderly population [31].

## Urine Cortisol Determination

24-hour urinary excretion of free cortisol is a good screening test. Specific structural-based assay techniques such as high-performance liquid chromatography (HPLC) and tandem mass spectrometry (TMS) are becoming the gold standard [31]. This method is integrated with plasma-free cortisol measurement. When cortisol secretion increases, exceeding the binding capacity of CBG results in an increase in urinary-free cortisol. Despite its widespread use, urinary-free cortisol is less sensitive than salivary cortisol and dexamethasone suppression tests. Due to patient errors in sample collection and episodic cortisol secretion, especially in adrenal adenomas, patients should collect two or three consecutive samples. Normal values can be found in 8-15% of patients with CS [29, 32]. Measurement of the cortisol/creatinine ratio in the first urine sample after waking up eliminates the need for time for sample collection and can be used as a screening test, especially when cyclic CS is suspected [33]. A cortisol/creatinine ratio above 25 nmol/mmol in repeated measurements is indicative of hypercortisolism [34].

### Dexamethasone Suppression Tests (DST)

1. Low-Dose Dexamethasone Suppression Tests.

In normal subjects, supraphysiologic doses of glucocorticoids result in suppression of ACTH and cortisol secretion. In CS, there is no suppression when low doses of dexamethasone are given, regardless of the cause [34].

2. High Dose Dexamethasone Suppression Tests.

2 mg dexamethasone is given every 6 hours for 48 hours, and plasma or urine-free cortisol is measured at 0 and 48 hours. Suppression of plasma cortisol by more than 50 percent is defined as a positive response [35].

### Adrenocorticotropic Hormone (ACTH)

This test distinguishes ACTH-dependent causes from ACTH-independent causes. It is not affected by cortisol-binding globulin (KBG) and is heat labile. If not collected on ice, it undergoes proteolysis, and its plasma value decreases. While cortisol is measured in serum, ACTH is measured in plasma. Measurement of ACTH in saliva has not been reported; frequent ACTH measurement may be useful in the evaluation of hypercortisolism. In the diagnosis of ACTH-independent CS, a morning ACTH level that cannot be measured by a sensitive method is valuable [36, 37].

### Inferior Petrosal Sinus Sampling (IPSS)

IPSS is considered the gold standard method in the differentiation of pituitary and ectopic ACTH-dependent Cushing's picture, but it requires experience because it is invasive [38]. After catheterization of both petrosal sinuses, CRH is administered intravenously at a dose of 100 μg. Blood is collected for ACTH measurement before and at 2, 5, and 10 minutes after CRH administration. If the central/peripheral ACTH ratio is >2 in basal measurement and >3 after CRH administration, it is interpreted in favor of CS [39].

## Metabolic Effects of Cushing's Syndrome

### *Cardiometabolic Complications in Cushing's Syndrome*

Elevated circulating endogenous glucocorticoids are associated with morbidity and mortality, including MetS, cardiovascular events, elevated blood glucose, bone fractures, neurovascular disorders, and psychiatric disorders. The elimination of hypercortisolemia may not always lead to remission of these clinical disorders [40].

In a study on mortality in cases with CS, cardiovascular diseases, malignancy, infections, and cerebrovascular accident (SVA) were reported to be 23.4%, 19%, 17%, and 12.8%, respectively, among the causes of mortality. As seen in the studies, cardiovascular diseases are the most important cause of mortality and morbidity in CS [41]. The increase in cardiovascular risks persisting 5 years after surgery is due to increased waist-to-hip ratio, diastolic hypertension, increased total/HDL ratio, and increased plasma fibrinogen.

### *Impact on Lipid Profile*

Dyslipidemia is important in terms of cardiovascular risks in patients with Cushing's syndrome and subclinical CS [42]. Its prevalence has been found to be 20-71% in patients with CS [43]. Triglyceride and total cholesterol levels are found to be increased in patients diagnosed with CS, whereas HDL levels have been found to vary. Direct and indirect effects of cortisol on lipolysis, free fatty acid production, VLDL production, and fat accumulation in the liver are responsible for the pathogenesis.

Glucocorticoids are involved in the differentiation, function, and distribution of adipose tissue. The effect of glucocorticoids on lipid metabolism is regulated in a controlled manner, both in the direction of lipolysis and lipogenesis. In addition, the effects of glucocorticoids on lipid metabolism may vary according to acute or chronic hypercortisolism [44].

Cortisol activates lipoprotein lipase activity in adipose tissue and lipolysis in visceral adipose tissue *in vitro*, thus increasing the circulation of free fatty acids. The increase in free fatty acids increases hepatic fat accumulation, resulting in decreased glucose uptake into the liver and activation of serine kinases, leading to a decrease in insulin signaling levels. Glucocorticoids have been shown to contribute to IR through this pathophysiologic mechanism in addition to IR due to their own effects. Studies on mouse liver models have shown that when liver-specific glucocorticoid receptors are blocked, steatosis regresses and hepatic triglyceride levels normalize. Hepatic steatosis of around 20% has been reported in patients with CS. While VLDL, LDL, triglyceride, and cholesterol levels were found to be high in patients with CS, no similar elevation was observed in HDL levels [42].

## Impact on Systemic Hypertension

Hypertension is a common manifestation of CS, with a prevalence of 70-85%. Factors such as the mineralocorticoid effect of cortisol, RAAS activation, and changes in vasoregulatory systems (increase in vasoconstriction, decrease in vasodilation) have been held responsible for the pathogenesis [45].

Considering these mechanisms, the mineralocorticoid effect of cortisol is thought to be majorly responsible for hypertension developing in hypercortisolism [43]. In healthy individuals, blood pressure has a diurnal rhythm, and blood pressure is expected to be lower at night in relation to sleep [46]. A decrease in blood pressure by 20-25% at night is called the 'Dipping Phenomenon'. It has been observed that this mechanism is preserved in many hypertensive patients. In hypertension seen in endogenous CS, the circadian rhythm of blood pressure, which is expected to be lower at night, is lost. The disruption of this diurnal rhythm of blood pressure has been associated with many undesirable effects, including stroke, increased target organ damage, faster progression to albuminuria, and left ventricular hypertrophy, which increases the risk of cardiovascular mortality [47]. It has been observed that the prevalence of hypertension is much lower in iatrogenic Cushing's cases in a dose-dependent manner [48]. The pathophysiology of hypertension in Cushing's syndrome is shown in Table5 [48].

**Table 5. Pathophysiology of hypertension in Cushing's syndrome.**

| |
|---|
| • Mineralocorticoid effect of cortisol. |
| • Inhibition of vasodilator systems. |
| • Activation of the RAA system. |
| • Increased cardiac output. |
| • Increased peripheral system resistance. |
| • Increased binding of cortisol to mineralocorticoid receptors. |
| • Insulin resistance and sleep apnea syndrome. |
| • Increased beta receptor sensitivity to catecholamines. |

Increased peripheral system resistance: Glucocorticoids increase the levels of ET1, a vasoconstrictor agent, and ET-1 levels have been found to be elevated in patients with CS. Glucocorticoids cause the downregulation of the Na-Ca pump in vascular smooth muscle, resulting in increased cytosolic Ca constriction and vasoconstriction. In addition, glucocorticoids increase EPO levels, which are known to have a direct vasoconstrictor effect. All these mediators are thought to play a role in the pathogenesis of cortisol-induced hypertension [48].

## Impact on metabolic syndrome and abdominal obesity

Visceral obesity, hypertension, IR, and dyslipidemia are common features in patients with CS. Abdominal obesity is associated with decreased peripheral insulin sensitivity and hepatic insulin secretion. IR is a prerequisite for the development of MetS. In the case of hypercortisolism, IR and abdominal obesity stimulate gluconeogenesis, leading to MetS. IR and MetS have been shown to be partially persistent after short and long-term disease remission. After disease remission in Cushing's disease, hypertension persists in 40% of patients, obesity or overweight in 70%, glucose intolerance or diabetes mellitus in 60%, and dyslipidemia in 30% [49 - 51].

Glucocorticoid excess has been shown to be associated with MetS. Increased glucocorticoid levels in the body have been shown to lead to metabolic disorders with MS components, such as central obesity, hypertension, hyperlipidemia, and glucose intolerance. These clinical findings suggest that glucocorticoids play a role in the pathogenesis of MetS [43]. It is observed that clinical findings such as obesity, hypertension, and glucose intolerance seen in CS are included in the diagnostic criteria for MetS. It has been observed that two-thirds of CS patients fulfill all 5 diagnostic criteria of MetS [52].

Abdominal visceral obesity is a common condition in patients with CS. It is characterized by an increased waist/hip circumference ratio and is considered an independent risk factor for cardiovascular disease and diabetes. In the pathogenesis of visceral obesity in CS, the role of glucocorticoids in adipocyte differentiation and their effects on lipoprotein lipase activity are more effective in visceral tissue adipocytes than in subcutaneous adipocytes [52 - 54].

## CONCLUSION

Technological advances during the past decade have greatly improved the biochemical and radiologic diagnosis of CS. Since the prevalence of MetS is estimated to be about one-fourth of the worldwide adult population, and CS is significantly rarer (estimated incidence of 2 per million), the presence of moon face, hirsutism, buffalo hump, central obesity, hypertension, hyperglycemia, mood disorders, psychosis, immunosuppression, osteoporosis, muscle weakness or peptic ulcer should suggest CS. No single symptom or finding is pathognomonic for CS, but the simultaneous presence of multiple signs or symptoms should be a warning sign. CS shares many features with a far more prevalent disorder, the MetS. Both syndromes are characterized by abdominal obesity, glucose impairment, insulin resistance, dyslipidemia, and arterial hypertension. These conditions may persist even after remission of CS and presumably contribute to maintaining, to some extent, the risk of cardiovascular morbidity. Efficient treatment of hypercortisolism helps to improve all the components of MetS.

## REFERENCES

[1]     Zimmet P, Magliano D, Matsuzawa Y, Alberti G, Shaw J. The metabolic syndrome: a global public health problem and a new definition. J Atheroscler Thromb 2005; 12(6): 295-300.
        [http://dx.doi.org/10.5551/jat.12.295] [PMID: 16394610]

[2]     Hruby A, Hu FB. The Epidemiology of Obesity: A Big Picture. PharmacoEconomics 2015; 33(7): 673-89.
        [http://dx.doi.org/10.1007/s40273-014-0243-x] [PMID: 25471927]

[3]     Decani S, Federighi V, Baruzzi E, Sardella A, Lodi G. Iatrogenic Cushing's syndrome and topical steroid therapy: case series and review of the literature. J Dermatolog Treat 2014; 25(6): 495-500.
        [http://dx.doi.org/10.3109/09546634.2012.755252] [PMID: 23210698]

[4]     Bovolini A, Garcia J, Andrade MA, Duarte JA. Metabolic Syndrome Pathophysiology and Predisposing Factors. Int J Sports Med 2021; 42(3): 199-214.
        [http://dx.doi.org/10.1055/a-1263-0898] [PMID: 33075830]

[5]     Executive Summary of the Third Report of the National Cholesterol Education Program (NCEP) Expert Panel on Detection, Evaluation, and Treatment of High Blood Cholesterol in Adults (Adult Treatment Panel III). JAMA 2001; 285(19): 2486-97.
        [http://dx.doi.org/10.1001/jama.285.19.2486] [PMID: 11368702]

[6]     The IDF consensus worldwide definition of the metabolic syndrome http://www.idf.org/webdata/docs/Metabolic_syndrome_definition.pdf

[7]     Alberti KG, Zimmet PZ. Definition, diagnosis and classification of diabetes mellitus and its complications. Part 1: diagnosis and classification of diabetes mellitus provisional report of a WHO consultation. Dia Med 1998; 15: 539e53.

[8]     Huang PL. A comprehensive definition for metabolic syndrome. Dis Model Mech 2009; 2(5-6): 231-7.
        [http://dx.doi.org/10.1242/dmm.001180] [PMID: 19407331]

[9]     Reincke M, Fleseriu M. Cushing Syndrome. JAMA 2023; 330(2): 170-81.
        [http://dx.doi.org/10.1001/jama.2023.11305] [PMID: 37432427]

[10]    Duan K, Hernandez KG, Mete O. Clinicopathological correlates of adrenal Cushing's syndrome. J Clin Pathol 2015; 68(3): 175-86.
        [http://dx.doi.org/10.1136/jclinpath-2014-202612] [PMID: 25425660]

[11]    Raff H, Sharma ST, Nieman LK. Physiological basis for the etiology, diagnosis, and treatment of adrenal disorders: Cushing's syndrome, adrenal insufficiency, and congenital adrenal hyperplasia. Compr Physiol 2014; 4(2): 739-69.
        [http://dx.doi.org/10.1002/cphy.c130035] [PMID: 24715566]

[12]    Reimondo G, Pia A, Bovio S, *et al.* Laboratory differentiation of Cushing's syndrome. Clin Chim Acta 2008; 388(1-2): 5-14.

[http://dx.doi.org/10.1016/j.cca.2007.10.036] [PMID: 18053807]

[13]    Kirk LF Jr, Hash RB, Katner HP, Jones T. Cushing's disease: clinical manifestations and diagnostic evaluation. Am Fam Physician 2000; 62(5): 1119-1127, 1133-1134. [published correction appears in Am Fam Physician 2002 Feb 1;65(3):386].
[PMID: 10997535]

[14]    Bertagna X, Guignat L, Groussin L, Bertherat J. Cushing's disease. Best Pract Res Clin Endocrinol Metab 2009; 23(5): 607-23.
[http://dx.doi.org/10.1016/j.beem.2009.06.001] [PMID: 19945026]

[15]    Buliman A, Tataranu LG, Paun DL, Mirica A, Dumitrache C. Cushing's disease: a multidisciplinary overview of the clinical features, diagnosis, and treatment. J Med Life 2016; 9(1): 12-8.
[PMID: 27974908]

[16]    Ohmori N, Nomura K, Ohmori K, Kato Y, Itoh T, Takano K. Osteoporosis is more prevalent in adrenal than in pituitary Cushing's syndrome. Endocr J 2003; 50(1): 1-7.
[http://dx.doi.org/10.1507/endocrj.50.1] [PMID: 12733704]

[17]    Wagner-Bartak NA, Baiomy A, Habra MA, *et al.* Cushing Syndrome: Diagnostic Workup and Imaging Features, With Clinical and Pathologic Correlation. AJR Am J Roentgenol 2017; 209(1): 19-32.
[http://dx.doi.org/10.2214/AJR.16.17290] [PMID: 28639924]

[18]    Saad-Omer SM, Kinaan M, Matos M, Yao H. Exogenous Cushing Syndrome and Hip Fracture Due to Over-the-Counter Supplement (Artri King). Cureus 2023; 15(7): e41278.
[http://dx.doi.org/10.7759/cureus.41278] [PMID: 37405128]

[19]    Braun LT, Riester A, Oßwald-Kopp A, *et al.* Toward a Diagnostic Score in Cushing's Syndrome. Front Endocrinol (Lausanne) 2019; 10: 766.
[http://dx.doi.org/10.3389/fendo.2019.00766] [PMID: 31787931]

[20]    Hoenig LJ. The Buffalo Hump of Cushing Syndrome. Clin Dermatol 2022; 40(5): 617-8.
[http://dx.doi.org/10.1016/j.clindermatol.2021.08.018] [PMID: 36509510]

[21]    Wright K, van Rossum EFC, Zan E, *et al.* Emerging diagnostic methods and imaging modalities in cushing's syndrome. Front Endocrinol (Lausanne) 2023; 14: 1230447.
[http://dx.doi.org/10.3389/fendo.2023.1230447] [PMID: 37560300]

[22]    Slagboom TNA, Stenvers DJ, van de Giessen E, *et al.* Continuing Challenges in the Definitive Diagnosis of Cushing's Disease: A Structured Review Focusing on Molecular Imaging and a Proposal for Diagnostic Work-Up. J Clin Med 2023; 12(8): 2919.
[http://dx.doi.org/10.3390/jcm12082919] [PMID: 37109254]

[23]    Bashari WA, Gillett D, MacFarlane J, *et al.* Modern imaging in Cushing's disease. Pituitary 2022; 25(5): 709-12.
[http://dx.doi.org/10.1007/s11102-022-01236-w] [PMID: 35666391]

[24]    Grigoryan S, Avram AM, Turcu AF. Functional imaging in ectopic Cushing syndrome. Curr Opin Endocrinol Diabetes Obes 2020; 27(3): 146-54.
[http://dx.doi.org/10.1097/MED.0000000000000541] [PMID: 32250975]

[25]    Hou G, Jiang Y, Li F, Cheng X. Use of [18]F-FDG PET/CT to Differentiate Ectopic Adrenocorticotropic Hormone-Secreting Lung Tumors From Tumor-Like Pulmonary Infections in Patients With Ectopic Cushing Syndrome. Front Oncol 2021; 11: 762327.
[http://dx.doi.org/10.3389/fonc.2021.762327] [PMID: 34692551]

[26]    Fleseriu M. Salivary Cortisol in the Diagnosis of Cushing Syndrome, Always More Than One! J Endocr Soc 2020; 4(10): bvaa109.
[http://dx.doi.org/10.1210/jendso/bvaa109] [PMID: 32939437]

[27]    Petersenn S. Biochemical diagnosis of Cushing's disease: Screening and confirmatory testing. Best Pract Res Clin Endocrinol Metab 2021; 35(1): 101519.

[http://dx.doi.org/10.1016/j.beem.2021.101519] [PMID: 33757676]

[28] Bäcklund N, Brattsand G, Israelsson M, *et al.* Reference intervals of salivary cortisol and cortisone and their diagnostic accuracy in Cushing's syndrome. Eur J Endocrinol 2020; 182(6): 569-82.
[http://dx.doi.org/10.1530/EJE-19-0872] [PMID: 32213657]

[29] Garrahy A, Forde H, O'Kelly P, *et al.* The diagnostic utility of late night salivary cortisol (LNSF) and cortisone (LNSE) in Cushing's syndrome. Ir J Med Sci 2021; 190(2): 615-23.
[http://dx.doi.org/10.1007/s11845-020-02334-z] [PMID: 32803648]

[30] Yaneva M, Mosnier-Pudar H, Dugué MA, Grabar S, Fulla Y, Bertagna X. Midnight salivary cortisol for the initial diagnosis of Cushing's syndrome of various causes. J Clin Endocrinol Metab 2004; 89(7): 3345-51.
[http://dx.doi.org/10.1210/jc.2003-031790] [PMID: 15240613]

[31] Liu H, Bravata DM, Cabaccan J, Raff H, Ryzen E. Elevated late-night salivary cortisol levels in elderly male type 2 diabetic veterans. Clin Endocrinol (Oxf) 2005; 63(6): 642-9.
[http://dx.doi.org/10.1111/j.1365-2265.2005.02395.x] [PMID: 16343098]

[32] Casals G, Hanzu FA. Cortisol Measurements in Cushing's Syndrome: Immunoassay or Mass Spectrometry? Ann Lab Med 2020; 40(4): 285-96.
[http://dx.doi.org/10.3343/alm.2020.40.4.285] [PMID: 32067427]

[33] Schäfer I, Rehbein S, Holtdirk A, *et al.* Diagnostic cut-off values for the urinary corticoid:creatinine ratio for the diagnosis of canine Cushing's syndrome using an automated chemiluminescent assay. Vet Clin Pathol 2023; 52(3): 443-51.
[http://dx.doi.org/10.1111/vcp.13219] [PMID: 37204225]

[34] Melmed S, Polonsky KS, Larsen PD, Kronenberg HM. Williams textbook of Endocrinology. In: Stewart PM, Newell-Price JDC, Eds. The Adrenal Cortex. 13th ed. Elsevier Canada 2016; pp. 489-555.

[35] Qiao J, Li J, Zhang W, *et al.* The usefulness of the combined high-dose dexamethasone suppression test and desmopressin stimulation test in establishing the source of ACTH secretion in ACTH-dependent Cushing's syndrome. Endocr J 2021; 68(7): 839-48.
[http://dx.doi.org/10.1507/endocrj.EJ20-0837] [PMID: 33790062]

[36] Cunningham JM, Buxton OM, Weiss RE. Circadian variation in Cushing's disease and pseudo-Cushing states by analysis of cortisol and adrenocorticotropin pulsatility. J Endocrinol Invest 2002; 25: 791-9.
[http://dx.doi.org/10.1007/BF03345514] [PMID: 12398238]

[37] Espinosa-Cardenas E, Garcia-Saenz M, de los Monteros-Sanchez ALE, Sosa-Eroza E. Non-Invasive Biochemical Testing of ACTH-dependent Cushing's Disease: Do We Still Need Petrosal Sinus Sampling? Arch Med Res 2023; 54(8): 102882.
[http://dx.doi.org/10.1016/j.arcmed.2023.102882] [PMID: 37749028]

[38] Detomas M, Ritzel K, Nasi-Kordhishti I, *et al.* Bilateral inferior petrosal sinus sampling with human CRH stimulation in ACTH-dependent Cushing's syndrome: results from a retrospective multicenter study. Eur J Endocrinol 2023; 188(5): 448-56.
[http://dx.doi.org/10.1093/ejendo/lvad050]

[39] Vassiliadi DA, Mourelatos P, Kratimenos T, Tsagarakis S. Inferior petrosal sinus sampling in Cushing's syndrome: usefulness and pitfalls. Endocrine 2021; 73(3): 530-9.
[http://dx.doi.org/10.1007/s12020-021-02764-4] [PMID: 34080096]

[40] Webb SM, Valassi E. Morbidity of Cushing's Syndrome and Impact of Treatment. Endocrinol Metab Clin North Am 2018; 47(2): 299-311.
[http://dx.doi.org/10.1016/j.ecl.2018.01.001] [PMID: 29754633]

[41] Arnaldi G, Angeli A, Atkinson AB, *et al.* Diagnosis and complications of Cushing's syndrome: a consensus statement. J Clin Endocrinol Metab 2003; 88(12): 5593-602.

[http://dx.doi.org/10.1210/jc.2003-030871] [PMID: 14671138]

[42]   Ivović M, Marina LV, Šojat AS, *et al.* Approach to the Patient with Subclinical Cushing's Syndrome. Curr Pharm Des 2020; 26(43): 5584-90.
[http://dx.doi.org/10.2174/1381612826666200813134328] [PMID: 32787757]

[43]   Pivonello R, De Martino MC, Iacuaniello D, *et al.* Metabolic Alterations and Cardiovascular Outcomes of Cortisol Excess. Front Horm Res 2016; 46: 54-65.
[http://dx.doi.org/10.1159/000443864] [PMID: 27212264]

[44]   Salehidoost R, Korbonits M. Glucose and lipid metabolism abnormalities in C ushing's syndrome. J Neuroendocrinol 2022; 34(8): e13143.
[http://dx.doi.org/10.1111/jne.13143] [PMID: 35980242]

[45]   Isidori AM, Graziadio C, Paragliola RM, *et al.* The hypertension of Cushing's syndrome. J Hypertens 2015; 33(1): 44-60.
[http://dx.doi.org/10.1097/HJH.0000000000000415] [PMID: 25415766]

[46]   Singh Y, Kotwal N, Menon AS. Endocrine hypertension - Cushing's syndrome. Indian J Endocrinol Metab. 2011;15 Suppl 4(Suppl4):S313-S316.

[47]   Pecori Giraldi F, Toja P, Martin M, *et al.* Circadian blood pressure profile in patients with active Cushing's disease and after long-term cure. Horm Metab Res 2007; 39(12): 908-14.
[http://dx.doi.org/10.1055/s-2007-992813] [PMID: 18046661]

[48]   Cicala MV, Mantero F. Hypertension in Cushing's syndrome: from pathogenesis to treatment. Neuroendocrinology 2010; 92 (Suppl. 1): 44-9.
[http://dx.doi.org/10.1159/000314315] [PMID: 20829617]

[49]   Chanson P, Salenave S. Metabolic syndrome in Cushing's syndrome. Neuroendocrinology 2010; 92 (Suppl. 1): 96-101.
[http://dx.doi.org/10.1159/000314272] [PMID: 20829627]

[50]   Pivonello R, Faggiano A, Lombardi G, Colao A. The metabolic syndrome and cardiovascular risk in Cushing's syndrome. Endocrinol Metab Clin North Am 2005; 34(2): 327-339, viii.
[http://dx.doi.org/10.1016/j.ecl.2005.01.010] [PMID: 15850845]

[51]   Feelders RA, Pulgar SJ, Kempel A, Pereira AM. MANAGEMENT OF ENDOCRINE DISEASE: The burden of Cushing's disease: clinical and health-related quality of life aspects. Eur J Endocrinol 2012; 167(3): 311-26.
[http://dx.doi.org/10.1530/EJE-11-1095] [PMID: 22728347]

[52]   Ferraù F, Korbonits M. Metabolic Syndrome in Cushing's Syndrome Patients. Front Horm Res 2018; 49: 85-103.
[http://dx.doi.org/10.1159/000486002] [PMID: 29894989]

[53]   Ferraù F, Korbonits M. Metabolic comorbidities in Cushing's syndrome. Eur J Endocrinol 2015; 173(4): M133-57.
[http://dx.doi.org/10.1530/EJE-15-0354] [PMID: 26060052]

[54]   Geer EB, Islam J, Buettner C. Mechanisms of glucocorticoid-induced insulin resistance: focus on adipose tissue function and lipid metabolism. Endocrinol Metab Clin North Am 2014; 43(1): 75-102.
[http://dx.doi.org/10.1016/j.ecl.2013.10.005] [PMID: 24582093]

# CHAPTER 21

# Non-Alcoholic Fatty Liver Disease as a Cause and Consequence of Metabolic Syndrome

**Esma Altinoglu**[1,*]

[1] *Department of Internal Medicine, School of Medicine, Bahcesehir University, Istanbul, Turkey*

**Abstract:** The prevalence of non-alcoholic fatty liver disease (NAFLD), one of the most common liver diseases, is rapidly increasing worldwide, parallel to the global obesity epidemic. NAFLD can progress to steatohepatitis, which is a more severe form of liver disease characterized by hepatocyte injury, inflammation, and fibrosis. NAFLD is closely related to metabolic syndrome (MetS)/insulin resistance, and these relationships are the subject of active research. Other than in MetS, visceral adiposity and pro-inflammatory state are also key in the development of NAFLD. In addition to human genetic variants linked to NAFLD risk to date are genes involved in the regulation of lipid metabolism, providing support for the hypothesis that NAFLD is fundamentally a metabolic disease.

**Keywords:** Insulin resistance, Metabolic syndrome, Non-alcoholic fatty liver disease.

## INTRODUCTION

Non-alcoholic fatty liver disease (NAFLD) is defined by the presence of steatosis in over 5% of hepatocytes, absence of hepatocellular injury, and notable alcohol consumption [1 - 3]. The association between diabetes, liver disease, and gout has been recognized for 120 years and is strongly linked to insulin resistance. However, NAFLD was not acknowledged as a clinical entity until the 1980s [4,5]. Presently, NAFLD is a complex liver condition, which is also a multisystemic disorder defined with metabolic irregularities [1, 6, 7].

NAFLD is a complex liver condition that is viewed as the hepatic demonstration of metabolic syndrome (MetS), encompassing elevated plasma triglycerides, low HDL cholesterol, impaired fasting glucose levels, an increased waist circumference, and elevated blood pressure. Additionally, NAFLD can represent another facet of MetS, such as hyperuricemia, systemic inflammation (CRP), and

---
* **Corresponding author Esma Altinoglu:** Department of Internal Medicine, School of Medicine, Bahcesehir University, Istanbul, Turkey ; E-mail: esmaaltunoglu@yahoo.com

**Hafize Uzun & Seyma Dumur (Eds.)**

microalbuminuria [4]. NAFLD and MetS exhibit an inverse and reciprocal correlation, where MetS acts as both a cause and an effect [1,8]. According to recent evaluations, the frequency of NAFLD in adults ranged between 25% and 32% from 2009 to 2019 [6]. This prevalence aligns closely with the frequency observed in cases of MetS. Leit *et al.* discovered that around two-thirds of individuals with obesity and type 2 diabetes (T2DM) displayed hepatic steatosis. Approximately 50% of patients with hyperlipidemia and 50% of patients with essential hypertension also exhibited hepatic steatosis [9,10]. NAFLD carries the potential for adverse outcomes such as cirrhosis, hepatocellular carcinoma, the necessity for liver transplantation, and mortality. Approximately 1/5$^{th}$ of patients with NAFLD have the potential to advance to severe liver disease, with T2DM serving as a significant prognostic factor for unfavorable results [6]. Furthermore, NAFLD is also a common chronic liver disease among pediatric and adolescent populations, notably in those who are obese. It has also been identified in infants born to mothers with gestational diabetes [4,11]. Liver biopsy is the benchmark method for diagnosing NAFLD. State–of-the-art imaging tools, such as magnetic resonance spectroscopy (MRS) and computed tomography (CT), have also been employed. In contrast to the invasive nature of biopsy and the associated costs of MRS and CT, ultrasonography emerges as a cost-effective and readily accessible alternative within clinical settings [12]. Demographic variants are beingdeveloped for NAFLD and MetS. The various demographic factors have been identified, with specific studies revealing a higher prevalence of NAFLD among males than females within the MetS population. Males exhibit a greater susceptibility to grade 2 fatty liver, while females are more inclined towards grade 1. Moreover, the prevalence of NAFLD in females increases notably after the age of 50, a phenomenon attributed to estrogenic action [1]. The prevalence of NAFLD is comparatively higher among urban populations. The level of education plays a pivotal role in influencing both the onset and prevention of NAFLD. Individuals with higher educational levels tend to exhibit fewer adverse factors, such as eating disorders and obesity [1].

Obesity and insulin resistance are major risk factors for NAFLD. Various blood parameters have been identified as being associated with NAFLD and MetS. These blood parameters include total cholesterol, low-density lipoprotein (LDL), very low-density lipoprotein (VLDL), high-density lipoprotein (HDL), triglycerides (TG), AST, ALT, and fasting blood sugar (FBS). There is a significant correlation between FBS, TG, HDL-C (homeostasis model assessment -estimated insulin resistance), HOMA index ratio, and adiponectin [1, 13]. Dyslipidemia acts as an independent element in the progression of NAFLD. Physical activity and dietary patterns also contribute to the development of NAFLD. Elevated levels of ALT, AST, LDL-C, TG, and FBS and diminished HDL-C levels serve as alarming indicators for identifying NAFLD [1]. The liver produces glucose and very low-density lipoproteins (VLDLs) containing the majority of triglycerides. This involvement means that MetS and NAFLD share the same risk profiles [12].

**Pathogenesis**

Currently, "multiple-hit hypothesis" provides a more solid description of the NAFLD pathogenesis [5, 13]. According to the "multiple-hit hypothesis", there needs to be a dysfunction in adipocyte tissue triggered by genetic predispositions, host metabolic disorders, and environmental factors leading to a reduction in insulin sensitivity. The reduction in insulin sensitivity causes a decrease in liver fatty acid oxidation and intrahepatic accumulation of triglycerides (IHTG). Insulin resistance also triggers adipose-derived cytokines and hormones like tumor necrosis factor-alpha, interleukin-6, leptin, adiponectin, resistin, *etc*. Insulin resistance promotes the activation of protein kinase C-Delta and nuclear factor-Kappa B by elevated FFA and IHTG levels, together with raised production of diacylglycerols and other lipotoxins, leading to liver inflammation. Moreover, nutritional factors and gut microbiota also contribute to liver inflammation [4, 5, 13 - 16].

Both NAFLD and T2DM demonstrate insulin resistance (IR) in muscle and adipose tissue, which increases ectopic fat accumulation, induces lipotoxicity, impairs beta cell function, and causes excess free fatty acids (FFAs). Mitochondrial dysfunction increases oxidative and endoplasmic reticulum stress, and uncoupled oxidative phosphorylation causes chronic liver disease, NASH, to advance [5].

Other factors that trigger the evolution and progression of NAFLD include specific genes (*e.g.*, PNPLA, TMSF2, MBOOAT7, GCKR, and HSD17B13), environmental factors (*e.g.*, deficiency in nutrient-dense foods and/or lack of safe areas for physical activity), immunity, race, gut microbiota, *etc*. Moreover, NAFLD is observed more frequently in insulin resistance-correlated conditions like obstructive sleep apnea, hyperuricemia, hypo-testosteronemia in men, and polycystic ovary syndrome in women [5, 17]. As insulin resistance is considered one of the diagnostic criteria for MetS, its exacerbation can initiate mechanisms involving renal sodium reabsorption and sympathetic nervous system activity. The deficiency of insulin signaling in the endothelium further triggers vasoconstriction, ultimately resulting in hypertension among patients with MetS.

**NAFLD-> MAFLD**

In 2020, an international panel of experts led a consensus (Delphi consensus) proposing the term "metabolic dysfunction-associated fatty liver disease"

(MAFLD) [18]. To diagnose MAFLD, three out of these seven risk factors must be present: waist circumference, blood pressure, plasma triglycerides, plasma high-density lipoprotein-cholesterol, prediabetes, homeostasis model assessment of insulin resistance score, and plasma high sensitivity C- reactive protein. MAFLD is more acceptable than NAFLD in diagnosing cardiovascular and metabolic diseases [19].

## Treatment

Common traits of individuals with NAFLD are unhealthy diet and lack of physical activity. Hence, the first action item in the treatment of patients with NAFLD is to strive for a 5-10% weight loss. As fructose triggers de novo lipogenesis, endoplasmic reticulum stress, and liver inflammation, contributing to insulin resistance and dyslipidemia, high fructose consumption should be avoided [20, 21]. Instead, the recommended approach is the adoption of the Mediterranean diet, characterized by the consumption of plant-based foods, whole grains, olive oil, and fish. Switching to a mediterranean diet diminishes the progression of NASH by 23% [22]. Increased physical activity like aerobic and stretching exercises enhances hepatic and peripheral insulin sensitivity. Furthermore, weight loss reduces proinflammatory and oxidative stress markers, decreases intrahepatic lipids, and improves the gut microbiome [6, 22-24]. As previously emphasized, a minimum of 150 minutes per week of physical activity is recommended. It is crucial to effectively manage the comorbidities linked with NAFLD, such as diabetes, hypertension, coronary artery disease, and high cholesterol [25].

## Medical Treatment

***Glucagon-like peptide-1 receptor agonists (GLP-1):*** Drugs like liraglutide, semaglutide, duraglutide, exenatide, *etc.*, delay gastric emptying, reduce weight gain, and improve insulin sensitivity; hence, they are beneficial in NAFLD treatment.

***Sodium-glucose cotransporter 2 inhibitors:*** New diabetic drugs like empaglifozin, ipragliflozin, dapagliflozin, and canagliflozin inhibit the reabsorption of glucose by kidneys, hence decreasing blood glucose levels, which improves NAFLD treatment.

***Thiazolidinediones:*** This drug regulates insulin resistance in Type II diabetes and is the only antidiabetic drug that is shown to improve NAFLD. In addition, it is recommended to be used in nondiabetic patients with NAFLD who suffer from insulin resistance. It also improves liver histology [23].

## CONCLUSION

NAFLD is a complicated multisystem disease that is progressively rising worldwide, aligning with the increasing rates of type 2 diabetes and obesity. NAFLD is commonly followed by a later diagnosis of MetS and T2DM, thus establishing a strong association between them. Many factors have been implicated in the progression from hepatic steatosis to NAFLD, including altered lipid metabolism, mitochondrial dysfunction, oxidative stress, inflammatory cytokines, immune response, alterations in the gut microbiome, and others.

The key drivers of the disease among these mechanisms remain unclear. Some individuals with NAFLD have developed advanced liver disease and HCC. Managing NAFLD requires aggressive intervention involving a multidisciplinary healthcare team to facilitate weight loss, increased physical activity, and the management of cardiometabolic comorbidities.

## REFERENCES

[1]     Zohara Z, Adelekun A, Seffah KD, *et al.* The prospect of non-alcoholic fatty liver diseas in adult patients with mtabolic syndrome:A systematic review. Cureus 2023; 15(7): e41959.
[PMID: 37588314]

[2]     Guo X, Yin X, Liu Z, Wang J. Non-alcoholic fatty liver disease pathogenesis and natural producs for prevention and treatment. Int J Mol Sci 2022; 23(24): 15489.
[http://dx.doi.org/10.3390/ijms232415489]

[3]     Gofton C, Upendran Y, Zheng MH, George J. MAFLD: How is it different from NAFLD? Clin Mol Hepatol 2023; 29 (Suppl.): S17-31.
[http://dx.doi.org/10.3350/cmh.2022.0367] [PMID: 36443926]

[4]     Jensen T, Abdelmalek MF, Sullivan S, *et al.* Fructose and sugar: A major mediator of non-alcoholic fatty liver disease. J Hepatol 2018; 68(5): 1063-75.
[http://dx.doi.org/10.1016/j.jhep.2018.01.019] [PMID: 29408694]

[5]     El Hadi H, Di Vincenzo A, Vettor R, Rossato M. Cardio-metabolic disorders in non-alcoholic fatty liver disease. Int J Mol Sci 2019; 20(9): 2215.
[http://dx.doi.org/10.3390/ijms20092215] [PMID: 31064058]

[6]     Younossi ZM, Henry L. Zobair M. Younossi, Linda Henry; Understanding the Burden of Nonalcoholic Fatty Liver Disease: Time for Action. Diabetes Spectr 15 February 2024; 37 (1): 9–19.
[http://dx.doi.org/10.2337/dsi23-0010]

[7]     Adams LA, Anstee QM, Tilg H, Targher G. Non-alcoholic fatyy liver disease and cardiovascular disease and other extrahepatic diseases. Gut 2017; 66: 1138-53.
[http://dx.doi.org/10.1136/gutjnl-2017-313884] [PMID: 28314735]

[8]     Lutsey PL, Steffen LM, Stevens J. Dietary intake and the development of the metabolic syndrome: the Atherosclerosis Risk in Communities study. Circulation 2008; 117(6): 754-61.
[http://dx.doi.org/10.1161/CIRCULATIONAHA.107.716159] [PMID: 18212291]

[9]     Lyu J, Lin Q, Fang Z, Xu Z, Liu Z. Complex impacts of gallstone disease on metabolic syndrome and nonalcoholic fatty liver disease. Front Endocrinol (Lausanne) 2022; 13: 1032557.
[http://dx.doi.org/10.3389/fendo.2022.1032557] [PMID: 36506064]

[10]    López-Suárez A, Guerrero JMR, Elvira-González J, Beltrán-Robles M, Cañas-Hormigo F, Bascuñana-Quirell A. Nonalcoholic fatty liver disease is associated with blood pressure in hypertensive and

nonhypertensive individuals from the general population with normal levels of alanine aminotransferase. Eur J Gastroenterol Hepatol 2011; 23(11): 1011-7.
[http://dx.doi.org/10.1097/MEG.0b013e32834b8d52] [PMID: 21915061]

[11]    Mosca A, Della Corte C, Sartorelli MR, *et al.* Beverage consumption and paediatric NAFLD. Eat Weight Disord 2016; 21(4): 581-8.
[http://dx.doi.org/10.1007/s40519-016-0315-3] [PMID: 27565159]

[12]    Yang KC, Hung HF, Lu CW, Chang HH, Lee LT, Huang KC. Association of Non-alcoholic Fatty Liver Disease with Metabolic Syndrome Independently of Central Obesity and Insulin Resistance. Sci Rep 2016; 6: 27034.
[http://dx.doi.org/10.1038/srep27034] [PMID: 27246655] [PMCID: 4887873]

[13]    Grander C, Grabherr F, Moschen AR, Tilg H. Noon-alcoholic fatty liver disease:cause or effect of metabolic syndrome. Visc Med 2016; 32(5): 329-34.
[http://dx.doi.org/10.1159/000448940] [PMID: 27921044]

[14]    Buzzetti E, Pinzani M, Tsochatzis EA. The multiple-hit pathogenesis of non-alcoholic fatty liver disease (NAFLD). Metabolism 2016; 65(8): 1038-48.
[http://dx.doi.org/10.1016/j.metabol.2015.12.012] [PMID: 26823198]

[15]    Fabbrini E, Sullivan S, Klein S. Obesity and nonalcoholic fatty liver disease: Biochemical, metabolic, and clinical implications. Hepatology 2010; 51(2): 679-89.
[http://dx.doi.org/10.1002/hep.23280] [PMID: 20041406]

[16]    Musso G, Gambino R, Cassader M, Pagano G. Meta-analysis: Natural history of non-alcoholic fatty liver disease (NAFLD) and diagnostic accuracy of non-invasive tests for liver disease severity. Ann Med 2011; 43(8): 617-49.
[http://dx.doi.org/10.3109/07853890.2010.518623] [PMID: 21039302]

[17]    Yim JY, Kim J, Kim D, Ahmed A. Serum testosterone and non-alcoholic fatty liver disease in men and women in the US. Liver Int 2018; 38(11): 2051-9.
[http://dx.doi.org/10.1111/liv.13735] [PMID: 29517842]

[18]    Eslam M, Newsome PN, Sarin SK, *et al.* A new definition for metabolic dysfunction-associated fatty liver disease: An international expert consensus statement. J Hepatol 2020; 73(1): 202-9.
[http://dx.doi.org/10.1016/j.jhep.2020.03.039] [PMID: 32278004]

[19]    Cabandugama PK, Gardner MJ, Sowers JR. The renin angiotensin aldosterone system in obesity and hypertension: roles in the cardiorenal metabolic syndrome. Med.Clin. Med Clin North Am 2017; 101(1): 129-37.
[http://dx.doi.org/10.1016/j.mcna.2016.08.009] [PMID: 27884224]

[20]    Coronati M, Baratta F, Pastori D, Ferro D, Angelico F, Del Ben M. Added fructose in non-alcoohoolic fatty liver disease and in metabolic syndrome:A narrative review. Nutrients 2022; 14(6): 1127.
[http://dx.doi.org/10.3390/nu14061127] [PMID: 35334784]

[21]    Bence KK, Birnbaum MJ. Metabolic drivers of non-alcoholic fatty liver disease. Mol Metab 2021; 50: 101143.
[http://dx.doi.org/10.1016/j.molmet.2020.101143] [PMID: 33346069]

[22]    Alkhouri N, Poordad F, Lawitz E. Management of nonalcoholic fatty liver disease: Lessons learned from type 2 diabetes. Hepatol Commun 2018; 2(7): 778-85.
[http://dx.doi.org/10.1002/hep4.1195] [PMID: 30027137]

[23]    Hashida R, Kawaguchi T, Bekki M, *et al.* Aerobic vs. resistance exercise in non-alcoholic fatty liver disease: A systematic review. J Hepatol 2017; 66(1): 142-52.
[http://dx.doi.org/10.1016/j.jhep.2016.08.023] [PMID: 27639843]

[24]    Della Pepa G, Russo M, Vitale M, *et al.* Pioglitazone even at low dosage improves NAFLD in type 2 diabetes: clinical and pathophysiological insights from a subgroup of the TOSCA.IT randomised trial. Diabetes Res Clin Pract 2021; 178: 108984.

[http://dx.doi.org/10.1016/j.diabres.2021.108984] [PMID: 34311022]

[25]    Guzmán A, Navarro E, Obando L, *et al.* Effectiveness of interventions for the reversal of a metabolic syndrome diagnosis: An update of a meta-analysis of mixed treatment comparison studies. Efectividad de las intervenciones para revertir el diagnóstico del síndrome metabólico: actualización de un metaanálisis de comparación mixta de tratamientos. Biomedica 2019; 39(4): 647-62.
[http://dx.doi.org/10.7705/biomedica.4684]

# CHAPTER 22

# Metabolic Syndrome and COVID-19

**Neval Elgörmüş**[1,*]

[1] *Department of Microbiology, Faculty of Medicine, Istanbul Atlas University, Istanbul, Turkey*

**Abstract:** Metabolic syndrome (MetS) is a condition of abdominal diseases characterised by insulin resistance, obesity, atherogenic dyslipidaemia, hypertension, and hypercoagulability and is a serious risk factor for the development of cardiovascular diseases (CVD) and type II diabetes mellitus (T2DM) [1]. The outbreak of SARS-CoV-2 infection has been named Coronavirus Disease 2019 (COVID-19) by the World Health Organisation (WHO). MetS is emerging as a significant risk factor for worse outcomes in people with COVID-19. Metabolic diseases, especially chronic diseases related to diabetes, lead to heart disease and some neurodegenerative diseases in old age. With SARS-CoV-2, researchers all over the world have investigated the relationship between metabolic diseases and the virus. In fact, COVID-19 management is not different from the management of patients with severe and serious diabetes and the management of other critical illnesses. In the mortality and morbidity of COVID-19, the presence of comorbid diseases, especially diabetes (hypertension, obesity, diseases and drugs affecting the immune system, cardiovascular diseases, *etc.*) and advanced age are determinants. It has also been shown that patients with poor metabolic health are more susceptible to complications such as seizures, strokes, and encephalitis during COVID-19 due to factors accompanying previous illness. Chronic diseases are diseases that progress slowly, last three months or longer, are caused by more than one risk factor, usually show a complicated course, and affect the quality of life of the person. The end of COVID-19 as a global health emergency does not mean 'the end of COVID-19 as a global health threat'. The threat of different COVID-19 variants emerging that could cause new increases in morbidity and mortality remains. Monitoring and management of chronic diseases will not only positively change the course of COVID-19 but will also make it possible to use the limited resources in the health sector in the right way.

**Keywords:** COVID-19, Comorbid diseases, Chronic diseases, Diabetes mellitus, Hypertension, Metabolic syndrome, Obesity.

---

* **Corresponding author Neval Elgörmüş:** Department of Microbiology, Faculty of Medicine, Istanbul Atlas University, Istanbul, Turkey; E-mail: neyelgormus@yahoo.com

**Hafize Uzun & Seyma Dumur (Eds.)**

## INTRODUCTION

Metabolic syndrome (MetS) is a condition characterised by insulin resistance (IR), obesity, atherogenic dyslipidaemia, hypertension (HT), and hypercoagulability and is a serious risk factor for the development of cardiovascular diseases (CVD) and type II diabetes mellitus (T2DM). MetS was defined for the first time by the World Health Organisation (WHO) in 1998; IR and hyperglycaemia were emphasised in this definition [2]. In the aetiology of MetS, factors such as a sedentary lifestyle and high-calorie foods in the diet, as well as genetic factors, are effective. Although prothrombotic and proinflammatory conditions are not included in the diagnostic criteria, they are included under the title of MetS. Compared to individuals without MetS, the risk of developing atherosclerotic cardiovascular disease in the later years of life in individuals with MetS is increased 2-fold, and the risk of T2DM is increased 5-fold. In addition, sleep apnoea syndrome, asthma, gastroesophageal reflux, non-alcoholic fatty liver disease, gallstones, and depression may develop in relation to MetS [2, 3].

Report of cases of viral pneumonia of unknown cause in Wuhan, China, in December 2019, research on a new coronavirus strain was detected. COVID-19 caused by SARS-CoV-2, the so-called new coronavirus (CoV) disease, is a disease that affects human health and a threatening global problem. Although CoV is known as a family of RNA viruses that usually cause cold-like symptoms in humans, Severe Acute Respiratory Syndrome (SARS)-CoV and Middle East respiratory syndrome (MERS)-CoV, which belong to the same family, have shown that this family of viruses can cause more serious diseases. word "corona" means crown in Latin due to the resemblance of rod-like extensions on its surface to a crown [3].

Since the data records and observations of nations around the world vary considerably, it is very difficult to clearly determine the prevalence of COVID-19. The most typical symptoms of COVID-19 known so far are high fever, dry cough, and fatigue. These symptoms usually appear on the fifth day of the disease; however, in different cases, they have been found to vary over a range from the second to the fourteenth day. More rarely, headache, nasal congestion, general pain, loss of sense of taste and smell, diarrhoea, rashes on the body, and discolouration of the fingers are also observed in some patients. Research shows that 80% of cases survive the disease in a way that does not require serious medical intervention; however, in severe cases, the disease can turn into pneumonia, and artificial respiration methods may be needed. For those who have a mild illness, resting at home, antipyretic measures, and fluid intake are important. One out of every five people in contact with the disease has a severe illness. Individuals with chronic diseases such as diabetes, high blood pressure, lung and heart diseases, and elderly people are in the risk group. Apart from the elderly, children and young people are also likely to be infected and spread the disease to their environment. Cases have been identified in which people in this age group also had severe illness [4].

## METABOLIC SYNDROME AND ITS COMPONENTS

Different definitions were established by many associations. But the MetS components used today were determined with the common opinion of many associations in 2009. National Cholesterol Education Program (NCEP) Adult Treatment Panel (ATP) III (NCEP-ATP III) is one of the most widely used definitions among MetS criteria in the World [5].

Hyperglycaemia/IR, abdominal obesity, dyslipidaemia, and HT are the key determinants of the definition. Diagnostic criteria for MetS are:

- Obesity-increased waist circumference (>88 cm in women, >102 cm in men),
- Increased fasting blood glucose level (>100 mg/dL) or receiving antidiabetes treatment,
- High blood pressure (>130/85 mmHg) or receiving HT treatment,
- Two criteria associated with dyslipidaemia; high triglycerides (TG) (>150 mg/dL),
- Low high-density lipoproteins (HDL) (<50 in women and <40 mg/dL in men) [5]. The presence of three of these five criteria leads to the diagnosis of MetS. Among these criteria, obesity is among the controllable risk factors since it is generally associated with excess calorie intake and insufficient physical activity [6]. Over this 20-year period, cardiometabolic health has also significantly worsened, primarily related to worsening levels of adiposity and glucose, as well as increasing blood pressure. In addition, recent evidence shows that worldwide, about 3% of children and 5% of adolescents have MetS [7].

## RELATIONSHIP BETWEEN COVID-19 AND COMORBID DISEASE

Chronic diseases are diseases that progress slowly, last three months or longer, are caused by more than one risk factor, usually show a complicated course, and affect the quality of life of the person. These diseases, which are risk factors that increase case fatality rates in the COVID-19 pandemic, have become the leading cause of death in all developed or developing countries all over the World [8]. In fact, chronic diseases have created a silent global epidemic, and the COVID-19 pandemic has prepared a ground that increases the effects of the epidemic. According to the WHO, noncommunicable diseases (NCD), primarily cardiovascular diseases, cancers, chronic respiratory diseases, and diabetes, are responsible for 63% of all deaths worldwide. 80% of NCD deaths occur in low- and middle-income countries. While the mortality rate remains high, NCDs are preventable through effective interventions that tackle shared risk factors [9].

The first data on COVID-19 have increased our knowledge about the clinical features of the disease. In a multicentre epidemiological study conducted with 1099 patients in China, it was found that the median age was 47 years. The disease was also more common in men, with 52.1% and 23.7% of patients having at least one concomitant chronic disease, such as HT, DM, chronic obstructive pulmonary disease (COPD). In the same study, it was reported that 2.3% of the patients required invasive mechanical ventilation, 5.1% needed intensive care unit (ICU), and 1.4% died [10].

Early data have noted that the disease is more common and more severe in individuals with chronic diseases. In a study published in Wuhan in January 2020, 51% of 99 patients were found to have at least one chronic disease, and the majority of these diseases were cardiovascular diseases (CVD), cerebrovascular diseases (CVD), and DM [11]. Similarly, in a retrospective, multicentre cohort study conducted in China, it was shown that 48% of patients had comorbidities, the most common of which were HT (30%), DM (19%), and coronary artery disease (CAD) (8%). In this cohort study, which included 813 patients hospitalised with a diagnosis of COVID-19, it was reported that in-hospital mortality was higher in patients with DM (OR 2.85) and CAD (OR 21.4) [12].

In the case-population study (1139 cases and 11390 population controls), 444 (39.0%) were female, and the mean age was 69.1 years (SD 15.4). Despite being matched on sex and age, a significantly higher proportion of cases had pre- existing CVD (OR 1.98, 95% CI 1.62–2.41) and risk factors (1.46, 1.23–1.73) compared to controls. In addition, it was shown that comorbid diseases such as HT (OR 1.27), COPD (OR 1.35), DM (OR 1.5), and heart failure (HF) (OR 2.18) were found more frequently in cases compared to controls [13].

In the mortality and morbidity of COVID-19, the presence of comorbid diseases, especially diabetes (hypertension, obesity, diseases and drugs affecting the immune system, cardiovascular diseases, *etc.*) and advanced age are determinants [14 - 19].

## Diabetes Mellitus (DM) and COVID-19

Diabetes is a chronic inflammatory disease characterised by metabolic and cardiovascular complications. There are many studies showing that viruses cause or trigger chronic diseases such as DM [20]. Patients with DM are well known to be more prone to infection [21]. According to the WHO, over 420 million people worldwide have been diagnosed with DM [22]. DM, another global outbreak, is a chronic disease affecting approximately 9.3% of the world population (463 million) in the 20-79 age group, according to 2019 data [23, 24]. This disease is classified as a chronic MetS. The coexistence of two pandemics (dual pandemic) results in a large number of patients affected by both pandemics and poor prognosis in these patients. It has been reported that the rates of infection with COVID-19 and the development of severe pneumonia in diabetics are higher than those without diabetes; thus, mortality rates are also high [10, 15, 25, 26]. In the report of 72,314 COVID-19 cases published by the Chinese Centre for Disease Control and Prevention, it was shown that mortality in people with diabetes (7.3%) was approximately three times higher than in people without diabetes (2.3%) [27].

T1DM and T2DM are associated with an increased risk of COVID-19-related hospitalisation and severe outcomes, including mortality, particularly in people with poor glycemic control. Recent data have suggested an increased risk associated with the development of new-onset diabetes following COVID-19 hospitalization; however, longer-term follow-up data will determine if diabetes is permanent. Observational studies show small differences in risks and benefits associated with certain glucose-lowering therapies, which are likely to be confounded by indication. Results from several ongoing research studies of glucose-lowering therapies in people with COVID-19 are awaited, and currently, there are no clear indications to change guideline-recommended glucose-lowering therapies [28].

T2DM may contribute to amplifying the severity of COVID-19, while the liability to COVID-19 may increase the risk for T2DM. COVID-19 and T2DM-related processes form a vicious cycle, augmenting each other. Patients with T2DM may have an increased risk for severe outcomes of COVID-19, and T2DM may be an integral part of the post-COVID syndrome [29]. Patients with DM and comorbid conditions are at high risk of progression and severe course of COVID-19. SARS-CoV-2 increases the level of inflammatory mediators in the blood and the production of reactive oxygen species, which leads to acute lung damage and acute respiratory distress syndrome (ARDS). In severe cases of COVID-19, insulin and dipeptidyl peptidase 4 inhibitors are recommended; metformin and sodiumglucose cotransporter 2 inhibitors should be discontinued. Patients with diabetes and COVID-19 should follow general prevention rules, monitor glucose levels more often, eat well, and control other risk factors [30].

There have been studies linking SARS-CoV-2 infection with the development of T1DM [31 - 38]. The elevation of newly diagnosed T1DM in children and an increase in diabetic ketoacidosis (DKA) after the pandemic have been reported [31, 32].

Interferon response is very important in the fight against viruses. In COVID-19 patients, early interferon responses are suppressed, and the secondary maladaptive delayed and exaggerated interferon response leads to a cytokine storm and causes organ damage. Hypercoagulability in the microvascular bed, together with impaired endothelial-epithelial barrier functions triggered by cytokine storm, is responsible for the poor prognosis of the disease [15]. When cellular mechanisms triggered by COVID-19 are combined with pathological changes in diabetes-specific organs, the likelihood of a cytokine storm resulting in organ damage increases exponentially in individuals with diabetes. Interleukin-6 (IL-6), fibrinogen, ferritin, D-dimer, and C-reactive protein levels were found to be significantly higher in COVID-19-infected diabetic individuals compared to non-diabetic individuals [15]. In particular, in diabetic patients, exaggerated increases in lactate dehydrogenase (LDH), CRP, ferritin, D-dimer, low lymphocyte counts, and more diffuse computer tomography (CT) findings are indicators of poor prognosis [10].

Guo *et al.* [15] reported that in 24 patients, whether or not other comorbidities were present, SARS-CoV-2 pneumonia patients with diabetes had a severe clinical picture in terms of organ damage, inflammatory factors or hypercoagulability, worsening the prognosis compared to patients without diabetes. It is evident that people with diabetes are at high risk for COVID-19 infection and disease-related medical complications. This situation shows that more sensitivity should be shown in the diagnosis, treatment, and follow-up for COVID-19 in the approach to diabetic patients [39]. During the pandemic period, many diabetic patients had to cancel their routine controls in diabetes clinics. This situation, together with increased stress associated with social isolation and lack of physical activity, has laid the groundwork for worsening glycaemic and blood pressure control, making diabetic patients even more susceptible to COVID-19 infections [39].

COVID-19 infection in diabetic patients is associated with increased mortality. In patients with diabetes, both glycaemic regulation and stabilisation of comorbid conditions such as concomitant heart disease or kidney disease should be ensured. Diabetic patients, especially those with comorbidities, should be warned to comply with social isolation and other preventive measures for COVID-19 infection. Patients should be aware of the risk of hyperglycaemia and informed about medication dose changes. Interdisciplinary counselling with diabetologists, nutritionists, including remote (internet and web-based, online) follow-up systems, should be organised.

In hyperglycaemia and IR, which are indicators of diabetes, the synthesis of glycation end products, pro-inflammatory cytokines, and oxidative stress levels increase, as well as adhesion molecules that mediate tissue inflammation. This inflammatory process is thought to be the mechanism underlying the higher tendency of patients with diabetes to COVID-19 infection [17, 40]. It was concluded that pancreatic beta cell damage, cytokine-induced IR, hypokalemia, and drugs used in the treatment of COVID-19 (such as corticosteroids, lopinavir/ritonavir) may contribute to worsening glucose control in diabetic patients. Accordingly, it was stated that glucose control of diabetic patients with COVID-19 would be difficult [41]. The lung function of T2DM patients is affected in relation to hyperglycaemia and IR levels. In COVID-19 patients with T1DM and T2DM, IR is generally thought to worsen in association with hypokalaemia. It has been reported that hypokalaemia may adversely affect glucose control in patients with T1DM and T2DM, associated with downregulation of pulmonary ACE-2, impairment of angiotensin-2, and increased aldosterone secretion. Viral infection is the major trigger of ketoacidosis in people with T1DM, an autoimmune disease. When T1DM and T2DM are compared, according to retrospective results, T1DM patients have a higher risk of infection. However, mortality rates due to infection have been described as similar for both diabetic conditions [40, 41]. In a cohort of 551 patients hospitalized for COVID-19 in Italy, the authors found that 46% of patients were hyperglycemic, whereas 27% were normoglycemic. Using clinical assays and continuous glucose monitoring in a subset of those patients, the authors detected altered glycometabolic control with IR and an abnormal cytokine profile [42]. Even normoglycemic individuals had evidence of IR and increased cytokine levels.

COVID-19 may increase glucose levels, aggravate IR, and cause new-onset IR and chronic metabolic disorders that did not exist before the COVID-19 infection [43 - 45].

Hba1c gives an idea about the 3-month average blood glucose level by measuring glucosylated hemoglobin and is an important test for diagnosis, treatment follow-up, and prediction of risk factors for diabetes. There is a significant correlation between high HbA1c levels and increased all-cause mortality in diabetic patients. In COVID-19 patients, HbA1c levels were associated with low PaO2, coagulation disorders, and inflammatory processes. Mortality was higher in diabetic COVID-19 patients. The evaluation of diabetic COVID-19 patients with HbA1c levels and other prognostic markers may lead to early and advanced treatment options, thus reducing the mortality rate in DM [46].

Since diabetic patients with COVID-19 have a high mortality rate compared to the normal population, controlling diabetes and preventing fluctuations in blood glucose levels should be one of the main goals. Endocrinologists, in line with the recommendations of nutritionists, should aim to monitor blood glucose monitoring more closely by providing adequate information about the regulation of food consumption during the pandemic and the doses of drug use in this process in which we are in social isolation [47].

## Obesity and COVID-19

Several hypotheses have been postulated regarding the prognosis in obese COVID-19 patients. Obese individuals are at a greater risk for chronic diseases that increase the severity of COVID-19 disease. Clinical parameters of MetS and IR are frequently observed in these individuals. Morbid obese individuals are among the risk groups defined by the Centers for Disease Control (CDC) for severe COVID-19 [48]. These individuals often have clinical parameters of CVD and T2DM [49]. In addition, obesity causes a decrease in innate and adaptive immune responses. Increased body weight and abnormal accumulation of adipose tissue lead to harmful health consequences. One of the reasons for these unfavourable conditions is the increase in inflammation along with adipose tissue. Obesity, which is characterised by an excessive increase in adiposity, leads to increased cytokine production from preadipocytes and macrophages, resulting in an inflammatory response [50].

Because both diabetes and obesity trigger mechanisms that will lead to a cytokine storm, a worse inflammatory effect will occur in obese diabetic patients with the presence of COVID-19 infection. As the cytokine storm will increase IR, the glycaemic status will worsen [51]. Obesity is also associated with increased coagulopathy and thrombosis. Similarly, COVID-19 infection is also linked to thrombotic mechanisms and coagulation disorders. In addition, diabetics infected with COVID-19 have a higher D-dimer level than non-diabetics. Therefore, in the case of being infected with SARS-CoV-2, the presence of both diabetes and obesity is associated with a worse prognosis [51, 52]. Cariou *et al.* [53] showed in the Coronado study that body mass index (BMI) is an independent prognostic factor for COVID-19 severity and hospitalisation in the population with diabetes. Cai *et al.* [54] analyzed data from obese and overweight COVID-19 patients (n=383) in Shenzhen/China. They concluded that obese and overweight patients showed 2.4-fold greater and 86% higher odds, respectively, for developing severe pneumonia compared with normal-weight patients. He and Li [55] reported that obesity was consistently a significant risk factor for COVID-19 severity. They also showed that 17 risk factors affected the disease severity in 98 patients with COVID-19.

Obesity is a risk factor for many acute and chronic diseases, as well as respiratory infections. Obesity may, therefore, also be a risk factor for more severe COVID-19 disease, associated with a low-grade inflammatory state and a weakened immune system. Some studies show that there is a high rate of obesity in COVID-19 patients admitted to ICU and that BMI and disease severity increase in direct proportion [56 - 60]. Garg *et al.* [61] found that the comorbidity rate of patients hospitalised due to COVID-19 was 89.3%, and HT (49.7%) and obesity (48.3%) were the most common causes of comorbidity. Peng *et al.* [62] reported obesity along with CVD among the main comorbidities associated with high mortality risk in COVID-19 patients. However, some studies have shown that individuals with obesity are more likely to be COVID-19 positive than non-obese individuals [63, 64]. ACE2 expression in adipose tissue is higher than that in the lung tissue, and this shared viral tropism for both tissues may favor prolonged SARS-CoV-2 shedding in obese individuals [65]. It is also thought that vaccines developed for COVID-19 may be less effective in obese individuals due to a weakened immune response [66]. All these data show the importance of obesity in COVID-19 disease severity.

## Hypertension and COVID-19

Hypertension (HT) is the most common comorbidity in many epidemiological studies published on COVID-19. Many studies have shown that mortality and morbidity increase in COVID-19 patients with HT [67 - 70].

In an observational cohort study in which 1004 COVID-19-suspected patients from 25 hospitals in China were examined, 12% of 188 patients diagnosed with COVID-19 were found to have HT, while this rate was 7% in 816 patients who were not diagnosed [71]. In a multicentre study examining the impact of chronic diseases in 1590 COVID-19 patients in China, mortality was found to be higher in patients with HT (10.4%) compared to those without HT (1.7%) [72]. In a meta-analysis of four case-control studies including 1352 patients, HT was found to be the most common comorbidity, and it was reported that the risk of ICU admission increased (OR 2.54) in patients with HT [73]. In a study conducted in the United States of America (USA), 89.3% of 1482 patients hospitalised due to COVID-19 in 14 states had at least one chronic disease, with HT ranking first with a frequency of 49.7% [74]. ARDS and mortality risk factors in a retrospective cohort study were examined in COVID-19 patients and 201 patients. HT was detected in 27.4% of patients who developed ARDS, while this rate was 13.7% in those who did not develop ARDS, but no statistically significant difference was shown [75].

Like SARS-CoV, SARS-CoV-2 enters target cells by binding to angiotensin-converting enzyme 2 (ACE2) expressed on epithelial cells of the lung, kidney, and blood vessels. ACE2 expression is increased in HT and DM patients treated with ACE inhibitors or receptor blockers [76]. The idea that this potential up-regulation increases the risk of COVID-19 by increasing the entry pathway of the virus into host cells has been raised by many authors. On the other hand, it has been shown in animal experiments that ACE2 forms angiotensin 1-7 from angiotensin 2 and that the vasodilator effect that occurs in this way can reduce lung damage in viral pneumonia [68]. Similarly, it has been suggested that ACE2, which is down-regulated by SARS-CoV-2 spike (S) protein, can be increased by renin-angiotensin aldosterone system (RAAS) blockade, thus antagonising the effects of SARS-CoV-2 [77]. Conflicting information has been presented in post-mortem studies showing reduced ACE2 activation on myositis in patients treated with angiotensin receptor blockers (ARBs) [78]. In a joint statement, the American Heart Association and the American College of Cardiology (AHA/ACC) recommended the continuation of RAAS antagonists, which have proven to be beneficial in diseases such as HF, ischaemic heart disease, and HT, in COVID-19 patients [79]. In a case population study published in Madrid, it was shown that there was no increase in the risk of hospitalisation due to COVID-19 in patients using RAAS inhibitors, and there was no significant difference between long-term and short-term drug use. One of the important findings of this study was that the risk of hospitalisation due to COVID-19 was found to be less in DM patients using RAAS inhibitors (OR 0.53, p= 0.004) [13]. However, the association between HT and severe COVID-19 is still inconclusive [80 - 86]. In a recently published systematic review and meta-analysis, pre-existing hypertension is not an independent predictor of mortality during SARS-CoV-2 infection. Further studies should nevertheless be carried out worldwide to evaluate this role, independent of, or in interaction with, other confounders that may affect the mortality risk [86].

COVID-19 patients with HT should be carefully monitored for the need for mechanical ventilation and intensive care. Patients with a long-term diagnosis of HT and target organ damage should be rapidly transferred to hospitals providing advanced life support. The course of infection in patients treated with RAAS inhibitors and the role of these drugs in the management of COVID-19 will be the subject of many pre-clinical and clinical studies in future discussions.

**Cardiovascular Diseases (CVD) and COVID-19**

In COVID-19 patients, CVDs have been reported to be decisive in the course and mortality of the infection, although their frequency is lower than DM and HT among the accompanying comorbidities. As with other respiratory infections, pre-existing CVD and risk factors can increase the severity of COVID-19, leading to exacerbation and decompensation of underlying chronic cardiac pathologies, as well as new cardiac complications with acute onset.

Cardiovascular symptoms are diverse in COVID-19 patients [3, 10 - 12, 67, 86]. The susceptibility to SARS-CoV-2 infection and outcomes of COVID-19 are closely associated with pre-existing CVD [87].

COVID-19 may present a wide range of disease perspectives, such as myocardial damage, arrhythmias, sudden cardiac arrest, hypertension, HF, acute coronary syndrome, myocarditis, and pericarditis. The first sign of COVID-19 may be cardiovascular symptoms. It has been reported that 7.3% of COVID-19 patients complain of heart palpitations as the first symptom [88]. In a retrospective study involving 1590 patients from 575 hospitals in China, 3.7% of patients were found to have CVD [89]. In a study of 5700 COVID-19 patients hospitalised in New York, where more than 30% of cases were seen in the USA, 595 (11.1%) patients had CAD, and 371 (6.9%) patients had congestive HF [90].

Heart failure (HF) is one of the common diseases in COVID-19 patients [74]. Emerging or pre-existing heart failure complicates treatment management, worsens the clinical condition, or adversely affects the prognosis in COVID-19 patients. Effective use of haemodynamic and diagnostic tests such as electrocardiography (ECG), echocardiography (ECHO), invasive arterial blood pressure monitoring, and urine output monitoring is essential for the appropriate management of these patients. Abnormal changes in cardiac biomarkers (troponin T and I, NT-probnp) can be observed in COVID-19 disease. The most likely mechanisms are ACE-2-mediated myocardial damage, myocarditis, abnormal thrombotic activity, stress cardiomyopathy, and increased sympathetic activation [91 - 93]. A cytokine storm may be responsible for many of the observed mechanisms and presentations. Both the drugs used in the treatment of COVID-19 and the interaction of drugs used in the treatment of heart failure should be well known. Optimising drug-drug interactions is required.

Although respiratory symptoms seem to be at the forefront in COVID-19 patients, it has been shown that severe cardiac damage occurs, and the risk of death increases in case of underlying CVD [94]. In a meta-analysis by Wang *et al.*, it was found that the risk of serious illness was 3-4 times higher in those with CVD [95]. Similarly, in a meta-analysis including 1527 SARS-CoV-2-infected patients, it was found that the relative risk of CVD (RR=3.30, 95% CI) was higher in those who needed intensive care than in those who did not require intensive care follow-up [96]. In a study conducted in Washington state with severe COVID-19 patients, it was reported that acute HF may also develop in patients without previously known left ventricular dysfunction. It was observed that cardiomyopathy developed even in patients without significant pulmonary involvement [97]. In a multicentre study involving 168 patients who died due to SARS-CoV-2 in Wuhan, 74.4% of the patients were found to be accompanied by at least one chronic disease, and 18.5% had ischaemic heart disease [34]. According to the data obtained from 44,672 COVID-19 patients in China, including asymptomatic cases, the fatal rate was 0.9% in those without comorbid diseases, while this rate increased to 10.5% in those with CVD [98].

There is an increase in troponin levels in relation to disease severity and mortality in COVID-19, and severe viral infections cause "Systemic Inflammatory Response Syndrome (SIRS)" and increase the risk of plaque rupture and thrombus formation [99]. In a study investigating the impact of cardiovascular events in COVID-19 patients, increased troponin levels were more common in those with underlying CVD (13.2-54.5%), and complications such as ARDS, malignant arrhythmia and acute kidney injury were more common in those with high troponin levels [100]. Studies showing that SARS-CoV2 primarily attacks pericytes in the heart may explain the capillary endothelial cell dysfunction and the increase in cardiac damage markers [77].

In Sars-CoV-2 infection, approximately 6-17% develop various cardiac arrhythmias. Although these arrhythmias include ventricular arrhythmias, the prevalence of arrhythmias may increase up to 44% in patients requiring intensive care hospitalisation [66]. Although arrhythmias are less likely in clinically stable patients, the risk of arrhythmias is much higher in critically ill patients [100, 101]. Cardiac arrhythmias, including life-threatening VAs, may develop due to the effects of COVID-19 infection directly, the effects of systemic disease, or the side effects of some medications used in the pandemic [102]. A meta-analysis of 17 retrospective cohort studies including 5.815 COVID-19 patients showed that the incidence of cardiac arrhythmia was 9.3% (5.7% for cardiac arrest) [103]. Among 700 COVID-19 patients (mean age 50 ± 18 years, 45% male, 45% male, 71% African American, 11% treated in intensive care), 9 cardiac arrests, 25 episodes of atrial fibrillation (AF), 9 bradyarrhythmias and 10 non-sustained ventricular tachycardias (NSVTs) were observed. Arrhythmias occurring in patients admitted to the intensive care unit included cardiac arrest (all 9 cardiac arrest events occurred in this group), AF (OR 4.68 *versus* non-ICU patients), and NSVT (OR 8.92). Cardiac arrests have been associated with in-hospital mortality [104].

Myocardial injury is a common complication in hospitalised patients with or without prior CVD and is associated with increased in-hospital mortality and poor prognosis. Serial troponin monitoring as a prognostic marker is clinically important. In addition, as shown in retrospective studies, myocardial injury is associated with severe ventricular dysfunction and ventricular arrhythmias, and early diagnosis and treatment are clinically essential. The presence of CVD in patients infected with SARS-CoV-2 stands out as a poor prognostic factor. It should be kept in mind that patients with severe disease may also have newly developing HF and acute ischaemic heart disease.

### Lymphadenopathy and Infectious Disease

Lymphadenopathy may be a finding that causes the patient to consult a doctor, or it may be detected incidentally during the examination. Lymph node enlargement should be evaluated together with other symptoms and findings, and the cause should be clarified by making a differential diagnosis. While most lymphadenopathies, especially in children and young adults, develop due to viral or local bacterial infections, causes such as malignant disease or metastasis are increasing.

In the diagnosis of malignant lymph nodes, laboratory tests are performed before excisional lymph node biopsy to establish the diagnosis. Among laboratory parameters, acute phase reactants such as WBC, CRP, and erythrocyte sedimentation rate (ERS) take precedence. In addition, parameters such as neutrophils, monocytes, and lymphocytes may be used for bacterial, parasitic, and viral infectious etiology [105].

### LONG COVID SYNDROME

Although COVID-19 causes many symptoms in the acute period, it causes multisystem effects, requiring inpatient treatment and may lead to death in complicated cases. Long COVID syndrome, known as post-COVID syndrome, persistent COVID, or Long-Term COVID, has been defined due to the prolonged effects it causes after the acute period ends.

- **Acute COVID-19:** Symptoms and signs for up to 4 weeks.

- **Prolonged symptomatic period:** Presence of symptoms and signs persisting for 4-12 weeks.

- **Post-COVID-19 syndrome**: Symptoms and signs lasting longer than 12 weeks after COVID-19 infection are considered to be the exclusion of other causes to explain this condition.

Although the pathogenesis of this period is not clear, persistent hyperinflammatory process, ongoing viral activity in the host viral reservoir, inadequate antibody response, and long-term consequences of tissue tropism are held responsible for post-COVID-19 syndrome. However, the presence and extent of organ damage, the variability of the time required for the recovery of all organ systems, intensive care syndromes, COVID-19-related complications in the acute period, and side effects of the drugs used are also factors. In addition, conditions such as deconditioning and post-traumatic stress disorder may cause symptoms or increase existing symptoms. Re-infections or co-infections should not be ignored during this period [106].

A certain number of risk factors have been identified for post-COVID syndrome. The most important of these risk factors are acute disease period with severe course, being over 50 years of age, and underlying chronic diseases. In addition, although it is 2 times more common in women, the presence of 5 or more of the symptoms during the acute COVID process shows that the risk of developing prolonged COVID is higher in these patients. The risk of prolonged COVID syndrome increases in chronic diseases. The prolongation of COVID-19 is associated with these problems. Long COVID is associated with new-onset IR, which may contribute to the onset of depressive symptoms due to long COVID by enhancing overall neurotoxicity [107].

Post-COVID syndrome, the incidence of which varies between 10% and 60% in the light of new studies, may have symptoms involving many systems, such as fatigue, chest pain, shortness of breath, cough, decreased exercise intolerance, headache, and loss of taste and smell. In addition, palpitations, joint pain, muscle pain and weakness, insomnia, diarrhoea, rash or hair loss, balance and gait disturbance, memory and concentration problems, and cognitive problems, including worsening quality of life, may be observed [108].

In a study of 1733 COVID patients 6 months after discharge, 66% of patients had fatigue and muscle weakness, 26% had sleep problems, 23% had anxiety and depression, and 76% of patients had at least one symptom persisting in the long term. Although cardiac imaging was not used in this study, cardiac events were thought to accompany some of the patients who described weakness and fatigue [109].

Various symptoms affecting different systems of the body, such as neurocognitive, autonomic, cardiac, gastrointestinal, respiratory, musculoskeletal, psychological, dermatological, thromboembolic, and metabolic disorders, have been reported in patients recovering from infection [110, 111]. However, high blood pressure, obesity, and mental health status are risk factors for persistent post-COVID symptoms. It has been reported that young people without underlying chronic disease and even those who have a mild illness do not return to normal health status weeks after the illness and have difficulty performing their daily activities of daily living [112]. There are many studies showing that there is a relationship between pre-COVID-19 comorbidities and post-COVID-19 complaints [112 - 116]. Different opinions come to the fore regarding which comorbidities are risk factors. In a study of 1077 patients in the UK, a correlation was found between post-acute complaints and the presence of two or more comorbidities [113]. In a study conducted in Egypt in which 287 cases were analysed, asthma, diabetes, and hypertension were found to be associated with post-acute complaints in 83.3% of moderate and severe cases [116]. In a prospective cohort study involving 4182 patients from the UK, USA, and Sweden, only asthma among comorbidities was found to be statistically significantly associated with post-COVID-19 complaints [117].

Vimercati *et al.* [114] found that being overweight or obese was correlated with post-acute symptoms. In a prospective cohort study including 277 patients in Spain, no significant association was found with any comorbidity [118]. In a review of 27 articles, comorbidities, especially asthma and hypertension, were found to be risk factors for post-COVID complaints [119]. In another study, factors associated with persistent post-COVID-19 symptoms were reported as HT, chronic lung diseases, and having any chronic disease [112]. In a meta-analysis by Ceban *et al.*, the correlation of pre-infection comorbidities with post-COVID symptoms and decreased quality of life was shown in 9 studies [115]. In studies, HT has emerged as one of the important factors affecting the prognosis of COVID-19. In a retrospective, multicentre cohort study conducted in China, HT was found to be the most common comorbidity [120]. In the acute COVID-19 period, hypertensive patients had a higher mortality rate than normotensive patients [121]. One of the potential mechanisms causing this is ACE-2 receptor activity and pro-inflammatory response [122].

In studies, the association of hypertension with symptoms in the post-acute period has been found to be statistically significant, but specific studies directly examining this relationship are few. In a case-control study, 287 hypertensives and 287 controls were examined an average of 7.2 months after discharge; hypertensives reported three or more symptoms at a higher rate than normotensives. Hypertensives had a higher number of post-COVID-19 symptoms than normotensives. The most common symptom was found to be fatigue and dyspnoea occurring at rest and with movement. Migraine-like headaches and decreased sleep quality were reported to be more common in hypertensive patients. No difference was found between the two groups in terms of depression and anxiety [110].

Although different opinions emerge in studies, it is generally observed that comorbidities are associated with post-COVID-19 complaints; among these comorbidities, obesity, HT, and DM are at the forefront.

Different epidemiological data on the prevalence of Long COVID have been reported from different countries of the world [123, 124].

• Objective diagnostic criteria are not available.
• Long-COVID definitions are different.
• No consensus on diagnostic algorithms.
• Follow-up period after acute infection is different.
• Recording and reporting in the health system are different.
• Health system capacity is different.

Long-COVID-19 still has a limited amount of evidence-based knowledge. Diagnosis, evaluation and treatment plan should be managed using a multidisciplinary approach.

## CLINICAL IMPLICATIONS

MetS, IR, visceral obesity, hyperglycaemia, atherogenic hyperlipidaemia, and high blood pressure, as well as other features such as vascular inflammation, microalbuminuria, hyperuricaemia, and tendency to atherothrombosis, are among the most important and frequent causes of metabolic, cardiovascular and renal complications. Lifestyle modification is the most prioritised and effective approach in the prevention and treatment of MetS. In addition, pharmacological agents that reduce insulin resistance, improve blood pressure and serum lipid profile, and have been proven to prevent the development of T2DM and/or atherothrombotic events have a place in treatment. COVID-19 directly or indirectly affects the cardiovascular system. It is the role of ACE-2 that is recognised to be of high importance in the pathogenesis of COVID-19 due to its cardiovascular effects. Direct damage to infected myocardial cells through ACE-2 receptors can lead to an inflammatory storm or cause ARDS, leading to an oxygen supply-demand imbalance [125, 126]. It has been reported that myocardial damage may occur with COVID-19 infection by causing cytokine storm, respiratory dysfunction, hypoxaemia, shock, or hypotension due to the over-stimulation of T-Helper 1 and T-Helper 2 cells. This may lead to heart failure, liver and kidney damage, ARDS, shock, multiple organ failure, and death [127]. Optimal glycaemic control of patients with diabetes and COVID-19 can reduce, if not completely eliminate, the risks.

# CONCLUSION

MetS and its risk factors are among the most significant health problems of the 2000s. Therefore, prevention of MetS by identifying high-risk groups in advance is of great importance. Adipocyte dysfunction and high-grade inflammation with comorbidities such as diabetes, obesity, HT, and ischaemic heart disease cause a cytokine storm in COVID-19. While each of these comorbidities is responsible for high mortality with cytokine storm, mortality rates increase exponentially when they are present together. DM patients infected with SARS-CoV-2 should be hospitalised and closely monitored in the presence of advanced age, other comorbidities, and poor glycaemic control. HT is strongly associated with SARS-CoV-2 infection, possibly due to the proinflammatory state of this chronic disease in addition to hypocytokinemia that occurs in COVID-19. Detailed studies are needed to clarify the underlying pathophysiology of comorbidities (HT, DM, obesity, chronic diseases,..) and post-acute COVID-19 and to analyse the outcomes.

## REFERENCES

[1]     Huang PL. A comprehensive definition for metabolic syndrome. Dis Model Mech 2009; 2(5-6): 231-7.
        [http://dx.doi.org/10.1242/dmm.001180] [PMID: 19407331]

[2]     Dragsbæk K, Neergaard JS, Laursen JM, *et al.* Metabolic syndrome and subsequent risk of type 2 diabetes and cardiovascular disease in elderly women. Medicine (Baltimore) 2016; 95(36): e4806.
        [http://dx.doi.org/10.1097/MD.0000000000004806] [PMID: 27603394]

[3]     Huang C, Wang Y, Li X, *et al.* Clinical features of patients infected with 2019 novel coronavirus in Wuhan, China. Lancet 2020; 395(10223): 497-506.
        [http://dx.doi.org/10.1016/S0140-6736(20)30183-5] [PMID: 31986264]

[4]     Panahi Y, Gorabi AM, Talaei S, *et al.* An overview on the treatments and prevention against COVID-19. Virol J 2023; 20(1): 23.
        [http://dx.doi.org/10.1186/s12985-023-01973-9] [PMID: 36755327]

[5]     Meigs   JB.   2019.https://www-uptodate-com.qulib.idm.oclc.org/contents/metabolic-syndrome-ins-lin-resistance-syndrome-or-synd-ome-x?search=metabolic+syndrome+criteria+atp+iii&topicRef=15278&source=see_link

[6]     Neeland IJ, Poirier P, Després JP. Cardiovascular and Metabolic Heterogeneity of Obesity. Circulation 2018; 137(13): 1391-406.
        [http://dx.doi.org/10.1161/CIRCULATIONAHA.117.029617] [PMID: 29581366]

[7]     Noubiap JJ, Nansseu JR, Lontchi-Yimagou E, *et al.* Global, regional, and country estimates of metabolic syndrome burden in children and adolescents in 2020: a systematic review and modelling analysis. Lancet Child Adolesc Health 2022; 6(3): 158-70.
        [http://dx.doi.org/10.1016/S2352-4642(21)00374-6] [PMID: 35051409]

[8]     Organization   WHO.   Noncommunicable   diseases   https://www.who.int/news-room/fac--sheets/detail/noncommunicable-diseases

[9]     https://care2communities.org/2017/02/10/innovation-prevents-noncommunicable-diseases/

[10]    Guan W, Ni Z, Hu Y, *et al.* Clinical characteristics of coronavirus disease 2019 in China. N Engl J Med 2020; 382(18): 1708-20.
        [http://dx.doi.org/10.1056/NEJMoa2002032] [PMID: 32109013]

[11]     Chen N, Zhou M, Dong X, *et al.* Epidemiological and clinical characteristics of 99 cases of 2019 novel coronavirus pneumonia in Wuhan, China: a descriptive study. Lancet 2020; 395(10223): 507-13.
[http://dx.doi.org/10.1016/S0140-6736(20)30211-7] [PMID: 32007143]

[12]     Zhou F, Yu T, Du R, *et al.* Clinical course and risk factors for mortality of adult inpatients with COVID-19 in Wuhan, China: a retrospective cohort study. Lancet 2020; 395(10229): 1054-62.
[http://dx.doi.org/10.1016/S0140-6736(20)30566-3] [PMID: 32171076]

[13]     de Abajo FJ, Rodríguez-Martín S, Lerma V, *et al.* Use of renin–angiotensin–aldosterone system inhibitors and risk of COVID-19 requiring admission to hospital: a case-population study. Lancet 2020; 395(10238): 1705-14.
[http://dx.doi.org/10.1016/S0140-6736(20)31030-8] [PMID: 32416785]

[14]     Maddaloni E, Buzzetti R. Covid-19 and diabetes mellitus: unveiling the interaction of two pandemics. Diabetes Metab Res Rev 2020; 36(7): e33213321.
[http://dx.doi.org/10.1002/dmrr.3321] [PMID: 32233018]

[15]     Guo W, Li M, Dong Y, *et al.* Diabetes is a risk factor for the progression and prognosis of COVID -19. Diabetes Metab Res Rev 2020; 36(7): e3319.
[http://dx.doi.org/10.1002/dmrr.3319] [PMID: 32233013]

[16]     Katulanda P, Dissanayake HA, Ranathunga I, *et al.* Prevention and management of COVID-19 among patients with diabetes: an appraisal of the literature. Diabetologia 2020; 63(8): 1440-52.
[http://dx.doi.org/10.1007/s00125-020-05164-x] [PMID: 32405783]

[17]     Hussain A, Bhowmik B, do Vale Moreira NC. COVID-19 and diabetes: Knowledge in progress. Diabetes Res Clin Pract 2020; 162: 108142.
[http://dx.doi.org/10.1016/j.diabres.2020.108142] [PMID: 32278764]

[18]     Grasselli G, Zangrillo A, Zanella A, *et al.* Baseline Characteristics and Outcomes of 1591 Patients Infected With SARS-CoV-2 Admitted to ICUs of the Lombardy Region, Italy. JAMA 2020; 323(16): 1574-81.
[http://dx.doi.org/10.1001/jama.2020.5394] [PMID: 32250385]

[19]     Kumar A, Arora A, Sharma P, *et al.* Is diabetes mellitus associated with mortality and severity of COVID-19? A meta-analysis. Diabetes Metab Syndr 2020; 14(4): 535-45.
[http://dx.doi.org/10.1016/j.dsx.2020.04.044] [PMID: 32408118]

[20]     Rajsfus BF, Mohana-Borges R, Allonso D. Diabetogenic viruses: linking viruses to diabetes mellitus. Heliyon 2023; 9(4): e15021.
[http://dx.doi.org/10.1016/j.heliyon.2023.e15021] [PMID: 37064445]

[21]     Muller LMAJ, Gorter KJ, Hak E, *et al.* Increased risk of common infections in patients with type 1 and type 2 diabetes mellitus. Clin Infect Dis 2005; 41(3): 281-8.
[http://dx.doi.org/10.1086/431587] [PMID: 16007521]

[22]     https://www.who.int/health-topics/diabetes#tab=tab_1

[23]     Cuschieri S, Grech S. COVID-19 and diabetes: The why, the what and the how. J Diabetes Complications 2020; 34(9): 107637.
[http://dx.doi.org/10.1016/j.jdiacomp.2020.107637] [PMID: 32456846]

[24]     Saeedi P, Petersohn I, Salpea P, *et al.* 2019.

[25]     Yan Y, Yang Y, Wang F, *et al.* Clinical characteristics and outcomes of patients with severe covid-19 with diabetes. BMJ Open Diabetes Res Care 2020; 8(1): e001343.
[http://dx.doi.org/10.1136/bmjdrc-2020-001343] [PMID: 32345579]

[26]     Wu Z, McGoogan JM. Characteristics of and Important Lessons From the Coronavirus Disease 2019 (COVID-19) Outbreak in China. JAMA 2020; 323(13): 1239-42.
[http://dx.doi.org/10.1001/jama.2020.2648] [PMID: 32091533]

[27]     Singh AK, Khunti K. COVID-19 and Diabetes. Annu Rev Med 2022; 73(1): 129-47.

[http://dx.doi.org/10.1146/annurev-med-042220-011857] [PMID: 34379444]

[28]　Cao H, Baranova A, Wei X, Wang C, Zhang F. Bidirectional causal associations between type 2 diabetes and COVID-19. J Med Virol 2023; 95(1): e28100.
[http://dx.doi.org/10.1002/jmv.28100] [PMID: 36029131]

[29]　Markin L, Fartushok T, Fartushok N, Soyka L, Fedevych Y. DIABETES MELLITUS AND COVID-19: TODAY'S CHALLENGES. Georgian Med News 2023; (337): 43-50.
[PMID: 37354672]

[30]　Unsworth R, Wallace S, Oliver NS, *et al.* New-Onset Type 1 Diabetes in Children During COVID-19: Multicenter Regional Findings in the U.K. Diabetes Care 2020; 43(11): e170-1.
[http://dx.doi.org/10.2337/dc20-1551] [PMID: 32816997]

[31]　Ambati S, Mihic M, Rosario DC, Sanchez J, Bakar A. New-Onset Type 1 Diabetes in Children With SARS-CoV-2 Infection. Cureus 2022; 14(3): e22790.
[http://dx.doi.org/10.7759/cureus.22790] [PMID: 35382205]

[32]　Marchand L, Pecquet M, Luyton C. Type 1 diabetes onset triggered by COVID-19. Acta Diabetol 2020; 57(10): 1265-6.
[http://dx.doi.org/10.1007/s00592-020-01570-0] [PMID: 32653960]

[33]　Hollstein T, Schulte DM, Schulz J, *et al.* Autoantibody-negative insulin-dependent diabetes mellitus after SARS-CoV-2 infection: a case report. Nat Metab 2020; 2(10): 1021-4.
[http://dx.doi.org/10.1038/s42255-020-00281-8] [PMID: 32879473]

[34]　Liu F, Long X, Zhang B, Zhang W, Chen X, Zhang Z. ACE2 Expression in Pancreas May Cause Pancreatic Damage After SARS-CoV-2 Infection. Clin Gastroenterol Hepatol 2020; 18(9): 2128-2130.e2.
[http://dx.doi.org/10.1016/j.cgh.2020.04.040] [PMID: 32334082]

[35]　Akarsu C, Karabulut M, Aydin H, *et al.* Association between Acute Pancreatitis and COVID-19: Could Pancreatitis Be the Missing Piece of the Puzzle about Increased Mortality Rates? J Invest Surg 2022; 35(1): 119-25.
[http://dx.doi.org/10.1080/08941939.2020.1833263] [PMID: 33138658]

[36]　Wu CT, Lidsky PV, Xiao Y, *et al.* SARS-CoV-2 infects human pancreatic β cells and elicits β cell impairment. Cell Metab 2021; 33(8): 1565-1576.e5.
[http://dx.doi.org/10.1016/j.cmet.2021.05.013] [PMID: 34081912]

[37]　Tang X, Uhl S, Zhang T, *et al.* SARS-CoV-2 infection induces beta cell transdifferentiation. Cell Metab 2021; 33(8): 1577-1591.e7.
[http://dx.doi.org/10.1016/j.cmet.2021.05.015] [PMID: 34081913]

[38]　Hill MA, Mantzoros C, Sowers JR. Commentary: COVID-19 in patients with diabetes. Metabolism 2020; 107: 154217.
[http://dx.doi.org/10.1016/j.metabol.2020.154217] [PMID: 32220611]

[39]　Peric S, Stulnig TM. Diabetes and COVID-19. Wien Klin Wochenschr 2020; 132(13-14): 356-61.
[http://dx.doi.org/10.1007/s00508-020-01672-3] [PMID: 32435867]

[40]　Pal R, Bhadada SK. COVID-19 and diabetes mellitus: An unholy interaction of two pandemics. Diabetes Metab Syndr 2020; 14(4): 513-7.
[http://dx.doi.org/10.1016/j.dsx.2020.04.049] [PMID: 32388331]

[41]　Montefusco L, Ben Nasr M, D'Addio F, *et al.* Acute and long-term disruption of glycometabolic control after SARS-CoV-2 infection. Nat Metab 2021; 3(6): 774-85.
[http://dx.doi.org/10.1038/s42255-021-00407-6] [PMID: 34035524]

[42]　Govender N, Khaliq OP, Moodley J, Naicker T. Insulin resistance in COVID-19 and diabetes. Prim Care Diabetes 2021; 15(4): 629-34.
[http://dx.doi.org/10.1016/j.pcd.2021.04.004] [PMID: 33849817]

[43]    He X, Liu C, Peng J, *et al.* COVID-19 induces new-onset insulin resistance and lipid metabolic dysregulation *via* regulation of secreted metabolic factors. Signal Transduct Target Ther 2021; 6(1): 427.
[http://dx.doi.org/10.1038/s41392-021-00822-x] [PMID: 34916489]

[44]    Abramczyk U, Nowaczyński M, Słomczyński A, Wojnicz P, Zatyka P, Kuzan A. Consequences of COVID-19 for the Pancreas. Int J Mol Sci 2022; 23(2): 864.
[http://dx.doi.org/10.3390/ijms23020864] [PMID: 35055050]

[45]    2020.https://www.cdc.gov/coronavirus/2 019-ncov/need-extra precautions/groups-at-higher risk.html

[46]    Unluguzel Ustun G, Keskin A, Aci R, Arslanbek Erdem M, Ari M. Association between Hb A $_{1c}$ and Severity of COVID-19 Patients. Hemoglobin 2021; 45(2): 124-8.
[http://dx.doi.org/10.1080/03630269.2021.1926278] [PMID: 34162301]

[47]    Bansal R, Gubbi S, Muniyappa R. Metabolic Syndrome and COVID 19: Endocrine-Immune-Vascular Interactions Shapes Clinical Course. Endocrinology 2020; 161(10): bqaa112.
[http://dx.doi.org/10.1210/endocr/bqaa112] [PMID: 32603424]

[48]    Andersen CJ, Murphy KE, Fernandez ML. Impact of Obesity and Metabolic Syndrome on Immunity. Adv Nutr 2016; 7(1): 66-75.
[http://dx.doi.org/10.3945/an.115.010207] [PMID: 26773015]

[49]    Frasca D, Diaz A, Romero M, Blomberg BB. Ageing and obesity similarly impair antibody responses. Clin Exp Immunol 2016; 187(1): 64-70.
[http://dx.doi.org/10.1111/cei.12824] [PMID: 27314456]

[50]    Kassir R. Risk of COVID-19 for patients with obesity. Obes Rev 2020; 21(6): e13034.
[http://dx.doi.org/10.1111/obr.13034] [PMID: 32281287]

[51]    Kaye SM, Pietiläinen KH, Kotronen A, *et al.* Obesity-related derangements of coagulation and fibrinolysis: a study of obesity-discordant monozygotic twin pairs. Obesity (Silver Spring) 2012; 20(1): 88-94.
[http://dx.doi.org/10.1038/oby.2011.287] [PMID: 21959347]

[52]    Cariou B, Hadjadj S, Wargny M, *et al.* Phenotypic characteristics and prognosis of inpatients with COVID-19 and diabetes: the CORONADO study. Diabetologia 2020; 63(8): 1500-15.
[http://dx.doi.org/10.1007/s00125-020-05180-x] [PMID: 32472191]

[53]    Cai Q, Chen F, Wang T, *et al.* Obesity and COVID-19 severity in a designated hospital in Shenzhen, China. Diabetes Care 2020; 43(7): 1392-8.
[http://dx.doi.org/10.2337/dc20-0576] [PMID: 32409502]

[54]    He Z, Li J. Comment on Cai *et al.* Obesity and COVID-19 severity in a designated hospital in Shenzhen, China. Diabetes Care 2020;43:1392–1398. Diabetes Care 2020; 43(10): e160-1.
[http://dx.doi.org/10.2337/dc20-1195] [PMID: 32958624]

[55]    Lighter J, Phillips M, Hochman S, *et al.* Obesity in patients younger than 60 years is a risk factor for Covid-19 hospital admission. Clin Infect Dis 2020; 71(15): 896-7.
[http://dx.doi.org/10.1093/cid/ciaa415] [PMID: 32271368]

[56]    Mahase E. Covid-19: most patients require mechanical ventilation in first 24 hours of critical care. BMJ 2020; 368: m1201.
[http://dx.doi.org/10.1136/bmj.m1201] [PMID: 32209544]

[57]    Simonnet A, Chetboun M, Poissy J, *et al.* High prevalence of obesity in severe acute respiratory syndrome coronavirus-2 (SARS-CoV-2) requiring invasive mechanical ventilation. Obesity (Silver Spring) 2020; 28(7): 1195-9.
[http://dx.doi.org/10.1002/oby.22831] [PMID: 32271993]

[58]    Zheng KI, Gao F, Wang XB, *et al.* Letter to the Editor: Obesity as a risk factor for greater severity of COVID-19 in patients with metabolic associated fatty liver disease. Metabolism 2020; 108: 154244.

[http://dx.doi.org/10.1016/j.metabol.2020.154244] [PMID: 32320741]

[59]   Petrilli CM, Jones SA, Yang J, *et al.* Factors associated with hospital admission and critical illness among 5279 people with coronavirus disease 2019 in New York City: prospective cohort study. BMJ 2020; 369: m1966.
[http://dx.doi.org/10.1136/bmj.m1966] [PMID: 32444366]

[60]   Garg S, Kim L, Whitaker M, *et al.* Hospitalization rates and characteristics of patients hospitalized with laboratory-confirmed coronavirus disease 2019—COVID-NET, 14 States, March 1–30, 2020. MMWR Morb Mortal Wkly Rep 2020; 69(15): 458-64.
[http://dx.doi.org/10.15585/mmwr.mm6915e3] [PMID: 32298251]

[61]   Peng YD, Meng K, Guan HQ, *et al.* [Clinical characteristics and outcomes of 112 cardiovascular disease patients infected by 2019-nCoV]. Zhonghua Xin Xue Guan Bing Za Zhi 2020; 48(6): 450-5.
[PMID: 32120458]

[62]   Gu T, Mack JA, Salvatore M, Sankar SP, Valley TS, Singh K, *et al.* COVID-19 outcomes, risk factors and associations by race: a comprehensive analysis using electronic health records data in Michigan Medicine. medRxiv 2020.
[http://dx.doi.org/10.1101/2020.06.16.20133140]

[63]   Giannouchos TV, Sussman RA, Mier JM, Poulas K, Farsalinos K. Retraction notice for: Characteristics and risk factors for COVID-19 diagnosis and adverse outcomes in Mexico: an analysis of 89,756 laboratory-confirmed COVID-19 cases Theodoros V. Giannouchos, Roberto A. Sussman, José M. Mier, Konstantinos Poulas and Konstantinos Farsalinos. *Eur Respir J* 2020; in press. Eur Respir J 2021; 57(3): 2002144.
[http://dx.doi.org/10.1183/13993003.02144-2020] [PMID: 32732325]

[64]   Kruglikov IL, Scherer PE. The role of adipocytes and adipocyte-like cells in the severity of COVID-19 infections. Obesity (Silver Spring) 2020; 28(7): 1187-90.
[http://dx.doi.org/10.1002/oby.22856] [PMID: 32339391]

[65]   Popkin BM, Du S, Green WD, *et al.* Individuals with obesity and COVID-19: A global perspective on the epidemiology and biological relationships. Obes Rev 2020; 21(11): e13128.
[http://dx.doi.org/10.1111/obr.13128] [PMID: 32845580]

[66]   Wang D, Hu B, Hu C, *et al.* Clinical Characteristics of 138 Hospitalized Patients With 2019 Novel Coronavirus-Infected Pneumonia in Wuhan, China JAMA. 2020; 323(11): 1061-1069.

[67]   Patel AB, Verma A. COVID-19 and Angiotensin-Converting Enzyme Inhibitors and Angiotensin Receptor Blockers. JAMA 2020; 323(18): 1769-70.
[http://dx.doi.org/10.1001/jama.2020.4812] [PMID: 32208485]

[68]   Zhang J, Dong X, Cao Y, *et al.* Clinical characteristics of 140 patients infected with SARS-CoV-2 in Wuhan, China. Allergy 2020; 75(7): 1730-41.
[http://dx.doi.org/10.1111/all.14238] [PMID: 32077115]

[69]   Deng SQ, Peng HJ. Characteristics of and public health responses to the coronavirus disease 2019 outbreak in China. J Clin Med 2020; 9(2): 575.
[http://dx.doi.org/10.3390/jcm9020575] [PMID: 32093211]

[70]   Mao B, Liu Y, Chai YH, *et al.* Assessing risk factors for SARS-CoV-2 infection in patients presenting with symptoms in Shanghai, China: a multicentre, observational cohort study. Lancet Digit Health 2020; 2(6): e323-30.
[http://dx.doi.org/10.1016/S2589-7500(20)30109-6] [PMID: 32501440]

[71]   Guan W, Liang W, Zhao Y, *et al.* Comorbidity and its impact on 1590 patients with COVID-19 in China: a nationwide analysis. Eur Respir J 2020; 55(5): 2000547.
[http://dx.doi.org/10.1183/13993003.00547-2020] [PMID: 32217650]

[72]   Roncon L, Zuin M, Zuliani G, Rigatelli G. Patients with arterial hypertension and COVID-19 are at higher risk of ICU admission. Br J Anaesth 2020; 125(2): e254-5.

[http://dx.doi.org/10.1016/j.bja.2020.04.056] [PMID: 32381262]

[73] Garg S, Kim L, Whitaker M, *et al.* Hospitalization rates and characteristics of patients hospitalized with laboratory-confirmed coronavirus disease 2019 - COVID-NET, 14 States, March 1-30, 2020. MMWR Morb Mortal Wkly Rep 2020; 69(15): 458-64.
[http://dx.doi.org/10.15585/mmwr.mm6915e3] [PMID: 32298251]

[74] Wu C, Chen X, Cai Y, *et al.* Risk Factors Associated With Acute Respiratory Distress Syndrome and Death in Patients With Coronavirus Disease 2019 Pneumonia in Wuhan, China. JAMA Intern Med 2020; 180(7): 934-43.
[http://dx.doi.org/10.1001/jamainternmed.2020.0994] [PMID: 32167524]

[75] Wan Y, Shang J, Graham R, Baric RS, Li F. Receptor recognition by the novel coronavirus from Wuhan: an analysis based on decade-long structural studies of SARS coronavirus. J Virol 2020; 94(7): e00127-20.
[http://dx.doi.org/10.1128/JVI.00127-20] [PMID: 31996437]

[76] Messerli FH, Siontis GCM, Rexhaj E. COVID-19 and Renin Angiotensin Blockers. Circulation 2020; 141(25): 2042-4.
[http://dx.doi.org/10.1161/CIRCULATIONAHA.120.047022] [PMID: 32282224]

[77] Thum T. SARS-CoV-2 receptor ACE2 expression in the human heart: cause of a post-pandemic wave of heart failure? Eur Heart J 2020; 41(19): 1807-9.
[http://dx.doi.org/10.1093/eurheartj/ehaa410] [PMID: 32383758]

[78] https://www.acc.org/latest-in-cardiology/articles/2020/03/17/08/59/

[79] Kow CS, Ramachandram DS, Hasan SS. Hypertension and severe COVID-19. Hypertens Res 2023; 46(5): 1353-4.
[http://dx.doi.org/10.1038/s41440-023-01207-z] [PMID: 36843117]

[80] Shibata S, Arima H, Asayama K, *et al.* Hypertension and related diseases in the era of COVID-19: a report from the Japanese Society of Hypertension Task Force on COVID-19. Hypertens Res 2020; 43(10): 1028-46.
[http://dx.doi.org/10.1038/s41440-020-0515-0] [PMID: 32737423]

[81] Iaccarino G, Grassi G, Borghi C, *et al.* Age and multimorbidity predict death among COVID-19 patients: results of the SARS-RAS Study of the Italian Society of Hypertension. Hypertension 2020; 76(2): 366-72.
[http://dx.doi.org/10.1161/HYPERTENSIONAHA.120.15324] [PMID: 32564693]

[82] McFarlane E, Linschoten M, Asselbergs FW, Lacy PS, Jedrzejewski D, Williams B. The impact of pre-existing hypertension and its treatment on outcomes in patients admitted to hospital with COVID-19. Hypertens Res 2022; 45(5): 834-45.
[http://dx.doi.org/10.1038/s41440-022-00893-5] [PMID: 35352027]

[83] Wang B, Li R, Lu Z, Huang Y. Does comorbidity increase the risk of patients with COVID-19: evidence from meta-analysis. Aging (Albany NY) 2020; 12(7): 6049-57.
[http://dx.doi.org/10.18632/aging.103000] [PMID: 32267833]

[84] Ran J, Song Y, Zhuang Z, *et al.* Blood pressure control and adverse outcomes of COVID-19 infection in patients with concomitant hypertension in Wuhan, China. Hypertens Res 2020; 43(11): 1267-76.
[http://dx.doi.org/10.1038/s41440-020-00541-w] [PMID: 32855527]

[85] D'Elia L, Giaquinto A, Zarrella AF, *et al.* Hypertension and mortality in SARS-COV-2 infection: A meta-analysis of observational studies after 2 years of pandemic. Eur J Intern Med 2023; 108: 28-36.
[http://dx.doi.org/10.1016/j.ejim.2022.11.018] [PMID: 36411156]

[86] Shi S, Qin M, Shen B, *et al.* Association of Cardiac Injury With Mortality in Hospitalized Patients With COVID-19 in Wuhan, China. JAMA Cardiol 2020; 5(7): 802-10.
[http://dx.doi.org/10.1001/jamacardio.2020.0950] [PMID: 32211816]

[87] Nasab EM, Aghajani H, Makoei RH, Athari SS. COVID-19's immuno-pathology and cardiovascular

diseases. J Investig Med 2023; 71(2): 71-80.
[http://dx.doi.org/10.1177/10815589221141841] [PMID: 36647329]

[88]   Liu K, Fang YY, Deng Y, *et al.* Clinical characteristics of novel coronavirus cases in tertiary hospitals in Hubei Province. Chin Med J (Engl) 2020; 133(9): 1025-31.
[http://dx.doi.org/10.1097/CM9.0000000000000744] [PMID: 32044814]

[89]   Liang W, Guan W, Li C, *et al.* Clinical characteristics and outcomes of hospitalised patients with COVID-19 treated in Hubei (epicentre) and outside Hubei (non-epicentre): a nationwide analysis of China. Eur Respir J 2020; 55(6): 2000562.
[http://dx.doi.org/10.1183/13993003.00562-2020] [PMID: 32269086]

[90]   Richardson S, Hirsch JS, Narasimhan M, *et al.* Presenting Characteristics, Comorbidities, and Outcomes Among 5700 Patients Hospitalized With COVID-19 in the New York City Area JAMA. 2020; 323(20): 2052-2059.

[91]   Zhao X, Nicholls JM, Chen YG. Severe acute respiratory syndrome-associated coronavirus nucleocapsid protein interacts with Smad3 and modulates transforming growth factor-beta signaling. J Biol Chem 2008; 283(6): 3272-80.
[http://dx.doi.org/10.1074/jbc.M708033200] [PMID: 18055455]

[92]   Cameron MJ, Ran L, Xu L, *et al.* Interferon-mediated immunopathological events are associated with atypical innate and adaptive immune responses in patients with severe acute respiratory syndrome. J Virol 2007; 81(16): 8692-706.
[http://dx.doi.org/10.1128/JVI.00527-07] [PMID: 17537853]

[93]   Wong CK, Lam CWK, Wu AKL, *et al.* Plasma inflammatory cytokines and chemokines in severe acute respiratory syndrome. Clin Exp Immunol 2004; 136(1): 95-103.
[http://dx.doi.org/10.1111/j.1365-2249.2004.02415.x] [PMID: 15030519]

[94]   Zheng YY, Ma YT, Zhang JY, Xie X. COVID-19 and the cardiovascular system. Nat Rev Cardiol 2020; 17(5): 259-60.
[http://dx.doi.org/10.1038/s41569-020-0360-5] [PMID: 32139904]

[95]   Wang X, Fang X, Cai Z, *et al.* Comorbid Chronic Diseases and Acute Organ Injuries Are Strongly Correlated with Disease Severity and Mortality among COVID-19 Patients: A Systemic Review and Meta-Analysis. Research 2020; 2020: 2020/2402961.
[http://dx.doi.org/10.34133/2020/2402961] [PMID: 32377638]

[96]   Li B, Yang J, Zhao F, *et al.* Prevalence and impact of cardiovascular metabolic diseases on COVID-19 in China. Clin Res Cardiol 2020; 109(5): 531-8.
[http://dx.doi.org/10.1007/s00392-020-01626-9] [PMID: 32161990]

[97]   Arentz M, Yim E, Klaff L, *et al.* Characteristics and Outcomes of 21 Critically Ill Patients With COVID-19 in Washington State. JAMA 2020; 323(16): 1612-4.
[http://dx.doi.org/10.1001/jama.2020.4326] [PMID: 32191259]

[98]   Epidemiology Working Group for NCIP Epidemic Response, Chinese Center for Disease Control and Prevention. [The epidemiological characteristics of an outbreak of 2019 novel coronavirus diseases (COVID-19) in China]. Zhonghua Liu Xing Bing Xue Za Zhi. 2020 Feb 10; 41(2): 145-151. Chinese.
[http://dx.doi.org/10.3760/cma.j.issn.0254-6450.2020.02.003] [PMID: 32064853]

[99]   Kang Y, Chen T, Mui D, *et al.* Cardiovascular manifestations and treatment considerations in COVID-19. Heart 2020; 106(15): 1132-41.
[http://dx.doi.org/10.1136/heartjnl-2020-317056] [PMID: 32354800]

[100]  Guo T, Fan Y, Chen M, *et al.* Cardiovascular Implications of Fatal Outcomes of Patients With Coronavirus Disease 2019 (COVID-19). JAMA Cardiol 2020; 5(7): 811-8.
[http://dx.doi.org/10.1001/jamacardio.2020.1017] [PMID: 32219356]

[101]  Sala S, Peretto G, De Luca G, *et al.* Low prevalence of arrhythmias in clinically stable COVID-19 patients. Pacing Clin Electrophysiol 2020; 43(8): 891-3.

[http://dx.doi.org/10.1111/pace.13987] [PMID: 32543745]

[102]   Naksuk N, Lazar S, Peeraphatdit TB. Cardiac safety of off-label COVID-19 drug therapy: a review and proposed monitoring protocol. Eur Heart J Acute Cardiovasc Care 2020; 9(3): 215-21.
[http://dx.doi.org/10.1177/2048872620922784] [PMID: 32372695]

[103]   Kunutsor SK, Laukkanen JA. Cardiovascular complications in COVID-19: A systematic review and meta-analysis. J Infect 2020; 81(2): e139-41.
[http://dx.doi.org/10.1016/j.jinf.2020.05.068] [PMID: 32504747]

[104]   Bhatla A, Mayer MM, Adusumalli S, *et al.* COVID-19 and cardiac arrhythmias. Heart Rhythm 2020; 17(9): 1439-44.
[http://dx.doi.org/10.1016/j.hrthm.2020.06.016] [PMID: 32585191]

[105]   Aslanov A, Uçaner B, Çiftçi MS, Buldanlı MZ. Can malignant lymphadenopathies be predicted? Analysis of clinical, ultrasonographic and laboratory data. Annals of Clinical and Analytical Medicine 2023; 14(9): 768-71.
[http://dx.doi.org/10.4328/ACAM.21513]

[106]   Nabavi N. Long covid: How to define it and how to manage it. BMJ 2020; 370: m3489.
[http://dx.doi.org/10.1136/bmj.m3489] [PMID: 32895219]

[107]   Al-Hakeim HK, Al-Rubaye HT, Jubran AS, Almulla AF, Moustafa SR, Maes M. Increased insulin resistance due to Long COVID is associated with depressive symptoms and partly predicted by the inflammatory response during acute infection. Rev Bras Psiquiatr 2023; 45(3): 205-15.
[http://dx.doi.org/10.47626/1516-4446-2022-3002] [PMID: 36917827]

[108]   Carod-Artal FJ. Post-COVID-19 syndrome: epidemiology, diagnostic criteria and pathogenic mechanisms involved. Síndrome post-COVID-19: epidemiología, criterios diagnósticos y mecanismos patogénicos implicados. Rev Neurol 2021; 72(11): 384-96.
[http://dx.doi.org/10.33588/rn.7211.2021230]

[109]   Huang C, Huang L, Wang Y, *et al.* RETRACTED: 6-month consequences of COVID-19 in patients discharged from hospital: a cohort study. Lancet 2021; 397(10270): 220-32.
[http://dx.doi.org/10.1016/S0140-6736(20)32656-8] [PMID: 33428867]

[110]   Fernández-de-las-Peñas C, Palacios-Ceña D, Gómez-Mayordomo V, Cuadrado ML, Florencio LL. Defining Post-COVID Symptoms (Post-Acute COVID, Long COVID, Persistent Post-COVID): An Integrative Classification. Int J Environ Res Public Health 2021; 18(5): 2621.
[http://dx.doi.org/10.3390/ijerph18052621] [PMID: 33807869]

[111]   Greenhalgh T, Knight M, A'Court C, Buxton M, Husain L. Management of post-acute covid-19 in primary care. BMJ 2020; 370: m3026.
[http://dx.doi.org/10.1136/bmj.m3026] [PMID: 32784198]

[112]   Galal I, Hussein M, Amin MT, *et al.* Determinants of persistent post-COVID-19 symptoms: value of a novel COVID-19 symptom score. Egypt J Bronchol 15, 10 2021.
[http://dx.doi.org/10.1186/s43168-020-00049-4]

[113]   Evans RA, McAuley HJC, Harrison EM, *et al.* Physical, cognitive, and mental health impacts of COVID-19 after hospitalisation (PHOSP-COVID): a UK multicentre, prospective cohort study. Lancet Respir Med 2021; 9(11): 1275-87.
[http://dx.doi.org/10.1016/S2213-2600(21)00383-0] [PMID: 34627560]

[114]   Vimercati L, De Maria L, Quarato M, *et al.* Association between Long COVID and Overweight/Obesity. J Clin Med 2021; 10(18): 4143.
[http://dx.doi.org/10.3390/jcm10184143] [PMID: 34575251]

[115]   Ceban F, Ling S, Lui LMW, *et al.* Fatigue and cognitive impairment in Post-COVID-19 Syndrome: A systematic review and meta-analysis. Brain Behav Immun 2022; 101: 93-135.
[http://dx.doi.org/10.1016/j.bbi.2021.12.020] [PMID: 34973396]

[116]   Kamal M, Abo Omirah M, Hussein A, Saeed H. Assessment and characterisation of post-COVID-19

manifestations. Int J Clin Pract 2021; 75(3): e13746.
[http://dx.doi.org/10.1111/ijcp.13746] [PMID: 32991035]

[117] Sudre CH, Murray B, Varsavsky T, *et al.* Attributes and predictors of long COVID. Nat Med 2021; 27(4): 626-31.
[http://dx.doi.org/10.1038/s41591-021-01292-y] [PMID: 33692530]

[118] Moreno-Pérez O, Merino E, Leon-Ramirez JM, *et al.* Post-acute COVID-19 syndrome. Incidence and risk factors: A Mediterranean cohort study. J Infect 2021; 82(3): 378-83.
[http://dx.doi.org/10.1016/j.jinf.2021.01.004] [PMID: 33450302]

[119] Aiyegbusi OL, Hughes SE, Turner G, *et al.* Symptoms, complications and management of long COVID: a review. J R Soc Med 2021; 114(9): 428-42.
[http://dx.doi.org/10.1177/01410768211032850] [PMID: 34265229]

[120] Guan WJ, Liang WH, Zhao Y, *et al.* Comorbidity and its impact on 1590 patients with COVID-19 in China: a nationwide analysis. Eur Respir J 2020; 55(5): 2000547.
[http://dx.doi.org/10.1183/13993003.00547-2020]

[121] Zuin M, Rigatelli G, Zuliani G, Rigatelli A, Mazza A, Roncon L. Arterial hypertension and risk of death in patients with COVID-19 infection: Systematic review and meta-analysis. J Infect 2020; 81(1): e84-6.
[http://dx.doi.org/10.1016/j.jinf.2020.03.059] [PMID: 32283158]

[122] Azevedo RB, Botelho BG, Hollanda JVG, *et al.* Covid-19 and the cardiovascular system: a comprehensive review. J Hum Hypertens 2021; 35(1): 4-11.
[http://dx.doi.org/10.1038/s41371-020-0387-4] [PMID: 32719447]

[123] Crook H, Raza S, Nowell J, Young M, Edison P. Long covid—mechanisms, risk factors, and management. BMJ 2021; 374(1648): n1648.
[http://dx.doi.org/10.1136/bmj.n1648] [PMID: 34312178]

[124] Raman B, Bluemke DA, Lüscher TF, Neubauer S. Long COVID: post-acute sequelae of COVID-19 with a cardiovascular focus. Eur Heart J 2022; 43(11): 1157-72.
[http://dx.doi.org/10.1093/eurheartj/ehac031] [PMID: 35176758]

[125] Khan IH, Zahra SA, Zaim S, Harky A. At the heart of COVID-19. J Card Surg 2020; 35(6): 1287-94.
[http://dx.doi.org/10.1111/jocs.14596] [PMID: 32369872]

[126] Tan ZC, Fu LH, Wang DD, Hong K. [Cardiac manifestations of patients with COVID-19 pneumonia and related treatment recommendations]. Zhonghua Xin Xue Guan Bing Za Zhi 2020; 48(0): E005.
[PMID: 32118392]

[127] Zaim S, Chong JH, Sankaranarayanan V, Harky A. COVID-19 and multiorgan response. Curr Probl Cardiol 2020; 45(8): 100618.
[http://dx.doi.org/10.1016/j.cpcardiol.2020.100618] [PMID: 32439197]

CHAPTER 23

# Metabolic Syndrome In Thyroid Disease

**Iskender Ekinci**[1,*]

[1] *Department of Internal Medicine, Faculty of Medicine, Bezmialem Vakıf University, Istanbul, Turkey*

**Abstract:** Thyroid diseases significantly influence metabolic parameters, including blood pressure regulation, glucose metabolism, obesity, hyperlipidemia, and non-alcoholic fatty liver disease (NAFLD). Hypothyroidism is often linked to hypertension, insulin resistance, and dyslipidemia, while hyperthyroidism may induce weight loss, insulin resistance, and dyslipidemia. Both hypo- and hyperthyroidism impact blood pressure regulation, glucose homeostasis, and adiposity. Dyslipidemia is frequently observed in thyroid disorders, with hypothyroidism associated with elevated cholesterol levels and hyperthyroidism with altered lipid profiles. Additionally, thyroid dysfunction contributes to the development of NAFLD. There is a close relationship between thyroid hormones and metabolic syndrome components, as well as the development of metabolic syndrome.

**Keywords:** Hypothyroidism, Hyperthyroidism, Metabolic syndrome, Thyroid diseases.

## INTRODUCTION

Metabolic syndrome (MetS), characterized by a cluster of metabolic abnormalities, including central obesity, insulin resistance, dyslipidemia, and hypertension, poses a substantial burden on global health due to its association with increased cardiovascular risk and type 2 diabetes mellitus [1]. Concurrently, thyroid diseases constitute a diverse spectrum of conditions affecting thyroid hormone production and regulation. These disorders encompass hypothyroidism, which is characterized by insufficient thyroid hormone levels, subclinical hypothyroidism, where thyroid hormone levels are slightly decreased but still within the reference range, and hyperthyroidism, which is marked by excessive thyroid hormone production. Thyroid hormones play a pivotal role in regulating metabolic processes throughout the body, influencing energy expenditure, lipid metabolism, glucose homeostasis, and cardiovascular function [2].

[*] **Corresponding author Iskender Ekinci:** Department of Internal Medicine, Faculty of Medicine, Bezmialem Vakıf University, Istanbul, Turkey; E-mail: driskenderekinci@gmail.com

**Hafize Uzun & Seyma Dumur (Eds.)**

The relationship between MetS and thyroid diseases involves complex interactions. Both hypothyroidism and hyperthyroidism have been associated with MetS, a cluster of conditions including obesity, insulin resistance, dyslipidemia, and hypertension. Furthermore, common underlying factors, such as chronic low-grade inflammation, oxidative stress, and adipose tissue dysfunction, may contribute to the overlapping pathogenesis of both MetS and thyroid diseases.

## THYROID HORMONE SYNTHESIS AND THE PHYSIOLOGICAL EFFECTS OF THYROID HORMONES

The thyroid gland, the body's largest endocrine organ, is situated in the anterior neck and weighs approximately 15–20 grams. Thyrotropin-releasing hormone (TRH) from the hypothalamus stimulates the release of thyroid-stimulating hormone (TSH) from the pituitary gland. TSH acts as a stimulatory agent for the thyroid gland, prompting the synthesis of thyroxine (T4) and triiodothyronine (T3) hormones. The intricate process of thyroid hormone synthesis involves tiroglobulin synthesis within thyroid follicles, iodine uptake, iodine oxidation, iodination of tyrosine, and subsequent secretion of iodotyrosines into the circulation following coupling. The primary hormone originating from the thyroid gland is T4, which undergoes conversion to both the bioactive form T3 and the inactive form rT3 in peripheral tissues through the action of deiodinase enzymes. Surplus thyroid hormones are sequestered within follicles in association with tiroglobulins. With profound effects on virtually all bodily organs and systems, thyroid hormones principally accelerate metabolism and thermogenesis while exerting influences on body growth and development [3].

Hypothyroidism is a disease characterized by metabolic slowdown due to insufficient thyroid hormone at the tissue level or rarely ineffective thyroid hormone. It can be due to primary (thyroid), secondary (pituitary), or tertiary (hypothalamus) causes, depending on the level of hormone synthesis defect. The prevalence of hypothyroidism is around 5% worldwide, with the majority being attributable to primary hypothyroidism [4]. More prevalent among women and rising with age, it typically peaks between the ages of 30 and 50 [5]. Laboratory tests are used for diagnosis since hypothyroidism lacks overt and pathognomonic symptoms and signs. Diagnosis is established when free T4 levels are low and TSH levels are high. In cases where there are no clinical findings and free T4 levels are low with a mildly elevated TSH value, subclinical hypothyroidism may be considered. Fatigue, abnormal weight gain, constipation, intolerance to cold, dry skin, forgetfulness, and loss of appetite constitute general symptoms and signs associated with hypothyroidism. Other clinical findings that may occur in hypothyroidism include decreased cardiac output, bradycardia, increased peripheral vascular resistance and hypertension, hypercholesterolemia associated with decreased cholesterol metabolism, and weight gain because of decreased metabolic rate, leading to non-alcoholic fatty liver disease [6].

Hyperthyroidism, characterized by an overactive thyroid gland and excess thyroid hormone production, accelerates metabolic processes and is often attributed to conditions such as Graves' disease, toxic nodular goiter, or thyroiditis. The clinical presentation of hyperthyroidism encompasses a spectrum of symptoms and signs indicative of the heightened metabolic state associated with excessive thyroid hormone activity. These include weight loss despite increased appetite, palpitations, heat intolerance, sweating, tremors, psychological symptoms such as anxiety, nervousness, or irritability, fatigue, diarrhea, muscle weakness, and menstrual irregularities in women. Furthermore, physical examination may reveal tachycardia, elevated blood pressure, a goiter, warm and moist skin, fine tremors of the extremities, manifestations of thyroid eye disease, alopecia or hair thinning, and excessive perspiration accompanied by flushed skin [7].

## METABOLIC SYNDROME

It manifests as a clinical amalgamation of various interconnected metabolic irregularities linked to heightened risks of atherosclerotic disease, type 2 diabetes mellitus, and mortality. This condition typically arises from excessive weight gain and inadequate physical activity in individuals with a genetic predisposition. Diagnosis of MetS commonly relies on diagnostic criteria outlined by the International Diabetes Federation (IDF) and the National Cholesterol Education Program (NCEPT) (Table 1) [8]. With the recent surge in obesity rates, the prevalence of MetS has also increased. Examination of U.S. data reveals a steady increase in the prevalence of MetS from 22% in 2002 to 37.6% in 2011 and finally to 41.8% in 2017 [9 - 11].

## THYROID HORMONES AND METABOLIC SYNDROME

Thyroid hormones play a crucial role in metabolic regulation through their numerous effects on lipid metabolism, glucose homeostasis, energy expenditure, and blood pressure control. In recent years, a growing body of evidence has shed light on the intricate relationship between MetS and thyroid disorders. This emerging research suggests bidirectional influences and shared pathophysiological mechanisms between these two entities. Notably, individuals with MetS are more prone to developing thyroid dysfunction, while thyroid disorders, in turn, may exacerbate metabolic disturbances characteristic of MetS [12].

**Table 1. Metabolic syndrome diagnostic criteria.**

| - | NCEPT-ATP3 | IDF |
|---|---|---|
| Obesity | Waist ≥102 cm (men) or ≥88 cm (women). | Waist ≥94 cm (men) or ≥80 cm (women). |
| Glucose | Fasting glucose ≥100 mg/dL or drug treatment for elevated blood glucose. | Fasting glucose ≥100 mg/dL or diagnosed diabetes. |
| HDL cholesterol | <40 mg/dL (men); <50 mg/dL (women) or drug treatment for low HDL cholesterol. | <40 mg/dL (men); <50 mg/dL (women) or drug treatment for low HDL cholesterol. |
| Triglycerides | ≥150 mg/dL or drug treatment for elevated triglycerides. | ≥150 mg/dL or drug treatment for elevated triglycerides. |
| Hypertension | ≥130/85 mmHg or drug treatment for hypertension. | ≥130/85 mmHg or drug treatment for hypertension. |

**NCEPT-ATP3:** National Cholesterol Education Program, **IDF:** International Diabetes Federation.

It is noted that in cases of thyroid hormone deficiency, there is an increased risk of developing obesity due to reduced energy expenditure, elevated lipid levels, and impaired blood pressure and glucose regulation, consequently increasing the likelihood of developing MetS [13]. This process is not only evident in overt hypothyroidism cases but also expected in cases of subclinical hypothyroidism [14]. In a study involving 3075 participants monitored for the development of MetS, each unit increase in TSH levels was associated with a 3% increase in the likelihood of developing MetS. This increase was more pronounced in the group with TSH levels within the normal range, and an increased risk of developing MetS was observed in cases with subclinical hypothyroidism as well [13]. In a study examining the relationships between thyroid functions and MetS parameters in a euthyroid population, the frequency of MetS was found to be 19.2% in men and 15.4% in women. In the same study, it was stated that thyroid function tests were associated with MetS parameters [15]. On the other hand, in a study examining the effects of MetS presence on thyroid functions, it was reported that, because of a 9-year follow-up, the presence of MetS was not associated with the development of thyroid dysfunction [16].

**Thyroid Hormones and Obesity**

Obesity stands as a metabolic disturbance characterized by excessive adipose tissue accumulation, posing detrimental effects on health and often exhibiting a progressive nature. It is categorized as "overweight" with a body mass index (BMI) ranging between 25-29.9 kg/m2, "obesity" with a BMI of ≥30 kg/m2, and "severe obesity" with a BMI of ≥40 kg/m2 or ≥35 kg/m2 accompanied by comorbidities. The prevalence of obesity has been steadily escalating, with overweight affecting 39% and obesity impacting 13% of adults aged 18 and above [17]. Obesity significantly heightens the susceptibility to various ailments, including type 2 diabetes mellitus, hypertension, dyslipidemia, and coronary artery disease, alongside elevating mortality rates [18].

Obesity development is influenced by genetic factors, environmental factors, dietary disorders, sedentary lifestyles, and some metabolic diseases. Among the metabolic disorders contributing to obesity development, hypothyroidism stands out. The relationship between obesity and hypothyroidism is thought to be bidirectional. Hypothyroidism predisposes to obesity by slowing down metabolism, while it is noted that TSH levels tend to increase in obese individuals [19].

Nutritional intake and energy expenditure balance in the body are controlled by two different neuron groups *via* TRH in the hypothalamic arcuate nucleus. Proopiomelanocortin decreases appetite and increases energy expenditure, while the neuropeptide Y/agouti-related peptide (AgRP) neuron group antagonizes its effects. Leptin and ghrelin also act by antagonizing POMC and AgRP neurons [20]. In hypothyroidism, resting energy expenditure, which accounts for more than half of the energy spent on metabolic processes required to maintain vital physiological functions (rest, awake, and fasted state in a thermoneutral environment), decreases [21]. Changes in thyroid hormone levels, even if not sufficient to cause hypothyroidism, can lead to weight gain secondary to decreased energy expenditure. In a study analyzing the relationship between thyroid hormone levels and body mass index (BMI) and obesity with more than 4000 participants in Denmark, it was reported that serum TSH levels were positively associated with BMI, while serum-free T4 levels were inversely associated with BMI. In the same study, it was observed that the group with higher serum TSH levels gained more weight in the last 5 years compared to the group with lower serum TSH levels [22].

While hypothyroidism has long been associated with an increased risk of obesity, recent observations indicate a reciprocal relationship: obesity also heightens the risk of developing hypothyroidism. There is a relationship between thyroid hormone levels and anthropometric measurements such as body weight, waist circumference, and hip circumference [23, 24]. The reason for the increased risk of hypothyroidism in obese individuals is not yet clear, but some studies attempt to explain this situation. In obesity, where chronic low-grade inflammation is present, increased cytokine release from adipose tissue may reduce iodine uptake in thyroid follicular cells, leading to vascular and morphological changes in thyroid tissue and resulting in vasodilation and increased permeability [25, 26]. Additionally, in obesity, leptin release from adipose tissue increases due to inflammation, which can reduce sodium/iodide symporter and thyroglobulin expression in thyroid tissue and cause morphological changes [27]. A meta-analysis of 22 studies reported that obesity increases the risk of both overt and subclinical hypothyroidism while also causing an uptick in anti-TPO levels. Within this review, it was noted that having a BMI of ≥ 28 kg/m2 heightens the risk of evident hypothyroidism, and obesity substantially raises the probability of subclinical hypothyroidism by 70%. However, no association was observed between obesity and the onset of hyperthyroidism [19].

The impact of hyperthyroidism on obesity encompasses a complex interplay of metabolic factors. Although hyperthyroidism typically induces weight loss owing to heightened metabolic activity and increased energy expenditure, paradoxically, weight gain can manifest in certain cases [28]. This phenomenon may stem from augmented appetite despite accelerated metabolism or alterations in body composition characterized by muscle wasting and redistribution of fat. Moreover, hyperthyroidism exerts influence on diverse metabolic pathways, including lipid metabolism and insulin sensitivity, potentially exacerbating changes in body weight and adiposity [12].

## Thyroid Hormones and Hyperlipidemia

The coordinated effects of thyroid hormones on hepatic and adipose tissue regulate cholesterol biosynthesis, clearance, and metabolism. Hypothyroidism predisposes individuals to hyperlipidemia due to aberrant thyroid hormone metabolism. Thyroid-stimulating hormone (TSH) directly stimulates hepatic gluconeogenesis and attenuates the phosphorylation of HMG-CoA reductase, contributing to hypercholesterolemia [29]. Thyroid hormone receptor beta-2 serves as the primary thyroid hormone receptor in hepatic and adipose tissue, and its absence in animal models results in upregulation of lipogenic genes and downregulation of fatty acid β-oxidation, leading to hepatic lipid accumulation [30]. Triiodothyronine regulates the expression of genes involved in both hepatic lipogenesis and free fatty acid oxidation while inducing lipolysis [31].

The underlying pathophysiological mechanisms behind the development of hyperlipidemia in hypothyroid patients include decreased LDL cell-surface receptor number and activity, reduced LDL catabolism, increased LDL oxidation, decreased secretion of LDL cholesterol into bile, decreased lipolysis in adipose tissue, reduced uptake of free fatty acids by the liver, decreased beta-oxidation of free fatty acids and triglyceride clearance, decreased cholesterol ester transfer, and triglyceride accumulation in the liver [32 - 37].

In a study involving 62,408 adults in China, a close relationship between thyroid hormone levels and lipid levels has been reported [24]. In this study, it was noted that in men, TG levels were high in subclinical hyperthyroidism, overt hyperthyroidism, and subclinical hypothyroidism, while HDL levels were low in subclinical hypothyroidism; in women, TG levels were high in both subclinical and overt hypothyroidism. The study also indicated that overt hyperthyroidism and subclinical hypothyroidism in men and overt hypothyroidism and subclinical hypothyroidism in women were more closely associated with metabolic status. In a separate investigation involving 295 hypothyroid patients, it was found that merely 8.5% of individuals exhibited no lipid abnormalities [38]. Another study focusing on the lipid profile of Hashimoto's thyroiditis sufferers revealed that serum levels of total cholesterol, LDL cholesterol, HDL cholesterol, non-HDL cholesterol, and triglycerides were positively associated with serum TSH levels but negatively correlated with free T4 levels [39]. In this study, it was reported that the prevalence of primary hypothyroidism in patients with hypercholesterolemia was 3.8% (overt hypothyroidism 1.4%, subclinical hypothyroidism 2.4%) and that of central hypothyroidism was 0.6%. The same study also observed lower lipid levels in cases of thyrotoxicosis, higher levels in overt hypothyroidism, and an improvement in lipid profiles following thyroid hormone replacement therapy among those with subclinical hypothyroidism [39]. In hypothyroid patients, it has been noted that levels of triglycerides, LDL cholesterol, total cholesterol, and apolipoprotein B decrease after levothyroxine treatment, while increased levels of HDL and apolipoprotein E do not decline [40]. In hypothyroidism, the prevalence of hyperlipidemia is reported to increase, while in hyperlipidemic patients, the frequency of hypothyroidism is said to rise due to the thyrotoxic effects of lipids. In two separate studies examining the frequency of hypothyroidism in hyperlipidemic patients, subclinical hypothyroidism was found to be 3.5% and 4.4%, and overt hypothyroidism was reported to be 1.7% and 2.8%, respectively [41, 42]. In the patient groups with hypercholesterolemia, the Series *et al.* study reported the frequency of subclinical hypothyroidism to be 8% and overt hypothyroidism to be 4.4%, whereas, in the study by Diekman *et al.*, these rates were found to be 1.9% and 0.7%, respectively [43, 44]. In patients with subclinical hypothyroidism, lipid levels are generally expected to be normal, but mild elevations in total cholesterol, LDL cholesterol, and triglyceride levels, as well as lower HDL levels, may be observed [45]. Pirich *et al.* reported a subclinical hypothyroidism rate of 0.8% in the normocholesterolemic group, while it was found to be 1.4% in hypercholesterolemic patients [46]. Following thyroid hormone replacement therapy in patients with subclinical hypothyroidism, a decrease in serum total cholesterol levels has been reported, with the extent of reduction being greater in those with higher initial total cholesterol levels [47].

Hyperthyroidism induces heightened hepatic synthesis of cholesterol and triglycerides, enhanced lipolysis, and fatty acid mobilization from adipose tissue, along with increased cholesterol clearance through augmented hepatic uptake, collectively contributing to the development of hyperlipidemia in affected individuals [12, 48]. Reduced thyroid hormone levels downregulated the expression of LDL receptors-related protein 1, resulting in diminished LDL degradation and ultimately contributing to the onset of hyperlipidemia [49]. In a cohort study including 13,667 hyperthyroid individuals, the prevalence of hyperlipidemia in hyperthyroid patients was found to be 18.7% and was considered higher compared to those without hyperthyroidism.

## Thyroid Hormones and High Blood Pressure

Hypertension is a commonly encountered condition worldwide, with approximately half of the cases being undiagnosed and only about one-fifth being adequately controlled. Most hypertensive patients have primary hypertension, while a portion presents with secondary hypertension [50]. Secondary hypertension can occur due to many diseases, including thyroid diseases [50].

The development of hypertension involves many risk factors, yet contemporary attention has focused on obesity and sedentary lifestyles as precipitating elements. Perturbations in thyroid hormone levels, which exert diverse effects on the cardiovascular system and participate in blood pressure homeostasis, contribute to heightened hypertension susceptibility. Both hyperthyroidism and hypothyroidism confer an elevated risk of hypertension. Hyperthyroidism engenders diminished systemic vascular resistance, augmented arterial stiffness, positive chronotropic effects, enhanced cardiac contractility and preload, left ventricular hypertrophy, heightened activation of the renin-angiotensin-aldosterone system, intensified sodium retention, and expanded plasma volume, all fostering the onset of hypertension [51]. Conversely, hypothyroidism manifests vasoconstriction, elevated systemic vascular resistance, increased arterial stiffness, reduced cardiac output, negative chronotropy, elevated noradrenaline levels, diminished vasodilation in skeletal muscle, hypercholesterolemia, reduced nitric oxide release, and chronic low-grade inflammation, all contributing to the genesis of hypertension [52]. In hypothyroid patients with established hypertension, there is a noted decrease in serum renin levels associated with increased systemic vascular resistance and heightened salt sensitivity [53]. Both in patients with subclinical hypothyroidism and individuals with TSH levels at the upper limit of the normal range, endothelial dysfunction has been reported to occur, characterized by impaired flow-mediated dilation. This condition has been associated with an increased risk of both atherosclerosis and hypertension development [54, 55].

In hypothyroid patients, the emergence of diastolic hypertension is expected to be prominent, accompanied by decreased pulse pressure. The prevalence of hypertension in hypothyroid patients is not clearly defined, with various frequencies reported in several studies. In a group with overt hypothyroidism, the prevalence of hypertension was found to be 14.8%, whereas in the euthyroid group, this rate was reported as 5.5% [56]. Additionally, it has been reported that hypertension regressed following T4 replacement therapy in a group of patients who developed hypertension after thyroidectomy [57].

In 40 patients, including 8 with systolic hypertension and 5 with diastolic hypertension during the thyrotoxic phase, it has been reported that blood pressure decreased after RAI treatment, and in 16 of those who developed hypothyroidism after RAI, diastolic hypertension occurred [58]. It has been reported that blood pressure tends to decrease after thyroid hormone replacement therapy. In another study, it was noted that diastolic blood pressure was higher in patients with subclinical hypothyroidism compared to euthyroid individuals, and these patients were more hyperlipidemic [59]. Individuals who underwent thyroid surgery for various types of thyroid cancer and subsequently developed hypothyroidism were found to experience elevated nocturnal systolic, diastolic, and mean blood pressure levels [60].

In a study investigating the relationship between thyroid hormone levels and blood pressure in a non-hypertensive population, it was observed that nearly half of the participants had elevated blood pressure, which was significantly associated with high levels of T3 and T4 but not with TSH [61]. Another investigation involving a large cohort revealed that serum TSH levels were found to be associated with existing high blood pressure but not with the development of new hypertension over a five-year follow-up period [62]. Moreover, in a population-based study involving individuals without prior thyroid disease, it was noted that an increase in serum TSH levels, even within the normal range, was associated with an increased risk of developing hypertension [63]. Additionally, a separate longitudinal study demonstrated that higher T4 levels were correlated with elevated blood pressure, while no such association was observed with TSH levels [64].

In the study by Saito *et al.*, it was reported that individuals with hyperthyroidism had higher systolic blood pressure compared to those without, with no significant changes in diastolic blood pressure; it was also noted that blood pressure elevation in hyperthyroid patients decreased after treatment [65]. Another study similarly reported that systolic blood pressure was particularly higher in hyperthyroid patients, especially in younger individuals, and decreased after treatment [56].

## Thyroid Hormones, Glucose Metabolism, and Insulin Resistance

Thyroid hormone influences glucose homeostasis by affecting pancreatic β-cell development and glucose metabolism through various organs, including the liver, gastrointestinal system, pancreas, adipose tissue, skeletal muscles, and central nervous system. Thyroid hormones exert multiple effects on various aspects of glucose homeostasis, including insulin secretion, tissue sensitivity to insulin, gluconeogenesis, glycogenolysis, metabolic rate, and lipid metabolism. Thyroid hormones augment gastrointestinal motility, boost beta cell development and function, stimulate insulin and glucagon secretion, enhance hepatic glucose output *via* the promotion of gluconeogenesis and glycogenolysis in the liver, which is attributed to increased hepatic expression of glucose transporter 2, and elevate fatty acid levels through increased lipolysis in adipose tissue [66]. The heightened gluconeogenesis and glycogenolysis in the liver, resulting from increased free fatty acids due to lipolysis in adipose tissue, lead to hyperinsulinemia and glucose intolerance, ultimately causing peripheral insulin resistance [67]. Besides that, thyrotoxicosis speeds up the breakdown of insulin and shortens its lifespan [68]. In hypothyroidism, disturbances in gastrointestinal glucose absorption, delayed peripheral glucose assimilation, diminished insulin sensitivity in skeletal muscle and adipose tissue, and reduced glucose disposal collectively elevate the risk of insulin resistance development [69, 70].

The risk of thyroid disorders is increased in diabetic patients, and likewise, the frequency of diabetes is elevated in thyroid patients. While the co-occurrence of type 1 diabetes mellitus and autoimmune thyroid diseases is attributed to their association with autoimmunity, the relationship between type 2 diabetes mellitus and thyroid disorders is more complex. Elevated blood glucose levels may affect the secretion of TSH by the hypothalamus and modulate the response of TSH to thyrotropin-releasing hormone, consequently influencing the conversion of free thyroxine to free triiodothyronine in peripheral tissues [71]. In a research study comprising 1,310 adult diabetic patients, thyroid disorders were identified in 31.4% of individuals with type 1 diabetes mellitus and 6.9% of those with type 2 diabetes mellitus, resulting in an overall prevalence of thyroid disease of 13.4%. Notably, a higher prevalence was observed among females, with rates of 16.8% compared to 8.8% among males [72]. The frequency of thyroid disease was found to be highest in female patients with type 1 diabetes and lowest in male patients with type 2 diabetes in this study, with subclinical hypothyroidism being the most common thyroid disorder identified. In a study examining the relationship between thyroid hormone levels and type 2 diabetes in a euthyroid population, it was reported that a decrease in T3 levels and the T3/T4 ratio, along with an increase in T4 levels, were associated with an increased risk of developing diabetes mellitus in both men and women. Additionally, it was noted that TSH levels exhibited an inverse relationship with the development of type 2 diabetes mellitus, specifically in men [73]. In another study conducted by Nederstigt *et al.*, autoimmune thyroid disease was detected in 10.3% of patients with type 1 diabetes [74]. In an observational cohort study comprising 2822 participants, it was indicated that individuals with hypothyroidism faced a 40% greater risk of developing diabetes mellitus compared to their counterparts without hypothyroidism [75]. In a cross-sectional study, it has been noted that both insulin levels and HOMA-IR values are higher in patients with both hypothyroidism and hyperthyroidism compared to euthyroid individuals; furthermore, a positive correlation between TSH and HOMA-IR values in hypothyroid patients and a negative correlation with TSH and HOMA-IR values in hyperthyroid patients has been reported [76]. In a study encompassing 2703 euthyroid subjects, a negative correlation between T4 levels and HOMA-IR, alongside a positive correlation between TSH levels and HOMA-IR, was delineated. Moreover, T4 levels exhibited notable associations with various components of MetS [15].

Both hypothyroidism and hyperthyroidism are intricately linked with insulin resistance. Although insulin resistance is a common feature of hyperthyroidism, the likelihood of developing MetS in this context is reduced due to the catabolic effects of excess thyroid hormones, which can impact factors like body weight and lipid levels and impaired glucose tolerance primarily linked to hepatic insulin resistance; nonetheless, subclinical manifestations of hyperthyroidism have been associated with a dysregulated metabolic state characterized by elevated blood sugar levels [77]. A study by Dimitriadis *et al.* found that individuals with hyperthyroidism exhibited increased insulin resistance compared to euthyroid controls [78]. Similarly, another study by Maratou *et al.* observed a significant correlation between insulin resistance and hyperthyroidism / subclinic hyperthyroidism, suggesting a potential link between excess thyroid hormone levels and impaired insulin sensitivity [79]. Furthermore, research by Gierach *et al.* highlighted the role of thyroid hormones in modulating glucose metabolism, with hyperthyroidism contributing to insulin resistance through various mechanisms, such as alterations in glucose transport and utilization [80].

**Thyroid Hormones and Non-alcoholic Fatty Liver Disease**

Non-alcoholic fatty liver disease (NAFLD) is characterized by excessive fat accumulation in the liver and is closely associated with insulin resistance and MetS. This pathology is defined as histopathological due to the presence of >5% steatosis in hepatocytes or >5.6% proton fraction in the fat fraction using proton magnetic resonance spectroscopy [81]. NAFLD manifests in four progressive stages: Simple steatosis, denoting hepatic lipid accumulation devoid of inflammation or hepatocellular compromise; NASH, featuring hepatic fat deposition accompanied by inflammatory infiltration and cellular injury; fibrosis, characterized by hepatic tissue fibrosis stratified into mild, moderate, and advanced grades; and liver cirrhosis, indicative of irreversible hepatocellular damage with nodular regenerative hyperplasia ensconced in fibrous septa, potentially culminating in hepatocellular carcinoma (HCC) development [82]. The escalating incidence of NAFLD, presently the most prevalent liver disorder with a nearly 30% prevalence rate, can be ascribed to its intimate connection with the escalating trends in insulin resistance, obesity, type 2 diabetes, hypertension, hyperlipidemia, and MetS.

Hypothyroidism heightens the risk of insulin resistance and obesity, as it fosters enhanced cholesterol absorption in the intestines and diminishes LDL cholesterol clearance, resulting in elevated LDL cholesterol levels in the bloodstream and triglyceride buildup in the liver, precipitating the onset of NAFLD and consequent hepatic insulin resistance [83]. Hepatic *de novo* lipogenesis and adipose tissue lipolysis are further stimulated by insulin resistance, resulting in heightened delivery of free fatty acids to the liver, which is accompanied by elevated plasma triglyceride levels and diminished plasma HDL levels, thus exacerbating the atherogenic dyslipidemia characteristic of NAFLD [84]. In an epidemiological study conducted among patients with NAFLD, the prevalence rates were found to be 42% for MetS, 69% for hyperlipidemia, 51% for obesity, 39% for hypertension, and 22% for diabetes [85]. In Pagadala *et al.*'s study, the frequency of hypothyroidism was elevated among individuals with NAFLD in comparison to controls, and it was further increased in those with NASH compared to NAFLD patients without NASH. Additionally, NAFLD and NASH were more prevalent in individuals with hypothyroidism [86]. In a meta-analysis conducted by He and colleagues incorporating 13 studies, both hypothyroidism and subclinical hypothyroidism were found to elevate the risk of NAFLD [87]. Another meta-analysis, encompassing 51,407 hypothyroid patients with a NAFLD prevalence of 28.2%, highlighted that increased TSH levels, advanced age, elevated BMI, and decreased T4 levels were associated with heightened NAFLD risk in hypothyroid patients, while no relationship was observed between T3 levels and NAFLD development [88]. Unlike these results, in a systematic review that examined 14 observational studies, no significant association was found between NAFLD and either overt hypothyroidism or subclinical hypothyroidism [89].

Evidence suggests that hyperthyroidism may confer a protective influence on the development of NAFLD. A modest cross-sectional investigation conducted in China revealed a NAFLD prevalence of 11.9% among individuals with hyperthyroidism, notably indicating that elevated T3 levels correlated with reduced hepatic fat accumulation and diminished susceptibility to NAFLD [90]. Subsequently, a comprehensive case-control study corroborated these observations, affirming an inverse relationship between hyperthyroidism and the risk of NAFLD [91].

## CONCLUSION

The intersection between thyroid diseases and MetS presents a compelling area of inquiry, with both conditions exerting significant impacts on each other's pathophysiology. While hypothyroidism and hyperthyroidism have distinct metabolic effects, ranging from dyslipidemia to insulin resistance, understanding the bidirectional relationship between these disorders is crucial for comprehensive patient care. Despite ongoing research efforts, gaps in knowledge persist, necessitating continued exploration into the underlying mechanisms and clinical implications of this intricate interplay.

## REFERENCES

[1]     Cornier MA, Dabelea D, Hernandez TL, *et al.* The metabolic syndrome. Endocr Rev 2008; 29(7): 777-822.
[http://dx.doi.org/10.1210/er.2008-0024] [PMID: 18971485]

[2]     Mullur R, Liu YY, Brent GA. Thyroid hormone regulation of metabolism. Physiol Rev 2014; 94(2): 355-82.
[http://dx.doi.org/10.1152/physrev.00030.2013] [PMID: 24692351]

[3]     Shahid MA, Ashraf MA, Sharma S. Physiology, Thyroid Hormone. StatPearls. Treasure Island, FL: StatPearls Publishing 2024. Updated 2023 Jun 5 Internet Available from: https://www.ncbi.nlm.nih.gov/books/NBK500006/

[4]     Chiovato L, Magri F, Carlé A. Hypothyroidism in Context: Where We've Been and Where We're Going. Adv Ther 2019; 36(S2) (Suppl. 2): 47-58.
[http://dx.doi.org/10.1007/s12325-019-01080-8] [PMID: 31485975]

[5]     Aoki Y, Belin RM, Clickner R, Jeffries R, Phillips L, Mahaffey KR. Serum TSH and total T4 in the United States population and their association with participant characteristics: National Health and Nutrition Examination Survey (NHANES 1999-2002). Thyroid 2007; 17(12): 1211-23.
[http://dx.doi.org/10.1089/thy.2006.0235] [PMID: 18177256]

[6]     Mantovani A, Nascimbeni F, Lonardo A, *et al.* Association Between Primary Hypothyroidism and Nonalcoholic Fatty Liver Disease: A Systematic Review and Meta-Analysis. Thyroid 2018; 28(10): 1270-84.
[http://dx.doi.org/10.1089/thy.2018.0257] [PMID: 30084737]

[7]     Bahn RS, Burch HB, Cooper DS, *et al.* Hyperthyroidism and other causes of thyrotoxicosis: management guidelines of the American Thyroid Association and American Association of Clinical Endocrinologists. Thyroid 2011; 21(6): 593-646.
[http://dx.doi.org/10.1089/thy.2010.0417] [PMID: 21510801]

[8]     Available from: https://www.uptodate.com/contents/metabolic-syndrome-insulin-resistance-synd-ome-or-syndro-
e-
x?search=metabolic%20syndrome&source=search_result&selectedTitle=1%7E150&usage_type=defa
ult&display_rank=1

[9]     Ford ES, Giles WH, Dietz WH: Prevalence of the metabolic syndrome among US adults: findings from the third National Health and Nutrition Examination Survey. JAMA 2002, 16; 287(3): 356-359.
[http://dx.doi.org/10.1001/jama.287.3.356]

[10]    Hirode G, Wong RJ: Trends in the Prevalence of Metabolic Syndrome in the United States, 2011-2016. JAMA 2020, 23; 323(24): 2526-2528.

[11]    Liang X, Or B, Tsoi MF, Cheung CL, Cheung BMY. Prevalence of metabolic syndrome in the United States National Health and Nutrition Examination Survey 2011–18. Postgrad Med J 2023; 99(1175): 985-92.
[http://dx.doi.org/10.1093/postmj/qgad008] [PMID: 36906842]

[12]    Teixeira PFS, dos Santos PB, Pazos-Moura CC. The role of thyroid hormone in metabolism and metabolic syndrome. Ther Adv Endocrinol Metab 2020; 11(11): 2042018820917869.
[http://dx.doi.org/10.1177/2042018820917869] [PMID: 32489580]

[13]    Waring AC, Rodondi N, Harrison S, *et al.* Thyroid function and prevalent and incident metabolic syndrome in older adults: the health, ageing and body composition study. Clin Endocrinol (Oxf) 2012; 76(6): 911-8.
[http://dx.doi.org/10.1111/j.1365-2265.2011.04328.x] [PMID: 22187968]

[14]    Ruhla S, Weickert MO, Arafat AM, *et al.* A high normal TSH is associated with the metabolic syndrome. Clin Endocrinol (Oxf) 2010; 72(5): 696-701.
[http://dx.doi.org/10.1111/j.1365-2265.2009.03698.x] [PMID: 20447068]

[15]    Roos A, Bakker SJL, Links TP, Gans ROB, Wolffenbuttel BHR. Thyroid function is associated with components of the metabolic syndrome in euthyroid subjects. J Clin Endocrinol Metab 2007; 92(2): 491-6.
[http://dx.doi.org/10.1210/jc.2006-1718] [PMID: 17090642]

[16]    Mehran L, Amouzegar A, Abdi H, *et al.* Incidence of Thyroid Dysfunction Facing Metabolic Syndrome: A Prospective Comparative Study with 9 Years of Follow-Up. Eur Thyroid J 2021; 10(5): 390-8.
[http://dx.doi.org/10.1159/000512665] [PMID: 34540709]

[17]    Available from: https://www.who.int/news-room/fact-sheets/detail/obesity-and-overweight

[18]    Jensen MD, Ryan DH, Apovian CM, *et al.* American College of Cardiology/American Heart Association Task Force on Practice Guidelines; Obesity Society. 2013 AHA/ACC/TOS guideline for the management of overweight and obesity in adults: a report of the American College of Cardiology/American Heart Association Task Force on Practice Guidelines and The Obesity Society. Circulation 2014, 24; 129(25 Suppl 2): S102-138.

[19]    Song RH, Wang B, Yao QM, Li Q, Jia X, Zhang JA. The Impact of Obesity on Thyroid Autoimmunity and Dysfunction: A Systematic Review and Meta-Analysis. Front Immunol 2019, 1; 10: 2349.
[http://dx.doi.org/10.3389/fimmu.2019.02349]

[20]    Iwen KA, Oelkrug R, Kalscheuer H, Brabant G. Metabolic Syndrome in Thyroid Disease. Front Horm Res 2018; 49: 48-66.
[http://dx.doi.org/10.1159/000485996] [PMID: 29895010]

[21]    Kim B. Thyroid hormone as a determinant of energy expenditure and the basal metabolic rate. Thyroid 2008; 18(2): 141-4.
[http://dx.doi.org/10.1089/thy.2007.0266] [PMID: 18279014]

[22]    Knudsen N, Laurberg P, Rasmussen LB, *et al.* Small differences in thyroid function may be important for body mass index and the occurrence of obesity in the population. J Clin Endocrinol Metab 2005; 90(7): 4019-24.
[http://dx.doi.org/10.1210/jc.2004-2225] [PMID: 15870128]

[23]    Bjergved L, Jørgensen T, Perrild H, *et al.* Thyroid function and body weight: a community-based longitudinal study. PLoS One 2014; 9(4): e93515.
[http://dx.doi.org/10.1371/journal.pone.0093515] [PMID: 24728291]

[24]    He J, Lai Y, Yang J, *et al.* The Relationship Between Thyroid Function and Metabolic Syndrome and Its Components: A Cross-Sectional Study in a Chinese Population. Front Endocrinol (Lausanne) 2021,

31; 12: 661160.
[http://dx.doi.org/10.3389/fendo.2021.661160]

[25] Fontenelle L, Feitosa M, Severo J, *et al.* Thyroid Function in Human Obesity: Underlying Mechanisms. Horm Metab Res 2016; 48(12): 787-94.
[http://dx.doi.org/10.1055/s-0042-121421] [PMID: 27923249]

[26] Longhi S, Radetti G. Thyroid function and obesity. J Clin Res Pediatr Endocrinol 2013; 5(Suppl 1) (Suppl. 1): 40-4.
[PMID: 23149391]

[27] Isozaki O, Tsushima T, Nozoe Y, Miyakawa M, Takano K. Leptin regulation of the thyroids: negative regulation on thyroid hormone levels in euthyroid subjects and inhibitory effects on iodide uptake and Na+/I- symporter mRNA expression in rat FRTL-5 cells. Endocr J 2004; 51(4): 415-23.
[http://dx.doi.org/10.1507/endocrj.51.415] [PMID: 15351798]

[28] Ríos-Prego M, Anibarro L, Sánchez-Sobrino P. Relationship between thyroid dysfunction and body weight: a not so evident paradigm. Int J Gen Med 2019; 12(12): 299-304.
[http://dx.doi.org/10.2147/IJGM.S206983] [PMID: 31692525]

[29] Li Y, Wang L, Zhou L, *et al.* Thyroid stimulating hormone increases hepatic gluconeogenesis *via* CRTC2. Mol Cell Endocrinol 2017; 446(446): 70-80.
[http://dx.doi.org/10.1016/j.mce.2017.02.015] [PMID: 28212844]

[30] Jornayvaz FR, Lee HY, Jurczak MJ, *et al.* Thyroid hormone receptor-α gene knockout mice are protected from diet-induced hepatic insulin resistance. Endocrinology 2012; 153(2): 583-91.
[http://dx.doi.org/10.1210/en.2011-1793] [PMID: 22147010]

[31] Huang YY, Gusdon AM, Qu S. Cross-talk between the thyroid and liver: a new target for nonalcoholic fatty liver disease treatment. World J Gastroenterol 2013, 7; 19(45): 8238-8246.
[http://dx.doi.org/10.3748/wjg.v19.i45.8238]

[32] Klieverik LP, Coomans CP, Endert E, *et al.* Thyroid hormone effects on whole-body energy homeostasis and tissue-specific fatty acid uptake *in vivo*. Endocrinology 2009; 150(12): 5639-48.
[http://dx.doi.org/10.1210/en.2009-0297] [PMID: 19854865]

[33] Nedvidkova J, Haluzik M, Bartak V, *et al.* Changes of noradrenergic activity and lipolysis in the subcutaneous abdominal adipose tissue of hypo- and hyperthyroid patients: an *in vivo* microdialysis study. Ann N Y Acad Sci 2004; 1018(1): 541-9.
[http://dx.doi.org/10.1196/annals.1296.067] [PMID: 15240413]

[34] Thompson GR, Soutar AK, Spengel FA, Jadhav A, Gavigan SJ, Myant NB. Defects of receptor-mediated low density lipoprotein catabolism in homozygous familial hypercholesterolemia and hypothyroidism *in vivo*. Proc Natl Acad Sci USA 1981; 78(4): 2591-5.
[http://dx.doi.org/10.1073/pnas.78.4.2591] [PMID: 6264482]

[35] Hoogerbrugge N, Jansen H, Staels B, Kloet LT, Birkenhäger JC. Growth hormone normalizes low-density lipoprotein receptor gene expression in hypothyroid rats. Metabolism 1996; 45(6): 680-5.
[http://dx.doi.org/10.1016/S0026-0495(96)90131-6] [PMID: 8637440]

[36] Costantini F, Pierdomenico SD, Cesare DD, *et al.* Effect of thyroid function on LDL oxidation. Arterioscler Thromb Vasc Biol 1998; 18(5): 732-7.
[http://dx.doi.org/10.1161/01.ATV.18.5.732] [PMID: 9598831]

[37] Friedman M, Byers SO, Rosenman RH. Changes in excretion of intestinal cholesterol and sterol digitonides in hyper and hypothyroidism. Circulation 1952; 5(5): 657-60.
[http://dx.doi.org/10.1161/01.CIR.5.5.657] [PMID: 14926049]

[38] O'Brien T, Dinneen SF, O'Brien PC, Palumbo PJ. Hyperlipidemia in patients with primary and secondary hypothyroidism. Mayo Clin Proc 1993; 68(9): 860-6.
[http://dx.doi.org/10.1016/S0025-6196(12)60694-6] [PMID: 8371604]

[39] Tagami T, Tamanaha T, Shimazu S, *et al.* Lipid profiles in the untreated patients with Hashimoto

thyroiditis and the effects of thyroxine treatment on subclinical hypothyroidism with Hashimoto thyroiditis. Endocr J 2010; 57(3): 253-8.
[http://dx.doi.org/10.1507/endocrj.K09E-315] [PMID: 20032565]

[40]   Jung KY, Ahn HY, Han SK, Park YJ, Cho BY, Moon MK. Association between thyroid function and lipid profiles, apolipoproteins, and high-density lipoprotein function. J Clin Lipidol 2017; 11(6): 1347-53.
[http://dx.doi.org/10.1016/j.jacl.2017.08.015] [PMID: 28958565]

[41]   Willard DL, Leung AM, Pearce EN. Thyroid function testing in patients with newly diagnosed hyperlipidemia. JAMA Intern Med 2014; 174(2): 287-9.
[http://dx.doi.org/10.1001/jamainternmed.2013.12188] [PMID: 24217672]

[42]   Tsimihodimos V, Bairaktari E, Tzallas C, Miltiadus G, Liberopoulos E, Elisaf M. The incidence of thyroid function abnormalities in patients attending an outpatient lipid clinic. Thyroid 1999; 9(4): 365-8.
[http://dx.doi.org/10.1089/thy.1999.9.365] [PMID: 10319942]

[43]   Series JJ, Biggart EM, O'Reilly DS, Packard CJ, Shepherd J. Thyroid dysfunction and hypercholesterolaemia in the general population of Glasgow, Scotland. Clin Chim Acta 1988, 15; 172(2-3): 217-221.
[http://dx.doi.org/10.1016/0009-8981(88)90326-9]

[44]   Diekman T, Lansberg PJ, Kastelein JJ, Wiersinga WM. Prevalence and correction of hypothyroidism in a large cohort of patients referred for dyslipidemia. Arch Intern Med 1995, 24; 155(14): 1490-1495.
[http://dx.doi.org/10.1001/archinte.1995.00430140052004]

[45]   Kung AWC, Pang RWC, Janus ED. Elevated serum lipoprotein(a) in subclinical hypothyroidism. Clin Endocrinol (Oxf) 1995; 43(4): 445-9.
[http://dx.doi.org/10.1111/j.1365-2265.1995.tb02616.x] [PMID: 7586619]

[46]   Pirich C, Müllner M, Sinzinger H. Prevalence and relevance of thyroid dysfunction in 1922 cholesterol screening participants. J Clin Epidemiol 2000; 53(6): 623-9.
[http://dx.doi.org/10.1016/S0895-4356(99)00187-0] [PMID: 10880781]

[47]   Tanis BC, Westendorp RGJ, Smelt AHM. Effect of thyroid substitution on hypercholesterolaemia in patients with subclinical hypothyroidism: a reanalysis of intervention studies Clin Endocrinol (Oxf) 1996; 44(6): 643-9.
[http://dx.doi.org/10.1046/j.1365-2265.1996.739560.x] [PMID: 8759176]

[48]   Ortiga-Carvalho TM, Chiamolera MI, Pazos-Moura CC, Wondisford FE. Hypothalamus-Pituitar--Thyroid Axis. Compr Physiol 2016, 13; 6(3): 1387-1428.
[http://dx.doi.org/10.1002/cphy.c150027]

[49]   Herz J, Strickland DK. LRP: a multifunctional scavenger and signaling receptor. J Clin Invest 2001; 108(6): 779-84.
[http://dx.doi.org/10.1172/JCI200113992] [PMID: 11560943]

[50]   Young WF Jr, Calhoun DA, Lenders JWM, Stowasser M, Textor SC. Screening for endocrine hypertension: an endocrine society scientific statement. Endocr Rev 2017; 38(2): 103-22.
[http://dx.doi.org/10.1210/er.2017-00054]

[51]   Berta E, Lengyel I, Halmi S, *et al.* Hypertension in Thyroid Disorders. Front Endocrinol (Lausanne) 2019, 17; 10:482.
[http://dx.doi.org/10.3389/fendo.2019.00482]

[52]   Cappola AR, Ladenson PW. Hypothyroidism and Atherosclerosis. J Clin Endocrinol Metab 2003; 88(6): 2438-44.
[http://dx.doi.org/10.1210/jc.2003-030398] [PMID: 12788839]

[53]   Gumieniak O, Perlstein TS, Hopkins PN, *et al.* Thyroid function and blood pressure homeostasis in euthyroid subjects. J Clin Endocrinol Metab 2004; 89(7): 3455-61.

[http://dx.doi.org/10.1210/jc.2003-032143] [PMID: 15240631]

[54]    Lekakis J, Papamichael C, Alevizaki M, *et al.* Flow-mediated, endothelium-dependent vasodilation is impaired in subjects with hypothyroidism, borderline hypothyroidism, and high-normal serum thyrotropin (TSH) values. Thyroid 1997; 7(3): 411-4.
[http://dx.doi.org/10.1089/thy.1997.7.411] [PMID: 9226212]

[55]    Cikim AS, Oflaz H, Ozbey N, *et al.* Evaluation of endothelial function in subclinical hypothyroidism and subclinical hyperthyroidism. Thyroid 2004; 14(8): 605-9.
[http://dx.doi.org/10.1089/1050725041692891] [PMID: 15320973]

[56]    Saito I, Samta T. Hypertension in thyroid disorders. Endocrinol Metab Clin North Am 1994; 23(2): 379-86.
[http://dx.doi.org/10.1016/S0889-8529(18)30103-8] [PMID: 8070428]

[57]    Fommei E, Iervasi G. The role of thyroid hormone in blood pressure homeostasis: evidence from short-term hypothyroidism in humans. J Clin Endocrinol Metab 2002; 87(5): 1996-2000.
[http://dx.doi.org/10.1210/jcem.87.5.8464] [PMID: 11994331]

[58]    Streeten DH, Anderson GH Jr, Howland T, Chiang R, Smulyan H. Effects of thyroid function on blood pressure. Recognition of hypothyroid hypertension. Hypertension 1988; 11(1): 78-83.
[http://dx.doi.org/10.1161/01.HYP.11.1.78] [PMID: 3338842]

[59]    Luboshitzky R, Aviv A, Herer P, Lavie L. Risk factors for cardiovascular disease in women with subclinical hypothyroidism. Thyroid 2002; 12(5): 421-5.
[http://dx.doi.org/10.1089/105072502760043512] [PMID: 12097204]

[60]    Botella-Carretero JI, Gómez-Bueno M, Barrios V, *et al.* Chronic thyrotropin-suppressive therapy with levothyroxine and short-term overt hypothyroidism after thyroxine withdrawal are associated with undesirable cardiovascular effects in patients with differentiated thyroid carcinoma. Endocr Relat Cancer 2004; 11(2): 345-56.
[http://dx.doi.org/10.1677/erc.0.0110345] [PMID: 15163309]

[61]    Gu Y, Zheng L, Zhang Q, *et al.* Relationship between thyroid function and elevated blood pressure in euthyroid adults. J Clin Hypertens (Greenwich) 2018; 20(10): 1541-9.
[http://dx.doi.org/10.1111/jch.13369] [PMID: 30260550]

[62]    Ittermann T, Tiller D, Meisinger C, *et al.* High serum thyrotropin levels are associated with current but not with incident hypertension. Thyroid 2013; 23(8): 955-63.
[http://dx.doi.org/10.1089/thy.2012.0626] [PMID: 23427935]

[63]    Åsvold BO, Bjøro T, Nilsen TIL, Vatten LJ. Association between blood pressure and serum thyroid-stimulating hormone concentration within the reference range: a population-based study. J Clin Endocrinol Metab 2007; 92(3): 841-5.
[http://dx.doi.org/10.1210/jc.2006-2208] [PMID: 17200168]

[64]    Abdi H, Gharibzadeh S, Tasdighi E, *et al.* Associations Between Thyroid and Blood Pressure in Euthyroid Adults: A 9-Year Longitudinal Study. Horm Metab Res 2018; 50(3): 236-41.
[http://dx.doi.org/10.1055/s-0044-101756] [PMID: 29523010]

[65]    Saito I, Ito K, Saruta T. The effect of age on blood pressure in hyperthyroidism. J Am Geriatr Soc 1985; 33(1): 19-22.
[http://dx.doi.org/10.1111/j.1532-5415.1985.tb02854.x] [PMID: 3965551]

[66]    Eom YS, Wilson JR, Bernet VJ. Links between Thyroid Disorders and Glucose Homeostasis. Diabetes Metab J 2022; 46(2): 239-56.
[http://dx.doi.org/10.4093/dmj.2022.0013] [PMID: 35385635]

[67]    Nishi M. Diabetes mellitus and thyroid diseases. Diabetol Int 2018, 9; 9(2): 108-112.
[http://dx.doi.org/10.1007/s13340-018-0352-4]

[68]    O'Meara NM, Blackman JD, Sturis J, Polonsky KS. Alterations in the kinetics of C-peptide and insulin secretion in hyperthyroidism. J Clin Endocrinol Metab 1993; 76(1): 79-84.

[PMID: 8421108]

[69]   Rochon C, Tauveron I, Dejax C, *et al.* Response of glucose disposal to hyperinsulinaemia in human hypothyroidism and hyperthyroidism. Clin Sci (Lond) 2003; 104(1): 7-15.
[http://dx.doi.org/10.1042/cs1040007] [PMID: 12519082]

[70]   Duntas LH, Orgiazzi J, Brabant G. The interface between thyroid and diabetes mellitus. Clin Endocrinol (Oxf) 2011; 75(1): 1-9.
[http://dx.doi.org/10.1111/j.1365-2265.2011.04029.x] [PMID: 21521298]

[71]   Biondi B, Kahaly GJ, Robertson RP. Thyroid Dysfunction and Diabetes Mellitus: Two Closely Associated Disorders. Endocr Rev 2019, 1; 40(3): 789-824.
[http://dx.doi.org/10.1210/er.2018-00163]

[72]   Perros P, McCrimmon RJ, Shaw G, Frier BM. Frequency of thyroid dysfunction in diabetic patients: value of annual screening. Diabet Med 1995; 12(7): 622-7.
[http://dx.doi.org/10.1111/j.1464-5491.1995.tb00553.x] [PMID: 7554786]

[73]   Gu Y, Li H, Bao X, *et al.* The Relationship Between Thyroid Function and the Prevalence of Type 2 Diabetes Mellitus in Euthyroid Subjects. J Clin Endocrinol Metab. 2017, 1; 102(2): 434-442.

[74]   Nederstigt C, Corssmit EPM, de Koning EJP, Dekkers OM. Incidence and prevalence of thyroid dysfunction in type 1 diabetes. J Diabetes Complications 2016; 30(3): 420-5.
[http://dx.doi.org/10.1016/j.jdiacomp.2015.12.027] [PMID: 26868720]

[75]   Thvilum M, Brandt F, Almind D, Christensen K, Brix TH, Hegedüs L: Type and extent of somatic morbidity before and after the diagnosis of hypothyroidism. a nationwide register study. PLoS One 2013, 16; 8(9): e75789.

[76]   Kapadia KB, Bhatt PA, Shah JS. Association between altered thyroid state and insulin resistance. J Pharmacol Pharmacother 2012; 3(2): 156-60.
[PMID: 22629091]

[77]   Mehran L, Amouzegar A, Azizi F. Thyroid disease and the metabolic syndrome. Curr Opin Endocrinol Diabetes Obes 2019; 26(5): 256-65.
[http://dx.doi.org/10.1097/MED.0000000000000500] [PMID: 31369412]

[78]   Dimitriadis G, Mitrou P, Lambadiari V, Maratou E, Raptis SA. Insulin effects in muscle and adipose tissue. Diabetes Res Clin Pract 2011; 93 (Suppl. 1): S52-9.
[http://dx.doi.org/10.1016/S0168-8227(11)70014-6] [PMID: 21864752]

[79]   Maratou E, Hadjidakis DJ, Peppa M, *et al.* Studies of insulin resistance in patients with clinical and subclinical hyperthyroidism. Eur J Endocrinol 2010; 163(4): 625-30.
[http://dx.doi.org/10.1530/EJE-10-0246] [PMID: 20643758]

[80]   Gierach M, Gierach J, Junik R. Insulin resistance and thyroid disorders. Endokrynol Pol 2014; 65(1): 70-6.
[http://dx.doi.org/10.5603/EP.2014.0010] [PMID: 24549605]

[81]   EASL–EASD–EASO Clinical Practice Guidelines for the management of non-alcoholic fatty liver disease. J Hepatol 2016; 64(6): 1388-402.
[http://dx.doi.org/10.1016/j.jhep.2015.11.004] [PMID: 27062661]

[82]   Wang J, He W, Tsai PJ, *et al*: Mutual interaction between endoplasmic reticulum and mitochondria in nonalcoholic fatty liver disease. Lipids Health Dis 2020, 13; 19(1): 72.
[http://dx.doi.org/10.1186/s12944-020-01210-0]

[83]   Mavromati M, Jornayvaz FR: Hypothyroidism-Associated Dyslipidemia: Potential Molecular Mechanisms Leading to NAFLD. Int J Mol Sci 2021, 26; 22(23): 12797.
[http://dx.doi.org/10.3390/ijms222312797]

[84]   Bugianesi E, Moscatiello S, Ciaravella MF, Marchesini G. Insulin resistance in nonalcoholic fatty liver disease. Curr Pharm Des 2010; 16(17): 1941-51.

[http://dx.doi.org/10.2174/138161210791208875] [PMID: 20370677]

[85]   Younossi ZM, Koenig AB, Abdelatif D, Fazel Y, Henry L, Wymer M. Global epidemiology of nonalcoholic fatty liver disease-Meta-analytic assessment of prevalence, incidence, and outcomes. Hepatology 2016; 64(1): 73-84.
[http://dx.doi.org/10.1002/hep.28431] [PMID: 26707365]

[86]   Pagadala MR, Zein CO, Dasarathy S, Yerian LM, Lopez R, McCullough AJ. Prevalence of hypothyroidism in nonalcoholic fatty liver disease. Dig Dis Sci 2012; 57(2): 528-34.
[http://dx.doi.org/10.1007/s10620-011-2006-2] [PMID: 22183820]

[87]   He W, An X, Li L, *et al*. Relationship between Hypothyroidism and Non-Alcoholic Fatty Liver Disease: A Systematic Review and Meta-analysis. Front Endocrinol (Lausanne) 2017; 8(8): 335.
[http://dx.doi.org/10.3389/fendo.2017.00335] [PMID: 29238323]

[88]   Zeng X, Li B, Zou Y: The relationship between non-alcoholic fatty liver disease and hypothyroidism: A systematic review and meta-analysis. Medicine (Baltimore) 2021, 30; 100(17): e25738.
[http://dx.doi.org/10.1097/MD.0000000000025738]

[89]   Jaruvongvanich V, Sanguankeo A, Upala S. Nonalcoholic Fatty Liver Disease Is Not Associated with Thyroid Hormone Levels and Hypothyroidism: A Systematic Review and Meta-Analysis. Eur Thyroid J 2017; 6(4): 208-15.
[http://dx.doi.org/10.1159/000454920] [PMID: 28868261]

[90]   Wang B, Wang B, Yang Y, *et al*: Thyroid function and non-alcoholic fatty liver disease in hyperthyroidism patients. BMC Endocr Disord 2021, 18; 21(1): 27.
[http://dx.doi.org/10.1186/s12902-021-00694-w]

[91]   Labenz C, Kostev K, Armandi A, Gallè PR, Schattenberg JM. Impact of thyroid disorders on the incidence of non-alcoholic fatty liver disease in Germany. United European Gastroenterol J 2021; 9(7): 829-36.
[http://dx.doi.org/10.1002/ueg2.12124] [PMID: 34288580]

# CHAPTER 24

# Metabolic Syndrome and Polycystic Ovary Syndrome

**Derya Aydın Sivri**[1,*]

[1] *Department of Obstetrics and Gynecology, Faculty of Medicine, Istanbul Atlas University, İstanbul, Turkey*

**Abstract:** Metabolic syndrome occurs at an early age in women with polycystic ovary syndrome (PCOS), particularly among women with the highest insulin levels and body mass index. Obesity is a common characteristic of PCOS and is more common in women with PCOS. Excessive weight gain may reveal the latent PCOS condition. Most women with PCOS are hyperinsulinemic and insulin-resistant. Insulin resistance (IR) is a major cause of metabolic manifestations and is known to be a common finding in PCOS. PCOS is also associated with an increased risk of impaired glucose tolerance, type 2 gestational diabetes mellitus, lipid and lipoprotein abnormalities, and nonalcoholic fatty liver disease. The presence of obesity, IR, impaired glucose tolerance, diabetes mellitus type 2, and dyslipidemia may predispose to coronary heart disease in women with PCOS.

**Keywords:** Insulin resistance, Metabolic syndrome, Polycystic ovary syndrome.

## INTRODUCTION

There are several definitions of metabolic syndrome. The National Cholesterol Education Program-(NCEP) Adult Treatment Panel III (ATP III) criteria are the most widely used. Any three of the following five criteria compose the diagnosis of metabolic syndrome, according to the 2005 NCEP, ATP III criteria. These criteria include:

1. Waist circumference over 40 inches (men) or 35 inches (women),

2. Blood pressure over 130/85 mmHg,

3. Fasting triglyceride (TG) level over 150 mg/dl,

* **Corresponding author Derya Aydın Sivri:** Department of Obstetrics and Gynecology, Faculty of Medicine, Istanbul Atlas University, İstanbul, Turkey; E-mail: deryasivri@hotmail.com

**Hafize Uzun & Seyma Dumur (Eds.)**

4. Fasting high-density lipoprotein (HDL) cholesterol levels less than 40 mg/dl (men) or 50 mg/dl (women) and

5. Fasting blood sugar over 100 mg/dl [1].

In the USA, 34.5% of adults (33.7% among men and 35.4% among women) met the National Cholesterol Education Program (NCEP) Adult Treatment Panel III (ATP III) criteria [2].

In addition to increased body weight, age, race, smoking, postmenopausal status, physical inactivity, high carbohydrate diet, low household income, and no alcohol consumption are the main risk factors for metabolic syndrome [3].

## Polycystic Ovary Syndrome (PCOS)

Polycystic ovary syndrome (PCOS) is the most common endocrine and metabolic disorder of reproductive-aged women, affecting approximately 9-18% of women in this age group, depending on the criteria used [4]. This syndrome is characterized by the polycystic appearance of the ovaries, chronic anovulation, and hyperandrogenism with variable clinical manifestations (oligo-amenorrhea, hirsutism, acne, and infertility) [5, 6].

PCOS is a multifactorial syndrome caused by the combination of many factors and is associated with multiple cardiometabolic outcomes, such as insulin resistance (IR), diabetes mellitus (both type 2 and gestational), obesity, atherogenic dyslipidemia, systemic inflammation, hypertension, coagulation disorders, and alcoholic fatty liver disease. Hyperandrogenemia plays a major role in the degree of these conditions.

The presence of IR plays an important role in the pathophysiology of metabolic syndrome, and hyperandrogenemia is an important cause of metabolic and reproductive disorders associated with PCOS, putting patients at increased risk of obesity, dyslipidemia, IR, type 2 diabetes, metabolic syndrome, and cardiovascular disease that may be important determinants of long-term health in this population [7].

Metabolic dysfunction, including hyperinsulinemia, IR, and type 2 diabetes of PCOS, overlap with components of the metabolic syndrome [4, 8 - 10].

More than 50% of women with PCOS are overweight or obese [11]. Abdominal visceral fat leads to IR, abnormal adipokine, and fatty acid enhancement [12]. Insulin resistance occurs in 50-70% of women with PCOS.

Metabolic syndrome occurs at an early age in women with PCOS, particularly among women with the highest insulin levels and BMI. Hyperinsulinemia, one of the main factors in the pathogenesis of PCOS, appears to be a common link between PCOS and metabolic syndrome. Strategies used in the treatment of IR have proven useful in the treatment of both syndromes. Whether these strategies will lead to a reduction in the risk of developing cardiovascular disease and type 2 diabetes remains to be proven. The metabolic syndrome is a common condition, especially in obese women with polycystic ovary syndrome (PCOS), particularly among women with the highest insulin levels and BMI. Hyperinsulinemia is a likely common pathogenetic factor for both PCOS and metabolic syndrome [13].

## Obesity and PCOS

Obesity is a common characteristic of PCOS and is more common in women with PCOS [11]. The prevalence of obesity in these women varies due to geographic, environmental, and population differences between studies. It is unclear whether PCOS causes obesity or PCOS development [14]. There is a bidirectional relationship between PCOS and obesity; furthermore, excessive weight gain may reveal the latent PCOS condition [14]. Obesity is generally associated with high circulating insulin levels, resulting in increased androgen production in the ovaries [15].

Although the role of androgens in the development of visceral adiposity is unclear, it is known that IR causes this issue in women with PCOS [16]. Visceral adiposity may be a factor that triggers the development of irregular menstruation.

In overweight or obese women with PCOS, weight loss of as little as 5% has been found to improve PCOS symptoms [17, 18].

It has been reported that at least 50% of women with PCOS are overweight or obese, and most of these women have abdominal adiposity [19].

The presence of obesity in women with PCOS worsens metabolic and reproductive features [20].

The risk of PCOS increases with the presence of obesity, and the metabolic complications of PCOS are worsened by the concomitant presence of obesity, but it is still unclear if obesity itself is causative [21, 22].

## Insulin Resistance and PCOS

Most women with PCOS are hyperinsulinemic and insulin-resistant compared with normal women, independent of obesity [23]. IR is a major cause of metabolic manifestations and is known to be a common finding in PCOS [23]. The estimated prevalence of IR is 30% and 70% in lean and obese women with PCOS, respectively [24], which may lead to additional metabolic and reproductive complications subsequently [25]. One study found that the severity of menstrual dysfunction is associated with greater IR [26].

Although the etiology of the increased IR in PCOS remains unclear, it is known that the theca cells in women with PCOS are hyperresponsive to the androgen secretory action of insülin and hyperinsulinemia contributes to hyperandrogenism by both stimulating androgen biosynthesis in theca cells and suppressing sex hormone binding globulin production [27].

The prevalence of impaired glucose tolerance is 23-35% and that of diabetes mellitus type 2 is 4-10% in women with PCOS [28, 29]. PCOS is also associated with an increased risk of gestational diabetes mellitus [30].

## Dyslipidemia and PCOS

Lipid and lipoprotein abnormalities associated with IR have been identified in women with PCOS [31]. The prevalence of these abnormalities has been reported to be 70% in PCOS women [32]. Dyslipidemia is characterized by increased levels of low-density lipoprotein (LDL), very low-density lipoprotein (VLDL), serum TG, and free fatty acid concentrations and decreased levels of HDL in PCOS [33].

## Nonalcoholic Fatty Liver Disease and PCOS

The prevalence of nonalcoholic fatty liver disease (NAFLD) appears to be increased in women with PCOS [34, 35]. IR appears to play the main pathogenic role in the development of NAFLD, independent of obesity [34]. In one study, 30% of women with PCOS had elevated serum alanine aminotransferase (ALT) concentrations [35].

## CONCLUSION

PCOS is a disease that causes chronic diseases such as diabetes, hypertension, and coronary artery disease at a young age, and all women with PCOS should be screened for metabolic syndrome.

## REFERENCES

[1]     Grundy SM, Cleeman JI, Daniels SR, *et al.* Diagnosis and Management of the Metabolic Syndrome. Circulation 2005; 112(17): 2735-52.
[http://dx.doi.org/10.1161/CIRCULATIONAHA.105.169404] [PMID: 16157765]

[2]     Ford ES. Prevalence of the metabolic syndrome defined by the International Diabetes Federation among adults in the U.S. Diabetes Care 2005; 28(11): 2745-9.

[http://dx.doi.org/10.2337/diacare.28.11.2745] [PMID: 16249550]

[3]     Park YW, Zhu S, Palaniappan L, Heshka S, Carnethon MR, Heymsfield SB. The metabolic syndrome: prevalence and associated risk factor findings in the US population from the Third National Health and Nutrition Examination Survey, 1988-1994. Arch Intern Med 2003; 163(4): 427-36.
[http://dx.doi.org/10.1001/archinte.163.4.427] [PMID: 12588201]

[4]     March WA, Moore VM, Willson KJ, Phillips DIW, Norman RJ, Davies MJ. The prevalence of polycystic ovary syndrome in a community sample assessed under contrasting diagnostic criteria. Hum Reprod 2010; 25(2): 544-51.
[http://dx.doi.org/10.1093/humrep/dep399] [PMID: 19910321]

[5]     Azziz R, Woods KS, Reyna R, Key TJ, Knochenhauer ES, Yildiz BO. The prevalence and features of the polycystic ovary syndrome in an unselected population. J Clin Endocrinol Metab 2004; 89(6): 2745-9.
[http://dx.doi.org/10.1210/jc.2003-032046] [PMID: 15181052]

[6]     Bozdag G, Mumusoglu S, Zengin D, Karabulut E, Yildiz BO. The prevalence and phenotypic features of polycystic ovary syndrome: a systematic review and meta-analysis. Hum Reprod 2016; 31(12): 2841-55.
[http://dx.doi.org/10.1093/humrep/dew218] [PMID: 27664216]

[7]     Legro RS, Urbanek M, Kunselman AR, Leiby BE, Dunaif A. Self-selected women with polycystic ovary syndrome are reproductively and metabolically abnormal and undertreated. Fertil Steril 2002; 78(1): 51-7.
[http://dx.doi.org/10.1016/S0015-0282(02)03153-9] [PMID: 12095490]

[8]     Haffner SM, Valdez RA, Hazuda HP, Mitchell BD, Morales PA, Stern MP. Prospective analysis of the insulin-resistance syndrome (syndrome X). Diabetes 1992; 41(6): 715-22.
[http://dx.doi.org/10.2337/diab.41.6.715] [PMID: 1587398]

[9]     Ford ES. The metabolic syndrome and mortality from cardiovascular disease and all-causes: findings from the National Health and Nutrition Examination Survey II Mortality Study. Atherosclerosis 2004; 173(2): 307-12.
[http://dx.doi.org/10.1016/j.atherosclerosis.2003.12.022] [PMID: 15064107]

[10]    Isomaa B, Almgren P, Tuomi T, *et al.* Cardiovascular morbidity and mortality associated with the metabolic syndrome. Diabetes Care 2001; 24(4): 683-9.
[http://dx.doi.org/10.2337/diacare.24.4.683] [PMID: 11315831]

[11]    Lim SS, Davies MJ, Norman RJ, Moran LJ. Overweight, obesity and central obesity in women with polycystic ovary syndrome: a systematic review and meta-analysis. Hum Reprod Update 2012; 18(6): 618-37.
[http://dx.doi.org/10.1093/humupd/dms030] [PMID: 22767467]

[12]    Lebovitz HE, Banerji MA. Point: visceral adiposity is causally related to insulin resistance. Diabetes Care 2005; 28(9): 2322-5.
[http://dx.doi.org/10.2337/diacare.28.9.2322] [PMID: 16123512]

[13]    Ehrmann DA, Liljenquist DR, Kasza K, Azziz R, Legro RS, Ghazzi MN. Prevalence and predictors of the metabolic syndrome in women with polycystic ovary syndrome. J Clin Endocrinol Metab 2006; 91(1): 48-53.
[http://dx.doi.org/10.1210/jc.2005-1329] [PMID: 16249284]

[14]    Lim SS, Norman RJ, Davies MJ, Moran LJ. The effect of obesity on polycystic ovary syndrome: a systematic review and meta-analysis. Obes Rev 2013; 14(2): 95-109.
[http://dx.doi.org/10.1111/j.1467-789X.2012.01053.x] [PMID: 23114091]

[15]    Rachoń D, Teede H. Ovarian function and obesity—Interrelationship, impact on women's reproductive lifespan and treatment options. Mol Cell Endocrinol 2010; 316(2): 172-9.
[http://dx.doi.org/10.1016/j.mce.2009.09.026] [PMID: 19818376]

[16] Tosi F, Di Sarra D, Kaufman JM, *et al.* Total body fat and central fat mass independently predict insulin resistance but not hyperandrogenemia in women with polycystic ovary syndrome. J Clin Endocrinol Metab 2015; 100(2): 661-9.
[http://dx.doi.org/10.1210/jc.2014-2786] [PMID: 25393642]

[17] Haqq L, McFarlane J, Dieberg G, Smart N. Effect of lifestyle intervention on the reproductive endocrine profile in women with polycystic ovarian syndrome: a systematic review and meta-analysis. Endocr Connect 2014; 3(1): 36-46.
[http://dx.doi.org/10.1530/EC-14-0010] [PMID: 24488490]

[18] Dokras A, Sarwer DB, Allison KC, *et al.* Weight Loss and Lowering Androgens Predict Improvements in Health-Related Quality of Life in Women With PCOS. J Clin Endocrinol Metab 2016; 101(8): 2966-74.
[http://dx.doi.org/10.1210/jc.2016-1896] [PMID: 27253669]

[19] Gambineri A, Pelusi C, Vicennati V, Pagotto U, Pasquali R. Obesity and the polycystic ovary syndrome. Int J Obes 2002; 26(7): 883-96.
[http://dx.doi.org/10.1038/sj.ijo.0801994] [PMID: 12080440]

[20] Carmina E, Koyama T, Chang L, Stanczyk FZ, Lobo RA. Does ethnicity influence the prevalence of adrenal hyperandrogenism and insulin resistance in polycystic ovary syndrome? Am J Obstet Gynecol 1992; 167(6): 1807-12.
[http://dx.doi.org/10.1016/0002-9378(92)91779-A] [PMID: 1471702]

[21] Álvarez-Blasco F, Botella-Carretero JI, San Millán JL, Escobar-Morreale HF. Prevalence and characteristics of the polycystic ovary syndrome in overweight and obese women. Arch Intern Med 2006; 166(19): 2081-6.
[http://dx.doi.org/10.1001/archinte.166.19.2081] [PMID: 17060537]

[22] Yildiz BO, Knochenhauer ES, Azziz R. Impact of obesity on the risk for polycystic ovary syndrome. J Clin Endocrinol Metab 2008; 93(1): 162-8.
[http://dx.doi.org/10.1210/jc.2007-1834] [PMID: 17925334]

[23] DeUgarte CM, Bartolucci AA, Azziz R. Prevalence of insulin resistance in the polycystic ovary syndrome using the homeostasis model assessment. Fertil Steril 2005; 83(5): 1454-60.
[http://dx.doi.org/10.1016/j.fertnstert.2004.11.070] [PMID: 15866584]

[24] Li W, Chen Q, Xie Y, Hu J, Yang S, Lin M. Prevalence and degree of insulin resistance in Chinese Han women with PCOS: Results from euglycemic-hyperinsulinemic clamps. Clin Endocrinol (Oxf) 2019; 90(1): 138-44.
[http://dx.doi.org/10.1111/cen.13860] [PMID: 30229990]

[25] Jeanes YM, Reeves S. Metabolic consequences of obesity and insulin resistance in polycystic ovary syndrome: diagnostic and methodological challenges. Nutr Res Rev 2017; 30(1): 97-105.
[http://dx.doi.org/10.1017/S0954422416000287] [PMID: 28222828]

[26] Wang YX, Shan Z, Arvizu M, *et al.* Associations of Menstrual Cycle Characteristics Across the Reproductive Life Span and Lifestyle Factors With Risk of Type 2 Diabetes. JAMA Netw Open 2020; 3(12): e2027928.
[http://dx.doi.org/10.1001/jamanetworkopen.2020.27928] [PMID: 33346844]

[27] Cassar S, Misso ML, Hopkins WG, Shaw CS, Teede HJ, Stepto NK. Insulin resistance in polycystic ovary syndrome: a systematic review and meta-analysis of euglycaemic–hyperinsulinaemic clamp studies. Hum Reprod 2016; 31(11): 2619-31.
[http://dx.doi.org/10.1093/humrep/dew243] [PMID: 27907900]

[28] Legro RS, Kunselman AR, Dodson WC, Dunaif A. Prevalence and predictors of risk for type 2 diabetes mellitus and impaired glucose tolerance in polycystic ovary syndrome: a prospective, controlled study in 254 affected women. J Clin Endocrinol Metab 1999; 84(1): 165-9.
[http://dx.doi.org/10.1210/jcem.84.1.5393] [PMID: 9920077]

[29]    Diamanti-Kandarakis E, Dunaif A. Insulin resistance and the polycystic ovary syndrome revisited: an update on mechanisms and implications. Endocr Rev 2012; 33(6): 981-1030.
[http://dx.doi.org/10.1210/er.2011-1034] [PMID: 23065822]

[30]    Yu HF, Chen HS, Rao DP, Gong J. Association between polycystic ovary syndrome and the risk of pregnancy complications. Medicine (Baltimore) 2016; 95(51): e4863.
[http://dx.doi.org/10.1097/MD.0000000000004863] [PMID: 28002314]

[31]    Robinson S, Henderson AD, Gelding SV, *et al.* Dyslipidaemia is associated with insulin resistance in women with polycystic ovaries. Clin Endocrinol (Oxf) 1996; 44(3): 277-84.
[http://dx.doi.org/10.1046/j.1365-2265.1996.674495.x] [PMID: 8729522]

[32]    Legro RS, Kunselman AR, Dunaif A. Prevalence and predictors of dyslipidemia in women with polycystic ovary syndrome. Am J Med 2001; 111(8): 607-13.
[http://dx.doi.org/10.1016/S0002-9343(01)00948-2] [PMID: 11755503]

[33]    Wild RA, Rizzo M, Clifton S, Carmina E. Lipid levels in polycystic ovary syndrome: systematic review and meta-analysis. Fertil Steril. 2011 Mar 1;95(3):1073-9.e1-11.
[http://dx.doi.org/10.1016/j.fertnstert.2010.12.027] [PMID: 21247558]

[34]    Macut D, Tziomalos K, Božić-Antić I, *et al.* Non-alcoholic fatty liver disease is associated with insulin resistance and lipid accumulation product in women with polycystic ovary syndrome. Hum Reprod 2016; 31(6): 1347-53.
[http://dx.doi.org/10.1093/humrep/dew076] [PMID: 27076501]

[35]    Schwimmer JB, Khorram O, Chiu V, Schwimmer WB. Abnormal aminotransferase activity in women with polycystic ovary syndrome. Fertil Steril 2005; 83(2): 494-7.
[http://dx.doi.org/10.1016/j.fertnstert.2004.08.020] [PMID: 15705403]

# SUBJECT INDEX

www.ingramcontent.com/pod-product-compliance
Lightning Source LLC
Chambersburg PA
CBHW050758220326
41598CB00006B/55